Cardiac Care

Cardiac Care

A Practical Guide for Nurses

Second Edition

Edited by

Angela M. Kucia
Adjunct Senior Lecturer, UNISA Clinical and Health Sciences
University of South Australia
South Australia, Australia

Clinical Nurse Consultant, Acute Cardiac Assessment
Lyell McEwin Hospital
South Australia, Australia

Ian D. Jones
Professor of Cardiovascular Nursing, School of Nursing and Allied Health
Liverpool John Moores University
Liverpool, UK

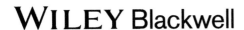

Registered Office(s)
John Wiley & Sons, Inc., 111 River Street, Hoboken, NJ 07030, USA
John Wiley & Sons Ltd, The Atrium, Southern Gate, Chichester, West Sussex, PO19 8SQ, UK

Editorial Office
9600 Garsington Road, Oxford, OX4 2DQ, UK

For details of our global editorial offices, customer services, and more information about Wiley products visit us at www.wiley.com.

Wiley also publishes its books in a variety of electronic formats and by print-on-demand. Some content that appears in standard print versions of this book may not be available in other formats.

Library of Congress Cataloging-in-Publication Data applied for

Paperback ISBN: 9781119117780

Cover Image: © Stocktrek Images/Getty Images
Cover Design by Wiley

Set in 9.5/12.5pt STIXTwoText by Straive, Pondicherry, India
Printed and bound by CPI Group (UK) Ltd, Croydon, CR0 4YY

C9781119117780_250822

Contents

List of Contributors

Barrett, David I.
Department of Paramedical
Perioperative and Advanced Practice
Faculty of Health Science
University of Hull
Hull, UK

Beltrame, John F.
Discipline of Medicine
The Queen Elizabeth Hospital
Adelaide, Australia

Faculty of Health and Medical Sciences
University of Adelaide
Adelaide, Australia

Translational Vascular Function Research
Collaborative
Basil Hetzel Institute for Translational Health
Research
Adelaide, Australia

Davidson, Patricia M.
Vice Chancellor Unit
University of Wollongong
Wollongong, New South Wales, Australia

Gloster, Annabelle S.
Faculty for Advancing Practice
Health Education England
Manchester, UK

Greaney, Brendan
Department of Nursing
Midwifery and Health
Faculty of Health & Life Sciences
Coventry University
Coventry, UK

Gregory, Pete
School of Allied Health and Midwifery
University of Wolverhampton
Walsall, UK

Hartley, Angela
Healthy Hearties
East Molesey
Surrey, UK. https://healthyhearties.co.uk/

Hassan, Salimah
Cardiology Department
Aintree University Hospital
Liverpool Foundation NHS Trust
Liverpool, UK

Horowitz, John D.
Cardiovascular Pathophysiology and
Therapeutics Group
Basil Hetzel Institute for Translational Health
Research
Adelaide, Australia

Jones, Ian D.
Cardiovascular Nursing
Liverpool John Moores University and
Liverpool Centre for Cardiovascular Sciences
Liverpool, UK

Keenan, Jan
Cardiology Ward
Oxford Heart Centre
Oxford University Hospital
John Radcliffe Hospital
Headington, Oxford, UK

Kucia, Angela M.
Department of Cardiology
Lyell McEwin Hospital
Elizabeth, Australia

UniSA Clinical and Health Sciences
University of South Australia
Adelaide, Australia

Board of Directors, Her Heart Ltd.,
Melbourne, Australia

Lotto, Robyn
Faculty of Health and Life Sciences
Liverpool John Moores University and
Liverpool Centre for Cardiovascular Sciences
Liverpool, UK

Nicholson, Christopher
Cardiology and Respiratory Directorate
East Lancashire Hospitals NHS Trust
Royal Blackburn Hospital, UK

Faculty of Health
Social Care and Medicine
Edge Hill University
Ormskirk, UK

Oldroyd, Carol
Faculty of Health and Life Sciences
Coventry University
Coventry, UK

Rabasse, Praba
Faculty of Health and Life Sciences
Liverpool John Moores University and
Liverpool Centre for Cardiovascular Sciences
Liverpool, UK

Rushton, Melanie
School of Health & Society
University of Salford
Manchester, UK

Ryan, Cassandra
Home Hospital, SA Health
Adelaide, Australia

Shepherd, Carolyn E.
Bristol Heart Institute
University Hospitals Bristol and Weston NHS
Bristol, UK

Tagney, Jenny
Bristol Heart Institute
University Hospitals Bristol and Weston NHS
Bristol, UK

Department of Nursing and Midwifery
University of the West of England
Bristol, UK

Thompson, David R.
School of Nursing and Midwifery
Queen's University Belfast
Belfast, UK

School of Nursing
Anhui Medical University
Hefei, People's Republic of China

School of Nursing
Midwifery and Health Systems
University College Dublin
Dublin, Ireland

Department of Psychiatry
University of Melbourne
Melbourne, Australia

School of Public Health
Monash University
Melbourne, Australia

School of Nursing and Midwifery
University of Queensland
Brisbane, Australia

School of Nursing and Midwifery
La Trobe University
Melbourne, Australia

Unger, Steven A.
Nuclear Medicine
The Queen Elizabeth Hospital and the Lyell
McEwin Hospital
Adelaide, Australia

Faculty of Health and Medical Sciences
University of Adelaide
Adelaide, Australia

Webster, Rosemary A.
Cardio-respiratory Directorate
Leicester Royal Infirmary
Leicester, UK

Williamson, Karen
Cardiology Department
Royal Bolton Hospital
Bolton, UK

Wright, Deborah
Department of Cardiology
The Queen Elizbeth Hospital
Woodville, South Australia
Australia

Zeitz, Christopher J.
Department of Cardiology
The Queen Elizabeth Hospital
Adelaide, Australia

Faculty of Health and Medical Sciences
University of Adelaide
Adelaide, Australia

Translational Vascular Function Research
Collaborative
Basil Hetzel Institute for Translational Health
Research
Adelaide, Australia

Foreword

It is my pleasure to write this Foreword for the follow up edition to *Acute Cardiac Care,* which has become an important seminal text and resource for Cardiovascular nurses. It is edited by two leading authorities in the field (Dr Angela Kucia and Prof Ian Jones) plus a series of other global experts from across the disciplines (nursing, medicine, psychology and others). The breadth and depth of each of the chapters is to be commended, plus the accessibility and readability of each chapter. I believe this allows nurses who work in diverse roles such as Nurse Practitioners, clinicians and managers to continue to remain up to date. The information supports evidence-based practice and can be used to inform clinical practice guidelines and policy.

As the roles of nurses expand so does the complexity of the technology that they face. There have also been unprecedented challenges such as the Pandemic and nurses have been at the forefront of this change. As Cardiovascular disease continues to be a leading cause of death, nurses who work in this area require up to date resources such as this invaluable text.

The areas covered are practical (from assessment through to knowledge implementation), they explore different aspects from assessing risk, detection and management including discharge planning and secondary prevention. There are also important sections divided into Acute as well as Chronic. The chapters around Non-obstructive coronary artery disease (MINOCA/INOCA) and risk assessment, plus Takotsubo Syndrome are important as they relate particularly to women. Globally we lose 1 in 3 women to heart disease and in Australia, that's one woman every hour. The literature around gender differences consistently show that women are under-diagnosed, under treated and have significantly worse outcomes than men. Cardiac nurses are in a unique position to raise awareness of these issues plus make a difference in assessment, intervene with any treatment and follow up care - not only with the patient but their carer.

Professor Linda Worrall-Carter
PhD, MEd(Prelim), BEd, R.N.,Coron Care Cert., FCSANZ
Founder & CEO Her Heart
July 2022

Preface

The development of the coronary care unit in the 1960s is often regarded as the foundation upon which modern-day cardiology was built. However, these specialist units that relied on highly skilled nurses to prevent and manage patients at risk of cardiac arrest also became one of the cornerstones of modern-day advanced nursing practice. The knowledge and skills gained in this specialist setting equipped nurses to lead care and has since led to the development of several specialist and advanced nursing roles in a plethora of cardio-vascular settings. From prevention to end of life care, nurses are undertaking increasingly complex roles supporting patients and families.

Most aspects of cardiac care are guided by clinical guidelines that are based on good evidence from clinical trials. Cardiac care guidelines continually evolve as new evidence becomes available. We have included many links to resources and guidelines in this book. The guidelines and links will be updated over time, but we have included them to bring to your attention the organisations that have a role in producing guidelines that guide cardiac care. Although weblinks may be superseded over time, you will be able to find these organisations in a web search where updated guidelines will be available in the future. Likewise, we have included links to some available resources such as YouTube videos that can enhance your learning. There is a great deal of information online that is useful, especially for visual learners, though caution must be taken in ensuring the sources are credible. As two cardiac nurses who have contributed to some of these developments over several decades, we are committed to advancing the profession whilst remaining true to our underpinning nursing principles. Ann Townsend, one of the leading figures in the early years of coronary care nursing one stated that "technical expertise without compassionate application is futile". It is upon this ethos that we present this text.

We would like to thank the authors of the chapters within the book whose knowledge and expertise shines through on every page. Finally we would like to thank our families and colleagues who have travelled with us upon our journey, and the patients who have helped us to understand how best to serve them over our long careers.

Part I

Knowledge for Practice

1

Mechanics of the Cardiovascular System

Brendan Greaney and Angela M. Kucia

Overview

The cardiovascular system consists of two primary components: the heart and blood vessels. The lymphatic system also has a cardiovascular exchange function but does not contain blood. This chapter will highlight the mechanics of the cardiovascular system and present an overview of the essential elements and structures involved in the flow of blood through the venous and arterial systems. It will also highlight how abnormalities in the mechanics of the cardiovascular system can result in cardiac disease states.

Learning Objectives

After reading this chapter, you should be able to:

- Identify the anatomical location of the heart and its basic function.
- Identify the key structures within the heart that are involved in the flow of blood through the heart and identify their specific function.
- Define the term 'cardiac cycle' and explain the key physiological changes that occur in the heart during this process.
- Define the terms 'cardiac output' (CO) and 'stroke volume' (SV) and explain their physiological significance in relation to the cardiac cycle.
- Define the terms 'preload', 'afterload' and 'contractility', and explain their physiological impact upon myocardial contraction.

Key Concepts

Cardiac cycle; cardiac output; cardiac chambers; cardiac valves; layers of the heart

---

Basic Heart Anatomy

The human heart is essentially a muscular pump which delivers blood containing oxygen, nutrients and other vital elements to the body tissues and major organs. The heart is conical in shape, about the size of a human fist and has an average weight in adults of 250 g in females and 300 g in males (Tortora and Derrickson 2018). The heart is located in the mediastinum, with one-third lying to the right of the sternum and two-thirds to the left. The top of the heart is known as the base, and this is located behind the sternum; the bottom of the heart, known as the apex, is located in the fifth intercostal space in the mid-clavicular line. The heart is a four-chambered structure: the upper chambers are known as the right and left atria, and the lower two chambers are known as the right and left ventricles (Figure 1.1a). The right- and left-sided chambers are divided by the septum.

The heart is predominantly composed of a thick contractile mass of cardiac muscle cells known as the myocardium (Figure 1.1d). It is the myocardium that provides the force of contraction to move blood out of the ventricles at the end of each cardiac cycle. Cardiomyocytes are the individual cells that make up the cardiac muscle (Figure 1.1d). Their primary function is to contract so that pressure is generated to pump blood through the circulatory system. Cardiomyocytes consist of chains of myofibrils, that in turn consist of repeating sections of sarcomeres (Figure 1.1c). Sarcomeres are the basic contractile units of cardiac muscle and are composed of thick and thin myofilaments: the thin filaments contain the protein actin, whereas the thicker filaments contain the protein myosin. The myofilaments slide past each other producing the formation of "cross-bridges," which causes contraction of the heart and generation and propagation of mechanical force. Between the actin strands are rod-shaped proteins known as tropomyosin to which the troponin complex is attached at regular intervals (see Figure 1.1a). The troponin complex is responsible for the regulation of actin–myosin function and is made up of three subunits: troponin-T (TN-T), troponin-C (TN-C) and troponin-I (TN-I).

> **Key Point**
>
> Troponin-I and troponin-T are released into the circulation when myocytes die and are used as diagnostic markers of myocardial infarction.

The plasma membrane of the myocyte is known as the sarcolemma (figure 1.1d). It is an excitable membrane that has extensions into the muscle fibre, known as T-tubules (transverse tubules). Excitation of the sarcolemma and T tubules causes Ca^{2+} release from the sarcoplasmic reticulum, the main intracellular calcium store, and initiation of contraction by the microfilaments (Deisch 2017).

Terminal cisternae are discrete regions of the sarcoplasmic reticulum surrounding the transverse tubule that store calcium and increase the capacity of the sarcoplasmic reticulum to release calcium (Figure 1.1e). The process resulting from the release of calcium from the sarcoplasmic reticulum when delivering an action potential to the muscle is called excitation-contraction coupling (Saxton et al. 2021). See Chapter 3 for information on cardiac electrophysiology and the action potential.

Mitochondria (Figure 1.1d) occupy a large portion of each myocyte and are located just below the sarcolemma to ensure efficient localised delivery of adenosine triphosphate (ATP), the cell's primary energy source needed to support contraction, metabolism, and ion homeostasis (Saxton et al. 2021).

Cardiac cells (myocytes) are connected by intercalated discs (Figure 1.1b). Intercalated discs are part of the sarcolemma and contain gap junctions and desmosomes that are important in cardiac muscle contraction (Figure 1.1b). Gap junctions form channels between adjacent cardiac muscle fibres to allow depolarizing current produced by cations to flow from one cardiac myocyte to the next, known as electrical coupling. Desmosomes anchor the ends of cardiac muscle fibres together so that the cells do not pull apart during contraction. Gap junctions and desmosomes facilitate quick transmission of action potentials and the coordinated contraction of the heart. This network of electrically connected cardiac muscle cells creates a functional unit of contraction called a syncytium.

The heart is surrounded by the pericardium, which is comprised of two principal layers that surround and protect the heart. The outer layer is known as the fibrous pericardium, which is made up of tough and fibrous connective tissue. This layer provides both protection and anchorage for the heart. The second layer, the serous pericardium, is a thinner, more delicate layer and forms two distinct layers around the heart. The outer parietal layer is adhered to the inner side of the fibrous pericardium, whilst the inner visceral layer, also known as the epicardium, is adhered tightly to the myocardium. Between these two layers there exists a potential space termed the pericardial cavity. Within this cavity is a very thin film of lubricating serous fluid known as pericardial fluid. The key function of this fluid is to reduce friction between the pericardial layers as the heart

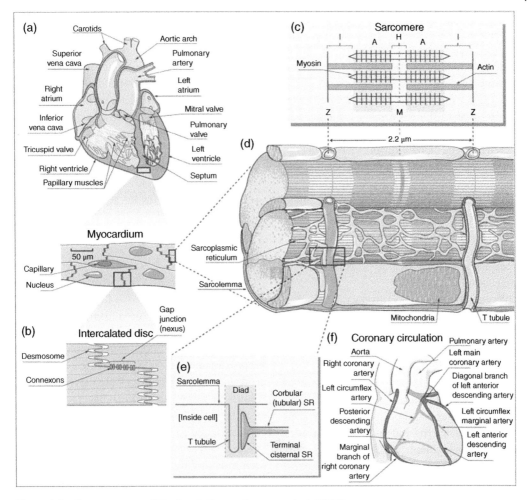

Figure 1.1 Gross anatomy of the heart. *Source:* Aaronson et al. (2012).

contracts. The inner layer lining the heart is a continuous sheet of squamous epithelium, continuing into the tunica intima of blood vessels, and is known as the endocardium.

The atria and ventricles are separated by the atrioventricular (AV) valves. The tricuspid valve separates the right atrium (RA) and right ventricle (RV) and the bicuspid valve or mitral valve separates the left atrium (LA) and left ventricle (LV) (Figure 1.1a). Attached to each AV valve are two structures: the chordae tendinae and the papillary muscles. These two structures are adhered to the walls of each ventricle (Figure 1.1a). Their function is to prevent the valve cusps inverting or swinging upward

into the atria during ventricular systole. The key function of the heart valves is to permit the flow of blood in one direction only as it flows through the heart.

The heart can be viewed functionally as two pumps serving the pulmonary and systemic circulations. The pulmonary circulation refers to the flow of blood within the lungs that is involved in the exchange of gases between the blood and the alveoli. Deoxygenated blood returns to the RA via the inferior and superior vena cavae. It then passes through the tricuspid valve to the RV before entering the pulmonary circulation via the pulmonary artery, where gases are exchanged. The pulmonary artery has a pulmonary valve or semilunar valve, which opens and closes during contraction and relaxation of the heart, again having a similar function to the AV valves, allowing the flow of blood in one direction only (Figure 1.1a). The systemic circulation consists of all the blood vessels within and outside of all organs excluding the lungs. Once oxygenated, the blood returns to the LA via the pulmonary veins and then passes through the mitral valve into the thicker-walled left ventricle, which ejects the oxygenated blood through the aortic valve into the aorta and into the systemic circulation. The aorta also has a valve, the aortic valve, which prevents the backflow of blood during myocardial contraction (Figure 1.1a).

Figure 1.1f shows the coronary circulation which is discussed in detail in Chapter 4.

The Cardiac Cycle

In simple terms, the heart is a pump that receives blood from the venous system at low pressure and generates pressure through contraction to eject the blood into the arterial system. The mechanical action of the heart is created by a synchronised contraction and relaxation of the cardiac muscle, referred to as systole and diastole. The actual mechanical function of the heart is influenced by pressure, volume and flow changes that occur within the heart during one single cardiac cycle.

When the heart muscle contracts (systole) and relaxes (diastole), sequential changes in pressure are produced in the heart chambers and blood vessels, which result in blood flowing from areas of high pressure to areas of lower pressure. The valves prevent backflow of blood. Under normal conditions, this cycle will take place in the human heart between 60 and 100 times/min.

Figure 1.2a demonstrates the seven phases of the cardiac cycle showing key events, heart pressures and volumes. Figure 1.2b shows the left ventricular pressure/volume loop and its relationship to events in the cardiac cycle.

Phase 1: Atrial Systole

Atrial systole (Figure 1.2a/A) begins after a wave of depolarisation passes over the atrial muscle. Atrial depolarisation is represented by the P wave on the electrocardiogram (ECG). As the atria contract, pressure builds up inside the atria forcing blood through the tricuspid and mitral valves into the ventricles. Atrial contraction causes a small increase in proximal venous pressure (in the pulmonary veins and vena cavae).

- Blood flows from the RA across the tricuspid valve into the RV.
- Blood flows from the LA through the mitral valve into the LV.

Pressure in the atria falls and the AV valves float upward. Ventricular volumes are now at their maximum (around 120 ml), and this is known as end diastolic volume (EDV). Left ventricular end diastolic pressure (LVEDP) is approximately 8–12 mm Hg; right ventricular end diastolic pressure (RVEDP) is usually around 3–6 mm Hg. A fourth heart sound (S4) may be heard in this phase if ventricular compliance is reduced, such as happens with ventricular hypertrophy, ischaemia or as a common finding in older individuals.

Ventricular filling occurs passively before the atria contract and is dependent upon venous return. When the body is at rest, atrial contraction accounts for around 10% of ventricular filling.

Key Point

Enhanced ventricular filling due to atrial contraction is sometimes referred to as the 'atrial kick'.

Learning Activity 1.1

As atrial contraction contributes little to ventricular filling under normal conditions, what do you think happens to ventricular filling during high heart rates and exercise?

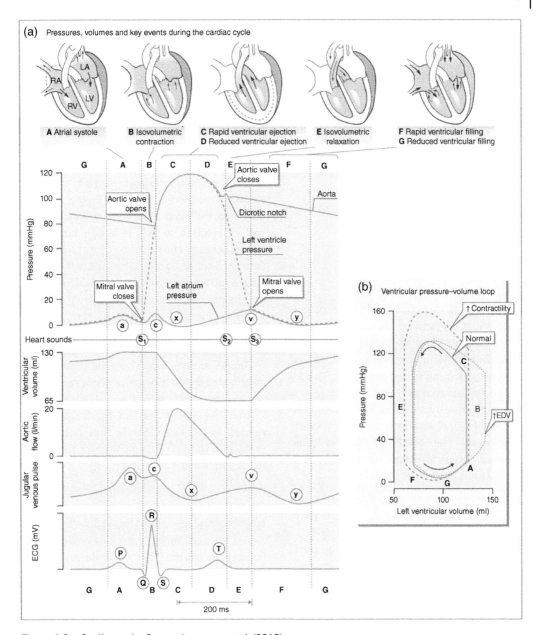

Figure 1.2 Cardiac cycle. *Source:* Aaronson et al. (2012).

Learning Activity 1.2

Although atrial contraction normally contributes little to cardiac output, consider what circumstances may lead to some patients becoming severely haemodynamically compromised with faster heart rates.

Phase 2: Isovolumetric Contraction

Isometric contraction (Figure 1.2a/B) coincides with the QRS complex on the ECG. The ventricle depolarises and initiates contraction of the myocytes, resulting in a rapid increase in ventricular pressure. This rise in pressure causes the AV valves to close. Closure of the AV valves generates the first heart sound (S1).

A split S1 may be heard as mitral valve closure precedes tricuspid valve closure by around 0.04 of a second, although usually only one sound can be heard through a stethoscope. The time between closure of the AV valves and opening of the semilunar valves is known as isovolumetric contraction because there is no change in the volume of blood in the ventricle at this stage, although the ventricle contracts and becomes more spheroid in shape. The pressure in the LV becomes maximal at this stage and is termed dp/dt (maximal slope of the ventricular pressure tracing/time) (Klabunde 2012).

Phase 3: Rapid Ventricular Ejection

Rapid ventricular ejection (Figure 1.2a/C) occurs when the ventricular pressure exceeds that of the aorta (around 80 mm Hg) and pulmonary arteries (around 10 mm Hg) causing the aortic and pulmonary valves to open and blood is ejected out of the ventricles. The LV has a thick muscular wall that allows it to generate high pressures during ventricular contraction. Maximal outflow velocity occurs early in the ejection phase, so the highest aortic and pulmonary artery pressures are reached at this time (Klabunde 2012).

- Blood is ejected from the RV across the pulmonic valve and into the pulmonary artery to the pulmonary circulation.
- Blood is ejected from the LV across the aortic valve and into the aorta to the systemic circulation.

Between 70 and 90 ml of blood is ejected with each stroke (stroke volume), but about 50 ml remains in each ventricle. The residual amount of blood left in the ventricle is known as the end-systolic volume (ESV). Stroke volume thus is the difference between EDV and ESV. Around 60% of the total volume of the ventricle is ejected in each cycle. To work out the ejection fraction of the ventricle, divide the stroke volume by the EDV. The normal left ventricular ejection fraction (LVEF) is above 55% (Klabunde 2012).

> **Key Point**
>
> In the healthy heart, no heart sounds should be heard during the ejection phase of the cardiac cycle. The presence of sounds during ejection likely indicates valve disease or intracardiac shunts (Klabunde 2012).

Phase 4: Reduced Ventricular Ejection

Reduced ventricular ejection (Figure 1.2a/D) occurs as the ventricle relaxes and causes the rate of ejection to fall, although kinetic or inertial energy continues to propel the blood forward into the aorta. This phase coincides with ventricular repolarisation, which occurs approximately 150–200 ms after the QRS complex and appears as the T wave on the ECG. Atrial pressure starts to rise during this phase due to venous return (Klabunde 2012).

The RA receives blood from the systemic circulation via the inferior and superior vena cavae at a low pressure (approximately 0–4 mm Hg).

After circulating through the lungs, blood returns to the heart via the four pulmonary veins into the LA. The pressure in the LA is usually between 8 and 12 mm Hg.

Phase 5: Isovolumetric Relaxation

Isovolumetric relaxation (Figure 1.2a/E) occurs as the pressure in the ventricles continues to fall and reaches the point where the pressure is less in the ventricles than that in the outflow tracts (aorta and pulmonary veins), the aortic and pulmonary valves close abruptly, causing a second heart sound (S2). Aortic and pulmonary artery pressures fall slowly due to a combination of stored energy in the elastic walls of these vessels, which controls pressure and flow, and because forward flow is impeded by systemic and pulmonic vascular resistance as blood is distributed through the systemic and pulmonary circulations (Klabunde 2012). As the aortic valve closes before the pulmonic valve, there is a physiological splitting of the S2 sound, and this may be heard with a stethoscope. Closure of the aortic and pulmonary valves result in a characteristic notch in aortic and pulmonary artery pressure tracings (Figure 1.2a).

Key Point

Identifying the aortic notch on the arterial waveform is important in setting timing for intra-aortic balloon counterpulsation.

Phase 6: Rapid Ventricular Filling

Low pressures in the heart allow blood to passively return to the atria. When the ventricular pressure falls below the atrial pressure, the AV valves open and the ventricles fill quickly. Blood flows into the atria and ventricles throughout diastole with the rate of filling decreasing as the amount of blood in the chambers distends the walls. About 70% of ventricular filling occurs passively at this time. No prominent heart sounds should be heard at this time. If a third heart sound (S3) is heard during ventricular filling in adults, it may indicate tensing of the chordae tendinae and AV ring, often associated with ventricular dilation. It is a normal finding in children.

Phase 7: Reduced Ventricular Filling

There is no clear demarcation as to when this phase begins, but this is a stage during diastole when passive ventricular filling is near completion. As the ventricles fill, they become less compliant, causing intraventricular pressure to rise and the rate of ventricular filling starts to fall. Immediately following this phase, atrial systole occurs following firing of the sino-atrial node.

Key Point

At slow heart rates, diastole is lengthened, resulting in increased filling time. In rapid heart rates, there is less filling time.

Cardiac Output

CO is an important index of cardiac function and refers to the amount of blood that is ejected with each contraction, or stroke volume (SV), multiplied by heart rate (HR): $CO = SV \times HR$. At typical resting values, if the heart rate is 75 beats/min and the average stroke volume is 70 ml/beat, the CO should equal 5.25 l/min. This volume is close to the total blood volume, which is about 5 l in a typical adult male (Tortora and Derrickson 2018). Factors that alter stroke volume or heart rate will alter CO and it can vary significantly during normal physical exercise, as well as in the setting of impaired cardiac function. Other factors such as preload, afterload, and contractility (inotropy) will indirectly affect CO.

Preload is described as the degree of stretch on the myocardium before it contracts (Tortora and Derrickson 2018). The greater the preload (the larger the amount of blood that has filled the heart during diastole), the greater the contraction will be. A simple analogy to explain this concept is that the further you stretch an elastic band prior to releasing it, the further it will recoil. The same principle applies here: the greater the stretch or tension on the myocardium, the greater the force of contraction. When venous return to the heart increases, ventricular filling and preload also increase. The Frank Starling Law of the Heart (Starling's Law) asserts that the more the ventricle is filled with blood during diastole (EDV), the greater the volume of blood that will be ejected (stroke volume) during the ensuing systolic contraction. Thus, altered preload is a mechanism by which the force of contractility can be affected (Klabunde 2012).

Contractility, also known as inotropy, is the ability of a cardiac myocyte to alter its tension development independently of preload changes (Klabunde 2012). Contractility is affected by autonomic innervation and circulating catecholamines (adrenaline, noradrenaline), and additionally changes in afterload and heart rate can augment contractility. A number of pharmacological agents can positively or negatively affect contractility. Agents that affect contractility are called positive or negative inotropes, depending upon whether they increase or decrease contractility. Loss of myocardial contractility results in heart failure.

Afterload is described as the pressure that must be exceeded before ejection of blood from the ventricles can occur (Tortora and Derrickson 2018). This force or pressure is constantly present in the arteries as arterial blood pressure. Therefore, any increase in systemic blood pressure will result in the left ventricular myocardium having to contract more forcefully to eject its volume of blood. Any increase in the pressure of the pulmonary circulation, such as pulmonary oedema, or the presence of any physical obstruction to the pulmonary circulation, such as lung scar tissue, will result in the right ventricular myocardium having to contract more forcefully. In the long term, this increased workload for the myocardium will eventually result in the abnormal enlargement of the myocardium (hypertrophy), which may in turn lead to heart failure. The myocardium requires oxygen to regenerate adenosine triphosphate (ATP) that is hydrolysed to produce energy during contraction and relaxation. Any change to the force or frequency of contraction will influence myocardial oxygen consumption (MVO_2) and demand.

Key Point

Imbalances in the supply and demand of oxygen to the myocardium may result in myocardial ischaemia or infarction.

This chapter has provided you with an overview of anatomical and physiological underpinnings underlying much of the assessment and nursing care of the patient with a cardiovascular disorder. When next you check a patient's heart rate or blood pressure, or listen to their heart sounds, consider in detail the anatomical and physiological determinants of those measures.

Learning Activity 1.3

Multiple Choice Questions

1) **What is a typical blood volume in a typical adult male?**
   (a) 6 l   (b) 5 l   (c) 7 l   (d) 6.5 l

2) **How many stages make up the cardiac cycle?**
   a) 5   (b) 6   (c) 8   (d) 7

3) **What is the key function of heart valves in the heart?**
   a) Separate key chambers of the heart
   b) Prevent backflow of blood
   c) Add stability to the myocardium
   d) Serve as an anchor for the hearts fibrous skeleton

4) **What is the function of the papillary muscles and chordae tendinae?**
   a) Provide support for the walls of the ventricles
   b) Prevent the valve cusps inverting or swinging upward into the atria
   c) Act as electrical conduction for the impulses as they pass through the ventricle
   d) Form an integral part of the ventricular walls

5) **Which of the following statements is true?**
   a) At slow heart rates, diastole is lengthened, resulting in increased filling time.
   b) At slow heart rates, diastole is shortened, resulting in increased filling time.
   c) At slow heart rates, diastole is lengthened, resulting in decreased filling time.
   d) In rapid heart rates, diastole is lengthened, resulting in increased filling time.

Suggested Resource
Cardiovascular system in under 10 min
CTE Skills.com (2015)
https://youtu.be/_lgd03h3te8

Learning Activity Answers

Learning Activity 1.1 Critical Thinking

Answer: At high heart rates, such as during periods of exercise, there is less time for ventricular filling. As long as the heart is in sinus rhythm and heart function is normal, compensatory mechanisms will maintain an adequate cardiac output for a period of time. These mechanisms include increased venous return, venous constriction, increased force of atrial and ventricular contraction (inotropy) and enhanced rate of ventricular relaxation (lusitropy) (Klabunde 2012).

Learning Activity 1.2 Relating Theory to Practice

Answer: The presence of pre-existing poor ventricular function is strongly associated with cardiovascular compromise in patients who develop fast heart rates. During periods of fast heart rates, atrial contraction can contribute up to 40% of ventricular filling. In rhythms such as rapid atrial fibrillation or ventricular tachycardia, the lack of coordinated atrial contraction (loss of "atrial kick") further compromises the patient. An example of this would be a patient with chronic heart failure and reduced ejection fraction, who develops rapid atrial fibrillation or ventricular tachycardia.

Learning Activity 1.3: Multiple Choice Questions

Answers: 1 (b); 2 (d); 3 (b); 4 (b); 5 (a)

References

Aaronson, P.I., Ward, J.P.T., and Connelly, M.J. (2012). The Cardiovascular System at a Glance, 4ee. Oxford: Wiley Blackwell.

Deisch, J.K. Nerve and muscle development in health and disease (2017) disease in Swaiman, K.F., Ashwal, S., Ferriero, D.M., Schor, N., Finkel, R.S., Gropman, A.L., ... & Shevell, M. (Eds). *Swaiman's Pediatric Neurology e-Book: Principles and practice* (6th edn). Elsevier Health Sciences. pp.1029–1037. https://doi.org/10.1016/B978-0-323-37101-8.00135-1

Klabunde, R. (2012). Cardiovascular Physiology Concepts, 2ee. Philadelphia: Lippincott Williams & Wilkins.

Saxton A, Tariq M.A., Bordoni B. Anatomy, Thorax, Cardiac Muscle. [Updated 2021 Aug 11]. In: StatPearls [Internet]. Treasure Island (FL): StatPearls Publishing; 2022 Jan-. https://www.ncbi.nlm.nih.gov/books/NBK535355/

Tortora, G.J. and Derrickson, B.H. (2018). Principles of Anatomy and Physiology, 15ee. Danvers, MA: Wiley.

2

Regulation of Cardiac and Vascular Function

Brendan Greaney and Angela M. Kucia

Overview

The regulation of cardiac and vascular function is complex, involving neural (autonomic) and humoral (circulating or hormonal) factors. You will hear this referred to as 'neurohumoral control of the cardiovascular system'. These mechanisms control cardiac output, blood pressure and local control of blood flow in response to physiological requirements and in the setting of adverse clinical events such as trauma, disease or stress. In turn, neurohumoral control is influenced by sensors that monitor blood pressure (baroreceptors), blood volume (volume receptors), blood chemistry (chemoreceptors) and plasma osmolarity (osmoreceptors). These sensors work together to maintain arterial pressure at a level that is adequate for organ perfusion (Klabunde 2021a). This chapter reviews the mechanisms involved in neurohumoral controls of the cardiovascular system.

- Describe the effects of sympathetic and parasympathetic stimulation on the cardiovascular system.
- Discuss the function of baroreceptors in the regulation of arterial pressure.
- Discuss the function of chemoreceptors in the regulation of respiratory activity and arterial pressure.
- List the chemicals that can stimulate the heart and cardiovascular system and describe their negative and positive effects.

Key Concepts

Neurohumoral control; sympathetic and parasympathetic nervous system; baroreceptors; chemoreceptors; blood pressure regulation

Learning Objectives

After reading this chapter, you should be able to:

- Describe the components of the autonomic nervous system that relate to cardiac function.

Central Nervous System Regulation of the Cardiovascular System

The central nervous system (CNS) controls the autonomic regulation of cardiovascular function. Autonomic refers to functions of the nervous system that are not under voluntary control (such as regulation of heart rate). The heart is innervated by both parasympathetic and sympathetic nerve fibres. These fibres together play a vital role in the control of heart rate and contractility, as well as regulation of blood pressure. Nervous system regulation of the heart originates in the medulla oblongata. This region of the brain stem, termed the cardiovascular centre, receives input from a variety of sensory receptors (Totora and Derrickson 2009). Parasympathetic innervation is associated with the cardioinhibitory centre of the cardiovascular centre, and sympathetic innervation is associated with the cardioacceleratory centre (also known as cardiostimulatory centre) of the cardiovascular centre.

The cardioinhibitory centre sends signals via parasympathetic fibres in the vagus nerve to the sino-atrial (SA) and atrio-ventricular (AV) nodes, conduction pathways, myocytes and coronary vasculature. The right vagus nerve predominantly innervates the SA node, and the left vagus nerve innervates the AV node and ventricular conduction system. Nerve fibres in the parasympathetic nervous system are cholinergic, which means they release acetylcholine. Acetylcholine binds to muscarinic receptors that are specifically associated with vagal nerve endings in the heart, resulting in negative chronotropy (decreased heart rate), negative inotropy (decreased contractility, more so in the atria than the ventricles) and negative dromotropy (decreased conduction velocity).

The cardioacceleratory centre sends signals by way of the thoracic spinal cord and sympathetic cardiac accelerator nerves to the SA node, AV node and myocardium. These nerves secrete norepinephrine, which binds to β-adrenergic receptors in the heart. The term 'pressor' is sometimes used to describe the responses associated with sympathetic stimulation on the heart, which are positive chronotropy (increased heart rate), positive inotropy (increased contractility, more so in the atria than the ventricles) and positive dromotropy (increased conduction velocity).

Key Point

The SA and AV nodes are autorhythmic: they fire at their own intrinsic rate. Therefore, if parasympathetic and sympathetic nerve fibres to these nodes were severed, the heart would continue to beat at its own intrinsic rate.

Parasympathetic activity, or vagal tone, is the dominant controlling factor of heart rate, and it inhibits the nodes to a normal rate of 70–80 bpm. Maximum vagal stimulation can reduce the heart rate to as low as 20 bpm! The cardiovascular centre receives both neural and chemical input from many sources. Stimuli such as exercise, anxiety, fear, pyrexia and pain will act upon the cardiovascular centre via higher centres in the brain such as the cerebral cortex, the limbic system and the hypothalamus. Several specific mechanisms exist at various locations in the body, which control and regulate the heart and vascular system in response to such factors. Sudden fear or emotion, for example, may cause vagal stimulation resulting in bradycardia, loss of vascular tone and fainting (vasovagal syncope) (Klabunde 2021a).

Suggested Resource

Autonomic nervous system effects on the heart
Khan Academy Health and Medicine (2012)
https://youtu.be/KiouveG278Y

Learning Activity 2.1

In some clinical situations, such as during an episode of pain, or whilst pressure is being applied during removal of a femoral arterial sheath, patients may have an exaggerated vagal response resulting in extreme sinus bradycardia and reduced blood pressure. How is this usually managed in your setting?

Vasomotor Control

As described, the CNS plays an important role in regulating systemic vascular resistance (SVR) and cardiac function, which in turn influence arterial blood pressure. The distribution of blood, as well as the control of arterial blood pressure, can be influenced by factors that control changes in the diameter of blood vessels. The vasomotor centre is located in the medulla of the brain and controls sympathetic activation of the vascular system. Sympathetic activation causes an impulse outflow via sympathetic fibres that terminate in the smooth muscle tissue of both resistance (arteries and arterioles) and capacitance (veins and venules) vessels, causing constriction. This increases SVR and thus arterial blood pressure.

Baroreceptors

Arterial blood pressure is regulated through a negative feedback system that uses pressure sensors, known as baroreceptors, located in the carotid sinus and aortic arch and the bifurcation of the subclavian artery (Bridges 2010). These baroreceptors are sensitive to changes in pressure or stretch in the vessel walls where they are located. They are also sensitive to the rate of pressure change and to a steady (mean) pressure. To understand how baroreceptors function, consider what happens in the physiologic circumstance of when a person suddenly changes from a reclining position to one of standing as in Figure 2.1.

Gravity and Venous Return

Forces of gravity affect venous return, CO, and arterial and venous pressures. Figure 2.1 shows the effect of gravity on venous return. When a person is supine, the gravitational force on the thorax, abdomen and legs is similar and venous

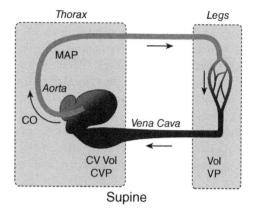

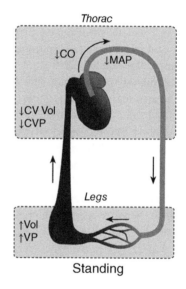

Figure 2.1 Effects of gravity on venous return. *Source:* Klabunde (2021b).

blood volumes and pressures are distributed evenly throughout the body. When a person who has been supine suddenly stands upright, gravity causes blood to accumulate in the lower extremities as venous compliance is high. Venous volume and pressure become very high in the feet and lower limbs when standing. Thoracic venous blood volume and CVP decrease, leading to a decrease in right ventricular filling pressure and reduction in SV. LV filling pressure also falls because of reduced pulmonary venous return (decreased left ventricular preload), and consequently CO and MAP fall (Klabunde 2021a).

Key Point

A fall in blood pressure on standing from a sitting or recumbent position can reduce cerebral blood flow resulting in syncope. This is known as postural or orthostatic hypotension. Postural hypotension is diagnosed when there is a drop in blood pressure (≥20 mmHg systolic and/or ≥10 mmHg diastolic) that occurs within 3 minutes of standing (Gilani et al. 2021).

Learning Activity

Compare the size of veins in the top of your feet while lying down and standing. Explain why this happens.

On standing, baroreceptor reflexes are rapidly activated to ensure that blood pressure does not substantially decrease. The mechanisms involved include increased systemic vascular resistance (sympathetic mediated), decreased venous compliance (due to sympathetic activation of veins), decreased stroke volume (due to decreased preload) and increased heart rate (baroreceptor-mediated tachycardia) (Klabunde 2021a).

Key Point

Patients with autonomic nerve dysfunction or hypovolemia will not be able to effectively utilise these compensatory mechanisms and therefore will display orthostatic hypotension (Klabunde 2021a).

In addition to arterial baroreceptors, there are stretch receptors located at the veno-atrial junctions of the heart that respond to atrial filling and contraction (Klabunde 2021a). Low-pressure baroreceptors are located in the atria, ventricles, pulmonary artery and veins that are sensitive to changes in transmural pressure in these chambers or vessels. Stimulation of certain mechanoreceptors (sensory receptors that respond to

mechanical pressure or distortion) and chemoreceptors in the heart and coronary arteries can result in a vagally mediated triad of bradycardia, apnoea and hypotension (Bridges 2010) known as the Bezold–Jarisch reflex. This happens commonly when dye is injected into the coronary arteries during coronary angiography or during ischaemia/reperfusion involving the inferoposterior wall of the left ventricle.

Key Point

Clinical states such as hypovolaemia may result in the vascular system recruiting blood from the reservoirs found in the venous plexuses and sinuses in the skin and abdominal organs, especially the liver and spleen (Thibodeau and Patton 2007). Blood can be shifted quickly out of these reservoirs to arteries that supply heart and skeletal muscles when increased activity demands.

Suggested Resources

Regulation of blood pressure with baroreceptors
Khan Academy Health and Medicine (2012)
https://youtu.be/ajLgwCygHsc

Baroreceptors and the Regulation of Blood Pressure
NurseMinder (2020)
https://youtu.be/_3hRHgA8CN0

Chemoreceptors

Chemoreceptors are specialised cells that have a significant role in the regulation of respiratory activity to maintain arterial blood PO_2, PCO_2 and pH within a physiologic range (Klabunde 2021a). These receptors are sensitive to small changes in oxygen levels but are more sensitive to abnormal carbon dioxide and hydrogen ion levels in the blood plasma. Abnormal levels of any of these substances trigger the chemoreceptors to send impulses to the cardiovascular centre. In response, the cardiovascular centre increases sympathetic stimulation to the smooth muscle of arterioles and veins, bringing about vasoconstriction and a subsequent increase in arterial blood pressure and heart rate, thus improving tissue perfusion. Peripheral chemoreceptors are located in the aortic arch (known as the aortic bodies) and in the carotid arteries (known as the carotid bodies) and are responsive to hypoxaemia (decreased arterial PO_2), hypercapnia (increased arterial PCO_2) and hydrogen ion concentration (acidosis). Central chemoreceptors are located within the medulla of the brain (central chemoreceptors) and are responsive to hypercapnia and acidosis but not directly to hypoxia (Klabunde 2021a). Stimulation of these receptors leads to hyperventilation and sympathetic activation causing vasoconstriction in most vascular beds except those of the brain and heart (Bridges 2010). Although the chemoreceptor reflex results in an increase in arterial blood pressure, this rise will be mediated by the baroreceptor response.

Key Point

Central and peripheral chemoreceptor responses may be enhanced in heart failure patients, resulting in increased sympathetic activation which may contribute to sleep apnoea in those patients and is associated with a poor prognosis (Javaheri 2003; Narkiewicz and Somers 2003).

Humoral Control

There are several naturally produced chemicals (humoral substances) in the body that significantly affect the action of the heart and vascular system. These can have both positive and negative effects. These include circulating catecholamines, the renin-angiotensin-aldosterone system (RAAS), atrial natriuretic peptide (ANP) and antidiuretic hormone (ADH) (vasopressin). Other substances such as thyroxine, oestrogen, insulin, and growth hormone also have direct or indirect effects on the cardiovascular system (Klabunde 2021a).

Epinephrine (adrenaline) and norepinephrine (noradrenaline) are classed as non-steroid hormones called catecholamines and are particularly potent cardiac stimulants. They are secreted by the adrenal medulla and cardiac accelerator nerves in response to arousal, stress (physical or emotional) and exercise and are associated with the body's 'fight and flight' reflex. Epinephrine accounts for about 80% of the adrenal medulla's secretions, the other 20% is norepinephrine (Thibodeau and Patton 2007). When secreted into the bloodstream, epinephrine prepares the body to respond to an acute stressor by increasing the supply of oxygen and glucose to the brain and muscles while suppressing other non-emergency bodily processes such as digestion (fight or flight mechanism). It binds to numerous adrenergic receptors (β_1, β_2, α_1 and α_2) throughout the body, although it has a greater affinity for β-adrenoreceptors than α-adrenoreceptors. Therefore, when plasma levels of epinephrine are low, it will bind preferentially to β-adrenoreceptors. This is important to know because heart rate, inotropy and dromotropy are mainly mediated by β_1-adrenoreceptors (Klabunde 2021a). Low-dose epinephrine binds to β_2-adrenoreceptors in skeletal muscle and splanchnic arterioles, triggering vasodilation. However, when epinephrine binds with α-adrenergic receptors that are found in smooth muscle in the walls of blood vessels, it causes vasoconstriction. Blood pressure is increased due to the resulting increase in cardiac output and SVR.

Key Point

When epinephrine is administered exogenously, its effects are dose related. Low-dose epinephrine stimulates the β-adrenoreceptors resulting in vasodilation and increased heart rate and contractility. Higher doses stimulate the α-adrenoreceptors, increasing vascular resistance and blood pressure. Thus, if the intent of epinephrine administration is vasoconstriction, it is important to administer a large enough dose to achieve this effect (Bridges 2010).

Circulating norepinephrine transiently increases heart rate and increases β_1-adrenoreceptor-mediated inotropy. It causes vasoconstriction in most systemic arteries and veins (α_1 and α_2 adrenoreceptors). The overall effect is increased cardiac output and SVR leading to an increase in arterial blood pressure. The initial increase in heart rate is not sustained due to activation of baroreceptors which cause vagal-mediated slowing of heart rate (Klabunde 2021a).

Learning Activity 2.2

β-Blockers are drugs that bind to β-adrenoceptors, blocking the ability of norepinephrine and epinephrine to bind to these receptors.

(a) The first generation of β-blocking drugs was 'non-selective'. What does this mean? What disadvantages do non-selective β-blockers have compared to later generation β-blockers?

(b) Second-generation β-blockers are said to be more 'cardioselective'. What does this mean?

(c) Third-generation β-blockers have vaso-dilator actions through blockade of α-adrenoreceptors. Which drugs are included in this class?

Make a table and list β-blockers in current use under non-selective, cardioselective and those with vasodilator actions. The article below will help you in completing the above activities.

Suggested Resource

Farzam K, Jan A. Beta Blockers. [Updated 2021 Dec 13]. In: StatPearls [Internet]. Treasure Island (FL): StatPearls Publishing; 2022 Jan-. https://www.ncbi.nlm.nih.gov/books/NBK532906/

Stoschitzky, K. (2010). E-journal of Cardiology Practice.

http://www.escardio.org/Guidelines-&-Education/Journals-and-publications/ESC-journals-family/E-journal-of-Cardiology-Practice/Volume-8/Betablockers-in-hypertension-acquiring-a-balanced-view

---

Arginine vasopressin (AVP), commonly known as antidiuretic hormone (ADH), is a peptide hormone produced in the hypothalamus and stored in the posterior pituitary gland and is mainly released into the bloodstream (and some directly into the brain) in response to increased plasma osmolality (detected by osmoreceptors in the hypothalamus). AVP may also be secreted in response to decreased blood volume or blood pressure (detected by baroreceptors), but this is a less-sensitive mechanism than osmolality. AVP causes the kidneys to conserve water (but not sodium) by concentrating the urine and reducing urine volume and elevates blood pressure through vasoconstriction.

Natriuretic peptides are hormones that are involved in the homeostatic regulation of blood pressure, volume, and electrolytes. Atrial natriuretic peptide (ANP) is released from the walls of the atria. Brain natriuretic peptide (BNP) is released from the walls of the ventricles in response to increased stretch or hormonal stimuli (angiotensin II, catecholamines, glucocorticoids, endothelin 1). C-type natriuretic peptide (CNP) is distributed throughout the heart, brain, lungs, kidneys, and endothelin and is released in response to stress. Natriuretic peptides increase excretion of sodium and water and inhibit sodium reabsorption, thereby reducing blood pressure. They also inhibit activation of the RAAS.

The RAAS is a hormone system that has a role in regulating long-term blood pressure and extracellular fluid volume. Several hormones and enzymes, which are significant in the RAAS, cause both vasodilation and vasoconstriction and therefore influence arterial blood pressure in specific clinical and associated disease states.

The RAAS has a cascade effect (Figure 2.2) that is triggered by renin release from the kidney in response to sympathetic nerve activation (acting via β_1-adrenoceptors); renal artery hypotension (caused by systemic hypotension or renal artery stenosis) or decreased sodium delivery to the distal

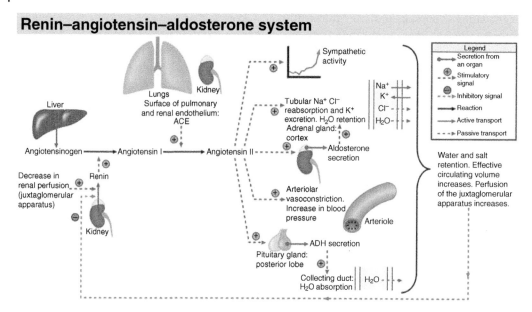

Figure 2.2 The renin–angiotensin–aldosterone system (RAAS). *Source:* Wikipedia (2022). Available under Creative Commons License BY-SA3.0 https://creativecommons.org/licenses/by-sa/3.0/

tubules of the kidney (Klabunde 2021a). When renin is released into the bloodstream, it acts upon a circulating substrate, angiotensinogen, which through the process of proteolytic cleavage becomes angiotensin I. Angiotensin-converting enzyme, found mainly in vascular endothelium in the lungs, converts angiotensin I to angiotensin II. Angiotensin II is a powerful substance that causes vasoconstriction in the resistance vessels leading to increased SVR and arterial pressure and stimulates the adrenal cortex to release aldosterone that acts on the kidneys to increase sodium and fluid retention. It also stimulates the posterior pituitary to release AVP (ADH) that acts on the kidneys to increase fluid retention, stimulates thirst centres within the brain and enhances sympathetic adrenergic function by facilitating the release of norepinephrine from sympathetic nerve endings and inhibiting its reuptake. The net effect of this cascade is to maintain blood pressure and volume. Natriuretic peptides modulate the function of the RAAS and have an important counter-regulatory influence (Klabunde 2021a).

> **Key Point**
>
> Knowledge of the RAAS pathway is necessary in understanding the action of drugs used to treat heart failure and hypertension, as the RAAS is often the target of therapeutic manipulation in treating these conditions.

> **Suggested Resource**
>
> Renin-angiotensin-aldosterone-system Mechanisms in Medicine (2012) https://youtu.be/bY6IWVgFCrQ

Electrolytes

Potassium, sodium, and calcium have an influence on heart rate and rhythm through their role in action potentials (see Chapter 3). Elevated blood levels of potassium and sodium decrease heart rate and the contractility of the heart, but a moderate increase in extracellular and intracellular calcium levels increases both heart rate and contractility (Totora and

Grabowski 2003). Potassium also appears to induce vasodilation, though its specific role in vaso-regulatory processes has not yet been fully elucidated (Berne and Levy 2001).

Suggested Resources

The heart, part 1 – Under pressure: crash course A&P #25 Crash Course (2015)
https://youtu.be/X9ZZ6tcxArI

Cardiovascular physiology concepts
Klabunde, R.E. (2021)
http://www.cvphysiology.com

Conclusion

This chapter has provided an overview of the regulation of cardiovascular function. The processes and mechanisms by which the cardiovascular system is regulated are many and complex. It is important for nurses to have a broad understanding of these mechanisms to recognise any disturbance in neurohumoral control that might compromise the patient and also to understand the actions of a number of pharmacological substances that are utilised to therapeutically manipulate neurohumoral processes.

Learning Activity 2.3

Multiple Choice Questions

1) The cardioacceleratory centre sends signals by way of the thoracic spinal cord and sympathetic cardiac accelerator nerves to the:
   a) SA node
   b) AV node
   c) myocardium
   d) all of the above

2) In the case of sinus bradycardia, atropine may be used to:
   a) increase parasympathetic activity
   b) increase sympathetic activity
   c) decrease parasympathetic activity
   d) decrease sympathetic activity

3) Which of these are classed as cardiac stimulants?
   a) Epinephrine
   b) Norepinephrine
   c) Vasopressin
   d) All of the above

4) Which of these are classed as hormones?
   a) Arginine vasopressin
   b) Atrial natriuretic peptide
   c) Angiotensin
   d) All of these

5) When plasma levels of epinephrine are low, which of the following will epinephrine preferentially bind to?
   a) Calcium channels
   b) α-Adrenoreceptors
   c) β-Adrenoreceptors
   d) Both b and c

Learning Activity Answers

Learning Activity 2.1 Relating Theory to Practice

Answer: The drug atropine, a vagal nerve blocker, may be used to block vagal stimulation on the heart, allowing sympathetic nerve fibres to be the dominant nervous stimulus, producing an increase in the heart rate.

Learning Activity 2.2 Critical Thinking

Answer: β_1-adrenergic receptors are located mainly in the heart and in the kidneys. β_2-adrenergic receptors are located mainly in the lungs, gastrointestinal tract, liver, uterus, vascular smooth muscle and skeletal muscle.

a) Non-selective β-blockers block both beta-1 (β_1) and beta-2 (β_2) adrenoceptors and will affect not only the heart but also affect kidneys, lungs, gastrointestinal tract, liver, uterus, vascular smooth muscle and skeletal muscle. Non-selective β-blockers are contraindicated in patients with asthma or chronic obstructive pulmonary disease as blockade of β_2 receptors can lead to bronchoconstriction. β_2-adrenoceptors normally stimulate glycogenolysis and pancreatic release of glucagon to increase plasma glucose. Blocking β_2-adrenoceptors lowers plasma glucose, resulting in hypoglycaemia. Therefore, non-selective β-blockers should be avoided in people with diabetes.

b) Cardio-selective β-blockers block only β_1 receptors and as such will mostly affect the heart and cardiac output.

c) Third-generation β-blockers have vasodilator actions through blockade of β-adrenoreceptors. Examples of these are carvedilol and nebivolol.

Learning Activity 2.3 Multiple Choice Questions

Answers: 1 (d); 2 (c); 3 (d); 4 (d); 5 (c)

References

Bridges, E.J. (2010). Regulation of cardiac output and blood pressure. In: *Cardiac Nursing*, 6ee (ed. S.L. Woods, E.S.S. Froelicher, S.A.U. Motzer and E.J. Bridges) 2010. Philadelphia: Wolters Kluwer Health/ Lippincott Williams & Wilkins.

Berne, R.M. and Levy, M.N. (2001). *Cardiovascular Physiology*, 8ee. Philadelphia: Mosby.

Gilani, A., Juraschek, S.P., Belanger, M.J. et al. (2021). Postural hypotension. *BMJ* 373: n922. https://doi.org/10.1136/bmj.n922 (accessed 23 April 2021).

Javaheri, S. (2003). Heart failure and sleep apnea: emphasis on practical therapeutic options. *Clinics in Chest Medicine* 24: 207–222.

Klabunde, R.E. (2021a). Cardiovascular physiology concepts. https://www.cvphysiology.com (accessed 10 June 2021).

Klabunde, R.E. (2021b). *Cardiovascular Physiology Concepts*. Wolters Kluwer https://

www.cvphysiology.com/Cardiac%20Function/ CF017 (accessed 8 March 2021).

Narkiewicz, K. and Somers, V.K. (2003). Sympathetic nerve activity in obstructive sleep apnoea. *Acta Physiologica Scandanavia* **177**: 385–390.

Thibodeau, G.A. and Patton, K.T. (2007). *Anatomy and Physiology*, 8ee. Philadelphia: Mosby.

Tortora, G.J. and Grabowski, S.R. (2003). *Principles of Anatomy and Physiology*. John Wiley & Sons Inc.: *New York*.

Totora, G.J. and Derrickson, B.H. (2009). *Principles of Anatomy and Physiology*, 12ee. Asia: Wiley.

Wikipedia Contributors (2022). Renin-angiotensin system. In *Wikipedia, The Free Encyclopedia*. https://en.wikipedia.org/w/index.php?title=Renin%E2%80%93angiotensin_system&oldid= 1065912430 (accessed 27 January 2022).

3

Cardiac Electrophysiology
Brendan Greaney and Angela M. Kucia

Overview

This chapter outlines the anatomy and physiology of the conduction system of the heart and the vital role it plays in the overall function of the heart. An understanding of cardiac electrophysiology will provide a basis for interpretation of the 12-lead electrocardiogram (ECG), and the impact that myocardial ischaemia and other metabolic derangements have upon the 12-lead ECG. This chapter will also facilitate an understanding of the electrophysiological basis of arrhythmia generation, the pharmacological actions of certain classes of medications and the underlying physiological concepts related to defibrillation and cardioversion.

Learning Objectives

After reading this chapter, you should be able to:

- Describe the structure and function of cardiac myocytes and autorhythmic cells.
- Describe the process of action potentials within the myocardium.
- Name the key components of the heart's conduction system.

- Describe the specific anatomical location of the key components of the heart's conduction system.
- Relate the specific electrophysiological events in the cardiac cycle to the generation of ECG waveforms.

Key concepts

Electrophysiology; automaticity; contractility; action potential; cardiac conduction system

---

Cardiac Cells

When referring to the electrophysiology of the heart, we are describing the overall electrical activity within the myocardium, which plays a vital role in the overall effective function of the heart. The conduction system is made up of a series of specific structures within the myocardium, which are still essentially part of the cardiac muscle, but are modified enough in their structure and function to be significantly different from ordinary cardiac muscle (Thibodeau and Patton 2007). The main function of the

---

Cardiac Care: A Practical Guide for Nurses, Second Edition. Edited by Angela M. Kucia and Ian D. Jones.
© 2022 John Wiley & Sons Ltd. Published 2022 by John Wiley & Sons Ltd.

cardiac cells is to contract. Contraction is initiated by electrical changes within the cardiac cells making up the cardiac muscle (myocardium). The myocardium is mainly composed of muscle cells, myocytes, that can be classified into two types: contractile cells that account for around 99% of cardiac cells, and autorhythmic cells that account for the remaining 1%. Autorhythmic cells have the ability to generate electrical activity without an external stimulus and are found in the sinoatrial (SA) node, atrioventricular (AV) node, bundles of His and Purkinje fibres.

The structure and function of contractile cells (myocytes) is discussed in Chapter 1.

Suggested Resource

Electrical System of the Heart Khanacademyofmedicine (2012) https://youtu.be/7K2icszdxQc

---

The Action Potential

All living cells in the body have an electrical potential across the cell membrane. This can be measured by inserting a microelectrode into the cell and measuring the electrical potential in millivolts (mV) inside the cell relative to that outside the cell. At rest, a ventricular myocyte has a membrane potential of around $-90\,mV$, and this is known as the resting membrane potential (Em). Em is determined by a combination of the concentrations of negatively and positively charged electrons across the cell membrane, the relative permeability of the cell membrane to these ions and the function of the ionic pumps that transport ions across the cell membrane (Klabunde 2021). The primary ions involved in the determination of cell membrane potential are sodium (Na^+), chloride (Cl), potassium (K^+) and calcium (Ca^{++}). The cardiac action potential is the electrical activity of the individual cells of the heart that occurs through changes in the cell membrane, permitting the inward and outward flow of ions, resulting in:

- depolarisation, which occurs when the interior of the cardiac cell is maximally charged with positive ions; and
- repolarisation, the process of restoration of a cell to its normal resting membrane polarity following depolarisation.

Cardiac action potentials act in a similar manner to other action potentials within the human body but have an extended contraction time that is needed to effectively move blood through the heart and lungs and into the systemic circulation. The duration of ventricular action potentials range from 200 to 400 ms, compared to 2–5 ms in skeletal muscle cells or 1 ms in a typical nerve cell (Klabunde 2021).

As outlined earlier in this chapter, there are two types of cells in the heart: myocytes (non-pacemaker cells) and autorhythmic (pacemaker) cells. These cells have different action potentials. Non-pacemaker action potentials are triggered by depolarisation currents from adjacent cells, whereas pacemaker action potentials are capable of spontaneous action potential generation, known as automaticity. Pacemaker cells have no true resting potential; instead, they generate regular, spontaneous action potentials (Klabunde 2021).

Suggested Resource

Cardiac Action Potential Kevin Gorman (2013) https://youtu.be/DSDf_dbWy_I

The Action Potential in Non-Pacemaker Cells

The action potential in non-pacemaker cells (atrial and ventricular myocytes and Purkinje cells) has five phases, numbered 0–4 (Figure 3.1).

- Phase 0 represents the rapid depolarisation phase where the fast sodium channels open and there is a rapid influx of Na^+ into the cell. Calcium moves slowly but steadily into the cell. The membrane potential moves from the negative charge of 85–90 mV to +10–20 mV. This creates a gradient with the surrounding cell membranes, allowing the electrical current to flow from the depolarised cell to the surrounding cells, propagating the impulse.

- Phase 1 represents an initial repolarisation of the cell caused by opening of special transient outward K^+ channels and the inactivation of the Na^+ channels. Cl^- ions re-enter the cell.
- Phase 2 represents the plateau phase where repolarisation is delayed because of the slow inward movement of Ca^{++} through long lasting (L-type) calcium channels.

Key Point

L-type calcium channels are blocked by pharmacological L-type calcium channel blockers such as verapamil, diltiazem and dihydropyridines such as nifedipine.

- Phase 3 is the final repolarisation phase. Ca^{++} channels close and K^+ flows rapidly out of the cell.
- Phase 4 refers to the phase where the cell is not stimulated (the resting membrane potential). This phase coincides with diastole. K^+

is restored to the inside of the cell and Na^+ to the outside by active transport through the sodium–potassium pump.

During phases 0, 1, 2 and part of phase 3, the cell is refractory (unexcitable, unresponsive) to the initiation of new action potentials. This is known as the effective refractory period (ERP). The ERP acts as a protective mechanism in the heart by limiting the frequency of action potentials (and therefore contractions) that the heart can generate, enabling the heart to have adequate time to fill and eject blood. At the end of ERP, the cell is in its relative refractory period, where suprathreshold depolarisation stimuli are required to elicit action potentials (Klabunde 2021).

Key Point

The electrophysiological properties of cardiac conducting tissue are strongly influenced by the relative concentrations of intracellular and extracellular potassium. It is therefore very important to maintain the intracellular and extracellular potassium gradient (He and MacGregor 2001). The potassium concentration within human cells is approximately 140 mmol/l, and extracellular potassium concentration is normally 3.5–5.0 mmol/l (Ingelfinger 2015).

Figure 3.1 Action potential in a cardiac cell.

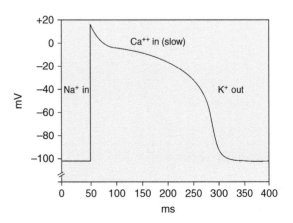

Learning Activity 3.1

a) What would you expect to happen to the action potential in hypokalaemia?

b) What ECG changes and abnormal cardiac rhythms might be associated with hypokalaemia?

c) Which class of drugs is commonly associated with hypokalaemia?

d) What would you expect to happen to the action potential in hyperkalaemia?

e) What ECG changes and abnormal cardiac rhythms might be associated with hyperkalaemia?

f) Which class of drugs is commonly associated with hyperkalaemia? What chronic disease processes are associated with hyperkalaemia?

The Cardiac Conduction System

Cells within the cardiac conduction system are described as autorhythmic or self-excitable, meaning they can repeatedly and rhythmically generate their own electrical impulses. The conduction system therefore forms a route or pathway for electrical impulses to travel through the myocardium, which in turn will initiate the mechanical contraction of the heart.

The sinoatrial (SA) node is often described as the natural pacemaker of the heart, as this is where initial electrical impulses arise. It is in the wall of the right atrium just below the opening of the superior vena cava. The SA node at rest generates impulses at an inherent rate of between 60 and 70 impulses per minute. This rate will increase in response to specific stimuli including exercise, stimulant drugs such as epinephrine, and pyrexia. Additionally, there are specific structures that link the SA node to the left atrium and the atrioventricular (AV) node to ensure rapid propagation of the electrical impulse throughout the atria (Figure 3.2).

These structures are termed the internodal tracts over which conduction proceeds more rapidly than in other areas of the atrial myocardium. The conduction of the electrical impulse throughout the right and left atria is seen on the ECG as the P wave and stimulates atrial contraction (Figure 3.3).

Key Point

If a rhythm originates from the sinus node at a rate less than 60 bpm, this is known as sinus bradycardia. If a rhythm originates from the sinus node at a rate greater than 100 bpm, this is known as sinus tachycardia.

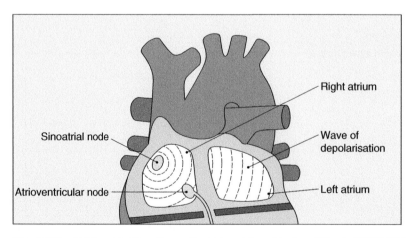

Figure 3.2 Atrial conduction. *Source:* Reproduced from Meek and Morris (2002). With permission from BMJ Publishing Group Ltd.

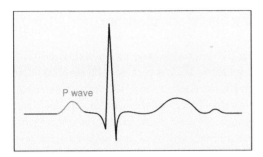

Figure 3.3 The P wave. *Source:* Reproduced from Meek and Morris (2002). With permission from BMJ Publishing Group Ltd.

Impulses from the SA node are received directly by the AV node via the internodal tracts. The AV node lies in the right atrium along the lower part of the interatrial septum and forms the only acceptable pathway between the atria and the ventricles. It delays passage of the impulse to the ventricles to allow time for ventricular filling. This delay is represented on the ECG by the P–R interval. Like the SA node, the AV node is autorhythmic and therefore generates its own impulses. At rest, the AV node generates impulses of 40–60 per minute. From the AV node, the impulses pass down the bundle of His, which is a direct extension of the AV node and thus often referred to as the AV bundle. It is located at the top of the ventricular septum and separates within the ventricular septum into two distinct divisions, termed the left and right bundle branches. They course through the interventricular septum towards the apex of the heart (Figure 3.4). These branches allow impulses to pass equally through both ventricles. In contrast to the right ventricle, the left ventricle constitutes a larger mass of myocardium due to the increased workload that is demanded of it; thus, the left bundle branch separates into two distinct fascicles termed the anterior and posterior fascicles, allowing impulses to pass effectively and evenly throughout the left ventricle.

At the apex of the ventricles, the left and right bundle branches separate further into a sheet of fibres termed the Purkinje fibres, or conduction myofibres which spread across the posterior of the left and right ventricles. These fibres come into contact with the myocardium

Figure 3.4 Wave of depolarisation through the ventricles giving rise to the QRS complex. *Source:* Reproduced from Meek and Morris (2002). With permission from BMJ Publishing Group Ltd.

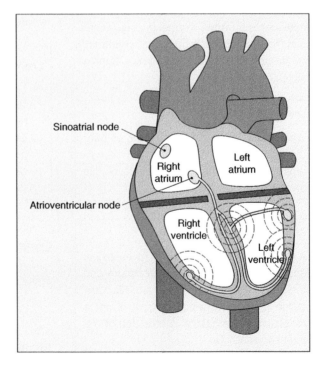

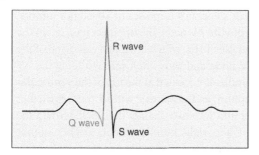

Figure 3.5 Components of the QRS complex. *Source:* Reproduced from Meek and Morris (2002). With permission from BMJ Publishing Group Ltd.

at the subendocardial regions, depolarising the myocardium. The papillary muscles contract first, followed by a wave of excitation and contraction which proceeds from endocardium to epicardium, and travels from the apex of the heart to the ventricular outflow tract, causing the ventricle to contract and expel blood into the systemic and pulmonary circulations. This part of the electrical impulse is represented by the QRS complex on the ECG (Figure 3.5). Both the Purkinje fibres and the left and right bundle branches intrinsically fire impulses at a much lower rate than the SA node and AV node (approximately 20–40 impulses per minute). Normal passage of electrical impulses through the entire conduction system or the cardiac cycle takes approximately 0.8 of a second.

Learning Activity 3.2

What is the physiological meaning of 'bundle branch block'?

What does a bundle branch block look like on the ECG?

Key Point

An ECG reflects the passage of electrical impulses throughout the myocardium and the process of depolarisation and repolarisation of the myocardial cells; it is not a reflection of mechanical contraction of the atria and ventricles.

The Electrocardiogram

The ECG is separated into a series of three distinct waveforms: the P wave, the QRS complex and the T wave. Each of these waveforms represents a specific phase in the passage of electrical impulses through the heart's conduction system and subsequently atrial and ventricular depolarisation as well as ventricular repolarisation.

The P wave represents depolarisation of the atria which is a result of the passage of an electrical impulse from the SA node through both atria The QRS complex represents depolarisation of the ventricles. Depolarisation of the ventricles is a process involving depolarisation of the interventricular septum and the subsequent spread of depolarisation by the Purkinje fibres through the lateral ventricular walls. The T wave represents repolarisation of the ventricles and the return of the ventricles to the resting membrane potential. Occasionally a U wave may be seen immediately following the T wave. The U wave is believed to result from late repolarisation of Purkinje fibres in the papillary muscle of the ventricular myocardium (Thibodeau and Patton 2007); however, there remains some contention as to its true origin.

Learning Activity 3.3

a) Can electrophysiological activity be seen in the heart in the absence of mechanical activity?

b) Can mechanical activity be seen in the heart in the absence of electrophysiological activity? What cardiac rhythm is likely to be associated with this syndrome?

Conclusion

This chapter has provided an overview of the anatomy and physiology of the conduction system of the heart, and the complex way it interacts and augments mechanical function. Disturbances of the conducting system can result in arrhythmias, which may result in sub-optimal mechanical function of the heart, and in some cases, death. It is therefore essential that nurses understand the principles of cardiac electrophysiology as a basis for early recognition and management of cardiac arrhythmias.

Learning Activity 3.4

Multiple Choice Questions

1) What is the inherent rate of impulse generation of the SA node at rest?
   a) 60–70
   b) 100
   c) 80–90
   d) 50–60

2) What is the ratio of contractile cells to autorhythmic cells in the myocardium?
   a) 3:1
   b) 50:50
   c) 99:1
   d) 5:1

3) Which of the following does the T wave represent?
   a) Contraction of the ventricles
   b) Repolarisation of the ventricles
   c) Depolarisation of the ventricles
   d) None of these

4) What important protein is important to initiate contraction in myocytes?
   a) Adenosine diphosphate
   b) Adenosine triphosphate
   c) Troponin
   d) All of these

5) Which phase in the action potential of the cardiac muscle represents the plateau phase?
   a) Phase 1
   b) Phase 3
   c) Phase 2
   d) Phase 4

Learning Activity Answers

Learning Activity 3.1 Relating Theory to Practice

Answer:
a) In hypokalaemia, the magnitude of the concentration gradient for potassium across the myocyte increaseses, thus increasing the resting membrane potential and speeding up conduction through the myocardium. Hypokalaemia may cause prolonged repolarisation. The myocardium is extremely sensitive to the effects of hypokalaemia, particularly if the patient has coronary artery disease or is taking digoxin (He and& McGregor 2001).
b) Hypokalaemia can produce ECG changes such as U-waves and T-wave flattening. The arrhythmias most commonly associated with hypokalaemia are torsades de pointes, polymorphic ventricular tachycardia, and ventricular fibrillation (Pezhouman, Singh, Song, et al. 2015).
c) Patients taking diuretics without potassium supplementation may be prone to hypokalaemia.
d) In hyperkalaemia, the magnitude of the concentration gradient for potassium across the myocyte diminishes, thus decreasing the resting membrane potential and slowing conduction through the myocardium (Parham et al., Mehdirad, & Biermann, 2006).
e) The first ECG sign of hyperkalaemia is peaked t waves. As hyperkalaemia becomes more severe, the P-wave will widen and flatten and PR segment lengthen until the P-waves eventually disappear. The QRS interval will become prolonged with bizarre QRS morphology and conduction blocks (bundle branch blocks, fascicular blocks). Bradycardia, possibly with a sine wave appearance, will develop, and cardiac arrest will eventuate due to pulseless

electrical activity, ventricular fibrillation or asystole (Parham et al., Mehdirad, & Biermann, 2006).

f) Patients taking renin–angiotensin-aldosterone system inhibitors may be at risk of hyperkalaemia (Kovesdy 2015). Hyperkalaemia is particularly common in patients with chronic kidney disease and those with heart failure (Ingelfinger 2015).

Learning Activity 3.2 Relating Theory to Practice

Answer: The normal sequence of cardiac conduction starts with an impulse that originates in the sinoatrial node (located in the right atrium), which first activates the right atrium then the left atrium. Conduction of the impulse to the ventricles is delayed in the atrioventricular node to allow the ventricular chambers to fill, and is then conducted rapidly through the ventricles via the bundle of His, the right and left bundles, and the Purkinje fibres. When either the left or right bundle branch is blocked (bundle branch block), impulses still travel from the atria to the ventricles so there is no complete block. The ventricles will still be driven by the SA node, but the sequence and duration of ventricular depolarisation will be altered as the impulse will have to travel

outside of the normal conducting pathway. As the impulse takes more time to travel through the ventricles, the QRS is wider than normal. Bundle branch block is diagnosed on the ECG when the QRS complex exceeds 120 ms (three small squares). You will learn more about ECG interpretation of bundle branch blocks in Chapter 9.

Learning Activity 3.3 Critical Thinking

Answer:

a) A lack of ventricular electrical activity always results in a lack of ventricular mechanical activity. The associated rhythm would be asystole.

b) Electrical activity can be present for a short period of time without associated mechanical activity. This is referred to as pulseless electrical activity (PEA), a clinical condition characterised by unresponsiveness and lack of palpable pulse in the presence of organised cardiac electrical activity. PEA has previously been referred to as electromechanical dissociation (EMD) (Shah & Shah 2018).

Learning Activity 3.4 Multiple Choice Questions

Answers: 1 (a); 2 (c); 3 (b); 4 (b); 5 (c)

References

He, F.J. and MacGregor, G.A. (2001). Beneficial effects of potassium. *British Medical Journal* **323** (7311): 497–501.

Ingelfinger, J.R. (2015). A new era for the treatment of hyperkalemia? *New England Journal of Medicine* **372** (3): 275–277.

Klabunde, R.E. (2021). Cardiovascular physiology concepts. https://www.cvphysiology.com (retrieved 10 June 2021).

Kovesdy, C.P. (2015). Management of hyperkalemia: an update for the internist. *The American Journal of Medicine*, **128** (12): 1281–1287.

Meek S, Morris F. Introduction. II – basic terminology. *BMJ*. 2002; **324** (7335): 470–473. doi:https://doi.org/10.1136/bmj.324.7335.470

Parham, W.A., Mehdirad, A.A., Biermann, K.M., & Fredman, C.S. (2006). Hyperkalemia revisited. *Texas Heart Institute Journal,* **33** (1), 40.

Pezhouman, A., Singh, N., Song, Z., Nivala, M., Eskandari, A., Cao, H., ... & Weiss, J.N. (2015). Molecular basis of hypokalemia-induced ventricular fibrillation. *Circulation*, **132** (16); 1528–1537.

Shah, S.N & Shah, A.N (2018). Pulseless electrical activity. *Medscape.* http://emedicine.medscape.com/article/161080-overview (retrieved 6th April 2022).

Thibodeau, G.A. and Patton, K.T. (2007). Anatomy and Physiology, 8ee. Philadelphia: Mosby.

4

The Coronary Circulation

Brendan Greaney and Angela M. Kucia

Overview

This chapter will outline the structure and function of the coronary circulation, describing the key coronary arteries and specific areas of the heart muscle supplied by each of these arteries. An understanding of the structure and function of the coronary circulation will be useful in the interpretation of cardiac catheterisation reports and assist the nurse in understanding the signs and symptoms that occur because of occlusion of a particular coronary artery, relative to the myocardial structures that it supplies.

Learning Objectives

After reading this chapter, you should be able to:

- List the components of the coronary circulation.
- Name the specific areas of the heart supplied by each of the coronary arteries.
- Describe the structure and function of the coronary arterial and venous circulation.
- Discuss the function of collateral vessels.
- Describe the function of the coronary microvascular system.

Key Concepts

Sub-epicardial arteries; collateral circulation; microvascular circulation; coronary dominance; coronary perfusion

The Coronary Circulation

To maintain the function of supplying all body organs and tissues with oxygen and nutrients, the heart requires an effective and reliable blood supply. Disruption to this blood supply has potentially catastrophic consequences. The coronary circulation has blood vessels that supply blood to and remove blood from the heart. The vessels that supply blood rich in oxygen to the heart are known as coronary arteries. The vessels that remove the deoxygenated blood from the heart are known as cardiac veins. When we think of the coronary arteries, we generally form a picture of the large arteries that run on the surface of the heart known as the epicardial or sub-epicardial arteries, which, in a healthy state, are capable of autoregulation to maintain coronary blood flow at levels appropriate to the needs of the myocardium at any given time. The other component to the normal coronary arterial circulation consists of high-resistance distal microvascular vessels that form the arteriolar–capillary network (Angelini et al. 2002).

The right and left coronary arteries branch from the ascending aorta and provide oxygenated blood supply to the myocardium (Tortora et al. 2009). The venous circulation returns to the right atrium through the coronary sinus, a large vein located on the posterior surface of the heart. The name and nature of a coronary artery is defined by the vessel's distal vascularisation pattern or territory rather than its origin (Pelech 2006). The exact anatomy of the myocardial blood supply varies considerably from person to person, but the common anatomical characteristics of the epicardial arteries are depicted in Figure 4.1.

The Left Main Coronary Artery

In most people, there is a left main coronary artery (LMCA or LMA) that originates from the ostium of the left sinus of Valsalva. Typically, it is 1–2 cm in length and 5–10 mm in diameter. The LMCA courses between the left atrial appendage and the pulmonary artery, before

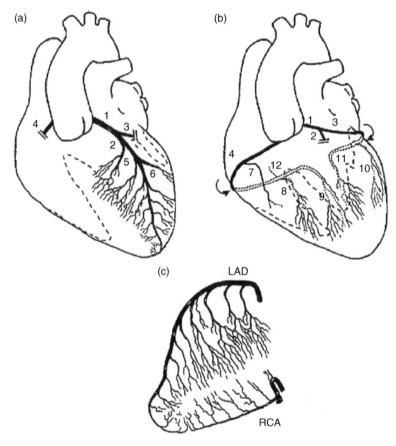

Figure 4.1 Coronary artery diagram. Coronary circulation: (a) territory of the LAD; (b) territory of the RCA and the LCX; (c) septal perfusion. The anterior part is perfused by the septal branches of the LAD and the inferior part by the septal branches of the posterior descending coronary artery (RCA or, less frequently, LCX). Numbers refer to the following elements: (1) left main trunk; (2) LAD; (3) LCX; (4) RCA; (5) first septal branch (S1); (6) first diagonal branch (D1); (7) RV branch; (8) posterior descending from the RCA; (9) posterolateral from the RCA; (10) obtuse marginal (OM) from the LCX; (11) posterobasal from the LCX; (12) AV node branch (RCA). *Source:* Bayes De Luna (2006).

reaching the left atrioventricular (AV) groove, where it bifurcates into the left anterior descending (LAD) and the left circumflex (LCX or CX) arteries. In some cases, an artery may arise from the LMCA between the LAD and LCX, and this may be referred to as the intermediate, ramus or optional diagonal coronary artery.

The Left Anterior Descending Artery

The LAD artery continues directly from the bifurcation of the LMCA down the anterior interventricular groove; its length is extremely variable. In most cases, it reaches the apex of the heart and supplies the anterolateral myocardium, apex and interventricular septum. Arteries branching from the LAD artery include the diagonals, septal perforators and right ventricular branches. There may be between two and six diagonals, which supply the anterior wall of the myocardium. The first diagonal is usually the largest of these vessels. The septal perforators are generally between two and six in number. The first of these vessels, the largest, originates just beyond the take-off of the first diagonal. The septal perforators supply the anterior two-thirds of the ventricular septum (Mill et al. 2003). In some cases, the LAD artery gives off right ventricular branches that supply the anterior surface of the right ventricle. The LAD artery may extend for several millimetres and wrap around the apex of the left ventricle to supply the apical portion of the inferior wall (Sadanandan et al. 2003). In rare cases, it may replace the posterior descending artery (PDA) (Mill et al. 2003).

The Left Circumflex Artery

The LCX artery runs across the left AV groove and gives off obtuse marginal (OM) branches that supply blood to the lateral wall of the left ventricle and the posteromedial papillary muscle. In 10–15% of cases, the LCX artery

continues to the crux of the heart and gives rise to the PDA and posterolateral artery (PLA). You may hear medical or nursing staff refer to a patient/client as being 'right or left dominant' in terms of their coronary blood supply. The artery that supplies the PDA and the PLA determines the coronary dominance. Thus, if the LCX artery supplies the PDA and PLA, the person is said to be 'left dominant'. When the LCX artery supplies the PDA, it also supplies the AV node. Additional branches supply blood to the left atrium and to the sinoatrial (SA) node in 40–50% of people (Mill et al. 2003).

The Right Coronary Artery

The right coronary artery (RCA) originates from the aorta, above the right cusp of the aortic valve and travels down the right AV groove. In the majority of people, the RCA crosses to the crux and makes a characteristic 'U turn' before bifurcating into the PDA and right PLA. The RCA gives off the PDA and PLA in 85% of people (right dominance). The PDA runs along the posterior intraventricular groove towards the apex of the heart and gives off perpendicular branches; the posterior septal perforators, which supply the posterior third of the ventricular septum. The right PLA gives rise to branches that supply the posterior surface of the left ventricle.

The first branch arising from the RCA is the conal or infundibular branch which courses anteriorly to supply the right ventricular outflow tract (Pelech 2006). The atria are supplied by the RCA, but the pattern of branches supplying them is highly variable. The RCA supplies the SA node in 50–60% of people. The acute marginal branches of the RCA supply the anterior wall of the right ventricle, and in 10–20% of people, one of the branches will course along the diaphragmatic surface of the right ventricle to supply the distal ventricular septum. The RCA supplies collaterals to the LAD artery through its septal perforators, and additionally, the conus branch may serve as a collateral to the LAD artery.

Learning Activity 4.1

Picking the culprit artery in acute myocardial infarction isn't always straightforward. Consider the following scenario:

A 53-year-old male patient presents with what appears on ECG to be an acute inferior myocardial infarction (ST-segment elevation in ECG leads II, III and aVF). There is also marked ST depression in all chest (v) leads. What do you think is the likely culprit artery?

Collateral Circulation

Blood flow to the myocardium can be influenced by the function of collateral vessels (Chilian 1997). Although they are present at birth, collateral vessels do not become functionally significant unless the myocardium experiences hypoxic or ischaemic insult (Woods et al. 2010). These small, normally closed vessels connect two larger arteries or different parts of the same artery. They can connect two branches of a single coronary artery or connect branches of the right coronary artery with the left (Woods et al. 2010). When blood flow to one of the major vessels is obstructed, the collaterals enlarge and the blood flow through them increases, providing an alternate blood supply. In the setting of a coronary occlusion, collaterals may provide sufficient perfusion to limit myocardial damage, and prevent myocardial infarction and/or sudden ischaemic death (Marcus 1983). Collaterals only become visible angiographically when coronary occlusion is complete or virtually complete (Chilian 1997). Collaterals may grow quite large in people with coronary artery disease. Although collaterals are present in all people, they do not necessarily open in all individuals (American Heart Association 2007).

Microvascular Circulation

The microcirculation is comprised of arterioles, capillaries, venules and terminal lymphatic vessels. The vessels in this system have a much higher resistance to blood flow compared with the epicardial arteries (Klabunde 2012). The microvascular arterioles are very sensitive to agents causing vasoconstriction. Tissue perfusion is regulated at the microvascular level: thus, any downstream resistance to flow due to vasoconstriction, microemboli or inflammation will have a strong influence on coronary perfusion (Becker and Armani 2003).

Learning Activity 4.2

In a first myocardial infarction, acute occlusion of which artery is most likely to cause a patient to present with acute pulmonary oedema? Give the rationale for your answer.

Coronary Venous Circulation

The venous circulation of the heart is essentially a venous drainage system from the myocardial capillary bed. The source of this capillary network within the myocardial fibres stems from the coronary arteries, which penetrate the myocardium and proliferate in a rich network of capillaries (Little and Little 1989). The venous drainage system from the myocardial capillary bed is drained via three major systems:

1) The thespian veins, which empty into the right and left atrium and a limited amount into the right ventricle.
2) The anterior cardiac veins, which empty into the right atrium.
3) The coronary sinus and its connecting coronary veins, which return blood to the right atrium.

Table 4.1 shows the regions of the heart that are supplied by the different coronary arteries in most people. It is important to know this anatomic distribution because these cardiac regions are assessed by 12-lead ECGs to help localise ischaemic or infarcted regions. Although cardiac regions can be loosely correlated with specific coronary vessels, because of variations (heterogeneity) in coronary vessels between people, actual vessel involvement in ischaemic conditions needs to be verified by coronary angiogram or other imaging techniques (Klabunde 2012).

Table 4.1 Anatomical correlation between anatomical region of the heart and most likely associated coronary artery.

Anatomic region of the heart	Most likely associated coronary artery
Inferior	RCA
Antero-septal	LAD
Antero-apical	LAD (distal)
Lateral	LCX
Posterior	RCA

Suggested Resource

Heart disease 9: coronary arteries
Dr. John Campbell (2014)
https://youtu.be/bpK-tb2hAf4

Suggested Resource

Coronary anatomy and anomalies
The Radiology Assistant (2008)
http://rad.desk.nl/en/48275120e2ed5

Learning Activity Answers

Learning Activity 4.1 Critical Thinking

Answer: Whilst it is logical that the presenting ECG changes are caused by acute occlusion to the right coronary artery, in this case, it was actually acute occlusion of the left anterior descending artery that had collateral supply from the right and circumflex coronary arteries. Sometimes it can be difficult to predict a culprit artery on the ECG, particularly if more than one artery is involved. Ischaemia due to causes other than acute coronary occlusion (such as severe anaemia often results in widespread ischaemic abnormalities on the ECG. For full details of this case, read the article below:

Suggested Resource

Honda, T., Fujimoto, K., Miyao, Y., Koga, H., & Ishii, M. et al. (2014). Acute myocardial infarction caused by left anterior descending artery occlusion presenting as inferior ST elevation and anterior ST depression. *Journal of Cardiology Cases* 9: 67–70.
https://www.journalofcardiologycases.com/article/S1878-5409(13)00136-9/fulltext

Learning Activity 4.2 Relating Theory to Practice

Answer: Acute pulmonary oedema (APO) in the setting of a first myocardial infarction usually caused by left ventricular (LV) failure resulting from anterior myocardial infarction. The largest arteries supplying the left side of the heart are the left main coronary artery and the left anterior descending (LAD) artery. These arteries are the most likely culprits, though this is not always the case.

References

American Heart Association (2007). Collateral circulation. http://www.americanheart.org/presenter.jhtml?identifier=4583 (accesed 17 October 2007).

Angelini, P., Velasco, J.A., and Flamm, S. (2002). Coronary anomalies: incidence, pathophysiology, and clinical relevance. *Circulation* **105**: 2449–2454.

Bayes De Luna, A., Fiol-Sala, M., and Antman, E.M. (2006). *The 12 Lead ECG in ST Elevation Myocardial Infarction*. Oxford: Blackwell Publishing.

Becker, R.C. and Armani, A. (2003). Linking biochemistry, vascular biology, and clinical events in acute coronary syndromes. In: *Management of Acute Coronary Syndromes*, 2ee (ed. C.P. Cannon). New Jersey: Humana Press.

Chilian, W.M. (1997). Coronary microcirculation in health and disease: summary of an NHLBI workshop. *Circulation* **95**: 522–528.

Klabunde, R. (2012). *Cardiovascular Physiology Concepts*. Philadelphia: Lippincott Williams & Wilkins.

Little, R.C. and Little, W.C. (1989). *Physiology of the Heart and Circulation*, 4ee. Chicago: Year Book Medical Publishers Inc.

Marcus, M.L. (1983). *The Coronary Circulation in Health and Disease*. New York: McGraw-Hill.

Mill, M.R., Wilcox, B.R., and Anderson, R.H. (2003). Surgical anatomy of the heart. In: *Cardiac Surgery in the Adult* (ed. L.H. Cohn and L.H.J. Edmunds), 3152. New York: McGraw Hill.

Pelech, A.N. (2006). Coronary artery anomalies. *eMedicine*. http://www.emedicine.com/ped/topic2506.htm (accesed 20 August 2007).

Sadanandan, S., Hochman, J.S., Kolodziej, A. et al. (2003). Clinical and angiographic characteristics of patients with combined anterior and inferior ST-segment elevation on the initial electrocardiogram during acute myocardial infarction. *American Heart Journal* **146**: 653–661.

Tortora, G.J., Derrickson, B., and Tortora, G.J. (2009). *Principles of Anatomy and Physiology*. Hoboken, NJ: Wiley.

Woods, S.L., Sivarajan Froelicher, E.S., Underhill Motzer, S., and Bridges, E.J. (2010). *Cardiac Nursing*, 6ee. Wolters Kluwer/Lippincott Williams & Wilkins.

Part II

Cardiovascular Disease Assessment

5

Risk Factors for Cardiovascular Disease

Angela M. Kucia and Angela Hartley

Overview

Cardiovascular disease (CVD) is the term used to describe diseases of the heart and blood vessels. CVD is caused by atherosclerosis. Atherosclerotic lesions consisting of fat, cholesterol, calcium, and other substances develop throughout the arterial system. Atherosclerosis most commonly manifests as coronary artery disease, peripheral vascular disease, and cerebrovascular disease.

CVD is a major cause of premature death and chronic disability. In 2015, there were an estimated 422.7 million cases of CVD (Roth et al. 2017). CVD was responsible for 17.9 million deaths in 2015, equating to around one third of all deaths globally (Roth et al. 2017). The development of CVD is associated with specific conditions and behaviours that are collectively known as 'cardiovascular risk factors'. The cardiovascular nurse must understand the interplay of cardiovascular risk factors and be able to identify individuals and groups who are most at risk of developing CVD to initiate primary and secondary prevention strategies for cardiac health. This chapter discusses factors that are associated with increased cardiovascular risk and outlines current recommendations for managing these conditions. See Chapter 18 for further information about the management of cardiovascular risk factors.

Learning Objectives

After reading this chapter, you should be able to:

- Identify non-modifiable and modifiable behavioural and biomedical risk factors associated with CVD.
- Discuss absolute and relative risk in relation to the development of CVD in individuals.
- Explain current management strategies for reducing the risk of CVD.

Key Concepts

Absolute risk; cardiovascular risk factors; modifiable and non-modifiable risk factors; biomedical and behavioural risk factors

Absolute Risk

Everyone can be at risk of a cardiac event at some point in their lives, but this risk is lower for some people than for others. For instance, a young person with no risk factors for CVD is less likely to have a CVD-related event in the next five years when compared with a 70-year-old person with high blood pressure, high cholesterol, and tobacco use. Health-related risk is often referred to in terms of absolute risk. Absolute risk refers to the likelihood of developing a disease over a certain time, based on the presence, intensity, and interplay of multiple risk factors. Absolute CVD risk is usually expressed as the numerical probability of a cardiovascular event occurring within a specific time (usually 5 or 10 years). CVD risk calculators combine several risk factors to calculate a risk score.

Learning Activity 5.1

Watch the video below which will explain how considering the interplay of cardiovascular risk factors is better at assessing absolute risk of developing cardiovascular disease compared with looking at cardiovascular risk factors individually.

Suggested Resource

Absolute risk and what it means in practice
Heart Foundation (2010)
https://vimeo.com/16198026

Learning Activity 5.2

Visit the two websites below and calculate your personal CVD risk.

Suggested Resources

SCORE2 and SCORE2-OP Heart score European Society of Cardiology (2021)
https://www.heartscore.org/en_GB/access-heartscore-quick-calculator

Australian absolute cardiovascular disease risk calculator
Australian Chronic Disease Prevention Alliance (ACDPA) (2022)
http://www.cvdcheck.org.au/

SCORE2 Working Group and ESC Cardiovascular Risk Collaboration (2021). SCORE2 risk prediction algorithms: new models to estimate 10-year risk of cardiovascular disease in Europe. *European Heart Journal* 42 (25): 2439–2454. https://doi.org/10.1093/eurheartj/ehab309

Learning Activity 5.3

You may see the term 'relative risk' used in scientific publications. Relative risk is generally used in medical research to compare risk in two different groups of people (or in the same group of people following an intervention).

Relative risk reduction is often misinterpreted in the media as a treatment or health strategy offering a greater benefit to the general population rather than a targeted group of people. Access the suggested resource below to get a better understanding of the differences between absolute and relative risk.

Suggested Resource

Absolute risk and relative risk
Patient (2018)
https://patient.info/news-and-features/calculating-absolute-risk-and-relative-risk

---

Classification of Risk Factors for CVD

Identified risk factors for the development of CVD are listed in Table 5.1. These risk factors can be classed as biomedical, behavioural and psychosocial. Biomedical risk factors can be further categorised as modifiable and non-modifiable. Modifiable biomedical risk factors include hypertension, dyslipidaemia, overweight/obesity, diabetes/insulin resistance and renal disease. Non-modifiable risks are age, gender and family history. Behavioural risk factors include tobacco smoking, physical inactivity, poor nutrition and excessive alcohol consumption. Psychosocial risk factors include depression, stress, anxiety and social isolation. Modifiable and behavioural risk factors are themselves strongly influenced by factors such as personal economic resources, education, living and working conditions, and

Table 5.1 Risk factors for the development of CVD.

Biomedical		Behavioural	Psychosocial
Non-modifiable	**Modifiable**	**Behavioural**	**Psychosocial**
• Age • Gender • Family history of CVD	• Hypertension • Dyslipidaemia • Overweight/obesity • Diabetes/insulin resistance • Renal disease	• Tobacco smoking • Physical inactivity • Poor nutrition • Excessive alcohol consumption	• Depression • Anxiety • Social isolation • Stress

access to health care and social services (Australian Institute of Health and Welfare [AIHW] 2015).

Biomedical Risk Factors

Non-modifiable risk factors are listed as age, gender and a family history of CVD. CVD predominantly affects middle-aged and older individuals. Men are at greater risk of CVD than women until the age of 65 due to the protective effects of oestrogen in younger women, but by the age of 65, women have a risk equal to that of men. The risk of developing CVD is increased if a first-degree relative is diagnosed with heart or blood vessel disease before the age of 60 (Boudi et al. 2015). Although age, gender and family history (genetics) are non-modifiable risk factors, awareness of these risks and their interplay with other CVD risk factors may encourage people to take positive steps in addressing risk factors that can be modified. A family history reflects a genetic component of risk, but shared family behavioural and environmental risk factors likely play a part (Mozaffarian et al. 2016).

Modifiable biomedical risk factors include hypertension, dyslipidaemia, diabetes and renal failure.

Hypertension

Hypertension remains a dominant risk factor for cardiovascular disease. It is estimated that 874 million people had a systolic blood pressure (SBP) of 140 mm Hg or higher in 2015. It is estimated that SBP of 140 mm Hg or higher was responsible for 14% of total deaths and 143 million disability-associated life-years worldwide (Forouzanfar et al. 2017).

Primary hypertension with no identifiable underlying cause is the most common form of hypertension. Secondary hypertension is associated with an underlying cause and occurs in around 5–10% of cases of hypertension. Hypertension is more likely to occur in those who are physically inactive, overweight or have high sodium intakes.

The risk of developing CVD due to hypertension is related to both elevated systolic and diastolic BP levels. Causes of hypertension are shown in Table 5.2.

Most people with hypertension exhibit additional risk factors for CVD. Hypertension and other cardiovascular risk factors may potentiate each other, leading to an increased total risk of developing CVD that is greater than the number (sum) of individual risk factors. All patients with hypertension should have a thorough clinical assessment to identify all cardiovascular risk factors; detect end-organ damage and related or comorbid clinical conditions and identify any causes of secondary hypertension (National Heart Foundation of Australia [NHFA] 2016). Classification of blood pressure differs slightly between organisations and countries. National guidelines for the management of hypertension state systolic and diagnostic

Table 5.2 Causes of hypertension.

Primary (essential) hypertension	Secondary hypertension
Cause unknown	Renal artery stenosis
	Chronic kidney disease
	Hyper/hypothyroidism
	Coarctation of the aorta
	Cushing syndrome
	Aldosteronism
	Hyperparathyroidism
	Obesity
	Pregnancy
	Preeclampsia
	High alcohol intake
	Medications/ supplements/illegal drugs
	Birth control pills
	Ginseng
	Licorice
	Ephedra
	Cocaine
	Methamphetamine

thresholds for diagnosis of hypertension and recommend that a decision to treat at lower BP levels should consider absolute CVD risk and/or evidence of end-organ damage, together with accurate BP assessment (Gabb et al. 2016). The American College of Cardiology/American Heart Association (Whelton et al. 2018) have recategorised the blood pressure ranges as shown below:

- Normal: Systolic less than 120 and diastolic less than 80
- Elevated: Systolic between 120 and 129 *and* diastolic less than 80
- Stage 1 hypertension: Systolic between 130 and 139 *or* diastolic between 80 and 89
- Stage 2 hypertension: Systolic 140 and above or diastolic 90 and above

Measuring BP

BP should be measured using standard measurement techniques on several occasions to obtain a realistic assessment and plan appropriate management. This should include measuring the blood pressure (BP) on both arms, and if there is a difference, using the arm with the higher reading thereafter. In patients who may have orthostatic hypotension BP should be measured. in the sitting position and repeat after the patient has been standing for at least 2 minutes (NHFA 2016).

> **Key Point**
>
> Patients should refrain from caffeine and smoking for at least 2 hours before BP measurement (NHFA 2016).

It may be necessary to monitor BP outside of the clinical setting, either by self-measurement or 24–48 hours ambulatory BP monitoring. For clients with unusual BP variability or a 'white coat' effect where BP becomes elevated primarily during visits to the health professional, it may be necessary to assess BP in the home or ambulatory setting, particularly in situations where there may be unusual variations in BP between clinic visits; hypertension that is resistant to medication; suspected hypotensive episodes; or a 'white coat' effect where BP becomes elevated primarily during clinic visits (NHFA 2016).

> **Suggested Resource**
>
> How to measure blood pressure
> British and Irish Hypertension Society (2017)
> https://bihsoc.org/resources/bp-measurement/measure-blood-pressure/

> **Key Point**
>
> Although automated non-invasive BP monitoring is widely used, a comparative baseline measurement with a mercury sphygmomanometer and an appropriately sized cuff (with the bladder length at least 80% and the width at least 40% of the circumference of the mid-upper arm) is recommended to ensure accuracy (NHFA 2016).

Dyslipidaemia

Dyslipidaemia is a metabolic derangement resulting from the elevation of plasma cholesterol and/or triglycerides (TGS), or a low high-density lipid (HDL) level that contributes to the development of atherosclerosis. Dyslipidaemia does not cause symptoms, but it leads to symptomatic vascular disease. Dyslipidaemia may be a hereditary (primary) or acquired (secondary) disorder. Primary causes of dyslipidaemia are genetic mutations that result in either overproduction or defective clearance of TGS and low-density lipid (LDL) cholesterol, or underproduction or excessive clearance of HDL (Goldberg 2015). Primary causes of dyslipidaemia are more common in children, but secondary causes are more common in adults, with the most common cause in developed countries being a sedentary lifestyle with excessive dietary intake of saturated fat, cholesterol and trans fatty acids (TFAs) (Goldberg 2015). Other causes include diabetes mellitus, alcohol overuse, chronic renal insufficiency and/or failure, hypothyroidism, primary biliary cirrhosis and other cholestatic liver diseases. Drugs such as thiazides, β-blockers, retinoids, highly active antiretroviral agents, anabolic steroids, amiodarone, thiazide diuretics, immunosuppressive drugs, oestrogen and progestins, and glucocorticoids may also cause, or contribute to, dyslipidaemia (Jacobson et al. 2014; Goldberg 2015). People with greater risk of dyslipidaemia include those with clinical evidence of vascular disease (including CVD, peripheral arterial disease, or stroke), diabetes mellitus, chronic kidney disease, and familial hypercholesterolaemia. See Chapter 18 for information about the management of hypertension.

> **Key Point**
>
> Indigenous populations such as Aboriginal and Torres Strait Islander people and Maori and Pacific Islanders and ethnic minority populations including South Asian and Middle Eastern people (Ray et al. 2014) and Asian and Mexican Americans (Frank et al. 2014) have an increased risk of dyslipidaemia.

People with diabetes (particularly type 2 diabetes) have a particularly atherogenic type of dyslipidaemia (diabetic dyslipidaemia or hypertriglyceridaemic hyperapo B), characterised by elevated TGS, which are thought to have atherogenic properties; low HDL cholesterol; shift in LDL particle density towards small, dense LDL (type B); and a tendency towards postprandial lipidaemia. Most patients with diabetes and dyslipidaemia will require pharmacological therapy to reach target lipid goals.

Familial hypercholesterolaemia (FH) is associated with a raised cholesterol concentration in the blood from birth and may lead to premature development of atherosclerosis and coronary heart disease (CHD) at a young age. FH is caused by an inherited genetic defect (Santos et al. 2016).

> **Key Point**
>
> Coronary heart disease risk estimation tools should not be used in people with FH as they are already at a high risk of premature coronary heart disease.

Measuring Lipids

Dyslipidaemia is diagnosed by measuring serum lipids. Lipids can be measured in the non-fasting state, but for consistency and accuracy, all patients should at some time have fasting serum lipids measured. A lipid panel typically includes:

- Total cholesterol
- High-density lipoprotein cholesterol (HDL-C)
- Triglycerides

HDL-C is often referred to as the 'good cholesterol' as it removes excess cholesterol and transports it to the liver for removal. LDL-C is referred to as the 'bad cholesterol' as it deposits excess cholesterol in the walls of blood vessels and can contribute to atherosclerosis.

Target lipid levels vary slightly according to the information source and an individual's absolute risk of developing CVD. Target lipid levels for those at high absolute risk of developing CVD or known to have CVD are more aggressively managed than for individuals with low risk for CVD. Normal lipid profile ranges can be found in Chapter 7. Further resources relating to dyslipdaemia can be found in Chapter 18.

Key Point

Fasting (except for water) is usually required for 9–12 hours prior to having blood taken for a lipid profile.

Diabetes Mellitus

Diabetes mellitus (DM) "is a group of metabolic disorders characterised by the presence of hyperglycaemia in the absence of treatment" (WHO 2020a, p.9) resulting from defects in insulin secretion, insulin action, or both. Diabetes may result from genetic predisposition and abnormalities, epigenetic processes, insulin resistance, autoimmunity, illness, inflammation, and environmental factors. The common characteristic to all forms of diabetes is the dysfunction or destruction of beta cells. Risk factors are similar to those for cardiovascular disease but also include ethnicity (South Asian, Afro-Caribbean, or Hispanic) (WHO 2020a). See Table 5.3 for classifications of diabetes mellitus.

CVD is the most common cause of death among adults with diabetes mellitus (Fox et al. 2015). Both type 1 and type 2 diabetes mellitus (T2DM) are independent risk factors for CVD (Vistisen et al. 2016), but the most prevalent form is T2DM, which typically manifests later in life and is associated with obesity, physical inactivity, hypertension, dyslipidaemia and thrombotic tendencies (NICE 2015).

Testing for Diabetes

The fasting blood glucose (FBG) and oral glucose tolerance test (OGTT) are blood tests used in the diagnosis of diabetes. Commonly used blood tests to diagnose diabetes are shown in Table 5.4. The OGTT measures the body's ability to metabolise glucose, or clear it out of the bloodstream, and although it is more time consuming than the FBG, it is a more sensitive measure and can be used to diagnose diabetes, gestational diabetes (diabetes during pregnancy) or pre-diabetes. Glycated haemoglobin (HbA1c) reflects average plasma glucose over the preceding 8–12 weeks and can be performed at any time of the day without any special preparation such as fasting. It is the preferred test for assessing glycaemic control in people with diabetes and as a diagnostic test for pre-diabetes (WHO 2020a; Fox et al. 2015).

Suggested Resource

Diagnosis and management of type 2 diabetes (HEARTS-D). Geneva: World Health Organization; 2020 (WHO/UCN/NCD/20.1). Licence: CC BY-NC-SA 3.0 IGO. https://www.who.int/publications/i/item/who-ucn-ncd-20.1

National Institute of Diabetes and Digestive and Kidney Diseases https://www.niddk.nih.gov/health-%AD information/diabetes

Diabetes Australia https://www.diabetesaustralia.com.au/

National Institute of Clinical Excellence (NICE). Type 2 diabetes in adults: management NICE guideline [NG28]Published: 02 December 2015 Last updated: 31 March 2022. https://www.nice.org.uk/guidance/ng28

Table 5.3 Diabetes mellitus classifications.

Diabetes mellitus

Type 1	Type 2	Pre-diabetes
The pancreas is unable to produce insulin because the pancreatic b-cells that make the insulin have been destroyed by the body's own immune system	Progressive condition in which the body becomes resistant to the normal effects of insulin and/or the pancreas loses the capacity to produce enough insulin	Also known as impaired glucose tolerance (IGT) or impaired fasting glucose (IFG). Occurs as a result of insulin resistance. Diagnosed when the blood glucose level (BGL) is higher than normal but not high enough to be classed as diabetes. Often progresses to type 2 diabetes
Accounts for around 10% of all cases of diabetes	Accounts for 85–90% of all cases of diabetes	
Previously known as juvenile onset or insulin-dependent diabetes	May be referred to as mature onset or non-insulin-dependent diabetes	
Is not caused by lifestyle factors	Being overweight and physically inactive are contributors to diabetes development	
Requires insulin injections or an insulin pump	Medication usually required	
One of the most common chronic childhood diseases in developed nations	Modifications to lifestyle such as improved levels of physical activity and diet are needed	

Table 5.4 Blood tests used to diagnose diabetes and their ranges.

Test	Test conditions	Normal	Pre-diabetes	Diabetes
Random	Nil	< 7.8 mmol/l (140 mg/dl)	7.8–11 mmol/l (140–199 mg/dl)	≥11.1 mmol/l (≥200 mg/dl)
FBG	Fasting	4.0–5.6 mmol/l (72–108 mg/dl)	5.6–6.9 mmol/l (100–125 mg/dl)	>7.0 mmol/l (≥126 mg/dl)
OGTT	Fasting; sample taken 2 hours after ingesting 75 g of glucose	Up to 7.8 mmol/l (140 mg/dl)	7.8–11 mmol/l (140–199 mg/dl)	≥11.1 mmol/l ≥200 mg/dl
HbA1c	Nil	<5.7%	5.7–6.4%	≥6.5% (48 mmol/mol)

Note that this is a general guide and that values will vary slightly between countries and pathology laboratories.

Kidney Disease

Chronic kidney disease (CKD) is closely associated with an increased incidence of CVD, and major cardiac events represent almost 50% of the causes of death in CKD patients, which may in part be explained by higher rates of diabetes, dyslipidaemia and HT in the CKD population. Vascular disease in people with CKD tends to be different from atherosclerotic CVD in the general population. In addition to the tradition CVD risk factors, people with CKD also have hyperphosphataemia, secondary hyperparathyroidism, endothelial dysfunction, chronic inflammation, oxidative stress and vascular calcification that directly affect arterial compliance and the coronary circulation (Di Lullo et al. 2015).

Suggested Resources

National Institute for Health and Care Excellence (NICE) (2021). Chronic kidney disease: assessment and management NICE guideline [NG203] Published: 25 August 2021. Last updated: 24 November 2021. https://www.nice.org.uk/guidance/ng203

Kidney Health Australia. https://kidney.org.au/

Key Point

Angiotensin-converting enzyme (ACE) inhibitors and angiotensin receptor blockers (ARBs) cause a reversible reduction in GFR when treatment is initiated. Monitor renal function, potassium and BP before starting, 7 days after commencement and regularly during treatment.

Behavioural Risk Factors

Several risk factors for CVD may have biomedical consequences but are often due to behavioural factors. Included in this group are obesity/overweight (which may be due to biomedical or behavioural factors), tobacco use, physical inactivity and alcohol use at harmful levels.

Overweight/Obesity

The WHO (2021a) defines overweight and obesity as 'abnormal or excessive fat accumulation that may impair health'. Worldwide obesity has more than doubled since 1980 and being overweight is a greater cause of mortality than being underweight. Overweight and obesity is a result of an energy imbalance between calories consumed and calories expended. Globally, overweight and obesity is influenced by a shift in diet towards increased intake of energy-dense foods that are high in fat and sugars but low in vitamins, minerals and other micronutrients. Furthermore, contemporary forms of work, modes of transportation and increasing urbanisation are of an increasingly sedentary nature.

Measuring Overweight and Obesity

Overweight and obesity can be crudely measured by body mass index (BMI), defined as a person's weight in kilograms divided by the square of his height in meters (kg/m^2).

Overweight is generally defined as a BMI equal to or more than 25 and obesity as a BMI equal to or more than 30, but these cutoff points may differ slightly in some populations. Using BMI to diagnose obesity in the elderly is suboptimal as changes in body composition with normal ageing leads to increased adiposity and decreased muscle mass (Batsis et al. 2016). Other measures that may be used are waist circumference (WC) or waist-to-height circumference (WtHC). WtHC appears to be superior to BMI and WC in predicting diabetes, dyslipidaemia, hypertension, and CVD risk in both sexes in populations of various nationalities and ethnic groups (Ashwell et al. 2012). For further information and resources on overweight and obesity in secondary prevention see Chapter 18.

Suggested Resource

Obesity
WHO (2021)
https://www.who.int/health-topics/
obesity#tab=tab_1

Tobacco Use

There are more than one billion smokers in the world, and whilst tobacco use is decreasing in high-income countries, overall global use of tobacco is increasing due to increased use in developing countries. Tobacco is one of the main risk factors for several chronic diseases, including CVD, and kills around half of those who use it (WHO 2021b). It is one of the most important causes of acute myocardial infarction globally, especially in men (WHO 2015). Cigarette smoke has both long- and short-term effects on the cardiovascular system and promotes the development of atherosclerosis, inflammation, vascular dysfunction, and thrombosis via several mechanisms (Table 5.5) (Willis et al. 2007). All forms of tobacco use (inhalation or ingestion) are harmful and both active and passive (environmental or second-hand) cigarette smoke exposure increases cardiovascular risk (Eriksen and Whitney 2013).

Key Point

E-cigarettes are devices which heat a liquid to create an aerosol which is then inhaled by the user. The longterm effects are not yet known but they are considered to be unsafe whether or not they contain nicotine (WHO 2021b).

Physical Inactivity and Sedentary Behaviour

The WHO (2020b) defines physical activity as being 'any bodily movement produced by skeletal muscles that requires energy expenditure'. Physical inactivity, or sedentary behaviour, is the fourth leading risk factor for global

Table 5.5 Cardiovascular effects of cigarette smoke.

Atherogenic effects
 Inflammation
 Modification of lipid profile (Campbell et al. 2008)
Thrombotic effects
 Platelet activation and aggregation
 Alterations in antithrombotic and prothrombotic factors Alterations in fibrinolysis (Barua and Ambrose 2013)
Endothelial dysfunction
 Increased oxidative stress
 Decreased nitric oxide availability
 Coronary vasospasm (Barua and Ambrose 2013)
Autonomic effects leading to increased myocardial workload
 Increased heart rate (Dinas et al. 2013)
 Increased BP
 Increased stroke volume
 Increased cardiac output (Smith and Fischer 2001)
Plaque instability
 Higher plaque extracellular lipid content
 Intraplaque inflammation
 Increased expression and activity of matrix metalloproteinases
 Involved in degradation of plaque matrix (Barua and Ambrose 2013)

mortality and is responsible for an estimated 3.2 million deaths globally (WHO 2020b). Physical inactivity is also a major risk factor for the development of CVD and contributes to the development of other CVD risk factors including obesity, hypertension, dyslipidaemia, and diabetes.

Sedentary behaviour may seem like the opposite of exercise, but it is an independent risk factor for certain chronic diseases and is therefore considered separately to physical activity, body weight, and diet. Common sedentary behaviours include watching television, reading, using a computer, and driving. Research in sedentary behaviour has been conducted in both adults and children, and clearly links sedentary behaviour with chronic disease, morbidity and mortality in adults (Tremblay et al. 2010; Grontved and Hu 2011; Proper et al. 2011). It is harder to determine the effects of sedentary behaviour on health in childhood since the relevant diseases generally do not surface until later in life; however, available evidence suggests that sedentary behaviour may also be a health risk in children and young people (Tremblay et al. 2011). It is especially important to discourage prolonged sedentary behaviour in children, since we know that sedentary behaviour increases with age, and a sedentary child is likely to become a sedentary adult (Biddle et al. 2010). For more information on physical activity see Chapter 18.

Key Point

The WHO (2020b) recommends that adults aged 18–64 years should do at least 150–300 minutes of moderately intense physical activity, or alternately at least 75–150 minutes of vigorous activity (or equivalent combination of moderate and vigorous activity) throughout the week and all activity should be performed in bouts of at least 10 minutes duration.

Alcohol Consumption

Habitual moderate alcohol intake (1–2 standard drinks/d) appears to confer some long-term cardiovascular benefits in terms of improvements in high-density lipoprotein cholesterol, heart rate variability, endothelial function, insulin sensitivity, and coagulation and fibrinolytic cascades, whereas heavy drinking (>3 drinks/d) is associated with a higher risk of HT, diabetes mellitus, and CVD. However, due to its physiological effects, alcohol may cause an immediate transient increase in CVD risk resulting from increases in heart rate, interatrial electromechanical delay, and plasminogen activator

inhibitor levels (Mostofsky et al. 2016). Any level of alcohol use can cause health problems in some people even moderate alcohol intake should not be promoted to patients as a good health strategy.

Psychosocial Risk Factors

Psychosocial functioning includes thinking, feeling and acting, and is strongly influenced by self-concept and self-esteem; relationships with others and the ability to engage in social interaction; the ability to cope with stress and adapt to change; and the capacity to develop values and beliefs. Internal factors such as genetics and physical health and fitness, and external factors such as culture, geography and socioeconomic status also have an influence on psychosocial health. Psychosocial factors may contribute to the development of CVD and lead to poorer outcomes following a cardiac event. Abnormal psychosocial functioning may be associated with stress-related disorders such as anxiety, depression, anger and hostility.

Psychological Stress

People often blame stress for causing illness. Stress results in increased output from the sympathetic nervous system and hypothalamic–pituitary–adrenal axis, resulting in a range of pathophysiologic responses such as autonomic nervous system dysfunction, hypertension, inflammation, platelet activation, insulin resistance, endothelial dysfunction and central obesity (Rozanski et al. 2005). Stress, anger, and depressed mood can act as acute triggers of acute cardiac events. Reactions to stress, such as depression, anger, fear, anxiety and sleeping disorders may compound psychological stress. The negative impact of psychological stress on cardiac outcomes has been suspected for some time, but has been somewhat overlooked as a significant risk factor for the development of CVD, and as a precursor of acute coronary events.

This may be due in part to the difficulty of defining or measuring perceptual aspects of stress in individuals. Stress may contribute to the development of heart disease across the lifespan, and also may also influence the development of risk factors for CVD, accelerating atherosclerosis. Even early-life stressors, such as childhood abuse and early socioeconomic adversity, can contribute to an increased risk of cardiovascular morbidity in adulthood (Steptoe and Kivimäki 2013).

Anxiety and Depression

Anxiety disorders are common in Western societies and have been associated with increased risk of cardiac mortality in medically healthy individuals, as well as CHD populations (Watkins et al. 2013). Anxiety disorders include conditions such as panic disorder, social anxiety disorder, specific phobias or generalised anxiety disorder.

Depression has a range of severity that can be as mild as a transient feeling of flat mood, through to serious clinical syndromes that can be severe, disabling, and recurrent, involving symptoms such as a loss of interest or pleasure in activities, sleep disturbance, constant fatigue or impaired concentration (Hare et al. 2014). Depression has for some time been known to be a risk factor for adverse medical outcomes in patients with acute coronary syndrome (ACS) and more recently has been found to be an important contributing factor in ACS presentations (Lichtman et al. 2014). Whilst a developmental mechanism for CHD is not yet fully understood, several possible mechanisms have been proposed including alterations in the function of coagulopathic factors, platelets, pro-inflammatory cytokines, the endothelium, neurohormonal factors and the autonomic nervous system (Hare et al. 2014) (see Figure 5.1).

Individuals with anxiety and depression are more likely to have a poor diet with increased dietary cholesterol and total energy intake, an increased prevalence of smoking and a sedentary lifestyle than non-anxious or non-depressed subjects (Boudi et al. 2015). Depression is also associated with behaviours that are known to increase cardiovascular risk, such as smoking, low levels of physical activity and poor adherence to medical treatment (Hare et al. 2014).

Anger and Hostility

Outbursts of anger have consistently been found to be associated with a transiently higher risk of an acute cardiovascular event, including acute myocardial infarction (AMI) (Mostofsky et al. 2016), ACS (Strike et al. 2006), and ventricular arrhythmias (Reich et al. 1981; Lampert 2010). A recent study by Mostofsky et al. (2016) found that the risk of AMI was around 2.5 times higher in the 2 hours after outbursts of moderate or extreme anger compared with at other times.

Mental Health

People with severe mental health problems are almost twice as likely to die from CVD compared with the general Western population (Laursen et al. 2012). They are also more likely to smoke, be overweight, have high blood pressure, insulin resistance or diabetes, high cholesterol, and metabolic syndrome. Reasons for this include symptoms such as low motivation levels; co-occurring mental health issues such as depression, anxiety and substance-use disorders; physical comorbidities; suboptimal lifestyle factors; low socioeconomic status and unemployment; suboptimal proactive treatment of CVD risk factors by health workers; and the adverse metabolic effects of antipsychotic and mood-stabilising agents used to treat severe mental health disorders (Gladigau et al. 2014). Mental illness is also associated with a high rate of medication non-compliance, and so individuals with mental illness and risk factors for CVD are less likely to comply with therapies to reduce risk (Jonsdottir et al. 2013).

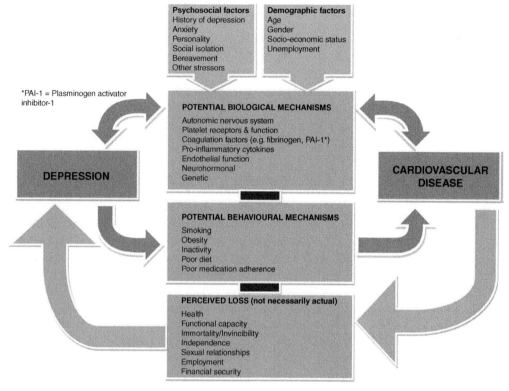

Figure 5.1 Factors that may explain the relationship between cardiovascular disease and depression. *Source:* Hare et al. (2014).

Health behaviours are very much influenced by social, material and cultural circumstances and can be difficult to change. Whilst changing people's health-related behaviour can have a major impact on cardiovascular mortality and morbidity, attempts to modify health behaviours are often unsuccessful. Strategies for risk factor reduction are covered in Chapter 18.

Suggested Resource

Heart disease and mental health disorders Centers for Disease Control and Prevention (2020)
https://www.cdc.gov/heartdisease/mental-health.htm

Conclusion

This chapter has outlined the common risk factors for CVD. Risk for CVD rises progressively according to the number of risk factors present in an individual. Individuals with CVD often have multiple risk factors which elevate their risk of an acute event exponentially. The application of risk assessment tools and identifying those individuals at greatest risk of CVD is dealt with in the next chapter. We do know that people with existing CVD are in the highest risk group for future cardiac events; so a stringent approach to risk factor management through pharmacological and lifestyle interventions will be required.

References

Ashwell, M., Gunn, P., and Gibson, S. (2012). Waist-to-height ratio is a better screening tool than waist circumference and BMI for adult cardiometabolic risk factors: systematic review and meta-analysis. *Obesity Reviews* **13** (3): 275–286.

Australian Institute of Health and Welfare (AIHW) (2015). *Cardiovascular Disease, Diabetes and Chronic Kidney Disease – Australian Facts: Risk Factors*. Australian Institute of Health and Welfare http://www.aihw.gov.au/publication-detail/?id=60129550538 (accessed 26 March 2015).

Barua, R.S. and Ambrose, J.A. (2013). Mechanisms of coronary thrombosis in cigarette smoke exposure. *Arteriosclerosis, Thrombosis, and Vascular Biology* **33** (7): 1460–1467.

Batsis, J.A., Mackenzie, T.A., Bartels, S.J. et al. (2016). Diagnostic accuracy of body mass index to identify obesity in older adults: NHANES 1999–2004. *International Journal of Obesity* **40** (5): 761–767. doi: 10.1038/ijo.2015.243. Epub 2015 Dec 1. PMID: 26620887; PMCID: PMC4854777.

Biddle, S., Pearson, N., Ross, G.M., and Braithwaite, R. (2010). Tracking sedentary behaviours of young people: a systematic review. *Preventative Medicine.* **51** (5): 345–351.

Boudi, B., Chowdhury, A., and Subhi, Y. (2015). Risk factors for coronary artery disease. http://emedicine.medscape.com/article/164163-overview (accessed 20 March 2016).

Campbell, S., Moffatt, R., and Stamford, B. (2008). Smoking and smoking cessation – the relationship between cardiovascular disease and lipoprotein metabolism: a review. *Atherosclerosis* **201**: 225–235.

Di Lullo, L., House, A., Gorini, A. et al. (2015). Chronic kidney disease and cardiovascular complications. *Heart Failure Reviews* **20** (3): 259–272.

Dinas, P., Koutedakis, Y., and Flouris, A. (2013). Effects of active and passive tobacco cigarette smoking on heart rate variability. *International Journal of Cardiology.* **163** (2): 109–115.

Eriksen, M. and Whitney, C. (2013). Risk factors: tobacco. In: *Global Handbook on Noncommunicable Diseases and Health Promotion* (ed. D.V. McQueen), 115–136. New York: Springer.

Forouzanfar, M.H., Liu, P., Roth, G.A. et al. (2017). Global burden of hypertension and systolic blood pressure of at least 110–115 mmHg, 1990–2015. *JAMA* **317** (2): 165–182.

Fox, C.S., Golden, S.H., Anderson, C. et al. (2015). Update on prevention of cardiovascular disease in adults with type 2 diabetes mellitus in light of recent evidence a scientific statement from the American Heart Association and the American Diabetes Association. *Circulation* **132** (8): 691–718.

Frank, A.T., Zhao, B., Jose, P.O. et al. (2014). Racial/ethnic differences in dyslipidemia patterns. *Circulation* **129** (5): 570–579.

Gabb, G.M., Mangoni, A.A., Anderson, C.S. et al. (2016). Guideline for the diagnosis and management of hypertension in adults – 2016. *Medical Journal of Australia* **205** (2): 85–89.

Gladigau EL, Fazio TN, Hannam JP, Dawson LM, Jones SG. Increased cardiovascular risk in patients with severe mental illness. *Internal Medicine Journal* 2014 Jan; **44** (1): 65-9. doi: https://doi.org/10.1111/imj.12319. PMID: 24383746.

Goldberg, A. (2015). Dyslipidemia (Hyperlipidemia). http://www.msdmanuals.com/eu-au/professional/endocrine-and-metabolic-disorders/lipid-disorders/dyslipidemia (accessed 20 March 2016).

Grontved, A. and Hu, F. (2011). Television viewing and risk of type 2 diabetes, cardiovascular disease, and all-cause mortality: a meta-analysis. *Journal of the American Medical Association.* **305**: 2448–2455.

Hare, D.L., Toukhsati, S.R., Johansson, P., and Jaarsma, T. (2014). Depression and cardiovascular disease: a clinical review. *European Heart Journal* **35** (21): 1365–1372.

Jacobson, T., Maki, K., Orringer, C. et al. (2014). National lipid association recommendations for patient-centred management of dyslipidemia: part 1 – executive summary. *Journal of Clinical Lipidology* **8** (5): 473–488.

Jonsdottir, H., Opjordsmoen, S., Birkenaes, A.B. et al. (2013). Predictors of medication adherence in patients with schizophrenia and bipolar disorder. *Acta Psychiatrica Scandinavica* **127** (1): 23–33.

Lampert, R. (2010). Anger and ventricular arrhythmias. *Current Opinion in Cardiology* **25** (1): 46.

Laursen, T.M., Munk-Olsen, T., and Vestergaard, M. (2012). Life expectancy and cardiovascular mortality in persons with schizophrenia. *Current Opinion in Psychiatry* **25** (2): 83–88.

Lichtman, J.H., Froelicher, E.S., Blumenthal, J.A. et al. (2014). Depression as a risk factor for poor prognosis among patients with acute coronary syndrome: systematic review and recommendations a scientific statement from the American Heart Association. *Circulation* **129** (12): 1350–1369.

Mostofsky, E., Chahal, H.S., Mukamal, K.J. et al. (2016). Alcohol and immediate risk of cardiovascular events a systematic review and dose – response meta-analysis. *Circulation* **133** (10): 979–987.

Mozaffarian, D., Benjamin, E.J., Go, A.S. et al. (2016). Heart disease and stroke statistics – 2016 update: a report from the American Heart Association. *Circulation* **133** (4): e38–e360.

National Heart Foundation of Australia (2016). *Guideline for the Diagnosis and Management of Hypertension in Adults – 2016*. Melbourne: National Heart Foundation of Australia https://www.heartfoundation.org.au/images/uploads/publications/PRO-167_Hypertension-guideline-2016_WEB.pdf (accessed 12 November 2016).

National Institute for Health and Care Excellence (NICE) (2015 (updated 2016). *Type 2 Diabetes in Adults: Management*. London: NICE https://www.nice.org.uk/guidance/ng28 (accessed 10 November 2016).

Proper, K., Singh, A., Van Mechelen, W., and Chinapaw, M. (2011). Sedentary behaviors and health outcomes among adults: a systematic review of prospective studies. *American Journal of Preventative Medicine* **40** (2): 174–182.

Ray, K.K., Kastelein, J.J., Boekholdt, S.M. et al. (2014). The ACC/AHA 2013 guideline on the treatment of blood cholesterol to reduce atherosclerotic cardiovascular disease risk in adults: the good the bad and the uncertain: a comparison with ESC/EAS guidelines for the management of dyslipidaemias 2011. *European Heart Journal* **35** (15): 960–968. https://doi.org/10.1093/eurheartj/ehu107.

Reich, P., DeSilva, R.A., Lown, B., and Murawski, B.J. (1981). Acute psychological disturbances preceding life-threatening ventricular arrhythmias. *JAMA* **246** (3): 233–235.

Roth GA, Johnson C, Abajobir A, et al. Global, Regional, and National Burden of Cardiovascular Diseases for 10 Causes, 1990 to 2015. *Journal of the American College of Cardiology* 2017; **70** (1): 1–25. doi:https://doi.org/10.1016/j.jacc.2017.04.052

Rozanski, A., Blumenthal, J.A., Davidson, K.W. et al. (2005). The epidemiology, pathophysiology, and management of psychosocial risk factors in cardiac practice: the emerging field of behavioral cardiology. *Journal of the American College of Cardiology* **45**: 637–651.

Santos, R.D., Gidding, S.S., Hegele, R.A. et al. (2016). Defining severe familial hypercholesterolaemia and the implications for clinical management: a consensus statement from the International Atherosclerosis Society Severe Familial Hypercholesterolemia Panel. *The Lancet Diabetes and Endocrinology* **4** (10): 850–861. doi: 10.1016/S2213-8587(16)30041-9. Epub 2016 May 27. Erratum in: *Lancet Diabetes Endocrinology* 2016; 4(8):e8. PMID: 27246162.

Smith, C.J. and Fischer, T.H. (2001). Particulate and vapor phase constituents of cigarette mainstream smoke and risk of myocardial infarction. *Atherosclerosis* **158**: 257–267.

Steptoe, A. and Kivimäki, M. (2013). Stress and cardiovascular disease: an update on current knowledge. *Annual Review of Public Health* **34**: 337–354.

Strike, P.C., Perkins-Porras, L., Whitehead, D.L. et al. (2006). Triggering of acute coronary syndromes by physical exertion and anger: clinical and sociodemographic characteristics. *Heart* **92** (8): 1035–1040.

Tremblay, M., Colley, R., Saunders, T. et al. (2010). Physiological and health implications of a sedentary lifestyle. *Applied Physiology, Nutrition and Metabolism* **12** (35): 725–740.

Tremblay, M., Leblanc, A., Kho, M. et al. (2011). Systematic review of sedentary behavior and health indicators in schoolaged children and youth. *International Journal of Behaviour, Nutrition and Physical Activity* **8**: 98. doi: 10.1186/1479-5868-8-98. PMID: 21936895; PMCID: PMC3186735.

Vistisen, D., Andersen, G.S., Hansen, C.S. et al. (2016). Prediction of first cardiovascular disease event in type 1 diabetes mellitus: the steno type 1 risk engine. *Circulation* **133** (11): 1058–1066.

Watkins, L.L., Koch, G.G., Sherwood, A. et al. (2013). Association of anxiety and depression with all-cause mortality in individuals with coronary heart disease. *Journal of the American Heart Association* **2** (2): e000068.

Whelton, P.K., Carey, R.M., Aronow, W.S. et al. (2018). 2017 ACC/AHA/AAPA/ABC/ACPM/ AGS/ APhA/ASH/ASPC/NMA/PCNA guideline for the prevention, detection, evaluation, and management of high blood pressure in adults: a report of the American College of Cardiology/American Heart Association Task Force on Clinical Practice Guidelines. *Journal of the American College of Cardiology* **71** (19): e127–e248.

Willis, C., Bodenmann, P., Ghali, W. et al. (2007). Active smoking and the risk of type 2 diabetes: a systematic review and meta-analysis. *Journal of the American Medical Association* **289**: 2654–2664.

World Health Organization (WHO) (2020a) Diagnosis and management of type 2 diabetes (HEARTS-D). Geneva]: (WHO/ UCN/NCD/20.1). Licence: CC BY-NC-SA 3.0 IGO.

World Health Organization (WHO) (2021a). Obesity and Overweight factsheet from the WHO. https://www.who.int/news-room/ fact-sheets/detail/obesity-and-overweight (Retrieved 6th April 2022).

World Health Organization (WHO) (2021b). WHO report on the global tobacco epidemic, 2015. https://www.who.int/news-room/ fact-sheets/detail/tobacco (Retrieved 6th April 2022).

World Health Organization (WHO) (2020b). Physical Activity. https://www.who.int/ news-room/fact-sheets/detail/physical-activity (Retrieved April 6th 2022).

6

Cardiovascular Assessment

Jan Keenan and Angela M. Kucia

Overview

Assessment data are obtained from a patient's history, physical examination and the appropriate use of diagnostic tests. The information is used to establish a clinical diagnosis, establish goals for care and management and to evaluate outcomes. Assessment is undertaken by various members of the health care team, and synthesis of the information allows development of a comprehensive plan of care for the patient that takes immediate and long-term health care needs into consideration. Immediate assessment of a patient with an acute or suspected acute cardiac condition will be different from that for patients presenting with chronic or stable disease because rapid assessment diagnosis and treatment will have a significant impact on outcomes for those with an acute condition.

This chapter outlines the components of assessment for a patient with a cardiac disorder. Chest pain assessment is discussed in detail in Chapter 14.

Learning Objectives

After reading this chapter, you will be able to:

- Describe the components of the cardiovascular history.
- Describe the steps of the cardiovascular physical examination.
- Explain the principles of accurate blood pressure measurement.
- Explain the steps in cardiac auscultation and the significance of abnormal heart sounds.
- Describe the aspects of cardiovascular examination that assess cardiac output and circulation.

Key Concepts

Health history; symptom history; precordial inspection; palpation; cardiac auscultation

Cardiac Care: A Practical Guide for Nurses, Second Edition. Edited by Angela M. Kucia and Ian D. Jones.

Health History

A health history provides physiological and psychosocial information that guides physical assessment, selection of diagnostic tests and the choice of investigation and potential treatment options. A health history is obtained from a patient, but supplementary information may be provided by secondary sources such as the patient's family or local doctor.

The history should focus on:

- A comprehensive history of the presenting problem
- Previous health history, including previous investigations
- Risk factors for cardiovascular disease (CVD)
- Medication history, including allergies and intolerance to medications
- Social and personal influences on cardiovascular health

Information about the patient's coping mechanisms, their perception of illness causation and impact on their life and activities is also relevant.

Presenting Problem

The patient is asked about the problem that has prompted them to seek care and about symptoms or problems associated with the chief complaint.

The nature of the problem will guide the development of further questions to explore the health issue.

Key Point

When taking a history of a problem that has subjective symptoms such as shortness of breath, a differentiation needs to be made between true dyspnoea that is an unpleasant subjective true difficulty in breathing and breathlessness, or a response to exertion or exercise.

Past Health History

Past history includes information about childhood and adult illnesses, accidents, injuries, operations, and interventions that may or may not be relevant to the current illness. It may be necessary to prompt the patient by asking questions such as 'have you ever been hospitalised for any reason?', or 'have you had any accidents illnesses or injuries?' as patients often relate only what they think may be relevant to the current health issue. The patient is also asked about current medication use and known allergies or intolerance to any previous medication.

Previous Illnesses and Operations

Previous illnesses and operations provide important clues to the current condition or offer potential alternative diagnoses where the problem is not clearly cardiac in nature. These include:

- History of cardiovascular disease, transient ischaemic attacks, stroke and peripheral arterial disease
- History of heart failure, cardiomyopathy or valvular disease
- History of peptic ulcer disease, gastro-oesophageal reflux or frequent ingestion of nonsteroidal anti-inflammatory drugs or steroids
- Recent operations (such as cardiothoracic surgery)
- History of pulmonary embolus or a long period of inactivity or immobility (such as a long journey, recent operation, or illness)
- History of arrhythmia or syncope (fainting)
- Recent viral illness
- Childhood illness or illnesses in later life such as rheumatic fever or a history of rheumatoid arthritis

Risk Factors for Cardiovascular Disease

It is important to assess for the presence of cardiac risk factors or diseases that are associated with an increased risk of CVD. These are discussed in detail in Chapter 5.

Medications

A comprehensive medication history should be obtained addressing the following elements:

- Identify prescribed medications currently taken including dosage, frequency, length of time taken, side effects and adherence to the medication including how it is taken and whether it is being taken at recommended timings dose and frequency
- Identify over-the-counter medications or alternative remedies/herbal preparations taken regularly or recently and the reason for use.
- Identify any known allergies or intolerances to medications.
- Identify any contraindications or cautions to medications that might be indicated, such as aspirin or beta blockers in asthmatics
- Identify any cautions to medication that may be prescribed, such as anti-platelet therapy where there may a bleeding risk
- identify any recreational drugs being used or addictions

Social and Personal History

Social and personal factors that affect cardiovascular health should be included in the patient's history. These include factors such as:

- Family composition/significant other support
- Living conditions
- Daily routine and activities
- Occupation and employment
- Cultural/religious beliefs
- Coping patterns

It is important to know the person, as well as the illness. These details will give some indication as to how the person will cope with illness, what support is available to them, what services need to be offered or put into place to assist the patient through the illness and achieve optimal health and involve the patient in formulating a plan of care that considers their individual needs and preferences.

Learning Activity 6.1

Culture refers to learned and transmitted knowledge of values, beliefs, rules of behaviour and lifestyle practices that guide a group of people in their thinking and actions. In our multicultural societies, health providers must provide person-centred care to people from a diverse range of cultural backgrounds with different languages, levels of acculturation and unique ways of understanding illness. When misunderstood, cultural influences and differences can adversely affect the patient (and family)–provider relationship, leading to mistrust and poor co-operation.

1) What is meant by the terms 'cultural awareness' and 'cultural competence'?
2) How might you implement culturally competent care in the cardiovascular setting?

Suggested Resource

How to improve cultural competence in health care
Tulane University (2021)
https://publichealth.tulane.edu/blog/cultural-competence-in-health-care/

Physical Examination

A baseline physical examination is obtained, and this will determine the requirement and timing of further assessment. Subsequent assessment can be compared with baseline to look for improvement or deterioration.

General Appearance

Information gathering about the patient starts from the first interaction and begins with first impressions from the patient's appearance. These include things such as whether the patient appears well groomed or unkempt and may have implications for the patient's ability or motivation to perform self-care activities. If obesity or cachexia is present, an observation is made about the patient's nutritional state. Facial expressions and body language are some of the first things that are noticed and may give an indication as to whether the patient is anxious, distressed or in pain. Their affect and how they interact will become evident as you introduce yourself and explain your intent in taking a history and examination. Observe if they make eye contact and respond appropriately to conversation. Other observations that can be made whilst taking a patient history are presence of pallor or cyanosis, diaphoresis, laboured breathing, coughing, vomiting, and a rapid circulatory assessment based on whether they are cool or warm to touch.

Precordial Inspection and Palpation

With the patient supine and the head of the bed raised at a 45° angle, inspect the precordium for any visible pulsations, masses, scars, lesions, signs of trauma or previous surgery (such as median sternotomy or pacemaker scar). Locate the angle of Louis (sternal angle) also known as the notch of Louis (sternal notch), the raised notch where the manubrium and the body of the sternum are joined. This notch is at the level of the second rib and can, therefore, be used as a reference point for locating intercostal spaces.

Palpate the areas of the valves for any thrills (a palpable vibration felt as a result of turbulent blood flow) that can best be felt with the flat of the hand, palpate for parasternal heaves (large movements are best felt with the heel of the hand at the sternal border).

Palpate the epigastrium for pulsations that might represent aortic pulsation. An abnormally large pulsation may suggest pathology such as an abdominal aortic aneurysm and will require further investigation.

Palpate the apex beat, also known as the 'point of maximal impulse', which is usually found in the fifth intercostal space and 1 cm medial to the midclavicular line. The apex beat should be no larger than the width of two fingertips and tapping in character.

The apex beat does not exactly correspond to the anatomical apex of the heart, so if the apex beat can be felt across a large area, feel for the most lateral and inferior position of pulsation. If the apex beat is located in the axilla, it would suggest cardiomegaly or mediastinal shift. Characteristics of the apex beat can be described using the mnemonic in Box 6.1.

Box 6.1	Characteristics of the apex beat	
S	Size	Is it larger than one intercostal space?
A	Amplitude	Is it strong or weak?
L	Location	Is it in the fifth intercostal space at the mid-clavicular line?
I	Impulse	Is it monophasic or biphasic?
D	Duration	Is it abnormally sustained?

Key Points

If you are having difficulty palpating the apex beat, keep the pads of your fingers in the position described earlier and ask the patient to roll on to their left side.

It may not be possible to palpate the apex beat in late pregnancy, in obese patients or those with emphysema.

Jugular Venous Pressure

The jugular venous pressure (JVP) is an indirect measure of central venous pressure (CVP). The height of the level of blood in the right internal jugular vein (IJV) is an indication of right atrial pressure because there are no valves or obstructions between the vein and the right atrium. The patient should be positioned in a semi-recumbent position at a 45° angle with the head turned slightly to the left. If possible, have a tangential light source that shines obliquely from the left. Look for the surface markings of the right IJV that runs from the medial end of the clavicle to the ear lobe. The JVP has a double waveform pulsation. Measure the level of the JVP by measuring the vertical distance between the sternal angle and the top of the JVP. This is usually less than 3–4 cm.

Distinguishing the JVP from Carotid Pulse

Unlike the carotid pulse, the JVP pulse is not palpable, is obliterated by pressure and decreases with inspiration. The JVP has a double-waveform pulsation (Figure 6.1). Time the jugular venous pulse waves by simultaneous palpation of the carotid arterial pulse. The *a* wave precedes the carotid arterial pulse, whereas the *v* wave closely follows the pulse.

To confirm that the pulsation observed is caused by the JVP, apply firm pressure on the liver using the palm of the hand on the right upper quadrant and a transient increase in the JVP will be seen in a normal patient. This is known as the 'hepatojugular reflex'. Sustained elevation of the JVP during compression with an abrupt decrease of at least 4 cm following release of pressure signifies a positive test and has been demonstrated to correlate with elevated right atrial pressure and pulmonary capillary wedge pressure (Clerkin et al. 2019).

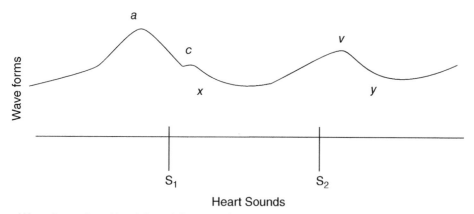

a Wave is produced by right atrial contraction.
c Wave represents tricuspid valve closure.
x Wave or *x* descent represents drop in pressure in the right atrium.
v Wave represents passive right atrial filling late in systole or by ballooning of the tricuspid valve during right venticular contraction.
y Wave or descent represents drop in pressure in the right ventricle.

Figure 6.1 Jugular venous pulse wave form.

Key Point

Kussmaul sign is a paradoxical increase in JVP occurring during inspiration and indicates an inability of the right side of the heart to handle an increased venous return. The Kussmaul sign is commonly found in severe heart failure, cor pulmonale (acute or chronic), restrictive cardiomyopathies, tricuspid stenosis and right ventricular infarction.

Pulses

The arterial pulses should be palpated using the pads of the fingers. In a full cardiovascular examination, the carotid, brachial, radial, femoral, popliteal, posterior tibial and dorsalis pedis pulses should be palpated. In a targeted examination (such as in an acute admission), the radial pulse is the usual site for assessing the arterial pulse. The pulse is assessed for rate and rhythm. Peripheral pulses are compared bilaterally for symmetry. The normal pulse is regular and between 60 and 100 bpm. The strength of the pulse is assessed, and this may be graded on a scale of 0–3 as described in Table 6.1.

The character of the pulse is described. A pulse that alternates in strength with alternate beats is known as pulsus alternans and

Table 6.1 Rating scale for strength of arterial pulses.

0	Absent
1	Weak, thready, easily obliterated
2	Normal
3	Strong, bounding, cannot be obliterated

invariably is associated with severe left ventricular systolic dysfunction and carries a poor prognosis (see Figure 6.2).

A pulse that reduces significantly in amplitude during inspiration but reappears during expiration is known as pulsus paradoxus. Mild pulsus paradoxus can be a normal finding. Changes in intrathoracic pressure during breathing are transmitted to the heart and great vessels, causing arterial blood pressure to fall with inspiration and rise with expiration. To determine if pulsus paradoxus is a pathological finding, use a sphygmomanometer and allow the cuff to deflate until the pulse is heard only during expiration and note the corresponding pressure. Continue to deflate the cuff. The point at which the pressure is heard throughout the inspiratory and expiratory cycle is noted. The second systolic pressure reading is subtracted from the first; if the difference is >10 mmHg during normal respirations, it is considered pathological (Morton and Tucker 2013).

Key Point

There are several pathologic causes of pulsus paradoxus. Cardiac causes include cardiac tamponade, percicardial effusion, constrictive pericarditis, restrictive cardiomyopathy, cardiogenic shock, right ventricular infarction, tricuspid atresia and superior vena caval syndrome. Pulmonary causes include severe obstructive pulmonary lung disease, tension pneumothorax, obstructive sleep apnoea, pulmonary embolism, bilateral pleural effusion and tracheal compression. Hypovolaemia and shock can also give rise to pulsus paradoxus (Raj 2014).

Figure 6.2 Pulsus alternans. *Source:* Wikipedia contributors (2021). Used under Creative Commons Attribution Share Alike 3.0 Unported License.

100

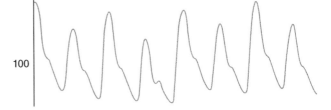

Peripheral Vascular System

Skin Temperature and Colour

The skin temperature and colour (including the peripheries) should be noted. Colour should be uniform. Note any areas of cyanosis. Central cyanosis reflects deoxyhaemoglobin from hypoxia and is generally distributed but best observed in the mucous membranes which appear dusky and bluish in colour. Central cyanosis is a sign of reduced oxygen concentration and is a late sign of hypoxia usually associated with heart or lung disease (Bickley 2013). Peripheral cyanosis, on the other hand, is localised in the extremities and protrusions (hands, feet, nose, ears and lips) and reflects impaired circulation.

Peripheral Oedema

Observe the legs and feet for oedema. Ask about the onset of oedema development and duration, and whether it is relieved by elevation of the limbs. In heart failure, oedema will usually be bilateral and pitting, resulting from water retention. It can also be caused by systemic diseases, pregnancy in some women, as well as directly or as a result of heart failure, or local conditions such as varicose veins or thrombophlebitis.

Peripheral Circulation

Look for any signs of thrombophlebitis, varicose veins, lesions and ulcers, and assess capillary filling time which will give an indication of the health of the peripheral arterial circulation. Do this bilaterally with both hands and feet and squeeze gently at the tip of the fingers or toes to blanch the skin. The time it takes for the skin to return to its normal colour reflects the capillary circulation, and in health this should be less than 2 seconds.

Blood Pressure

Comprehensive assessment of blood pressure (BP) should include multiple measurements taken on separate occasions, at least twice, one or more weeks apart. In a full cardiovascular examination, an initial BP assessment should be undertaken in lying and standing positions and in both arms. If postural hypotension is suspected, the patient should lie for 5–10 minutes before obtaining the BP and heart rate (HR); then BP and HR should be assessed again 2 minutes after standing (National Heart Foundation Australia [NHFA] 2016).

Key Points

A variation in BP by 5–15 mmHg in the setting of dizziness or syncope may indicate postural (orthostatic) hypotension.
A difference of systolic BP >15 mmHg between the left and right arms may indicate an increased risk of vascular disease and death and may identify persons who need further vascular assessment (Clark et al. 2016).

Learning Activity 6.2

Few clinicians observe the principles of accurate BP measurement. Consider whether you may need to update your practice. The following resources may be useful:

Suggested Resources

Hypertension and clinical management guidelines.
https://www.heartfoundation.org.au/Conditions/Hypertension
National Institute for Health and Clinical Excellence (2019; updated 2022). *Hypertension in Adults: Diagnosis and Management*. NICE guideline (NG136). https://www.nice.org.uk/guidance/ng136

There are several methods of measuring BP.

- The auscultatory method requires a sphygmomanometer and stethoscope. The sphygmomanometer is composed of an inflatable cuff that is inflated just enough to occlude the brachial artery. The cuff pressure is slowly released until the pressure in the cuff is equal to that of the patient's systolic BP, at which point first Korotkoff sound will be heard with the stethoscope over the brachial artery. The examiner notes the pressure at this point on the manometer, giving the systolic BP measurement. Deflation of the cuff continues until there is no longer any restriction to blood flow and no turbulence, so no audible sound is produced. The pressure reading on the manometer is noted at this point, and this is the diastolic BP measurement.
- Automated BP measurement devices are being increasingly used in hospitals and primary care and are reasonably accurate, but they rely on a constant pulse volume and may be inaccurate in some patients.
- The palpatory method requires the cuff to be inflated whilst palpating the radial pulse. When deflating the cuff, a pulsatile thrill can be palpated. The pressure at which the thrill appears is the systolic pressure and the disappearance of the thrill is the diastolic pressure. This method is not as accurate as using a sphygmomanometer or automated BP device, but may be useful when a quick estimate of systolic BP is required.

Key Point

Automated devices may have difficulty in 'reading' the BP and will continue to inflate and deflate, which will cause discomfort to the patient and can cause bruising to patients on antiplatelet or anticoagulation therapy.

Learning Activity 6.3

We use several devices in cardiovascular assessment. Understanding how these devices work helps us to ensure that we use them properly in order to get an appropriate result or reading. Obtaining a BP is something that we take for granted, but manual and automated methods of obtaining BP can be subject to operator error or equipment malfunction.

1) Consider factors that may contribute to an incorrect BP measurement when using automated devices.
2) What can you do to minimise errors in BP measurement?

Suggested Resource

The suggested resource from Learning Activity 6.1 can be used for this activity. See pages 15–25 of the resource

---

Cardiac Auscultation

With the availability of technological investigations, such as echocardiography, clinicians are becoming more dependent on technology and less skilled at auscultating heart sounds. This is an essential skill for nurses working in the cardiac environment. A good quality stethoscope is needed for cardiac auscultation. When using the diaphragm, it should be placed firmly on the chest wall to create a tight seal, and it is used to hear high-frequency sounds such as the first and second heart sounds (S1, S2), friction rubs, systolic murmurs and diastolic insufficiency murmurs. When using the bell, it should be placed lightly on the chest wall and is used to detect low-frequency sounds such as the third and fourth heart sounds (S3, S4) and the diastolic murmurs of mitral and tricuspid stenosis. The physiology behind heart sounds is demonstrated in Table 6.2.

The patient should be positioned in a semi-recumbent position with the head of the bed elevated 30–45°. Systematic auscultation of the

Table 6.2 Heart sounds.

Sound	Cause
First heart sound (S_1)	A normal heart sound timed with closure of mitral and tricuspid valves at the beginning of ventricular systole. Mitral closure is responsible for most of the sound produced, and so S_1 is best heard in the mitral area (apex). If the valves do not close at the same time, a 'split' S_1 sound may be heard. This may be physiological in a healthy individual (in conditions such as normal variant right bundle branch block) or might be pathological; right ventricular strain can give rise to right bundle branch block and can lead to splitting of S1, for example, in pulmonary embolism and the presenting history will guide the suspicion of a normal or pathological split. A split S_1 is best heard in the tricuspid area.
Second heart sound (S_2)	A normal heart sound produced by closure of the aortic and pulmonic valves at the beginning of diastole and best heard at Erb's Point. With inspiration, the pulmonic valve closes a bit later than the aortic valve, producing a split S_2 sound known as 'physiological splitting' which is best heard on inspiration with the stethoscope placed in the pulmonic area. The intensity of S_2 may be increased in the presence of aortic or pulmonic valvular stenosis or in pulmonary or systemic hypertension.
Third heart sound (S_3)	Low-frequency sound that occurs during the early, rapid-filling phase of ventricular diastole. May be a normal finding in children or young adults. In older adults, S_3 is associated with ventricular failure and is a sound caused by a non-compliant or failing ventricle that cannot distend to accept the rapid inflow of blood. The resulting turbulent flow causes vibration of the atrioventricular valvular structures or the ventricles themselves, producing a low-frequency sound. A left ventricular S_3 is best heard at the apex with the stethoscope bell. A right ventricular S_3 is heard best at the xiphoid or lower left sternal border and varies in intensity with respiration, becoming louder on inspiration (Morton and Tucker 2013).
Fourth heart sound (S_4)	An S_4, sometimes known as an atrial gallop, is a low-frequency sound heard late in diastole, just before S_1. The sound is produced by atrial contraction forcing blood into a non-compliant ventricle that is resistant to filling. Causes include systemic hypertension, acute myocardial ischaemia or infarction, cardiomyopathy and aortic stenosis (AS). S_4 is best heard with the bell of the stethoscope at the apex. Conditions affecting right ventricular compliance, such as pulmonary hypertension or pulmonic stenosis, may produce a right ventricular S_4 heard best at the lower left sternal border, where the sound is likened to the rhythm of the word 'Ten-ness-see' where the S4 represents the 'Ten. . .' and becomes louder on inspiration (Morton and Tucker 2013).
Summation gallop	As ventricular diastole is shortened in rapid heart rates, if S_3 and S_4 are both present, they may fuse together and become audible as a single diastolic sound called a summation gallop, because of the sound's likeness to a 'gallop'. This sound is loudest at the apex and is heard best with the stethoscope bell while the patient lies turned slightly to the left side (Morton and Tucker 2013).
Heart murmurs	Sounds produced either by the forward flow of blood through a narrowed or constricted valve into a dilated vessel or chamber, or by the backward flow of blood through an incompetent valve or septal defect. The sound produced is described as blowing, harsh, rumbling or musical and the intensity or loudness of a murmur is described using the following grading system: • Grade I: faint and barely audible • Grade II: soft • Grade III: audible but not palpable • Grade IV and V: associated with a palpable thrill • Grade VI: is audible without a stethoscope

Table 6.2 (Continued)

Sound	Cause
	Systolic murmurs are heard between S_1 and S_2 and the timing can be established during auscultation best when palpating a central pulse.

- Stenosis of the aortic or pulmonic valve results in an ejection systolic murmur. The quality of these murmurs is harsh and of medium pitch. AS is heard best in the aortic area and may radiate into the neck following the path of the carotid arteries; pulmonic stenosis is heard best over the pulmonic area.
- Mitral or tricuspid valvular insufficiency (regurgitation) or a ventricular septal defect (VSD) produces systolic murmurs caused by the backward flow of blood from an area of higher pressure to an area of lower pressure, which are harsh and blowing in quality. The sound is described as holosystolic (the murmur begins immediately after S_1 and continues throughout systole up to S_2). Mitral regurgitation (MR) is best heard at the apex and radiating to the left axilla. Tricuspid regurgitation (TR) is best heard at the left sternal border and increases in intensity during inspiration. This murmur may radiate to the cardiac apex.
- A VSD produces a harsh, blowing holosystolic sound caused by blood flowing from the left to the right ventricle through a defect in the septal wall during systole. This murmur is heard best from the fourth to sixth intercostal spaces on both sides of the sternum and is accompanied by a palpable thrill (Morton and Tucker 2013).

Diastolic murmurs occur after S_2 and before the onset of the following S_1.

- Aortic or pulmonary valvular insufficiency (regurgitation) produces a blowing diastolic murmur that begins immediately after S_2 and decreases in intensity as regurgitant flow decreases through diastole. These murmurs are described as early diastolic decrescendo murmurs. Aortic regurgitation (AR) is best heard in the aortic area and may radiate along the right sternal border to the apex. Pulmonic valve regurgitation is best heard in the pulmonic area.
- Mitral or tricuspid stenosis produces a diastolic murmur. This murmur decreases in intensity from its onset and then increases again as ventricular filling increases because of atrial contraction; this is termed decrescendo–crescendo. Mitral stenosis (MS) is best heard at the apex with the patient turned slightly to the left side. Tricuspid stenosis increases in intensity with inspiration and is loudest in the fifth intercostal space along the left sternal border (Morton and Tucker 2013).

Friction rubs	A pericardial friction rub may be heard anywhere over the pericardium with the diaphragm of the stethoscope. The rub may be accentuated by having the patient lean forward and exhale and, unlike a pleural friction rub, does not vary in intensity with respiration (Morton and Tucker 2013).

Suggested Resources

Heart Murmurs-Heart Sounds
Practical Clinical Skills (2017)
https://www.practicalclinicalskills.com/heart-murmurs
Systolic murmurs, diastolic murmurs, and extra heart sounds - Part 1

Khanacademymedicine (2014)
https://youtu.be/6YY3OOPmUDA
Systolic murmurs, diastolic murmurs, and extra heart sounds - Part 2
Khanacademymedicine (2014)
https://youtu.be/ZUHpAaVpiY8

precordium with the stethoscope diaphragm follows the following pattern:

- Right sternal border in the second intercostal space referred to as the aortic area.
- Left sternal border in the second intercostal space referred to as the pulmonic area.
- Left sternal border in the third intercostal space referred to as Erb's point where S_2 is best heard.
- Left sternal border in the fifth intercostal space referred to as the tricuspid area.
- Mid-clavicular line in the fifth intercostal space at the apex of the heart, which may be referred to as the mitral area where S_1 is the loudest.
- This pattern is then repeated with the stethoscope bell. Figure 6.3 shows the positions in which to place the stethoscope.

In each of the positions auscultated, the normal heart sounds S_1 and S_2 should be identified. The intensity of the sound, respiratory variation and splitting should be noted. After S_1 and S_2 are identified, listen for the presence of any extra sounds, first in systole, then in diastole. Each area is auscultated for the presence of murmurs and friction rubs (Morton and Tucker 2013). To help hear abnormal sounds, the patient may be asked to roll partly onto the left side to help bring the left ventricle closer to the chest wall. Quiet sounds over the aortic area can be amplified by sitting the patient forward and listening to the heart sounds through the respiratory cycle. If the patient holds their breath following expiration, this can amplify the murmurs associated with aortic stenosis or regurgitation. The apex should be auscultated during inspiration and

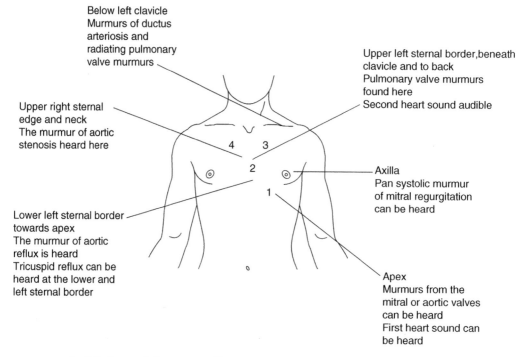

1 – Mitral regurgitation: apex, axilla
2 – Aortic regurgitation: lower left sternal border
3 – Pulmonary stenoses: upper left sternal border/clavicle
4 – Aortic stenoses: apex, upper right sternal border, neck

Figure 6.3 Sites for cardiac auscultation. *Source:* Chizner (2008). Used with permission.

expiration to differentiate between murmurs arising from the left or right side of the heart. Deep inspiration increases venous return to the right side of the heart and thus augments the intensity of right-sided murmurs while having little or no effect on murmurs arising from the left side of the heart.

Respiratory Assessment

A respiratory assessment should be undertaken to detect evidence of heart failure or other respiratory pathology.

Ask the patient about any symptoms of dyspnoea to establish whether:

- it occurs on exertion or at rest;
- the patient experiences orthopnoea – asking the patient how many pillows they use to sleep is often useful to establish whether orthopnoea is present;
- there is any evidence of paroxysmal nocturnal dyspnoea (PND);

Ask the patient about any symptoms of cough or sputum production. Observe the patient's pattern and cycle of breathing, including:

- The respiratory rate – in a healthy adult, inaudible respirations should occur between 12 and 20 times/min.
- The duration of the inspiratory/expiratory cycle, noting whether there is any difficulty in expelling air. Expiration [E] should take around twice as long as inspiration [I], giving an I:E ratio of 1:2.
- Use of accessory muscles of respiration, including the sternocleidomastoid, spinal, neck and abdominal muscles.
- Intercostal retractions, visible indentations between the ribs as the intercostal muscles aid in breathing.
- Nasal flaring, observed as intermittent outward movements of the nostrils.
- Pursed lip breathing (partial closure of the lips to allow air to be expired slowly).

Note the patient's posture, including whether the patient needs to sit upright and is unable to tolerate lying down. Auscultate the patient's posterior chest, beginning with the areas above the scapulae. Move downward in a stair-step fashion, comparing your findings from one side with those from the other side. Listen to the character of the breath sounds. Normal vesicular breath sounds are heard over most lung fields. See Table 6.3 for types and causes of abnormal (known as adventitious) breath sounds.

Key Point
As part of a respiratory assessment, look for signs of cyanosis, conscious level and mentation. An altered state of consciousness, anxiety, restlessness, confusion or other changes in mental status are important signs of potential respiratory problems.

Table 6.3 Abnormal breath sounds.

Type of breath sound	Nature of the sound	Potential causes
Crackles (rales)	Discontinuous breath sounds that sound like crinkling plastic wrap or can be simulated by rubbing strands of hair together between two fingers near one's ear. May be further described as: - Fine crackles are short high-pitched sounds - Coarse crackles are longer-lasting low-pitched sounds	Signify distension of fibrotic lung tissue or opening of collapsed alveoli most commonly with atelectasis and alveolar filling processes such as: - Pulmonary oedema - Interstitial lung disease

(Continued)

Table 6.3 (Continued)

Type of breath sound	Nature of the sound	Potential causes
Rhonchi	Low-pitched respiratory sounds that can be heard during inspiration or expiration	Probably relate to variations in obstruction as airways distend with inhalation and occur in a variety of conditions including: • Chronic bronchitis Pneumonia and infections of the lungs
Wheezes	Whistling, musical breath sounds that are worse during expiration than inspiration and are commonly associated with dyspnoea. May be audible without a stethoscope	• Asthma or chronic obstructive pulmonary (airways) disease (COPD) • Acute allergic reaction
Stridor	High-pitched, predominantly inspiratory sound that can normally be heard without a stethoscope formed by extrathoracic upper airway obstruction	It is a serious finding and often signifies a life-threatening upper airway obstruction
Decreased breath sounds	Poor air movement in airways	Usually caused by disease processes or mechanisms limiting airflow. May signify: • Bronchospasm • Pleural effusion • Pneumothorax • Asthma or COPD
Bronchial breath sounds	Louder, harsher and higher pitched than normal breath sounds	• Normal finding over trachea • May be caused by lung consolidation in conditions such as pneumonia
Bronchophony	Clear transmission of the patient's spoken voice through the chest wall	Results from alveolar consolidation such as in pneumonia
Egophony	Occurs when a patient says the letter 'e' and the examiner hears the letter 'a' on auscultation	Any condition that results in pulmonary consolidation such as pneumonia
Whispered pectoriloquy	Transmission of the patient's whispered voice through the chest wall at an increased volume	Pneumonia
Friction rubs	Grating or creaking sounds that fluctuate with the respiratory cycle	Sign of pleural inflammation associated with: • Pleurisy • Post thoracotomy • Empyema

---

Key Point

Auscultation and recognition of abnormal breath sounds takes practice. There is no substitute for practice, so make a habit of auscultating lung fields in the patients for whom you are caring.

A pulse oximeter is a computerised device that measures peripheral capillary oxygen saturation (S_pO_2). Pulse oximeters can distinguish oxygenated haemaglobin (Hb) from deoxygenated Hb (Chan et al. 2013) via a probe that is attached to the patient's finger or ear lobe. The device has a visual display and an audible situations in which oxygen is used (Beasley et al. 2015). A target S_pO_2 of 94–98% is suitable for most adult patients, although patients with long-standing respiratory or congenital heart disease may have lower readings reflecting the underlying severity of the disease. In patients with chronic obstructive pulmonary disease and other conditions associated with chronic respiratory failure, oxygen should only be administered if the S_pO_2 is less than 88% and titrated to a target S_pO_2 range of 88–92% (Beasley et al. 2015).

It should be remembered that pulse oximetry gives no information about the level of CO_2 and therefore has limitations in the assessment of patients developing respiratory failure due to CO_2 retention.

Table 6.4 Causes and mechanisms of unreliable SpO_2 readings.

1) Causes of intermittent dropouts or inability to read SpO_2
   - Poor perfusion due to a number of causes, e.g. hypovolaemia, vasoconstriction, etc.
2) Causes of falsely normal or elevated SpO_2
   - Carbon monoxide poisoning
   - Sickle cell anaemia vaso-occlusive crises (overestimation of FO_2Hb and underestimation of SaO_2)
3) Causes of falsely low SpO_2
   - Venous pulsations
   - Excessive movement
   - Intravenous pigmented dyes
   - Inherited forms of abnormal haemoglobin
   - Fingernail polish
   - Severe anaemia (with concomitant hypoxemia)
4) Causes of falsely low or high SpO_2
   - Methemoglobinaemia
   - Sulfhemoglobinaemia
   - Poor probe positioning
   - Sepsis and septic shock
5) Causes of falsely low FO_2Hb as measured by a co-oximeter
   - Severe hyperbilirubinaemia
   - Fetal Hb (HbF)

Source: Chan et al. (2013).

When using devices in cardiovascular assessment, nurses should be aware of situations that may affect the accuracy or reliability of the device. A pulse oximeter may not give accurate readings some situations (see Table 6.4). Therefore, the presence of a normal S_pO_2 does not always negate the need for blood gas measurements because S_pO_2 on pulse oximetry may appear to be normal in a patient with normal oxygen tension but abnormal blood pH or pCO_2 or with low blood oxygen content due to anaemia.

Conclusion

Cardiovascular assessment is a systematic process that involves a thorough history and examination of the patient. In emergency situations, a targeted history and examination may be needed, and further information is obtained when the patient is stabilised. Many of the skills required to perform cardiovascular assessment need to be practiced, and so every opportunity should be taken to perfect the techniques required.

References

Beasley, R., Chien, J., Douglas, J. et al. (2015). Thoracic Society of Australia and New Zealand oxygen guidelines for acute oxygen use in adults: 'swimming between the flags'. *Respirology* **20** (8): 1182–1191. https://doi.org/10.1111/resp.12620.

Bickley, L. (2013). *Bates' Pocket Guide to Physical Examination and History Taking*, 7ee. Philadelphia: Lippincott Williams and Wilkins.

Chan, E.D., Chan, M.M., and Chan, M.M. (2013). Pulse oximetry: understanding its basic principles facilitates appreciation of its limitations. *Respiratory Medicine* **107** (6): 789–799.

Chizner, M.A. (2008). Cardiac auscultation: rediscovering the lost art. *Current Problems in Cardiology* **33** (7): 326–408.

Clark, C.E., Taylor, R.S., Butcher, I., Stewart, M.C., Price, J., Fowkes, F.G.R., Shore, A.C. and Campbell, J.L., 2016. Inter-arm blood pressure difference and mortality: a cohort study in an asymptomatic primary care population at elevated cardiovascular risk. *British Journal of General Practice*, **66** (646), pp. e297-e308. doi: https://doi.org/10.3399/bjgp16X684949.

Clerkin, K.J., Mancini, D.M., and Lund, L.H. (2019). *Chapter 6: diagnosis of heart failure*. In: *Heart Failure* (ed. D.S. Feldman and P. Mohacsi). Springer International Publishing Imprint: Springer. https://doi.org/10.1007/978-3-319-98184-0.

Morton, P.G. and Tucker, T. (2013). *Critical Care Nursing: A Holistic Approach*, 10ee. Philadelphia: Lippincott Williams & Wilkins.

National Heart Foundation of Australia (2016). *Guideline for the Diagnosis and Management of Hypertension in Adults – 2016*, 15–25. Melbourne: National Heart Foundation of Australia https://www.heartfoundation.org.au/images/uploads/publications/PRO-167_Hypertension-guideline-2016_WEB.pdf (accessed 15 November 2016).

Raj, B. 2014. *Pulsus paradoxus*, emedicinelive. http://emedicinelive.com/?q=pulsus-paradoxus (accessed 14 November 2016).

Wikipedia contributors (2021). Pulsus alternans. In: *Wikipedia, The Free Encyclopedia*. Wikipedia https://en.wikipedia.org/w/index.php?title=Pulsus_alternans&oldid=1033588148 (accessed 23 September 2021).

7

Laboratory Tests Used in Acute Cardiac Assessment

David I. Barrett and Angela M. Kucia

Overview

Whenever you care for a patient with a cardiac condition, one of the initial elements of your assessment is a full set of serum laboratory (blood) tests. A great deal of useful information about physiological and biochemical states can be derived from blood tests: they can be used to assess organ function, help in the identification of the presence or progress of certain disease states, and monitor the effectiveness of treatment.

In this chapter, we explore commonly used laboratory tests in patients with a cardiac-related illness.

Learning Objectives

By the end of this chapter, you will be able to:

- Discuss the reasons for performing standard blood tests in patients with cardiac disorders.
- Recognise the diagnostic importance of specific biochemical markers in patients with acute coronary syndrome.
- Describe the significance of natriuretic peptide measurement in patients with heart failure.
- Discuss some of the limitations of laboratory tests.

Key Concepts

Serum testing; haematological examination; coagulation studies; screening; therapeutic monitoring

Generic Laboratory Tests

Most patients who come under your care will have a range of standard laboratory investigations performed. For patients with new or existing cardiac conditions, these tests are vitally important for three reasons: (i) aiding diagnosis; (ii) providing information that will help tailor the management of cardiac problems; and (iii) providing a baseline against which changes in health status can be tracked.

Common Laboratory Tests Used in Cardiovascular Disease

Electrolytes

Serum electrolytes are obtained via a venous blood sample and are electrically charged elements found in blood and body tissues in the form of dissolved salts. They are important in

Cardiac Care: A Practical Guide for Nurses, Second Edition. Edited by Angela M. Kucia and Ian D. Jones.
© 2022 John Wiley & Sons Ltd. Published 2022 by John Wiley & Sons Ltd.

maintaining fluid balance and play a role in stabilising the body's pH. There are four main electrolytes in the body:

- Sodium (Na^+), found mainly in plasma and interstitial fluid.
- Potassium (K^+), found mainly in cells but also in smaller amounts in plasma and interstitial fluid. Abnormalities in K^+ levels can cause life-threatening arrhythmias, so it is important to keep K^+ within normal parameters.
- Chloride (Cl^-) shifts in and out of cells to maintain electrical neutrality. Levels of Cl^- are often related to levels of Na^+.
- Bicarbonate, which helps to maintain a stable pH level (acid–base balance) through excretion and reabsorption via the kidneys.

Common components of a serum electrolyte screen and their normal ranges are shown in Table 7.1.

Key Point

Abnormal levels of K^+ and magnesium (Mg^{2+}) increase susceptibility to arrhythmias. Alterations in levels of K^+ and/or Mg^{2+} may result from disease processes or from prescribed treatment. Renal failure, for example, may lead to hyperkalaemia and hypermagnesaemia. Conversely, loop diuretics such as furosemide may cause hypokalaemia and hypomagnesaemia. These conditions can cause fatal arrhythmias and must be identified and promptly corrected.

Renal Function

Together with electrolytes, measurement of creatinine, urea and estimated glomerular filtration rate (eGFR) will give useful information about renal function (see Table 7.2). These tests are important, as impaired renal

Table 7.1 Components and normal value of a serum electrolytes screen (**normal values may differ between laboratories**).

Component	Reference range
Sodium	135–145 mmol/l
Potassium	3.8–4.9 mmol/l
Chloride	95–110 mmol/l
Bicarbonate	22–29 mmol/l
Calcium	2.1–2.55 mmol/l
Magnesium	0.8–1.0 mmol/l
Phosphate	0.80–1.50 mmol/l
Serum osmolality	280–300 mmol/kg water

Table 7.2 Renal function tests and normal reference ranges (normal **values may** differ **between** laboratories).

Test/component	Reference range
Creatinine	60–110 µmol/l (0.7–1.2 mg/dl) for men 45–90 µmol/l (0.5–1.0 mg/dl) for women
Urea	3.0–8.0 mmol/l
eGFR	>90 ml/min/1.73 m^2

function is closely associated with an increased risk of mortality in patients with cardiac disorders.

- Creatinine is a waste product of creatine phosphate metabolism in muscles. It is produced at a relatively constant rate and excreted almost exclusively by the kidneys, so serum levels of creatinine provide a good approximation of renal function. References ranges for creatinine vary according to age and sex. Increasing serum creatinine levels not only indicate worsening renal function but are also associated with higher mortality rates in patients with ACS (Marenzi et al. 2015).
- Urea is formed as a waste product of protein metabolism and is released into the bloodstream and transported to the kidneys where

it is filtered and excreted. A rise in urea levels can suggest renal failure and, as with raised Creatinine levels, is an indicator of increased mortality risk in cardiac patients (Kawabe et al. 2014).

- Measurement of a patient's actual GFR is a relatively complex process that would not usually be carried out during the assessment of a patient with an acute cardiac condition. However, the ability to calculate an eGFR based on the patient's creatinine, age, sex, and ethnicity provides a simple indicator of renal function (Thomas 2014).

Key Point

Many commonly used cardiac medications may need to be avoided or dose-adjusted in the setting of reduced renal function. Several investigative and therapeutic agents used in cardiac care can impact on renal function including radio-opaque contrast used during interventional cardiac procedures, angiotensin-converting-enzyme inhibitors (ACE-Is), angiotensin-receptor-blockers (ARBs), beta-blockers, digoxin, potassium-sparing diuretics, sotalol and statins. GPIIb/IIIa inhibitors and low molecular weight heparins (LMWH) are associated with increased bleeding risk in the setting of impaired renal function. Some medications used in diabetes (metformin) may need to be held and insulin used temporarily when percutaneous procedures are planned.

Learning Activity 7.1

Many people, particularly those of older age, take regular medications. It is important that you recognise which medications can affect renal function, and when medications may need to be reduced or ceased to protect renal function. Visit the resources below to work out which drugs may affect your patient's renal function.

Suggested Resources

Stefani, M., Singer, R. F., & Roberts, D. M. (2019). How to adjust drug doses in chronic kidney disease. Australian prescriber, 42(5), 163. https://www.nps.org.au/australian-prescriber/articles/how-to-adjust-drug-doses-in-chronic-kidney-disease

Veterans' Medicines Advice and Therapeutics Education Services (2012). *Therapeutic Brief 30 – Know your Patient's Renal Function – An Important Prescribing Consideration.* https://www.veteransmates.net.au/VeteransMATES/documents/module_materials/M30_TherBrief.pdf

Veteran's Mates
Australian Government Department of Veteran's Affairs
https://www.veteransmates.net.au/

Glucose Measurement

Glucose is the main source of energy for the body and needs to be maintained at a certain level for normal cellular function. Insulin, a hormone produced by the pancreas, is needed to transport glucose into the cells and to stimulate glycogen synthesis. Amounts of glucose and insulin must be balanced to prevent hyperglycaemia or hypoglycaemia, both of which can be acutely life threatening if severe. Chronically high blood glucose levels, such as that which occurs in uncontrolled diabetes, can cause progressive damage to the heart, blood vessels and kidneys. Normal ranges for blood glucose tests are shown in Table 5.4 (Chapter 5).

Key Point

For people presenting with a cardiovascular event, fasting blood glucose and HBA1C should be measured to exclude the presence of diabetes and an oral glucose tolerance test (OGTT) should be added if the others are inconclusive (Cosentino et al. 2020).

As diabetes is a strong risk factor for cardiovascular disease, cardiac patients should be screened for diabetes, ideally using a fasting glucose test. Initial blood glucose measurement in a patient with suspected cardiac problems may be by serum laboratory testing or by a capillary sample using a point-of-care (bedside) device. Samples taken in an acute presentation are often non-fasting samples. When screening for glucose intolerance or diabetes, it is recommended that the patient fasts (no food or drink other than water) for at least 8 hours prior to a laboratory blood sample being taken. The patient then drinks a liquid containing a specified amount of glucose and subsequent blood samples are taken at specified intervals for comparison.

Lipid Profiles

Dyslipidaemia is a major risk factor for cardiovascular disease. Screening for dyslipidaemia involves obtaining a lipid profile through a venous blood sample in acute settings but can be obtained using a point-of-care device and a capillary (finger prick) sample. The point-of-care device method is usually used during community screenings. The lipid profile (Table 7.3) includes:

- Total cholesterol (TC).
- High-density lipoprotein (HDL) cholesterol, which has a role in the removal and disposal of excess cholesterol.
- Non-HDL cholesterol. Increased levels of these different types of cholesterol are associated with increased risk of coronary heart

Table 7.3 Lipid profile normal ranges (**normal values may differ between laboratories**).

Test/component	Reference range
TC	< 5.18 mmol/l
HDL	>1.0 mmol/l for men
	>1.3 mmol/l for women
LDL	2.59–3.34 mmol/l
Fasting triglycerides	<1.70 mmol/l
TC/HDL ratio	<5:1

disease. Non-HDL cholesterol includes low-density lipoprotein (LDL) cholesterol which is harmful in excess as it is deposited in the walls of the blood vessel, thereby contributing to atherosclerosis.

- Triglycerides are the body's storage form of fat and are found mainly in the adipose tissue. As with non-HDL cholesterol, increased levels of triglycerides are associated with increased cardiovascular risk.
- TC/HDL ratio is a calculated value that provides an indicator of cardiovascular risk – the higher the ratio, the higher the risk.

Target lipid profiles for people with cardiovascular disease are discussed in Chapter 5.

Key Point

Triglyceride levels increase and cholesterol levels (TC, LDL and HDL) decrease in inflammatory states such as ACS. These changes usually only become apparent after 24–48 hours, so lipid profiles taken in the first day following onset of and ACS should be reliable. Changes to lipid profiles after ACS become most pronounced after 4–7 days but may be present for up to a few months (Balci 2011).

Complete Blood Count

The complete blood count (CBC), also called the full blood count (FBC), is one of the most frequently ordered blood tests. Parameters

Table 7.4 Complete blood count (normal **values may** differ **between** laboratories).

Component	Reference range
Red blood cell (RBC)	M: $4.5–6.5 \times 10^{12}/l$ F: $3.8–5.8 \times 10^{12}/l$
Haemoglobin (Hb)	M: $130–180\,g/l$ F: $115–165\,g/l$
Haematocrit (Hct) – (percentage of RBCs in the plasma)	M: 40–50% (0.40–0.54 l/l) F: 37–47% (0.37–0.47 l/l)
RBC indices	
Mean corpuscular volume (MCV)	80–100 fl
Mean corpuscular Hb	27–32 pg
Mean corpuscular Hb concentration (MCHC)	300–350 g/l
White blood cells	
White cell count (WCC)	$4.0–11.0 \times 10^9/l$
Differential count[a]	
Neutrophils	$2.0–7.5 \times 10^9/l$
Lymphocytes	$1.5–4.0 \times 10^9/l$
Monocytes	$0.2–0.8 \times 10^9/l$
Eosinophils	$0.04–0.4 \times 10^9/l$
Basophils	$< 0.1 \times 10^9/l$
Platelets	
Platelet count	$150–400 \times 10^9/l$

M: male; F: female.
[a] The proportion of each of the five types of white cells in a WCC sample is known as a differential count. The differential is usually needed to make a diagnosis in the setting of an abnormal WCC.

measured in the CBC are shown in Table 7.4. It is a useful test in patients with a known or potential acute cardiac problem such as ACS or heart failure. Anaemia, detected by measuring haemoglobin (Hb) levels, can be linked to myocardial ischaemia and/or heart failure. Infections, such as pneumonia, or inflammatory processes, such as endocarditis, may have similar presentations to ACS or heart failure, but elevated levels of white blood cells may assist diagnosis. A CBC also gives information about platelet levels, which can be important in the monitoring of antiplatelet therapy.

Clotting Screen

Acute coronary syndrome usually involves the disruption of an unstable plaque in a coronary artery, resulting in the formation of a blood clot. As a result, treatment regimens normally include the use of drugs that interfere with normal clotting mechanisms; thus, careful monitoring of clotting function is essential. The main measurements are:

- Activated partial thromboplastin time (APTT), which is used in the setting of abnormal clotting and in therapeutic monitoring of anticoagulation with unfractionated heparin (UFH). APTT is of no value in monitoring the dosage of low-molecular-weight heparin (LMWH).
- The International normalised ratio (INR), which is particularly useful for testing clotting in patients who are receiving oral anticoagulation with warfarin.
- Activated coagulation time (ACT) provides a rapid, point-of-care assessment of clotting. One of its uses is establishing whether clotting has recovered sufficiently to remove an arterial sheath following percutaneous cardiac intervention.

Biochemical Markers

There are two main types of biochemical markers used in the assessment of cardiac patients. Firstly, there are those that detect damage to the heart muscle – sometimes referred to as biochemical markers (biomarkers) of myocardial necrosis (Thygesen et al. 2019). These tend to be utilised whenever an ACS is suspected. The second type is those markers used in heart failure, known as the cardiac natriuretic peptides.

Markers of Myocardial Necrosis

When a cardiac cell dies (becomes necrotic), the cell membrane becomes disrupted, allowing the contents of the cell to leak into the bloodstream.

Creatine Kinase

Creatine kinase (CK) is an enzyme that is mostly found in skeletal muscles (CK-MM), heart muscle (CK-MB),and, to a lesser extent, in brain tissue (CK-BB). Serum CK and CK-MB were used to test for myocardial necrosis; however, the sensitivity of troponin, and particularly high sensitivity troponin (hsTnT), which is now commonly used, has resulted in CK and CK-MB becoming largely obsolete in the context of acute coronary syndrome (ACS) assessment.

Troponin T and I

Of the commonly used markers of myocardial necrosis, the cardiac forms of the proteins troponin I and troponin T are the most sensitive and specific to myocardial injury. Since the development of troponin testing, there has been much discussion about the level at which a rise becomes clinically significant. Myocardial injury is defined as being present when blood levels of cTn are increased above the 99th percentile upper reference limit. The injury may be acute, as evidenced by a newly detected dynamic rising and/or falling pattern of cTn values above the 99th percentile URL, or chronic, in the setting of persistently elevated cTn levels (Thygesen et al. 2019). Troponin assays in different hospital laboratories will have slightly different reference levels. Though actual cut-off levels for a 'positive' troponin may therefore vary slightly between clinical settings, there remains no doubt that an increase in troponin levels is associated with an increased risk of death following an ACS (Roffi et al. 2015).

Patients with suspected ACS have serum troponin levels (either I or T) measured to aid in confirming or refuting a diagnosis of acute myocardial infarction (MI) and to inform the risk stratification process. In most areas, a baseline troponin level is established on initial presentation, followed by another measurement at 3–6 hours or at a predetermined time interval based on the ACS risk algorithm used. High-sensitivity (hs) cardiac troponin (cTn) assays are now commonly used and can expedite the evaluation of patients with possible ACS in the emergency department. Various rapid screening protocols utilising hscTn in conjunction with other clinical variables and the ECG have been proposed for patients in whom ruling-in or ruling-out acute MI is the primary focus (Vasile and Jaffe 2018).

Though troponin is an extremely sensitive marker of myocardial necrosis, it can be influenced by conditions other than those related to coronary artery disease. Chronic or acute heart failure can cause myocardial damage, which may in turn lead to troponin elevation. Cardiac conditions such as myocarditis and pericarditis, in addition to non-cardiac disorders such as pulmonary embolism and stroke, may also cause troponin levels to rise (Collet et al. 2021). HscTn testing should therefore be considered as just one element of assessing patients with acute cardiac disorders: results should be evaluated in association with the clinical history, physical examination, and ECG findings to reach a definitive diagnosis.

Key Point

Most patients with ACS will have a rising or falling pattern of hscTn values, with the rise being more rapid than the fall. This should be considered when evaluating patients who present more than 12 hours after onset of symptoms (Vasile and Jaffe 2018).

Cardiac Natriuretic Peptides

Cardiac natriuretic peptides are hormones that are produced in response to increased pressures within the heart. Atrial natriuretic peptide (ANP), as the name suggests, is secreted predominantly from atrial cells, as a response to atrial walls being stretched. Secretion of two other peptides – B-type natriuretic peptide (BNP) and N-Terminal proBNP (NT-proBNP) – is stimulated by stretching or tension of the myocardial wall, notably that of the left ventricle.

The primary role of natriuretic peptide testing in the clinical setting remains the diagnosis of heart failure. For patients who attend an emergency department with shortness of breath, BNP/NT-proBNP levels may assist in differentiating between those with heart failure and those with dyspnoea not of cardiac origin (Mueller 2014). Serum BNP/NT-proBNP levels are also helpful as an adjunct to other diagnostic tests for distinguishing between Takotsubo syndrome and ACS. BNP/NT-proBNP are exponentially elevated in Takotsubo syndrome.

Laboratory Specimen Collection

Nurses often have a role in obtaining blood for testing and there are some general considerations to ensure a cost-effective and timely return of results. Laboratory sampling can be costly, particularly when inappropriate tests are ordered or duplicated. Sample labeling errors put patients at risk of transfusion-related death, medication errors, misdiagnosis, delay in treatment, and patient mismanagement (Sandhu et al. 2017) as well as the added cost and discomfort to the patient from repeat testing. Haemolysis is a common cause of laboratory rejection of specimens as it may cause inaccuracy in interpretation of some analytes, such as K+. Haemolysis refers to the breakage of the red blood cell membrane, causing release of haemoglobin and other cell components into the surrounding fluid. Haemolysis may occur due to improper specimen collection, specimen processing, or specimen transport (see Table 7.5).

Table 7.5 Potential causes of haemolysis of blood specimens.

Inappropriate preparation and/or site selection	• Selection of puncture site distal to the antecubital fossa is more likely to be associated with haemolysis. • Not allowing the site to dry after cleansing with alcohol prior to venepuncture may cause haemolysis. • Drawing blood from a peripheral IV catheter with a loose connection of the blood collection assemblies which causes frothing of the blood and haemolysis.
Inappropriate needle bore size	• Use of a small-bore needle resulting in a large vacuum force causing shear stress and rupture of RBCs. • Use of a large bore needle resulting in faster and more forceful flow of blood through the needle causing haemolysis.
Poor venepuncture technique	• Prolonged application of the tourniquet causes the interstitial fluid to leak into the tissue causing haemolysis. Slow blood flow may indicate occlusion due to the lumen of the needle being too close to the inner wall of the vein causing haemolysis. • Pulling the plunger of a syringe back too far while using a large bore needle, may cause enough pressure for haemolysis
Inappropriate processing and handling	• Transferring blood by pushing down on the syringe plunger to force blood into a tube may cause haemolysis. • Vigorous mixing or shaking of a specimen may cause haemolysis. • Exposure to excessive heat or cold can cause RBC rupture and haemolysis
Transfer issues	• Delay in processing resulting in prolonged contact of serum or plasma with cells may result in haemolysis. • Pneumatic tube systems may cause mechanical trauma during transport resulting in haemolysis. (Arzoumanian 2003)

Suggested Resource

Lab Tests Online (UK)
https://labtestsonline.org.uk/

Lab Tests Online (AU)
https://www.labtestsonline.org.au/

Conclusion

For patients suffering from an acute cardiac condition, several laboratory investigations are required. Some basic laboratory investigations such as CBC, urea, electrolytes, and blood glucose are necessary to exclude any underlying pathology and guide therapy. Specific markers such as markers of myocardial necrosis or dysfunction (troponin I and T) and BNP/NT-proBNP may assist in the diagnosis and management of relevant conditions. It is important to remember that laboratory tests only form a part of the clinical assessment in addition to history, physical examination and other investigations. Like any investigation, laboratory tests have their strengths and weaknesses, and results should always be considered in the context of other aspects of patient history and assessment.

References

Arzoumanian, L. (2003). What is hemolysis? *BD Tech Talk* **2** (2): 1.

Balci, B. (2011). The modification of serum lipids after acute coronary syndrome and importance in clinical practice. *Current Cardiology Reviews* **7**: 272–276.

Collet, J.P., Thiele, H., Barbato, E. et al. (2021). 2020 ESC Guidelines for the management of acute coronary syndromes in patients presenting without persistent ST-segment elevation: the task force for the management of acute coronary syndromes in patients presenting without persistent ST-segment elevation of the European Society of Cardiology (ESC). *European Heart Journal* **42** (14): 1289–1367.

Cosentino, F., Grant, P.J., Aboyans, V. et al. (2020). 2019 ESC Guidelines on diabetes, pre-diabetes, and cardiovascular diseases developed in collaboration with the EASD: the task force for diabetes, pre-diabetes, and cardiovascular diseases of the European Society of Cardiology (ESC) and the European Association for the Study of Diabetes (EASD). *European Heart Journal* **41** (2): 255–323.

Kawabe, M., Sato, A., and Hoshi, T. (2014). Impact of blood urea nitrogen for long-term risk stratification in patients with coronary artery disease undergoing percutaneous coronary intervention. *IJC Heart and Vessels* **4**: 116–121.

Marenzi, G., Cabiati, A., and Cosentino, N. (2015). Prognostic significance of serum creatinine and its change patterns in patients with acute coronary syndromes. *American Heart Journal* **169** (3): 363–370.

Mueller, C. (2014). Acute dyspnoea in the emergency department. In: *The ESC Textbook of Intensive and Acute Cardiovascular Care* (ed. M. Tubaro and P. Vranckx) Editors in Chief, 65–74. Oxford: Oxford University Press. Chapter 9.

Roffi, M., Patrono, C., Collet, J.P. 2015 ESC Guidelines for the management of acute coronary syndromes in patients presenting without persistent ST-segment elevation.

European Heart Journal DOI: https://doi.
org/10.1093/eurheartj/ehv320.

Thomas, N. (2014). Chronic kidney disease. In:
Renal Nursing (ed. N. Thomas), 116–135.
Oxford: Wiley-Blackwell. Chapter 6.

Thygesen, K., Alpert, J.S., Jaffe, A.S. et al. (2019).
Fourth universal definition of myocardial
infarction (2018). *European Heart Journal* **40**
(3): 237–269.

Vasile, V. and Jaffe, A. (2018). High-sensitivity
cardiac troponin in the evaluation of possible
AMI. *American College of Cardiology: Latest in
Cardiology. American College of Cardiology
Foundation* https://www.acc.org/latest-in-
cardiology/articles/2018/07/16/09/17/
high-sensitivity-cardiac-troponin-in-the-
evaluation-of-possible-ami (accessed 23
June 2021).

8

Diagnostic Procedures

Steven A. Unger and Angela M. Kucia

Overview

The diagnosis of acute cardiac conditions requires a multimodal approach that involves a thorough patient history and physical examination, laboratory tests and diagnostic procedures. There are many diagnostic procedures that can be utilised for assessing cardiac anatomy and physiology and pathophysiological conditions. Nurses require knowledge of the most common diagnostic tests to be able to assist with preparing the patient for the test, inform them about what to expect during the test and be aware of the care required following the test. Nurses must also know the implications of the test results to provide the most appropriate nursing care and support to the patient.

This chapter provides an overview of the basic concepts of diagnostic cardiac procedures, as well as the clinical indications for each procedure, and the role of the nurse in caring for clients undergoing diagnostic procedures.

- Explain the indications for each diagnostic procedure.
- Discuss the preparation and management of the patient undergoing each diagnostic procedure.
- Describe potential adverse outcomes resulting from diagnostic tests used in the cardiac patient.
- Identify strategies to maximise safety for patients and staff associated with diagnostic tests.

Key Concepts

Diagnostic imaging; radiological examination; exercise tolerance testing; myocardial perfusion imaging

Purpose of Diagnostic Tests

A diagnostic test should help the physician to revise disease probability for a patient and is selected for one of the following purposes:

- Establish a diagnosis in a symptomatic patient
- Screen for disease in an asymptomatic patient
- Provide prognostic information in a patient with established disease

Learning Objectives

After reading this chapter, you should be able to:

- Describe diagnostic procedures available for the assessment of heart disease.

- Monitor therapy by detecting either benefits or side effects
- Confirm that a person is free from a disease (rule out a disease) (Abram and Valesky 2019).

Preparation for Diagnostic Procedures

Diagnostic testing occurs in many environments and vary in complexity. There are some common nursing care actions that are (or may be) required when preparing patients for diagnostic procedures, and these are shown in Table 8.1.

Information and Consent to Diagnostic Procedures

As with any aspect of health care delivery, the patient must be informed about the indication for the diagnostic or laboratory test; how to prepare for the test; what to expect during the test; potential adverse outcomes; available alternatives to the test; and how the information from the test may influence their medical management and health outcomes.

Many diagnostic tests will require written informed consent from the patient, and so the nurse should check whether this is required in

Table 8.1 General preparation for cardiac diagnostic tests.

Checklist	Preparation
Assessment	Assessment and review of the patient's health history is required before ordering a diagnostic test to ensure that the test is appropriate for the patient
Ability to communicate	Ensure that the patient can communicate clearly – if not, an interpreter should be used to explain the procedure and be present during the procedure if required
Correct identification	At least three approved patient identifiers are used when providing care, therapy or services. These identifiers may include patient name (family and given names); date of birth; gender; address; and medical record number or individual health care identifier (Australian Commission on Safety and Quality in Health Care 2012)
Education	Education about the procedure may take the form of printed material or verbal information. Check that the patient understands their responsibilities during the procedure and is aware of reportable symptoms
Informed consent	This may be written or verbal. Check your institutional policy. Give the patient an opportunity to ask questions
Allergies	Clearly document and hand over to all staff involved in care, particularly during transfer of care
Appropriate dress	Provide a hospital gown to patients for any test that requires the patient to fully or partially undress.
Pregnancy check	You may need to check that a female is not pregnant prior to procedures using radiation, drugs or contrast. A urine sample may be required to conduct a pregnancy test
Diabetes care	Fasting for diagnostic tests for patients with diabetes may require adjustments to diabetes medication regimen and blood glucose levels to be checked more frequently
Removal of metal objects	For some tests, it may be necessary to ask the patient to remove metal objects such as jewellery, and body piercings
ECG electrode placement	If the test involves recording or monitoring the ECG, the patient's skin is prepared and electrodes attached in a manner that will optimise skin contact and quality of the ECG trace.

their institution. In preparation for any of the tests listed below, it is assumed that the nurse will ensure that the patient has received appropriate information and consented (either verbally or in writing) prior to the test.

Medical Imaging Tests

Cardiac Catheterisation and Coronary Angiography

Cardiac catheterisation is undertaken for the diagnosis of a variety of cardiac diseases and allows for intra-cardiac pressure measurements and measurements of oxygen saturation and cardiac output. Haemodynamic measurements are usually coupled with left ventriculography for the evaluation of left ventricular (LV) function and coronary angiography (Olade 2016). Coronary angiography (angiogram) is still considered to be the 'gold' standard for diagnosing coronary artery disease (CAD) as it delineates coronary anatomy and shows the site, severity and morphology of

coronary lesions. It also provides a qualitative assessment of coronary blood flow and identification of collateral vessels. When combined with left ventriculography, it provides an assessment of global and regional LV function and assists in identification of potentially viable areas of the myocardium that may benefit from a revascularisation procedure (Olade 2016). The limitation of coronary angiography is that it only produces a silhouette of the inner coronary artery and does not distinguish between stable and vulnerable plaques. The indications for cardiac catheterisation are shown in Table 8.2.

Cardiac catheterisation is performed using a percutaneous (through the skin) approach from the radial, femoral or brachial artery. The transradial approach (TRA) requires greater operator proficiency but is associated with fewer vascular complications, greater comfort for patients (early mobilisation), shortened hospital stay and lower healthcare costs. A femoral approach (FA) is widely used for ease and safety, particularly if the operator is not proficient with the TRA approach or the TRA approach carries

Table 8.2 Indications for coronary catheterisation.

Acute coronary syndromes	Assessment of ST-elevation acute coronary syndrome (STEAC) and non-STEACS prior to planned percutaneous intervention (PCI) Following failed thrombolysis (prior to rescue PCI)
Post-revascularisation ischaemia	Suspected abrupt closure or suspected in-stent thrombosis. Recurrent angina following revascularisation
Known or suspected CAD	Assess for presence of CAD in patients with (i) chest pain of uncertain origin; (ii) categorised as high risk of CAD following non-invasive testing; and (iii) following successful resuscitation from sudden cardiac death
	Assess the extent and severity of known CAD
	Evaluate LV function
	Angina refractory to adequate medical therapy or recurrent symptoms following stabilisation with medical therapy
	Collection of data to confirm and complement non-invasive studies
Assessment of valve disease and cardiomyopathies	Assessment of the severity of valve disorders such as aortic stenosis and/or insufficiency, mitral stenosis and/or insufficiency to determine the need for surgical correction (Ahmed and Hajouli 2020)
	Identification of Takotsubo Syndrome

more risk in an individual patient. The use of vascular closure devices (VCDs) allow for closure to be performed immediately following a procedure via the FA and allows for early mobilisation. If a brachial approach (BA) is used, it is usually percutaneous using a 5F or 6F sheath in the brachial artery. Surgical exposure of the brachial artery is rarely used.

If catheter access to the right side of the heart or pulmonary arteries is required, right heart catheterisation can be performed from the femoral, internal jugular or subclavian veins using percutaneous access (Olade 2016).

The risk of a procedure-related major complication is less than 1–2%. There are relatively few contraindications for coronary angiography that cannot be corrected prior to the procedure (Olade 2016). Table 8.3 shows risks related to cardiac catheterisation with some common causes.

Table 8.3 Procedural complications of cardiac catheterisation.

Complication	Incidence	Causes
Allergic reaction	≈1%	Local anaesthetics, iodinated contrast agents, protamine sulphate, latex atopic disorders (Olade 2016)
Arrhythmias		
Atrial		Irritation of the right atrium by the catheter during right heart catheterisation (Tavakol et al. 2012)
Bradycardia	Common	Vasovagal reaction; injection of contrast directly into a coronary artery or bypass graft; right coronary artery injection of high osmolar agent (Olade 2016)
Conduction disturbance	Rare <1%	Pre-existing left bundle branch block (Olade 2016)
Ventricular tachycardia or fibrillation	Rare <1%	Administration of local anaesthesia in the groin; catheter manipulations irritating ventricle; vigorous contrast injection into the conus branch of the right coronary artery (Olade 2016)
Chest pain	Common	Sensitivity to vasodilatory effects of the contrast medium (Olade 2016)
Congestive heart failure		Osmotic effects of the contrast agents; IV fluid used during the procedure; poor LV function (Olade 2016)
Death	Rare <1%	Embolism (air; atheroembolism); pre-existing cardiac disease (Olade 2016)
Heparin-induced thrombocytopenia	≈1–3%	Prior exposure to heparin (Tavakol et al. 2012)
Hypotension	Common	Right coronary artery injection; large volumes of ionic contrast agent used; low ventricular filling pressures; nitroglycerin use; occult blood loss from a retroperitoneal haematoma; poor fluid intake/fasting prior to the procedure (Olade 2016)
Infection	<1%	BA; existing femoral bypass grafts (Olade 2016)
MI	<1% (Olade 2016)	
Procedural failure	7.2%TRA; 2.4% FA	Prior coronary artery bypass grafting (CABG) short stature (Olade 2016)
Renal dysfunction	≈5%	Pre-existing renal insufficiency and diabetes mellitus; dehydration; taking nephrotoxic medications (Olade 2016)

(Continued)

Table 8.3 (Continued)

Complication	Incidence	Causes
Stroke	<1%	Dislodgement of thrombus debris or thrombus formation at catheter and guidewire tips (Taylor and Khatri 2016)
Vascular complications FA		
Haematoma and retroperitoneal bleed	≈3%	Use of drugs affecting coagulation; (Bashore et al. 2012) poorly controlled haemostasis following femoral sheath removal; femoral artery puncture above the inguinal ligament; traumatic femoral insertion; inadequate period of manual compression; vessel tortuosity (Tavakol et al. 2012).
Pseudoaneurysm	Up to 2%	
Arterio-venous fistula	≈1%	
Femoral/ iliac artery dissection	<1%	
Thrombosis and distal embolisation	<1%	Small vessel lumen, peripheral arterial disease; placement of a large diameter catheter or sheath (intraaortic balloon pump); long catheter dwell-time (Tavakol et al. 2012)
Vascular complications TRA		
Radial artery spasm/ occlusion	5% (Manda and Baradhi 2020)	Operator inexperience (Romagnoli et al. 2012); inadequate anticoagulation
Radial artery perforation	<0.1–1%	Operator inexperience; vessel tortuosity (Trayor and Sanghvi 2013)

Source: Adapted from Olade (2016); Tavakol et al. (2012); Taylor and Khatri (2016); Bashore et al. (2012); Manda and Baradhi (2020); Romagnoli et al. (2012); Trayor and Sanghvi (2013).

Patient preparation for cardiac catheterisation

In addition to general preparation for cardiac diagnostic tests listed in Table 8.1, there are several activities to be undertaken to prepare patients for cardiac catheterisation.

- Ascertain whether the patient has any allergies to radio-iodinated contrast material or drugs that may be given during the procedure.
- The written consent should also have details of the potential need for required additional procedures or emergency surgery.
- Through history and detailed physical examination should include the usual admission baseline observations. As part of the preparation for coronary angiogram, the nurse should check and document the status of the peripheral pedal pulses, presence or absence, colour, warmth, movement and sensation of the lower limbs distal to the proposed puncture site.
- Routine laboratory tests should include haemoglobin, platelet count, electrolytes, prothrombin time and creatinine obtained within 2–4 weeks of the procedure and repeated prior to the procedure if there has been a clinical or medication change or recent contrast exposure.
- Fasting is not routinely undertaken prior to elective PCI due to concern about dehydration. If the patient is fasting, it should not be for more than 2 hours prior to procedure for clear liquids or 4–6 hours after a light meal.
- Use electric clippers to remove hair from the planned arterial puncture site. The use of razors should be avoided. If a TRA is planned, the other wrist and groin areas should be prepared as alternative access sites in case of access problems (Gomes 2015).
- Cleanse the site to be used for catheter insertion as per hospital policy.

Additional preparation considerations for a TRA:

- Peripheral intravenous (IV) cannula sites should be in the opposite arm from that designated for the procedure. If the IV must be placed in the procedural arm, it should be proximal to the wrist to prevent occlusion following the procedure by the haemostasis device.
- A modified Allen's test should be performed prior to TRA.

Potential arterial access sites should be carefully assessed prior to coronary angiography. If the current practice is to use femoral arterial access, the femoral pulses should be palpated bilaterally and distally. Pulses should be auscultated for the presence of bruit, a vascular murmur that might suggest partial obstruction or turbulent flow, creating potential access problems.

If radial access is likely, then the Allen test should be used to assess the radial and ulnar circulation to the hands as follows:

- Palpate the radial and ulnar pulses.
- Ask the patient to make a tight fist and occlude both radial and ulnar arteries with your thumbs.
- Ask the patient to open and relax their hand.
- Release the pressure over one artery and the palm should flush within a few seconds.
- Repeat with the other artery.

The circulation from both the ulnar and radial arteries to the hand needs to be unimpeded to minimise arterial complications from radial access angiography. Alternately, a modified Allen's test can be performed using pulse oximetry (see Box 8.1)

Key Point

For a TRA, it is essential to ensure that the patient has dual circulation in the hand, so that if blood flow is impeded due to radial artery damage during the procedure, adequate circulation to the hand can be maintained by the ulnar artery alone.

Suggested Resource

How to perform a modified Allen's test
The Apprentice Corp (2013)
https://youtu.be/gdgomN6TsuE

Key Point

Cardiac catheterisation involves radiation exposure for staff. Staff working in the cardiac catheterisation laboratory wear lead jackets or aprons and have radiation badges to cumulatively monitor their exposure to radiation. Radiographic/fluoroscopic systems may be equipped with movable lead shields that can be placed between staff members and the source of radiation during the procedure. Catheterisation laboratories have a warning sign or light that indicates fluoroscopic activity and staff that are not protected by lead should not enter the laboratory at this time.

Post-Procedural Care

Immediate assessment should take place when the patient returns from the cardiac investigation unit. This will include level of pain, ECG, vital signs, oxygenation level, urine output, cardiac and respiratory assessment. Particular attention must be paid to the arterial puncture site for any evidence of outward bleeding or haematoma formation. Neurovascular assessment of the lower extremities including colour, warmth, sensitivity, movement, pulses and capillary return should be conducted on the affected limb and the other limb for comparison. Pain or change in sensation at the puncture site or of the affected limb should be assessed. These observations continue at 15–30 minutes intervals until the sheath is removed and for 2 hours following sheath removal (or according to unit policy).

The patient may have the arterial and venous (if used) sheaths removed soon after the procedure or may return to the ward with the sheaths

---

Box 8.1   How to perform a modified Allen's test using pulse oximetry.

Modified Allen's test using pulse oximetry

- Step 1: Place the oximetry probe on either the thumb or first finger of the hand designated for the procedure (usually the right).
- Step 2: Record the baseline oximetry reading and the pulse strength for post-procedure comparison. Manually occlude the radial and ulnar arteries until the oximetry waveform is lost.
- Step 3: Release pressure over the ulnar artery, recording the saturation level with the radial still occluded.
- Step 4: Repeat step 2.
- Step 5: Release the pressure over the radial artery, recording its saturation level indicated by the return of a uniform waveform (Gomes 2015).

The modified Allen's test is considered abnormal if the waveform does not return within a matter of seconds, or if saturation levels between the radial and ulnar arteries differ by more than a few percentage points (Durham 2012). It should be noted that the pulse oximetry waveform resulting from release of the ulnar artery has a smaller amplitude than that of the initial pulse oximetry wave form.

---

in situ. Often, this depends upon the clotting time, which is generally assessed by measuring the activated clotting time (ACT) as patients are often given large doses of heparin during the procedure, and the clotting time will need to be below a certain level to decrease the risk of bleeding when the sheath is removed. For patients who have had a femoral arterial puncture and have a sheath in situ should be placed on bed rest with the head of the bed elevated no higher than 30°. Immediately following removal of the sheath, the patient must lie flat until haemostasis is achieved. The patient should be reminded to limit movement in the bed and to keep the affected limb straight. Advise the patient to apply pressure to the puncture site whilst coughing, sneezing or urinating and to notify nursing staff if any ooze, swelling or feeling of warmth or wetness at the puncture site occurs. Patients become incapable of maintaining self-care because of having to be supine for 2–4 hours (and sometimes longer if the sheath is not removed immediately following the procedure or if the patient is on high-dose anticoagulation or bleeding complications occur). The goal of nursing intervention is to move a patient towards responsible self-care by reducing discomfort due to prolonged bed rest.

Post-Procedural Complications

It is not uncommon for patients to experience a vasovagal reaction, characterised by hypotension and bradycardia with symptoms of yawning, nausea and sweating, during or soon after sheath removal. This is precipitated by the application of pressure to obtain femoral artery haemostasis and can be aggravated by fasting from fluids for a number of hours prior to the procedure or poor oral fluid intake due to maintaining a supine position for patients with sheaths in situ for a prolonged period of time. The management for vasovagal reaction is intravenous fluids and atropine if required. Pre-medication with narcotics prior to sheath removal may reduce potential for vagal reaction (Bashore et al. 2012).

Bleeding is the most common vascular complication following coronary angiography using a FA. If the patient starts to bleed outwardly or a haematoma starts to form around the puncture site, pressure should be applied on the femoral artery above the puncture site until haemostasis is achieved.

Retroperitoneal bleeding can result from a high needle puncture above the inguinal ligament, where blood can enter the retroperitoneum. Typically, the patient complains of abdominal or back pain without any obvious haematoma formation in the groin, and severe back or loin pain after cardiac catheterisation should alert the clinician to this possibility. Retroperitoneal bleed can be life-threatening and result in severe blood loss in the absence of pain. Unexplained hypotension should alert the nurse to the possibility of retroperitoneal haematoma formation. A diagnostic abdominal ultrasound or computerised tomography (CT) scan should be performed if there is suspicion of retroperitoneal bleed.

Another potential source of bleeding is through the development of a pseudoaneurysm, which can develop if a connection persists between a haematoma and the arterial lumen. It presents as a pulsatile mass, sometimes with a systolic bruit and requires a duplex ultrasound for confirmation of the diagnosis. Pseudoaneurysms may be managed conservatively using prolonged compression or thrombin injection in selected patients, but surgical correction may be necessary for large pseudoaneurysms with a wide connection to the parent artery.

An arteriovenous fistula may occur if bleeding from the arterial puncture tracks into the adjacent venous puncture. These are usually small and resolve spontaneously, but surgical repair may be required to fix enlarging fistulae.

Changes to neurovascular observations and ability to palpate pulses should be reported immediately as it may represent serious arterial occlusion, which is a vascular emergency. The patient may experience pain, numbness or tingling if this occurs. The patient should be encouraged to commence oral fluids to aid contrast dye removal from the kidneys. A light diet may be given. Maintain the patient on hourly fluid intake and output.

Chest X-ray

A simple chest X-ray (CXR) is the most performed imaging procedure. It is diagnostically useful, relatively inexpensive and readily available in most acute health care settings. CXRs are usually performed by a radiographer. Ultimately, the findings are reported by a radiologist, though they may be viewed and interpreted by nursing and medical staff prior to a formal report being available. Radiology imaging results are usually available via intranets in larger organisations. A CXR is generally a safe procedure, using a small amount of radiation. Cumulative doses of radiation can be of concern, particularly if the patient has undergone several radiological procedures. The scientific unit of measurement for radiation dose is the millisievert (mSv). If you would like to know more about the radiation dose used in common radiological procedures, visit the website below:

Suggested Resource

Radiation dose in X-Ray and CT exams
Radiologyinfo.org – For Patients (2016)
https://www.radiologyinfo.org/en/info/safety-xray

Penetration of X-ray through the body is inversely proportional to tissue density. The chest has four levels of density: gas or air, water, fat and bone. X-ray beams pass easily through air-filled tissue such as the lung and appear black on the film. Dense matter such as bone is more difficult for the X-ray beam to penetrate and therefore appears white or opaque. A CXR can be obtained from the standard postero-anterior (PA) position, anterior–posterior (AP) position (which is the position used by portable X-ray machines) and lateral (left or right) positions. The PA position is preferred as the X-ray beam travels from the posterior to the anterior of the chest and puts the heart closer to the film allowing the cardiac outline to be seen more clearly (Huseby and Ledoux 2010). A portable CXR can be taken when a patient is acutely unwell and is unable to be transported to the radiology department but difficulty in positioning the patient often affects the quality of the X-ray and makes it diagnostically less useful.

Key Point

If a patient with suspected or known ACS needs to be transported to another area or department for a CXR, consideration should be given to ensuring safe transport with a suitably qualified nurse and monitoring defibrillation and resuscitation equipment.

Suggested Resource

X-ray (Radiography) – Chest Radiologyinfo.org – For Patients (2016) https://www.radiologyinfo.org/en/info/chestrad

---

Interpretation of the CXR

The CXR (Figure 8.1) should always be compared to previous films. The CXR is useful in examining anatomical structures in the chest, including cardiac and mediastinal contours and pulmonary vascular markings, but the

(a)

(b)

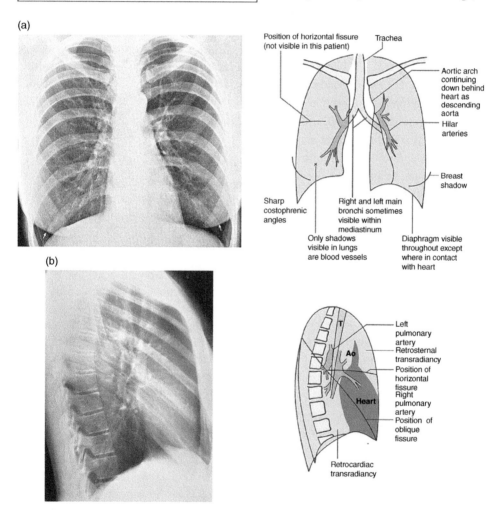

Figure 8.1 Normal chest X-ray. Normal chest X-ray of a female patient. (a) posterior–anterior view; (b) lateral view. *Source:* Rockall et al. (2013).

interior chambers of the heart and arteries are not visualised. The CXR assists in identification of conditions such as cardiomegaly, dissection or dilatation of the aorta, pericardial effusions and calcification of the heart valves or pericardium. It is also useful in evaluating placement of devices such as pacemakers, defibrillators, invasive catheters and chest tubes.

Cardiomegaly

Cardiomegaly can be detected by assessing the cardiothoracic ratio (CTR), which is the widest diameter of the heart compared to the widest internal diameter of the ribcage. The widest diameter of the heart should be no more than 50% of the widest internal diameter of the ribcage.

Key Points

X-rays are subject to divergence and reflection, which makes structures more distant from the film appear magnified and less distinctly outlined. The heart is distant from the film when a CXR is taken on a portable X-ray machine in the AP position and may make the heart appear to be enlarged when, in fact, it is normal (Huseby and Ledoux 2010). The heart appears larger in expiration than inspiration. In conditions such as pregnancy, obesity or ascites, the ability to take a full inspiratory breath is impaired, making the heart look bigger than it is.

Left Ventricular Failure

There are several radiological signs associated with left ventricular (LV) failure. Pulmonary venous congestion occurs initially in the upper zones (referred to as upper lobe diversion or congestion). The upper zone vessels are normally smaller than the lower zone vessels, but as pulmonary venous pressure increases, the upper zone vessels are the same size or larger than the lower zone vessels. As pulmonary venous congestion continues to increase, fluid or cellular infiltration into the interstitium of the lungs occurs and Kerley B lines may be evident. These are short parallel lines, usually less than 1 cm in length, representing interlobular septa. Kerley B lines are parallel to one another at right angles to the pleura and are most frequently observed at the costophrenic angles on the PA view. As pulmonary oedema progresses, fluid accumulates in the alveoli, giving a bilateral fluffy appearance often referred to as 'bats wings' or a 'butterfly effect'. Pleural effusions may also occur.

Suggested Resource

This short video goes through how to report a CXR. Chest X-rays (CXR) Made Easy! Ollie Burton (2019)
https://youtu.be/3Ok6wIiu0zk

Learning Activity 8.1

There are many resources online to help you recognise abnormalities in a CXR. See examples below:

Suggested Resources

DRSABCDE of CXR Interpretation
Life in the Fast Lane (LITFL)
https://litfl.com/drsabcde-of-cxr-interpretation/

Radiology Assistant
Chest X-ray
https://radiologyassistant.nl/chest/chest-x-ray

Computerised Tomography (CT)

Computerised tomography (CT) combines data from several X-rays to produce a detailed image of the heart and blood vessels. Tomography refers to imaging by sections: a CT imaging system produces cross-sectional images or 'slices' of anatomy, like the slices in a loaf of bread. Through combining the images obtained during the scan, a computer can produce a three-dimensional (3D) model of the heart and other body structures. CT scanning can be used to detect problems with heart function and valves; abnormalities such as hypertrophy and intraventricular thrombus; and pericardial disease such as pericardial effusions, pericardial thickening and calcification. CT is also used to detect conditions affecting the aorta, such as aortic dissection or aneurysm; pulmonary embolism and to further investigate abnormalities found on the CXR.

Suggested Resource

Basic CT anatomy of the heart and coronary arteries CTCUS (2010)
https://youtu.be/jGRdn-5RrPg

CT Coronary Angiogram (CTCA)

CT coronary angiogram (CTCA) uses computed tomography (CT) scanning to image the coronary arteries of the beating heart. Angiography refers to X-ray imaging of blood vessels using contrast agents that are injected directly into the bloodstream. The contrast agent (contrast medium) is injected into a vein (usually in the arm). Contrast agents increase the density of the blood in the vessels and allow inner and outer structures of blood vessels to be clearly visualised on the CT angiogram images. CTCA is usually used in patients presenting with chest pain who have an intermediate pre-test probability of having obstructive coronary artery disease. It is quicker, non-invasive, involves less risk and is more cost-effective than percutaneous angiography (Ramjattan et al. 2020), but a percutaneous procedure may be indicated if there is significant disease found on CTCA. See Box 8.2 for a summary of indications, contraindications, and relative contraindications for CTCA.

Box 8.2   Indications, contraindications and relative contraindications for CTCA.

Indications

- patients with suspected CAD who have a low to intermediate risk of CAD based on standard risk assessment criteria (see Chapter 5).

Absolute contraindications

- severe renal impairment (high risk of contrast-induced nephropathy)
- severe or anaphylactic reaction to iodinated contrast
- inability to cooperate with scan protocols
- haemodynamic instability
- decompensated heart failure
- acute myocardial infarction

Relative contraindications

- pregnancy (radiation risk)
- inability to tolerate glyceryl trinitrate
- inability to tolerate beta blockers
- recent phosphodiesterase inhibitor use
- severe aortic stenosis
- bronchospastic disease
- morbid obesity (impaired image quality and CT scanner table weight limits)

(Ramjattan et al. 2020)

Source: Adapted from Ramjattan et al. (2020).

Key Point

Patients with known CAD or at high risk of CAD should not have CTCA as if percutaneous intervention is subsequently required, the patient will then receive another substantial dose of radiation.

Suggested Resource

The following video by Derriford Hospital provides an excellent patient explanation

and rationale for preparation for a Cardiac CT scan:
Cardiac CT scan
PHNTNHSURL
https://youtu.be/6f8Ry2Z6Hj0

Potential Complications Associated with CTCA

There are a few potential adverse effects associated with CTCA:

- Severe contrast allergy has the potential to be life-threatening and adequate medical assistance must be available should this occur.
- Contrast-induced nephropathy.
- Side effects from beta-blocker medications and sublingual nitroglycerin if used.
- Incorrect treatment because of over-estimation of CAD due to low specificity of the test.

If beta-blockers are used for the procedure, a short period of post-CTCA observation (around 30 minutes) is required to ensure that there are no adverse effects, particularly on the patient's blood pressure.

CT Coronary Calcium Scoring Scan

A CT coronary calcium (CTCC) scoring scan can be used to evaluate CAD and calcium build up in the coronary arteries. A coronary calcium scan is a CT scan of the heart that detects and measures the amount of calcium in the walls of the coronary arteries. When used in conjunction with evaluation of traditional cardiovascular risk factors, it enhances the ability to predict the likelihood of future cardiovascular events (Dewey 2014).

Indications and Contraindications for CTCC Scoring Scan

A CTCC scoring scan is unlikely to be diagnostically helpful in people deemed to be at high or low risk of a cardiovascular event using CVD risk assessment calculators such as the 'Australian Absolute Cardiovascular Disease Risk Calculator' or the European Systemic Coronary Risk Evaluation (SCORE) tools and is most useful in those at intermediate risk. Those assesses as being at intermediate risk who are subsequently shown to have a low calcium score have been shown to have similar cardiovascular event rates to those who have been assessed as low risk using conventional risk calculators (Dewey 2014).

The calcium scan does not use contrast dye and will take about 10–15 minutes to complete. A coronary calcium scan has few risks but due to the small dose of radiation, there is a slight risk of developing cancer, particularly in people younger than 40 years old. As with all tests using radiation, pregnant women should not have a CT scan unless it is unavoidable, and this should be discussed with the physician (Dewey 2014).

Echocardiography

Echocardiography is a procedure that uses ultrasound to examine the heart and is one of the most used diagnostic tools in patients with cardiac disorders. A normal echocardiogram will provide information about the anatomy and haemodynamic function of the heart's chambers and valves, intracardiac and extracardiac masses and fluid collections (Kaddoura 2016).

There are primarily three imaging modes used in echocardiography.

2D Mode

Most cardiac images are observed in 2D mode. 2D imaging produces a cross-sectional view of the heart, chambers and blood vessels. 2-D imaging is based on reflection of transmitted ultrasound waves. 2D echocardiography enables calculation of the ejection fraction of the left ventricle and the stroke volume, which can be used to calculate the cardiac output when the heart rate is known. Newer technology, 3D echo (known as 4D echo when the picture is moving), can provide patient-specific three-dimensional modeling of the heart and enables detailed anatomical assessment of cardiac pathology such as valvular defects and cardiomyopathies.

Motion Mode (M-mode)

M-mode is used to assess valve motion, chamber sizes, aortic root size, wall thickness and ventricular function.

Doppler Echo

Doppler analysis is based on the scattering of ultrasound waves from moving blood cells and is used to determine the velocity of blood within the heart. Ultrasound is reflected by moving red blood cells to provide haemodynamic information. It can be used to measure the severity of valvular stenosis or regurgitation and detect intracardiac shunts such as ventricular and atrial septal defects. Commonly used Doppler techniques are:

- a combination of continuous wave Doppler and pulsed-wave Doppler known as spectral Doppler, which together allow a geographical representation of velocity against time;
- colour flow mapping, which is an automated 2D version of pulse wave Doppler that calculates blood velocity and direction at multiple points. Velocities and directions of flow are colour coded, with blood flow away from the transducer coded blue and blood flow towards the transducer coded red (Kaddoura 2016).

Indications for Echocardiography

There are several indications for echocardiography in both acute and chronic cardiac disorders. Indications for echocardiography in acute cardiac conditions are listed in Table 8.4.

Table 8.4 Indications for echocardiography.

Indication	Clinical features
Chest pain assessment	Suspected acute myocardial ischaemia when baseline ECG and laboratory markers are non-diagnostic (if the echo can be obtained during pain or within a few minutes of pain resolution)
	Suspected aortic dissection
	Severe haemodynamic instability
	Clinical evidence of valvular, pericardial or primary myocardial disease
	Left bundle branch block (LBBB) or paced rhythm
Risk stratification	Identify areas of reversible ischaemia and myocardial viability using stress echo
Assessment of mechanical function following MI	Infarct size
	Mechanical complications (mitral regurgitation, ventricular septal defect, cardiac tamponade)
	Baseline LV function required
	Guide for further therapy or assess effect of intervention such as drug therapy; implantable cardiac defibrillator insertion; and cardiac resynchronisation therapy
	Prior to coronary artery bypass surgery
Arrhythmia	Clinical suspicion of structural heart disease in proven arrhythmia
	Assessment of ventricular function for primary prevention of SCD following MI
	Syncope in a patient with clinically suspected heart disease
Heart failure	Clinical or radiographic signs of heart failure
	Periodic evaluation of cardiac function
	Unexplained shortness of breath in the absence of clinical signs of heart failure if ECG/CXR is abnormal

Transthoracic Echocardiography

The most used form of echocardiography is the transthoracic echo (TTE). TTE is an ultrasound of different frequencies that are transmitted from a transducer (probe), which is placed on the patient's anterior chest wall. The transducer transmits high-pitched sound waves to heart structures and picks up echoes of the sound waves as they bounce off the heart structures, providing moving images of the heart. Bone and air do not transmit ultrasound waves well, so specific 'echo windows' (apical, parasternal, subcostal and suprasternal) are used to obtain different views or axes of the heart by placing the transducer in specific positions. 'Axes' refer to the plane in which the ultrasound beam travels through the heart. Patient preparation for TTE is summarised in Box 8.3.

Transoesophageal Echocardiography

Examining the heart with a transducer in the oesophagus is called transoesophageal echocardiography (TOE). The procedure is similar to that of an endoscopy and the benefit is that visualisation of the heart is clearer as it is not obscured by the lungs, chest wall and ribs as with TTE. TOE enables high-resolution imaging of the aorta, the left atrium (including the left atrial appendage) and the mitral valve. Disadvantages are that it is invasive, uncomfortable for the patient and not without risk, including potential oesophageal trauma, problems associated with intravenous sedation and aspiration of stomach contents into lungs. Preparation for TOE is summarised in Box 8.4

Box 8.3   Patient preparation for transthoracic echocardiogram (TTE).

In addition to general preparation for cardiac diagnostic tests listed in Table 8.1, there are some activities to be undertaken to prepare patients for TTE:

- TTE is a non-invasive procedure, but some patients may find the pressure from the probe on the chest wall uncomfortable. They may need some simple analgesia prior to the procedure.
- The patient usually lies in the left lateral position during the procedure, which assists in obtaining quality images because the heart falls forward and the lungs are out of view and the patient's left arm is positioned above the head to aid in the separation of the ribs.
- If the patient is short of breath, they may not be able to tolerate this position and the test may need to be rescheduled.

Box 8.4   Patient preparation for transesophageal echocardiogram (TOE/TEE).

In addition to general preparation for cardiac diagnostic tests listed in Table 8.1, there are some activities to be undertaken to prepare patients for TOE/TEE:

- The patient should be fasted for at least four hours prior to the procedure.
- A short-acting sedative is generally used, and a local anaesthetic is sprayed directly on the patient's pharynx.
- The patient is placed in the left lateral position during the procedure with the neck fully flexed to allow easy insertion of the transducer.
- Oxygen, suction and continuous ECG monitoring should be available. Post-procedure, the patient will be drowsy and have a numb throat.
- Nursing care involves airway protection.
- The patient should not eat or drink for at least one hour after the procedure in case of aspiration.

Magnetic Resonance Imaging (MRI)

Magnetic resonance imaging (MRI) is a non-invasive test that relies upon a powerful magnetic field, radio waves and a computer to produce detailed images. The MRI scanner unit is a closed cylindrical magnet (long tube) within which the patient lies as still as possible on a moveable bed within the magnet. The procedure takes generally between 30 and 75 minutes, depending on the extent of the imaging needed. The magnetic field is produced by passing an electric current through wire coils to send and receive radio waves that are analysed by a computer to produce a series of images of the body.

Cardiac Magnetic Resonance (CMR)

Cardiac magnetic resonance (CMR) imaging provides superior detailed images of the heart as it is beats, creating moving images of the heart, including chambers and valves, throughout the cardiac cycle. The added advantage of this test is that is does not use ionising radiation. CMR is more expensive that echocardiography, CT or SPECT, but not as expensive as coronary angiography (Lipinski et al. 2013).

Indications for CMR

Indications for CMR include:

- assessment of cardiac structures if echocardiographic images are non-diagnostic;
- adjunct to other imaging methods for anatomical and functional evaluation of congenital heart disease (Fratz et al. 2013);
- evaluation of the extent of myocardial scarring and area of non-viable myocardium following myocardial infarction;
- assessment of myocardial perfusion and function using pharmacologic stress agents, particularly when other stress imaging methods (stress echo or myocardial perfusion imaging) are non-diagnostic;
- diagnostic evaluation of Takotsubo Syndrome.

Risks of MRI

The strong magnetic field in the MR environment presents unique safety hazards for patients with implants, external devices and accessory medical devices.

Key Point

Prior to undergoing an MRI procedure, the person must complete a screening tool to ensure that there are no known risks for an adverse event due to the procedure.

Risks associated with MRI arise from four mechanisms:

1) The static magnetic field has the potential to move, rotate, dislodge or accelerate a ferromagnetic object creating a 'projectile effect' towards the magnet that could lead to significant patient injury and damage to the magnetic resonance (MR) system. It also has the potential to alter device function (such as pacemakers and implantable defibrillators). It is important to know if the patient has had any procedures or injuries

in the past that have resulted in metal or magnetic implants or devices such as vascular clips used for cerebral aneurysm surgery, embedded metal objects such as shrapnel or bullets, insulin or narcotic pumps, prosthetic hip joints, implanted nerve stimulators or cochlear implants (Expert Panel on MR Safety et al. 2013).

2) Radiofrequency (RF) energy is 'pulsed' into the body to generate the MR image. Whilst the body absorbs most of the heat produced in this process, some metallic devices such as pacemaker leads or Swan–Ganz (pulmonary artery) thermodilution catheters may concentrate this RF energy and potentially cause a burn to the patient. Tattoo pigments may contain metal substances that create an electric current that can cause redness and swelling like a first degree burn at the site of the tattoo or permanently implanted eye makeup. Medication patches or clothing containing metallic fibres or backing can also cause RF-induced patient injury (Expert Panel on MR Safety et al. 2013).

Key Point

MR-safe ECG electrodes and leads should be used as conventional electrodes and leads may not be safe because of their incorporation of low-impedance conductors and/or ferromagnetic components, which can cause skin heating or burns. ECG leads should not be allowed to form loops and should not be positioned along the sides of the scanner bore or close to the body (Brau et al. 2015).

3) Gradient magnetic fields are weaker than static magnetic fields but are repeatedly turned on and off, which can induce electrical currents in electrically conductive devices, potentially causing arrhythmia, and may also excite peripheral nerves causing an unpleasant sensation (Brau et al. 2015).

4) Most scans involve intravenous injection of MRI contrast (gadolinium) to visualise myocardial perfusion, extent of myocardial scarring or fibrosis and proximal coronary arteries. Gadolinium contrast administration can lead to severe nephrotoxicity and nephrogenic systemic fibrosis, particularly if used in high doses or in patients with at least moderate underlying renal dysfunction (Expert Panel on MR Safety et al. 2013).

Many patients suffer a fear of enclosed spaces and cannot tolerate being enclosed within the MRI scanner. This is a contraindication to having MRI unless anxiety can be managed with sedation.

Suggested Resources

MRI safety
MRIPETCTSOURCE (2021)
https://youtu.be/DKy8DCJjnwl

MRI safety
Christiane Sarah Burton (2020)
https://youtu.be/LS2hwW6Ihj4

MRI Following Device Implant

Most coronary and peripheral vascular stents exhibit non-ferromagnetic or weakly ferromagnetic characteristics. Most prosthetic heart valves, annuloplasty rings and sternal suture wires and left atrial appendage occluder devices are unlikely to pose a threat to the patient during MRI but may be labelled 'MR conditional' (see Table 8.5).

Active implants, including permanent cardiac pacemakers or implantable cardioverter defibrillators (ICDs), contain metal with various ferromagnetic properties and complex electrical circuits, and use leads implanted into the myocardium. There is potential during the MR exam for movement or damage of the device, inhibition of pacing output, activation of tachyarrhythmia therapy or heating of the electrodes, leading to serious clinical consequences,

Table 8.5 Current terminology used for labelling implanted devices for MR safety.

Terminology	Symbol	Definition
MR safe	MR	Poses no known hazards in all MRI environments
MR conditional	MR	Poses no known hazards in a <u>specified</u> MR environment with <u>specified conditions of use</u>
MR unsafe	MR	Poses hazards in all MRI environments

Key Point

Medical devices labelled with old terminology 'MR safe' or 'MR compatible' prior to 2005 are safe or compatible when used according to the list of conditions under which the device had been tested at that time

---

including changes in pacing or defibrillation thresholds, arrhythmia or death. Older pacemakers and ICDs have therefore been considered a contra-indication to MRI (Brau et al. 2015). Newer developments in technology have led to the development of some MR conditional pacemakers and ICDs designed for use under specific conditions.

Key Point

Regulatory approvals for MR conditional pacemakers and ICDs vary by device manufacturer and by region, and it is important to follow institutional protocols and consult the device manufacturer's imaging guidelines for a particular device (Brau et al. 2015).

Insertable loop recorders (implanted devices with surface electrodes that continuously record the patient's ECG to detect arrhythmia) contain no lead wires and are normally labelled 'MR conditional'. However, any ECG data acquired during MR scanning should be considered unreliable due to excessive artefact during the procedure, and any stored ECG data should be downloaded before the MR exam (Brau et al. 2015).

Critically ill patients are not good candidates for MRI because of the large amount of equipment such as continuous monitoring systems and life-support ventilators that cannot be bought near the scanner. Use of haemodynamic support devices such as ventricular assist devices and intra-aortic balloon pumps are a contraindication for CMR unless the devices have been certified as MR safe by manufacturers. Devices incorporating cardiovascular catheters, such as pulmonary artery, haemodynamic monitoring and thermodilution catheters and temporary transvenous cardiac pacing devices may be prone to overheating and are considered 'MR unsafe' unless otherwise indicated by the manufacturer (see Table 8.5) (Brau et al. 2015). Preparation for MRI is summarised in Box 8.5.

Key Point

In case of cardiac or respiratory arrest or other medical emergency in the MRI room, appropriately trained and certified MR personnel should immediately initiate basic life support or CPR as required while the patient is being moved rapidly and safely to a magnetically safe location (Expert Panel on MR Safety et al. 2013).

Box 8.5   Patient preparation for MRI.

In addition to general preparation for cardiac diagnostic tests listed in Table 8.1, there are some activities to be undertaken to prepare patients for MRI:
• The patient should complete the pre-procedure check list for MRI, and this should be checked by staff conducting the MRI.

- Inform the ordering physician if the patient suffers from claustrophobia or confusion in case sedation is required.
- Devices or implants may be a contraindication for MRI, and all devices and implant need to be declared.
- Any metal fragments that may have been retained in the body (shrapnel, splinters of steel) can cause damage to the person.
- For large tattoos, a cold compress on that area may need to be applied to prevent heating.
- Metal objects (including body-piercing jewellery) should be removed from the patient before an MRI scan (Kucia 2017).

Learning Activity 8.3

Consider accompanying a monitored cardiac patient for an MRI scan and some of the issues you would face. Review your own institutional policies and procedures and how you might manage some of these issues in your own practice. The following website may help you:

Suggested Resource

MRISafety.com
http://www.mrisafety.com

Electrocardiography Tests

Electrocardiography (ECG or EKG) refers to a test that records the electrical activity of the heart over a period of time through electrodes placed on the skin. The electrodes detect the electrical changes in the myocardium arising from depolarisation and repolarisation during the cardiac cycle. A few cardiac diagnostic tests utilise electrocardiographic monitoring during the procedure.

12-Lead Electrocardiogram (ECG)

The 12-lead ECG has been used for over 100 years and is among the most useful diagnostic tests in clinical medicine. The ECG is and is still the most commonly used test to detect conditions such as myocardial injury, ischaemia, presence of prior infarction and disorders of the cardiac rhythm. It is also used in the evaluation of primary and secondary cardiomyopathies; syncope; metabolic disorders; effects and side effects of pharmacotherapy; and the function of implantable cardiac devices. The main indications for performing a 12-lead ECG are listed in Table 8.6.

There are no absolute contraindications to performing an ECG other than patient refusal. Some patients may have a sensitivity to the adhesive electrodes used to affix the leads, in which case a hypoallergenic alternative electrode can be used.

Detailed information about obtaining a 12-lead ECG and ECG interpretation can be found in Chapter 9.

Ambulatory Monitoring

For information about Holter monitoring, event recorders, implantable loop recorders, refer to Chapter 12.

Physiological Testing

Electrophysiological Studies

For information about electrophysiological studies, refer to Chapter 12.

Tilt Table Testing

Tilt-table testing (TTT) is a simple, noninvasive diagnostic test that is usually performed in EP departments for patients with signs or symptoms suggestive of orthostatic hypotension, vasodepressor or vasovagal syncope, postural orthostatic tachycardia or when other causes of syncope have been eliminated

Table 8.6 Indications for performing a 12-lead ECG.

Signs/symptoms/indications	Possible cause/finding
• Chest pain • New onset dyspnoea • Abnormal assessment findings (for example, third/fourth heart sound or murmur)	• Myocardial ischaemia or infarction • Structural heart disease • Pulmonary embolism • Arrhythmia
• Conscious or unconscious collapse • Seizures • Palpitations or abnormal pulse	• Arrhythmia • Myocardial ischaemia or infarction • Structural heart disease • Pulmonary embolism
• Ongoing assessment of known conditions	• Coronary heart disease • Structural heart disease • Arrhythmia • Conduction abnormalities caused by medications • Electrolyte abnormalities • Pacemaker function
• Screening	• Conditions causing sudden death (for example, hypertrophic cardiomyopathy, long QT and Brugada syndromes) • Pre-operative assessment for cardiac abnormalities

---

Box 8.6   Indications for tilt table testing.

Unexplained hypotension
Tachycardia when standing
Pallor when upright
Orthostatic palpitations
Unexplained dizziness or lightheadedness
History of frequent unexplained falls
History of episodes of fainting or loss of consciousness (Talano 2016).

Source: Based on Talano (2016).

Box 8.7   Patient preparation for tilt table testing.

In addition to general preparation for cardiac diagnostic tests listed in Table 8.1, there are some activities to be undertaken to prepare patients for a tilt table test:

Avoid dehydration on the day of the study in patients who have been fasting or receiving diuretic therapy.

Some medications may need to be held on the day of the procedure prior to the study to increase the sensitivity of the study. If diuretic or antihypertensive medications are a suspected contributor to syncopal episodes, the patient may be required to take these medications as usual.

Obtain IV access and start a maintenance IV fluid drip if ordered.

(Talano 2016). Indications for TTT are listed in Box 8.6.

The patient is initially positioned supine and horizontal on a flat table with a foot support. Blood pressure, heart rate and rhythm, and oxygen saturation is measured whilst the table is tilted by degrees to a completely vertical, upright position with the aim of causing the patient to faint, indicating a positive test result. Patient preparation for TTT is summarised in Box 8.7.

TTT is a relatively safe procedure, but patients can experience some complications including vasospasm (associated with isoproterenol administration during the procedure, and arrhythmias. Decreased perfusion of the brain during the procedure may also lead to seizures from prolonged hypotension, transient ischaemic attacks or stroke; transient mental confusion or nonspecific symptoms such as nausea or anxiety.

Suggested Resource

Zysko, D., Jamil, R.T., and Anilkumar, A.C. (2021). Tilt Table. [Updated 2021]. In: StatPearls [Internet]. Treasure Island (FL): StatPearls Publishing. https://www.ncbi.nlm.nih.gov/books/NBK482320/

Stress Testing

Exercise Stress Test

The exercise stress test (EST), also known as the exercise tolerance test, is a commonly used cardiac assessment technique used to assess the cardiac response to exercise. During exercise, coronary blood flow must increase to meet the higher metabolic demands of the myocardium. Coronary flow reserve (CFR) is the maximum increase in blood flow through the coronary arteries above the normal resting volume. It is determined by the capacity of components of the coronary vascular system, particularly the microvascular coronary arterial bed, to dilate to achieve maximal blood flow in response to hyperaemic stimulation such as exercise. For patients with normal coronary arteries, the coronary arteries will dilate as heart rate and blood pressure increase. For regions of myocardium that are supplied by an artery with significant stenosis, the artery is unable to dilate sufficiently in response to increasing myocardial work, resulting in inadequate blood flow to that region. Limitations to coronary blood flow due to narrowing or stenoses of coronary arteries may result in changes in the ECG, heart rate, blood pressure and cause angina. The EST can be used to determine functional capacity, assess the probability and extent of coronary disease, assess the effects of therapy and estimate prognosis. The most common indications for EST are listed in Box 8.8.

Box 8.8   Indications for exercise stress test (EST).

- Symptoms suggesting myocardial ischaemia
- Assessment of acute chest pain in patients in whop acute coronary syndrome (ACS) has been excluded
- Recent ACS treated without coronary angiography or incomplete revascularization
- Known CAD with worsening symptoms
- Assessment of patients who have had prior coronary revascularisation
- Valvular heart disease (to assess exercise capacity and need for surgical intervention)
- Certain cardiac arrhythmias to assess chronotropic competence
- Newly diagnosed heart failure or cardiomyopathy (Vilcant and Zeltser 2020; Chareonthaitawee and Wells Askew 2020).

Usefulness of Exercise Stress Testing

The diagnostic accuracy of EST varies with age, gender and clinical characteristics of the patient. EST is probably more useful in confirming CAD than excluding it. A positive EST is better at discriminating presence of CAD in younger patients and in men than in older patients and women (Banerjee et al. 2012).

Key Point

Pre-test probability is the probability of a patient having the target disorder/disease prior to the diagnostic test result being known. Due to ease of use and ready availability, EST is commonly used without due consideration of pre-test probability and may lead to unnecessary further testing when the EST is equivocal, falsely positive or the patient is unable to complete the test due to issues such as muscle fatigue.

Safety

The EST is a relatively safe procedure, but myocardial infarction and death have been reported to occur at a rate of one incident per 2500 tests; thus, careful patient selection is required. Table 8.7 lists absolute and relative contraindications for EST. Relative contraindications may be superseded by an experienced physician if the benefits of exercise outweigh the risks (Akinpelu 2018).

The most common method of ETT is for the patient to exercise on a treadmill with progressive increases in the speed and elevation of the treadmill (see Figure 8.2). A 12-lead ECG is

Table 8.7 Absolute and relative contraindications for exercise testing.

Absolute contraindications	Relative contraindications
Acute MI (within 2 days)	Known or suspected severe left main stenosis
Unstable angina (not stabilised by drug therapy)	Moderate stenotic valvular heart disease
Untreated life-threatening arrhythmia, complete heart block or rapid atrial arrhythmia	Uncontrolled hypertension (systolic blood pressure >220 mmHg, diastolic >120 mmHg)
Severe aortic stenosis	Recent stroke or transient ischaemic attack
Uncontrolled heart failure	Tachyarrhythmias or bradyarrhythmias
Acute pulmonary embolus or pulmonary infarction	Hypertrophic cardiomyopathy and any other forms of outflow tract obstruction
Acute myocarditis or pericarditis	Mental or physical impairment leading to an inability to exercise adequately
Acute aortic dissection/recent aortic surgery	High-degree atrioventricular (AV) block
Acute systemic infection	Underlying medical condition that may affect cardiac rhythm and/or haemodynamic stability (anaemia, electrolyte imbalance, hyperthyroidism, etc.)
Deep vein thrombosis	

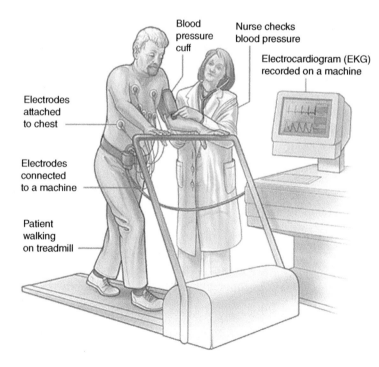

Blood pressure cuff

Nurse checks blood pressure

Electrocardiogram (EKG) recorded on a machine

Electrodes attached to chest

Electrodes connected to a machine

Patient walking on treadmill

Figure 8.2 Exercising on the treadmill. *Source:* National Heart, Lung, and Blood Institute; National Institutes of Health; U.S. Department of Health and Human Services.

recorded during the test, along with continuous monitoring of heart rate, heart rhythm and blood pressure.

The Bruce Protocol is the most widely adopted protocol for exercise testing using a treadmill. The protocol has seven stages and each stage lasts for three minutes. The speed and incline of the treadmill increase with each stage of the protocol. Exercise duration is dependent on the age and gender of the patient. To complete the test, the patient should exercise for the calculated exercise duration and reach 85% of their maximum predicted heart rate (MPHR). MPHR is defined as:

- 220 minus age for males
- 210 minus age for females

A modified Bruce protocol starts at a lower workload than the standard test and is typically used for exercise testing for elderly or sedentary patients. Other common modalities for EST are treadmill echo, bicycle ECG, bicycle echo and myocardial perfusion imaging. Patient preparation for EST is summarised in Box 8.9. Medication considerations for patients undertaking EST are summarised in Box 8.10.

Key Point

Patients scheduled to undertake an EST may be asked to avoid caffeine intake for 12–24 hours prior to the EST in case they are unable to complete a diagnostic EST and require a pharmacological single-photon-emission computed-tomography (SPECT) imaging study.

An EST may need to be terminated before the patient reaches the calculated exercise duration or target MPHR for reasons such as moderate to severe angina, haemodynamic compromise, ECG changes suggesting obstructive CAD or patient unable/unwilling to continue. A full list of absolute and relative

---

Box 8.9 Patient preparation for exercise stress testing (EST).

In addition to general preparation for cardiac diagnostic tests listed in Table 8.1, there are some activities t o be undertaken to prepare patients for an EST:

- The patient should be dressed in loose clothing/hospital gown that does not impede lead placement or quality of ECG recording.
- Ensure the patient is wearing footwear for the procedure.
- The patient should be assessed by an appropriate health practitioner as suitable for EST.
- Ensure that the patient's weight is compatible with treadmill manufacturer's recommendations and that the patient has no mobility restrictions that will impede their ability to exercise on the treadmill.
- There may be a variation required to a patient's medications prior to EST. Check that medications have been administered/withheld as ordered (see Box 8.10).
- Some centres advise patients not to eat or drink fluids other than water for 2–4 hours prior to the test due to concern that a vagal response on completing the test may result in dizziness or syncope (particularly in young people).
- The appropriate exercise protocol is chosen for the patient (usually Bruce or modified Bruce).
- ECG leads are attached and a strap applied to secure the acquisition module to patient to minimise movement of the ECG leads. Obtain an ECG trace to check the quality of the ECG recording.
- Check and record the patient's manual blood pressure (BP) and heart rate (HR) and baseline resting ECGs in the lying and standing positions.

Box 8.10   Medication considerations for patients undertaking EST.

Medication variations may include:

- Pre-test omission of nitrates
- Pre-test omission of beta-blockers
- Pre-test omission of calcium channel blockers
- Pre-test omission of diuretics
- Alterations in dose of diabetes medication

Patients with hypertension should take their antihypertensive medication unless advised by the physician not to do so. Poorly controlled hypertension may preclude the patient from being able to undertake or complete the EST.

Patients who take inhalers for asthma or airways disease should bring their inhalers with them to the test appointment.

Variation to normal medication regimes should only be undertaken following discussion with the physician.

---

indications to cease an EST can be found in the suggested resource below.

Interpretation of the EST

Clinical findings suggesting that the EST is positive for ischaemia include:

- exercise-induced hypotension
- exercise-induced angina or anginal equivalents
- appearance of an S_3, S_4 or heart murmur during exercise.

Horizontal or down-sloping ST segment depression or ST segment elevation in adjacent ECG leads is generally a reliable indicator of exercise-induced ischaemia (see Chapter 9).

Repolarisation and conduction abnormalities and some medications preclude accurate interpretation of the EST (see Box 8.6). If these abnormalities are present, other forms of exercise testing should be used. Confounders of EST interpretation are listed in Box 8.11.

A normal EST is one in which the person (i) achieves 85% of the maximum predicted heart rate with a physiological response in blood pressure and no associated ST segment depression on the ECG; and (ii) experiences no angina (or angina equivalent symptoms).

Suggested Resource

Exercise Tolerance Test
Chest Heart & Stroke Scotland (2013)
https://youtu.be/4-jS6BKaVSY

Myocardial Perfusion Imaging

A radionuclide stress test is a myocardial perfusion imaging technique that involves intravenous injection of a radiopharmaceutical agent (typically thallium 201 or ^{99m}Technetium sestamibi or ^{99m}Technetium tetrofosmin) to detect the distribution of nutritional blood flow in the myocardium. These radiopharmaceutical agents (isotopes) are often called 'tracers' because they can be traced as they move through the body. Perfusion imaging provides information about LV chamber size, global and regional LV function, location, size and extent of areas of reduced myocardial blood flow that are associated with ischaemia or infarction and scar. Perfusion can be assessed at rest, during periods of cardiovascular stress (induced by an acute coronary syndrome or exercise) or both.

In diagnostic perfusion imaging with treadmill EST, nuclear images are typically obtained immediately following an EST, and

---

Box 8.11   Confounders of EST interpretation.

Atrial repolarisation abnormalities
Left bundle branch block
LVH
Resting ST depression
Digoxin

---

if abnormal, a second scan is performed in the resting condition, often later the same day. The two sets of images are then compared. If there is a blockage in a coronary artery that results in diminished blood flow to a region of the cardiac muscle during exercise, there will be a diminished concentration of the radiopharmaceutical agent in the region of decreased perfusion known as a 'perfusion defect'. Following a period of rest, if coronary perfusion is adequate, the perfusion defect is not obvious. This is known as a 'reversible defect' and is indicative of reversible ischaemia during the stress test. Data from the test are presented as views from several axes. The tracer is injected at peak exercise and the single-photon emission computed tomography (SPECT) images are acquired soon after exercise and at least 3 hours later at rest. The procedure for the patient is like that of a standard EST but involves one or two scans and more time. The location and size of a reversible defect guides further treatment strategy in patients with CAD.

Although radionuclide stress testing is more time-consuming and expensive compared to an ordinary EST, it enhances the accuracy in diagnosing CAD and is useful in making decisions regarding coronary revascularisation. Preparation is similar to that for EST but has some additional considerations. Ensure that females undergoing this procedure are not pregnant. Patients may be asked to fast for 3–6 hours prior to the procedure to minimise gastric blood flow and gastric uptake of radionuclides. As the ability to exercise adequately may be underestimated by the referring clinician, pharmacologic stress may be required, and so all patients should abstain from caffeine intake for a minimum of 12 hours.

Pharmacologic Stress Test

Some patients, including those with severe pulmonary disease, arthritis, amputation, neurological disease, may be unable to undertake physical exercise. In this case, the heart can be subjected to chemical 'stressors'. There are two types of pharmacologic agents that are useful to stress the heart to evaluate myocardial perfusion:

- Vasodilator agents (dipyridamole and adenosine), which produce coronary hyperaemia
- Ino/chronotropic adrenergic agents (dobutamine) that increase myocardial oxygen demand.

For patients undergoing pharmacologic stress testing with dipyridamole or adenosine, caffeine-containing beverages should not be taken for at least 12 hours before pharmacologic stress imaging. A caffeinated beverage or IV aminophylline may be used after testing to reverse the effect of dipyridamole. Adenosine is shorter acting and so this is not usually necessary.

Stress Echocardiography

Stress echocardiography (SE), using a transthoracic approach, is an established method for the diagnosis and prognostic stratification of CAD and is particularly useful when a patient has had a prior non-diagnostic EST or there is a high likelihood of a false-positive result from an ECG EST. SE may be conducted using exercise, pharmacological stress using dobutamine or temporary cardiac pacing. Echocardiographic images in several views are obtained at rest and during or within 1–2 minutes of peak exercise.

Key Point

Inducible regional wall motion abnormalities resolve rapidly after stress and so for patients undergoing a stress test on a treadmill, it is preferable for echo images to be obtained within a minute of peak exercise.

Myocardial contractility normally increases with exercise, whereas ischaemia causes hypokinesis, akinesis or dyskinesis of affected segments. An exercise or stress echocardiogram is considered positive if regional wall motion abnormalities develop with exercise in previously normal segments or when pre-existing wall motion abnormalities become more severe (Fletcher et al. 2013).

Additionally, SE has a role in the assessment and evaluation of coronary microvascular disease, dilated cardiomyopathy, systolic and diastolic heart failure, hypertrophic cardiomyopathy, athletes' hearts, valvular heart disease, congenital heart disease and pulmonary hypertension. It may also be used in the assessment of some patients after heart transplantation preoperative risk assessment and in evaluation of athletes and persons who are submitted to extreme physiology, such as high altitudes or diving (Kossaify et al. 2020).

Key Point

Patients with permanent pacemakers are better assessed with stress echocardiography because paced rhythms produce apical and septal wall motion abnormalities. Pharmacologic stress echocardiography using dobutamine is also useful for individuals who have poor exercise capacity but is not useful in patients who are beta-blocked.

Generally, echocardiography is a safe addition to EST. The limitation of this procedure is that it is operator-dependant with regard to the quality of the images obtained and is subject to inter-interpreter variability.

Stress Cardiac Magnetic Resonance Imaging (CMR)

Stress cardiac magnetic resonance imaging (CMR) using a vasodilator or dobutamine is increasingly being used to assess chest pain in patients with known or suspected CAD. CMR is also useful in assessing left ventricular function and presence of structural or valvular heart disease. CMR may also have a role in the assessment for residual ischaemia due to coronary stenoses in noninfarct-related arteries after ST-segment elevation myocardial infarction (Lipinski et al. 2013). See the section below for further information on use of MRI in cardiovascular assessment.

Conclusion

This chapter presents an overview of some of the more commonly used diagnostic techniques that are currently available to assess cardiac structure and function. The determination of which diagnostic procedure to use depends on the clinical condition of the patient, the preference of the patient where there is more than choice and the availability of the test. Information required, expense, availability of expertise and organisational preferences are also factors that influence the choice of procedure.

Major advancements in diagnostic testing in cardiology continue to be made and evaluation of these technologies needs to be closely monitored to ensure patients receive the best options for diagnostic testing and management.

References

Abram, E. and Valesky, W.W. (2019). Rational Use of Screening and Diagnostic Tests. *Medscape*. https://emedicine.medscape.com/article/773832-overview (accessed 29 June 2021).

Ahmed, I. and Hajouli, S. (2020). Left Heart Cardiac Catheterization. [Updated 2020 December 25]. In: StatPearls [Internet]. Treasure Island (FL): StatPearls Publishing; 2021 January-. https://www.ncbi.nlm.nih.gov/books/NBK564323 (accessed 1 July 2021).

Akinpelu, D. (2018). Treadmill Stress Testing. *Medscape*. https://emedicine.medscape.com/article/1827089-overview (accessed 1 July 2021).

Australian Commission on Safety and Quality in Health Care (2012). *Safety and Quality Improvement Guide Standard 5: Patient Identification and Procedure Matching* (October 2012. Sydney: ACSQHC https://www.safetyandquality.gov.au/sites/default/files/migrated/Standard5_Oct_2012_WEB.pdf (accessed 1 July 2021).

Banerjee, A., Newman, D.R., Van den Bruel, A., and Heneghan, C. (2012). Diagnostic accuracy of exercise stress testing for coronary artery disease: a systematic review and meta-analysis of prospective studies. *International Journal of Clinical Practice* **66** (5): 477–492.

Bashore, T.M., Balter, S., Barac, A. et al. (2012). 2012 American College of Cardiology Foundation/Society for Cardiovascular Angiography and Interventions expert consensus document on cardiac catheterization laboratory standards update: a report of the American College of Cardiology Foundation Task Force on expert consensus documents. *Journal of the American College of Cardiology* **59** (24): 2221–2305.

Brau, A.C., Hardy, C.J., and Schenck, J.F. (2015). MRI safety. In: *Basic Principles of Cardiovascular MRI* (ed. M.A. Syed, S.V. Raman and O.P. Simonetti), 115–127. Cham: Springer.

Chareonthaitawee, P. and Wells Askew, J. (2020). Exercise ECG testing: Performing the test and interpreting the ECG results. UpToDate. https://www.uptodate.com (accessed 1 July 2021).

Dewey, M. (2014). *Cardiac CT*. Springer.

Durham, K.A. (2012). Cardiac catheterization through the radial artery. *AJN The American Journal of Nursing* **112** (1): 49–56.

Expert Panel on MR Safety, Kanal, E., Barkovich, A.J. et al. (2013). ACR guidance document on MR safe practices: 2013. *Journal of Magnetic Resonance Imaging* **37** (3): 501–530. doi: 10.1002/jmri.24011. Epub 2013 Jan 23. PMID: 23345200.

Fletcher, G.F., Ades, P.A., Kligfield, P. et al. (2013). Exercise standards for testing and training: a scientific statement from the American Heart Association. *Circulation* **128** (8): 873–934.

Fratz, S., Chung, T., Greil, G.F. et al. (2013). Guidelines and protocols for cardiovascular magnetic resonance in children and adults with congenital heart disease: SCMR expert consensus group on congenital heart disease. *Journal of Cardiovascular Magnetic Resonance* **15** (1): 1–26.

Gomes, B.R. (2015). Care of the patient undergoing radial approach heart catheterization: implications for medical-surgical nurses. *Medsurg Nursing* **24** (3): 173.

Huseby, J.S. and Ledoux, D. (2010). Radiologic examination of the chest. In: *Cardiac Nursing*, 6ee (ed. S.L. Woods, E.S.S. Froelicher, S.U. Motzer and E.J. Bridges), 267–376. Philadelphia: Lippincott Williams and Wilkins.

Kaddoura, S. (2016). *Echo Made Easy*, 3ee. Edinburgh: Churchill Livingstone Elsevier.

Kossaify, A., Bassil, E., and Kossaify, M. (2020). Stress echocardiography: concept and criteria, structure and steps, obstacles and outcomes, focused update and review. *Cardiology Research* **11** (2): 89. https://dx.doi.org/10.14740%2Fcr851.

Kucia, A.M. (2017). Diagnostic testing. In: *Kozier & Erb's Fundamentals of Nursing*, 4ee (ed. B. Kozier, G. Erb, A. Bermann, et al.). NSW: Pearson Australia.

Lipinski, M.J., McVey, C.M., Berger, J.S. et al. (2013). Prognostic value of stress cardiac magnetic resonance imaging in patients with known or suspected coronary artery disease: a systematic review and meta-analysis. *Journal of the American College of Cardiology* **62** (9): 826–838.

Manda, Y.R. and Baradhi, K.M. (2020). Cardiac Catheterization Risks and Complications. [Updated 2020 June 22]. In: StatPearls [Internet]. Treasure Island (FL): StatPearls Publishing; 2021 January-. https://www.ncbi.nlm.nih.gov/books/NBK531461 (accessed 1 July 2021).

Olade, R. (2016). Cardiac catheterization (left heart). Medscape. http://emedicine.medscape.com/article/1819224-overview (accessed 1 July 2021).

Ramjattan, N.A., Lala, V., Kousa, O. et al. (2020). Coronary CT Angiography. [Updated 2020 August 22]. In: StatPearls [Internet]. Treasure Island (FL): StatPearls Publishing; 2021 January-. https://www.ncbi.nlm.nih.gov/books/NBK470279 (accessed 1 July 2021).

Rockall, A.G., Hatrick, A., Armstrong, P., and Wastie, M. (2013). *Diagnostic Imaging*. Wiley.

Romagnoli, E., Biondi-Zoccai, G., Sciahbasi, A. et al. (2012). Radial versus femoral randomized investigation in ST-segment elevation acute coronary syndrome: the RIFLE-STEACS (Radial Versus Femoral Randomized Investigation in ST-Elevation Acute Coronary Syndrome) study. *Journal of the American College of Cardiology* **60** (24): 2481–2489.

Talano, J.V. (2016). Tilt table testing. Medscape. http://emedicine.medscape.com/article/1839773-overview (accessed 1 July 2021).

Tavakol, M., Ashraf, S., and Brener, S.J. (2012). Risks and complications of coronary angiography: a comprehensive review. *Global Journal of Health Science* **4** (1): 65.

Taylor, R.A. and Khatri, P. (2016). Stroke after cardiac catheterization. *UpToDate*, Waltham, MA. https://www-uptodate-com/contents/stroke-after-cardiac-catheterization?source=see_link (accessed 1 July 2021).

Trayor, T. and Sanghvi, K. (2013). Complications of transradial catheterization series: radial perforation. *Cath Lab Digest* **21**: 9. http://www.cathlabdigest.com/articles/Complications-Transradial-Catheterization-Series-Radial-Perforation (accessed 1 July 2021).

Vilcant, V., Zeltser, R. (2020). Treadmill Stress Testing. [Updated 2020 July 26]. In: StatPearls [Internet]. Treasure Island (FL): StatPearls Publishing; 2021 January-. https://www.ncbi.nlm.nih.gov/books/NBK499903 (accessed 1 July 2021).

Part III

Detection and Management of Heart Rhythm Disturbances

9

Electrocardiogram (ECG) Interpretation

Carol Oldroyd and Angela M. Kucia

Overview

Electrocardiography has been used diagnostically for over a 100 years. It is non-invasive, easy to perform, readily accessible and inexpensive. The ECG provides useful information about heart rate, rhythm, electrocardiographic intervals, electrical axis, bundle branch block (BBB) and hypertrophy. The ECG is used to detect conduction system abnormalities including pre-excitation, long QT syndromes and structural abnormalities including atrial abnormalities and ventricular hypertrophy. It is central to the diagnosis of myocardial ischaemia and infarction and is useful in detecting conditions such as drug toxicity, electrolyte imbalance and pericarditis. The ability to interpret an electrocardiogram (ECG) is a useful skill for most nurses and a 'must have' skill for nurses working in a cardiac environment. ECG abnormalities can only be appreciated when one is familiar with the range of normal findings. The theoretical basis of electrocardiography and practical applications will be discussed in this chapter, including normal ECG parameters and causes of abnormal ECG findings.

Learning Objectives

After reading this chapter, you should be able to:

- Identify the anatomical zones of the heart associated with the 12 ECG leads.
- Describe the ECG changes associated with acute myocardial ischaemia and evolving myocardial infarction (MI).
- Explain the term 'electrical axis' and calculate the electrical axis using Leads I and aVF.
- Identify the electrocardiographic features of left and right BBB, atrial and ventricular hypertrophy, pericarditis and changes due to drug toxicity and electrolyte imbalance.
- Describe the procedure for obtaining a 12-lead ECG.

Key Concepts

ST-segment changes; T-wave changes; bundle branch block; electrical axis; atrial and ventricular hypertrophy

Cardiac Care: A Practical Guide for Nurses, Second Edition. Edited by Angela M. Kucia and Ian D. Jones.
© 2022 John Wiley & Sons Ltd. Published 2022 by John Wiley & Sons Ltd.

Normal Sequence of Depolarisation and Repolarisation

The normal sequence of myocardial depolarisation and repolarisation was discussed in Chapter 3. To recap, the heart has specialised conduction cells that are designed to rapidly transmit electrical activity through the heart. This electrical activity produces sequential characteristic waveforms on the 12-lead ECG.

Figure 9.1 shows the elements of the ECG complex, which represent one cardiac cycle (one heartbeat).

The P-Wave

Under normal conditions, the sinoatrial (SA) node is the most rapidly depolarising tissue, and thus sets the heart rate. The electrical impulse then spreads via the internodal tracts throughout the left and right atria, before moving down to the atrioventricular (AV) node. As the SA node is located at the superior right border of the heart, the direction of the impulse tends to be downward and to the left. The atrial walls have little muscle mass, thus the electrical activity produced by their depolarisation causes only a small deflection on the 12-lead ECG. This is known as the P-wave (Figure 9.1).

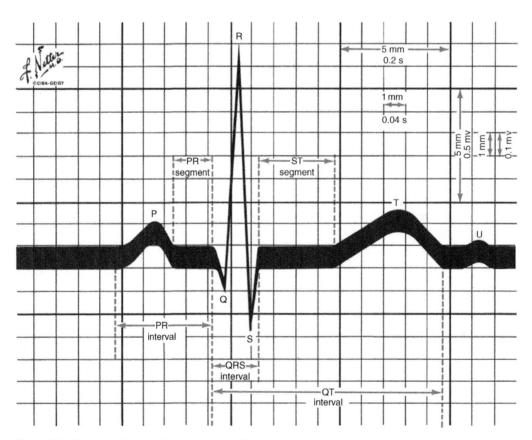

Figure 9.1 Electrocardiographic waveforms and intervals. *Source:* From Scheidt (1986). Copyright Novartis A.G. Used with permission.

Learning Activity 9.1

If cardiac cells must sequentially depolarise and repolarise to transmit a cardiac impulse, why is atrial depolarisation not seen on the 12-lead ECG?

The answer is at the back of the book.

The PR-interval

In the normal heart, the only pathway for the electrical impulse to travel from the atria to the ventricles is via the AV node. There is a short delay whilst the impulse is transmitted through the AV node, before travelling down the common bundle of His and the bundle branches. This is represented on the ECG as the PR-interval (Figure 9.1).

The QRS Complex

As the wave of depolarisation passes through the bundle branches, the septum begins to depolarise from left to right, and in a slightly downward direction. Septal depolarisation produces a characteristically small deflection (small negative deflection in Lead I and small positive deflection in V1). As the impulse spreads through the distal bundle branches and Purkinje fibres, the larger bulk of the ventricular myocardium depolarises from the septum to the apex and then the left and right free ventricular walls. As depolarisation of the left and right ventricles is meant to happen simultaneously, the left bundle branch divides into anterior and posterior fascicles to enable the impulse to be transmitted quickly throughout the larger bulk of the left ventricular myocardium. Given that the left ventricle is about 10 mm thick, compared with 3 mm for the right ventricle, the left ventricle generates substantially greater electrical activity; thus, the QRS complex, which denotes ventricular depolarisation on the ECG, is largely a reflection of left ventricular electrical activity when conduction is normal (Figure 9.1).

The ST-Segment

The period between the QRS ending and the T-wave beginning is known as the ST-segment (Figure 9.1). It represents the interval between ventricular depolarisation and repolarisation.

The T-Wave

Repolarisation of the ventricles begins from endocardium to epicardium and appears on the ECG as the T-wave (Figure 9.1).

Suggested Resource

ECG for beginners. Understanding the waves of ECG, P-wave, QRS complex. Critical Care Survival Guide 2020 (2017) https://youtu.be/1Q8YSpMcO-8

Theoretical Basis of Electrocardiography

Electrical changes resulting from the depolarisation and repolarisation of myocardial cells are recorded using electrodes that are placed in specific positions on the limbs and chest wall. These electrical changes are then transcribed on to graph paper to produce a 12-lead ECG. Electrical activity is recorded on the ECG as a positive or negative deflection (Figure 9.2).

ECG Leads

The 12 ECG leads all record the same electrical events within the heart at a given time, but each of the leads looks at a different view.

Limb Leads

The standard limb leads (II, III and aVF) are obtained by using three bipolar electrodes:

- Lead I records the electrical potential between the left arm (LA) electrode, which

P-wave	QRS complex	T-wave	Explanation

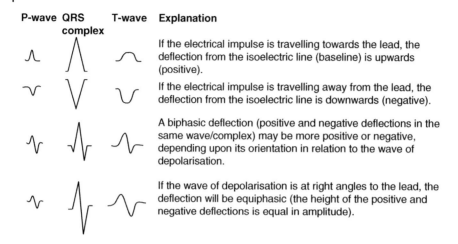

If the electrical impulse is travelling towards the lead, the deflection from the isoelectric line (baseline) is upwards (positive).

If the electrical impulse is travelling away from the lead, the deflection from the isoelectric line is downwards (negative).

A biphasic deflection (positive and negative deflections in the same wave/complex) may be more positive or negative, depending upon its orientation in relation to the wave of depolarisation.

If the wave of depolarisation is at right angles to the lead, the deflection will be equiphasic (the height of the positive and negative deflections is equal in amplitude).

Figure 9.2 ECG deflections.

is designated to be the positive pole in this lead, and the right arm (RA) electrode, which is the negative pole in this lead.

- Lead II records the electrical potential between the left leg (LL), which is designated as the positive pole in this lead, and the RA electrode, which is the negative pole in this lead.
- Lead III records the electrical potential between the LL electrode, which is the positive pole in this lead, and the LA electrode, which is the negative pole in this lead.

Where a fourth lead is attached to the right leg (RL), this is used as a ground electrode and is not represented on the 12-lead ECG.

Augmented Limb Leads

Leads aVR, aVL and aVF are referred to as the augmented limb leads. These leads measure the electric potential at one point with respect to zero potential. Zero potential means that no significant variation in electric potential is registered during contraction of the heart. It is obtained by comparing the electrical potential of one of the leads against the sum electrical potential of the other two leads. For example, in Lead aVF, the electric potential of the LL is compared to zero potential, which is obtained by adding together the potential of

Leads aVR and aVL. The positive pole of aVR is at the right arm, the positive pole of aVL is at the LA, and the positive pole of aVF is at the LL. Bipolar and augmented limb leads are frontal plane leads. If the three bipolar and three augmented limb leads are superimposed on a single diagram, they encompass a 360° circle (Figure 9.3). Conventionally, the positive pole of Lead I is taken as 0° and coordinates are measured at 30° intervals. This becomes important when determining the cardiac axis.

Precordial Leads (V leads)

The precordial leads (V1–V6) examine cardiac electrical activity in the horizontal plane (from sternum to vertebral column) (Figure 9.4).

R-Wave Progression

In a normal ECG, R-waves progressively increase in amplitude from V1 to V5 and then slightly decrease in V6. This is known as 'normal R-wave progression'. The R-wave in V1 starts off being very small in amplitude (or in some people non-existent) and progressively becomes larger throughout the precordial leads to the point where the R-wave is larger than the S-wave in lead V4. Poor R-wave progression may be associated with anterior myocardial infarction, left bundle branch block, left anterior fascicular block (left axis deviation), Wolff-Parkinson-White (WPW) syndrome and right or left ventricular hypertrophy.

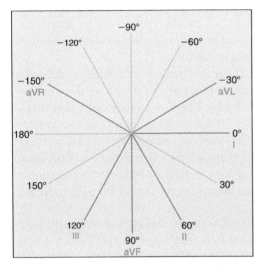

Figure 9.3 The hexaxial reference system. *Source:* Reproduced from Meek and Morris (2002). With permission from BMJ Publishing Group Ltd.

Key Point

A tall R-wave in V1 may occasionally be found as a normal variant but is generally an abnormal finding. The first thing to check is whether the precordial leads have been misplaced. A tall R-wave in V1 can be associated with the following: right bundle branch block, posterior myocardial infarction, progressive muscular dystrophy, right ventricular hypertrophy, acute right ventricular dilation, Type A WPW syndrome, ventricular ectopy/rhythm, hypertrophic cardiomyopathy, and dextrocardia.

Suggested Resource

EKG/ECG R-wave progression. The ECG Guy (2019)
https://youtu.be/uax1sYyl0Dw

Suggested Resource

Electrocardiography (ECG/EKG) – Basics Osmosis (2017)
https://youtu.be/xIZQRjkwV9Q

Figure 9.4 Vertical and horizontal perspective of the leads. The limb leads 'view' the heart in the vertical plane and the chest leads in the horizontal plane. *Source:* Reproduced from Meek and Morris (2002). With permission from BMJ Publishing Group Ltd.

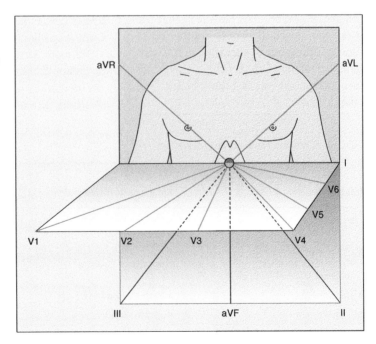

The Cardiac Axis

The flow of electrical current in the normal heart tends to be uniform as it follows a well-defined conduction pathway. The cardiac axis represents the mean direction that the electrical impulse takes as it spreads through the myocardium, which is usually from 11 o'clock to 5 o'clock.

The mean QRS axis represents the direction of electrical activity as seen from the frontal plane leads. Electrical activation is considered to occur from a point within the centre of a circle, and in addition to the radii representing the six limb leads, six further radii are produced. This is known as the hexaxial reference system (Figure 9.3). The axis is determined using this hexaxial reference system, with Lead I designated as 0°. An axis lying above this line is described as a negative number up to −180°, and an axis below as positive up to +180°. A normal axis lies between −30° and +90°. An axis greater than −30° is referred to as a left axis deviation (LAD), whereas an axis of greater than +90° is referred to as a right axis deviation (RAD).

Key Point

An axis deviation does not mean that the heart has moved to point in another direction. It represents an alteration in the general direction that the wave of depolarisation takes as it flows through the ventricles.

Determining the Axis

Axis determination is useful in the diagnosis of a variety of conditions including broad complex tachycardias, pre-excitation syndromes such as WPW syndrome, pulmonary embolism, conduction defects (hemi-blocks) and congenital heart disease. In some cases, an axis deviation can be normal for an individual. Common causes of axis deviation are summarised in Table 9.1.

There are various ways of calculating the cardiac axis, some of which are more precise than others. In most cases, a rough approximation is sufficient to detect an abnormality which can then be referred on to a specialist for more accurate determination. One quick and easy method of determining the cardiac axis involves using Leads I and aVF. Referring to the hexaxial reference system (Figure 9.3), the circle can be divided into quadrants (four equal parts) and labelled as normal (0 to +90°), left axis (0–90°), right axis (+90 to +180°) and extreme left or right (−90° to ±180°) also referred to colloquially as 'No man's land'. By looking at the directions of Leads I and aVF on the 12-lead ECG, it is possible to place the axis within one of the quadrants, thereby providing a rough indication at a glance as to whether the cardiac axis lies within normal limits.

If a more accurate estimate is required, it is necessary to examine all six limb leads. A positive deflection on an ECG indicates that the electrical current is moving towards that lead

---

Table 9.1 Common causes of axis deviation.

Left axis deviation (>−30°)	Right axis deviation (>+90°)	Extreme axis deviation (No man's land)
• Left anterior hemi-block	• Right ventricular hypertrophy	• Ventricular tachycardia
• WPW syndrome with right-sided, accessory pathway	• WPW with left-sided, accessory pathway	• ECG leads incorrectly applied
• Inferior MI	• Anterolateral MI	
	• Dextrocardia	
	• Left posterior hemi-block	

and a negative deflection indicates that the current is moving away from that lead; so if Lead I is the most positive limb lead, it can be assumed that the axis is bearing in that direction, which corresponds to 0° on the hexaxial reference system. A lead that lies at 90° (perpendicular to the current) will appear on the ECG as equiphasic, and this information can be used to as follows to determine the cardiac axis more precisely:

Identify the most equiphasic limb lead. The axis lies at 90° to the right or left of this lead. If, for example, Lead II is considered to be the most equiphasic lead, it can be assumed that the axis is running perpendicular to this lead and lies at either +150° or −30°.

Looking back at the hexaxial diagram, identify which leads lie at 90° to the equiphasic lead and decide whether this lead is positive or negative on the ECG. If Lead II was identified as the most equiphasic, the lead lying at 90° is aVL. If aVL is positive on the ECG, then the axis lies at −30° since the current must be travelling towards this electrode to produce a positive deflection. If aVL is negative, then the current must be moving away from the electrode and lies at +150° (Meek and Morris 2002).

This more-precise estimate can be useful for nurses working in specialist areas such as coronary care units and cardiothoracic centres, but for most nurses it is sufficient to simply be able to identify if the axis is normal or abnormal and understand the implications.

Suggested Resource

ECG interpretation for beginners. Different leads and axis deviation. Critical Care Survival Guide 2020 (2017)
https://youtu.be/SliVBwdBLMk

Determination of Heart Rate and Electrocardiographic Intervals

The horizontal axis on ECG paper represents time. The ECG is normally recorded on standard paper that travels at a speed of 25 mm/s, although this can be generally changed in most machines if required. The ECG paper is divided into large squares with darker lines, each of which is 5 mm wide and equates to 0.2 seconds. Each of these large squares has five smaller squares within it. These small squares are 1 mm wide and equivalent to 0.04 seconds (see Figure 9.1).

The vertical axis on the ECG paper represents voltage amplitude. Electrical activity detected by the ECG machine is measured in millivolts. ECG machines are calibrated so that a signal with an amplitude of 1 mV moves the recording stylus vertically 1 cm; therefore 0.1 mV = 1 mm (one small square).

Key Point

Several conditions can influence amplitude in ECG leads. Ventricular hypertrophy is likely to result in increased amplitude of the ECG waveform due to increased muscle mass. ECG leads may also have increased amplitude if people who are very thin as there is little impedance in ECG signal transmission from muscle or fat. If ECG signal transmission is impeded through tissue, such as occurs with pericardial fluid build-up, pulmonary emphysema or obesity, the waveform amplitude is likely to be reduced.

Heart Rate

Most modern ECG machines and monitors display or record the ventricular heart rate. Some will also include printouts of other electrocardiographic intervals. There may be times when you want to calculate atrial rate which may be different to the ventricular rate. In regular rhythms, calculating heart rate (atrial or ventricular) is a simple process. One large box represents 0.2 seconds; thus, there are five large boxes in a second. Count how many complexes are there in a second and multiply by 60. That will give you the heart rate. This method is not reliable for irregular heart rates. For irregular heart rates, it is suggested that the heart rate is calculated by counting the complexes that occur over 6 seconds (30 large boxes) and multiply by 10. This gives an estimate of the heart rate but is not an accurate measure.

Heart Rhythm

The normal heart rhythm is sinus rhythm. The rate should be between 60 and 100 beats/min. A normal P-wave should precede each QRS complex, and the PR interval should be of normal duration. Refer to Table 9.2 for normal criteria for these waveforms and intervals. Arrhythmia interpretation is dealt with in more detail in Chapter 11.

Suggested Resource

ECG interpretation. Time and the ECG-Part 1. ECG Teacher (2013)
https://youtu.be/FX49ccF5Kso

Learning Activity 9.2

Watch the video above. Collect rhythm strips and practice calculating the heart rate.

Electrocardiographic Waveforms and Intervals

Standard electrocardiographic intervals provide useful information about conduction (Table 9.2).

We refer to ventricular depolarisation as the QRS complex on the ECG, but there is not always an identifiable Q, R and S waves in every complex.

- Some complexes will just have a Q-wave before the stylus returns to baseline – there is no R- or S-wave.
- In some leads, you will see that the first deflection from the isoelectric line is upward rather than downwards. If the first deflection is upwards it is an R-wave and there is no Q-wave (Figure 9.5).
- In right bundle branch block, there is an initial R-wave, followed by an S-wave, and then a second R-wave, This QRS pattern is referred to as 'rSR'.

Key Point

You may see in some publications that lowercase and capital letters are used to describe QRS components, depending on the relative size of each wave. For example, an Rs complex would be positively deflected, while an rS complex would be negatively deflected. If both complexes were labelled RS, it would be impossible to appreciate this distinction without viewing the actual ECG.

Suggested Resource

Intro to EKG interpretation – Waveforms, segments and intervals
Strong Medicine (2013)
https://youtu.be/gvutn7fYvl0

Learning Activity 9.3

After viewing the video above, obtain a 12-lead ECG and look at the QRS complexes. Identify the QRS waveforms in all 12 leads.

Chamber Enlargement

Atrial Abnormalities

P-wave abnormalities suggestive of atrial enlargement are found by examining the amplitude (height), duration and contour of the P-wave.

In right atrial enlargement (RAE) or hypertrophy, the P-wave is characteristically tall and peaked, and this can be best seen in Leads II, III and aVF. Criterion for RAE is P-wave amplitude >2.5 mm. RAE is usually caused by pressure or volume overload in the right atrium, commonly associated with primary hypertension and conditions resulting in pulmonary hypertension.

Left atrial enlargement (LAE) or hypertrophy is associated with (i) a wide P-wave >0.11 seconds in duration; (ii) a notch in the top of the

Table 9.2 Normal waveforms and electrocardiographic intervals.

Waveform/Interval	Significance	Normal interval
P-wave	Represents atrial depolarisation. Measured from the first upward deflection from baseline to return to baseline	Width <0.11 s (3 small squares)
PR interval	Represents the delay between conduction from atria to ventricles through the AV node. Measured from the end of the P-wave to the beginning of the QRS complex	Width 0.12–0.20 s (3–5 small squares)
QRS interval	Represents ventricular depolarisation. Measured from the first upward/downward deflection from baseline until return to baseline	Width 0.06–0.10 s (1.5–2.5 small squares)
J point	The point at which the QRS complex ends and the ST segment begins	The J point may deviate from the baseline due to: • early repolarisation • epicardial or endocardial ischaemia or injury • pericarditis • bundle branch block • ventricular hypertrophy • digitalis effect
ST segment	Represents the time between ventricular depolarisation and ventricular repolarisation. Measured from the end of the QRS to the beginning of the T-wave.	Width dependent upon heart rate.
T-wave	Represents ventricular repolarisation. Measured from the first upward/downward deflection to return to baseline.	
QT interval	Measured from the first upward/downward deflection of the QRS complex to return of the T-wave to baseline.	Width markedly affected by heart rate (HR). The corrected QT (QTc) is commonly calculated using Bazett's formula and should be between 0.3 and 0.44 s.
U-wave	Thought to represent afterdepolarisations which interrupt or follow repolarisation and are more prominent at slower heart rates	

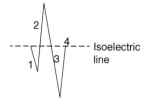

1. If the first deflection is downward from the isoelectric line, it is known as a Q-wave.
2. If the deflection crosses the isoelectric line, it is known as an R-wave.
3. If there is a third deflection that crosses the isoelectric line, it is known as an S-wave.
4. Point 4 is the ECG stylus returning to the baseline and does not represent an electrical event.

Figure 9.5 Waveforms in the QRS complex.

P-wave with the two peaks being >0.04 seconds apart in any lead and (iii) a negative deflection in the terminal end of the P-wave in V1 >1 mm deep and >1 mm wide. LAE is commonly the result of mitral valve insufficiency or stenosis. It is often associated with an increased workload in filling the left ventricle and is commonly associated with left ventricular hypertrophy (LVH) resulting from systemic hypertension, aortic valvular disease, hypertrophic cardiomyopathy and other conditions that reduce left ventricular compliance (Scheidt 1986).

Key Point

It is important to note that P-wave abnormalities are not reliable for both detection and prediction of anatomic atrial enlargement. Hence, ECG findings that are associated with atrial hypertrophy are usually referred to as 'atrial abnormalities'.

Ventricular Hypertrophy

Evidence of ventricular enlargement is found by examining the amplitude of components of the QRS complex.

Right ventricular hypertrophy (RVH) is characterised by (i) R-wave in V1 >7 mm that exceeds the S-wave depth in V1; (ii) right axis deviation; (iii) relatively taller R-waves in the right precordial leads and relatively deeper S-waves in the left precordial leads than normally seen. RVH may be due to abnormalities of the pulmonary valve (uncommon in adults), congenital lesions such as atrial or ventricular septal defect, tricuspid regurgitation or by

primary hypertension and conditions resulting in pulmonary hypertension.

Several methods have been proposed for ECG diagnosis of left ventricular hypertrophy (LVH). The Cornell voltage criteria (Casale et al. 1987) provide a relatively simple ECG diagnostic criterion for LVH and are based upon echocardiographic correlative studies designed to detect a left ventricular mass index >132 g/m^2 in men and >109 g/m^2 in women. The voltage criteria are as follows:

- For men: S in V3 + R in aVL >2.8 mV (28 mm)
- For women: S in V3 + R in aVL >2.0 mV (20 mm)

Conditions resulting in LVH include systemic arterial hypertension, aortic stenosis or insufficiency, and other conditions resulting in volume or pressure overload of the left ventricle.

Suggested Resource

ECG 12 lead chamber enlargement
Chris Touzeau (2014)
https://youtu.be/3RoIZsHbNgw

Bundle Branch Block

Bundle branch block can occur in either the right or left bundle branches. Ventricular depolarisation is abnormal in complete right or left bundle branch block as conduction is not facilitated across specialised conduction fibres within the His–Purkinje system, and the impulse has to travel to various parts of the myocardium via the myocardial cells, resulting in a widened QRS.

Right bundle branch block (RBBB) is characterised by a widened QRS and has the following diagnostic criteria:

- The heart rhythm must be supraventricular in origin.
- The QRS duration must be >0.12 seconds (three small squares).
- There should be a terminal R-wave in Lead V1 (usually has an 'rSR' pattern).
- There should be a slurred S-wave in Leads I and V6.

In RBBB, the T-wave generally is deflected in the opposite direction of the QRS complex. This is known as appropriate T-wave discordance with bundle branch block (Figure 9.6). A T-wave that deflects in the same direction of the QRS complex may suggest ischaemia or MI. RBBB generally is due to degenerative conduction system disease and ischaemic heart disease in the anterior septum.

Key Point

In some cases, the QRS has an 'rSR' pattern in V1 and is just above the normal duration of the QRS (<0.10 s), but under the RBBB criteria of >0.12 s duration. The ECG is sometimes interpreted as having an 'incomplete' or 'borderline' RBBB, but this does not necessarily reflect the anatomical abnormality; rather it is a description of the ECG. This type of abnormality may also be referred to as intraventricular conduction delay (IVCD) or right ventricular conduction delay (Scheidt 1986).

In left bundle branch block (LBBB), the ventricle cannot be depolarised normally from the left bundle; so, depolarisation must proceed down the right bundle, across the intraventricular septum to the left ventricle. As the wave of depolarisation has a right to left orientation (as is the case in normal depolarisation), the QRS complex, though wide, has the same general directional orientation as a normally conducted complex on the 12-lead ECG. Several variations in shape can be seen in the QRS complex in LBBB and the complex is usually notched. The following criteria should be used to diagnose LBBB on the ECG:

- The heart rhythm must be supraventricular in origin.
- The QRS duration must be >1.2 seconds (three small squares).
- There should be a QS or RS complex in Lead V1.
- There should be a monophasic R-wave in Leads I and V6.

The LBBB generally indicates widespread myocardial disease due to degenerative conduction disease, ischaemic heart disease and conditions that produce LVH, but in some people, it can develop in the absence of any apparent heart disease (Scheidt 1986). As with RBBB, the T-wave generally is deflected in the opposite direction of the QRS complex.

Left Anterior Hemi-Block (Left Anterior Fascicular Block)

A block in the left anterior fascicle is known as left anterior fascicular block (LAFB) or left anterior hemi-block (LAHB). In LAFB, the heart must be depolarised from areas other than the normal conduction pathway. In hemi-blocks, the spread of depolarisation is not greatly delayed and thus the duration of the QRS complex is within normal limits and generally, is of normal shape, without the characteristic notching found in complete LBBB. However, the axis is shifted to the left, and diagnosis of LAFB is made on LAD. LAFB is commonly caused by degenerative conduction disease or ischaemic heart disease. Unless it occurs in the setting of acute MI (AMI), it is usually benign and only rarely is a precursor of complete LBBB in the short term (Scheidt 1986).

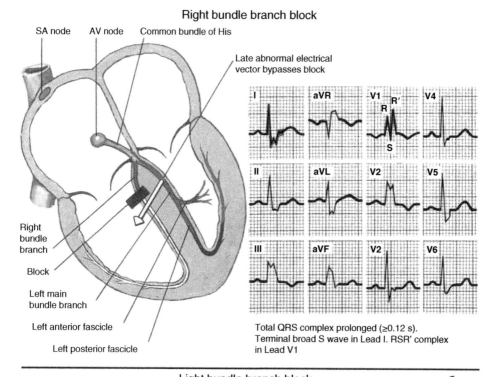

Right bundle branch block

SA node   AV node   Common bundle of His

Late abnormal electrical
vector bypasses block

I   aVR   V1   R'   V4
          R
          S

II   aVL   V2   V5

III   aVF   V2   V6

Right
bundle
branch

Block

Left main
bundle branch

Left anterior fascicle

Left posterior fascicle

Total QRS complex prolonged (≥0.12 s).
Terminal broad S wave in Lead I. RSR' complex
in Lead V1

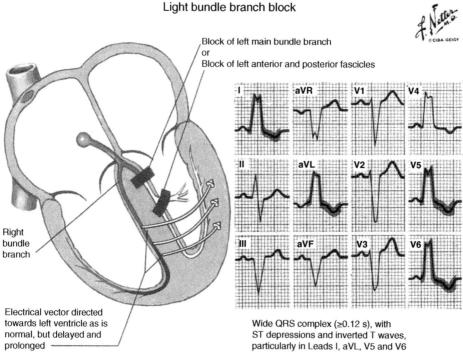

Light bundle branch block

Block of left main bundle branch
or
Block of left anterior and posterior fascicles

I   aVR   V1   V4

II   aVL   V2   V5

III   aVF   V3   V6

Right
bundle
branch

Electrical vector directed
towards left ventricle as is
normal, but delayed and
prolonged

Wide QRS complex (≥0.12 s), with
ST depressions and inverted T waves,
particularly in Leads I, aVL, V5 and V6

Figure 9.6   Right and left bundle branch block. *Source:* From Scheidt (1986). Courtesy of Novartis.

Left Posterior Hemi-Block (Left Posterior Fascicular Block)

As with LAFB, left posterior fascicular block (LPFB) or left posterior hemi-block (LPHB) does not result in a prolonged QRS, but in this case, the electrical axis is shifted to the right. It is more difficult to recognise than LAFB as the axis, although orientated towards the right, often remains within normal limits. LPHB is uncommon and rarely diagnosed on a routine ECG. The causes and prognostic significance of LPHB are similar to that of LAHB.

Bifascicular and Trifascicular Block

The left bundle branch divides into the left anterior fascicle and the left posterior fascicle. As the RBBB has one fascicle and the LBBB has two fascicles, there are three pathways through the ventricles for AV conduction. This gives rise to the notion of trifascicular conduction. A block in conduction in two fascicles is often referred to as 'bifascicular block' and in clinical practice usually involves an LAFB plus RBBB. Bifascicular and trifascicular blocks are common ECG findings. Some patients with these findings develop severe AV conduction abnormalities whilst others develop no further problems (Scheidt 1986).

Key Point

In clinical practice, the term 'trifascicular block' is often used to describe bifascicular block associated with first-degree AV block or second-degree AV block (usually LAFB plus RBBB plus first-degree AV block). This term is inaccurate, as the conduction delay resulting in PR interval prolongation usually occurs in the AV node, not in the third remaining fascicle (Larkin and Buttner 2021).

Suggested Resource

Intro to EKG interpretation – Bundle branch blocks
Strong Medicine (2012)
https://youtu.be/nKohbPclvbk

Learning Activity 9.4

Locate an ECG with a paced rhythm. In what ways does this resemble a BBB pattern and why? How might the type of pacemaker and lead placement change the QRS configuration?

ECG Changes Related to Myocardial Ischaemia and Infarction

The 12-lead ECG is the single-most important source of data in the assessment of patients with a potential acute coronary syndrome (unstable angina pectoris or MI). Acute myocardial ischaemia or infarction causes characteristic changes in the ST-segment and T-wave that are related to repolarisation abnormalities. Progressive development of Q-waves or loss of R-waves in infarct-related leads can often be detected as an MI evolves.

Sub-endocardial Ischaemia

Myocardial ischaemia usually occurs first in the sub-endocardial region as these deeper myocardial layers are farthest from the blood supply and have greater intramural tension and need for oxygen. Repolarisation normally proceeds in an epicardial-to-endocardial direction, and delayed recovery in the sub-endocardial region due to ischaemia does not reverse the direction of repolarisation but merely lengthens it. Thus, sub-endocardial ischaemia prolongs local recovery time, resulting in a prolonged QT-interval and/or increased amplitude of the T-wave in the electrodes overlying the ischaemic region on the 12-lead ECG. In the setting of severe ischaemia, injury to the myocardial cells results, and is manifested on the ECG by ST-segment depression.

Sub-epicardial or Transmural Ischaemia

Transmural ischaemia refers to sub-epicardial ischaemia, which has a more visible effect on recovery of sub-epicardial cells compared with sub-endocardial cells. Recovery is more delayed in the sub-epicardial layers than in sub-endocardial muscle fibres. Repolarisation is endocardial-to-epicardial, resulting in inversion of the T-waves in leads overlying the ischaemic regions. In the setting of severe ischaemia, injury to the myocardial cells results and is manifested on the ECG by ST-segment elevation.

Myocardial Infarction

Myocardial infarction refers to necrosis (death) of myocardial cells. The left ventricle is the predominant site for MI, but the right ventricle can also be involved. The process of MI involves various stages of ischaemia. There is usually a central area of necrosis that is generally surrounded by an area of injury, which in turn is surrounded by an area of ischaemia. Depending upon the presence or absence of ST elevation in the presence of elevated cardiac enzymes, MI may also be referred to as:

- ST-elevation MI (STEMI) or ST-elevation acute coronary syndrome (STEAC)
- Non-ST-elevation MI (non-STEMI) or non-ST-elevation acute coronary syndrome (NSTEAC)

Key Point

The distinction between ischaemia and necrosis is whether the phenomenon is reversible or not. Transient reversible ischaemia appears on the ECG as T-wave changes, and sometimes ST-segment changes, which can be reversed without producing permanent damage or serum enzyme elevation. Elevation of serum enzymes is expected in infarction. In the absence of enzyme elevation, ST- and T-wave abnormalities are interpreted as due to injury or ischaemia rather than infarction.

The ST-Segment

The ST-segment may become depressed or elevated during episodes of myocardial ischaemia or infarction. Taken in context with a patient history and examination, ST-segment elevation is usually the product of intense transmural ischaemia indicating MI. ST-segment elevation represents the most severe condition in the acute coronary syndrome spectrum and carries the poorest prognosis. Prompt management with pharmacological or percutaneous reperfusion is critical.

Commonly used criteria to identify ST-segment elevation MI are:

- >0.1 mV (one small square in height) of ST-segment elevation in two or more limb leads; or
- >0.2 mV (two small squares in height) of ST-segment elevation in two or more contiguous precordial leads (GUSTO Investigators 1993).

Persistent ST elevation can occur in the presence of ventricular aneurysm following an MI. This is generally associated with Q-waves in the infarct-related leads.

Suggested Resource

ECG for beginners. ECG diagnosis of ST Elevation Myocardial Infarction (STEMI) Critical Care Survival Guide 2020 (2020) https://youtu.be/uqNQvKxAiuo

---

Pericarditis

Another cause of ST-segment elevation is pericarditis. A thorough history of the features of associated chest pain must be obtained to differentiate between pericarditis and MI. Pericarditis is usually a generalised pathophysiological process; thus, the ST elevation associated with pericarditis is often widespread

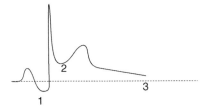

Figure 9.7 Acute ECG abnormalities in pericarditis.

on the ECG (Figure 9.7), involving more than one area of the heart. Another ECG characteristic that may differentiate pericarditis from AMI is PR interval depression in the setting of diffuse ST-segment elevation. ECG abnormalities associated with pericarditis often progress over four stages:

Stage I: This is the acute phase with concave upward ST-segment elevation and PR-segment depression that is usually diffuse. Spodick's sign may be present.

Stage II: ST-segment elevation and PR-segment depression have resolved. T-waves may be normal or flattened.

Stage III: T-waves are inverted. The ECG is otherwise normal.

Stage IV: T-waves return to the upright position. The ECG is normal.

Key Point

'Spodick's sign' refers to a down-sloping TP-segment that is present in some patients affected with acute pericarditis (stage 1). The sign is often best visualised in lead II and lateral precordial leads (Chabbra and Spodick 2012).

Early Repolarization Abnormality

A normal variant known as early repolarisation (sometimes called high take-off) can be seen in asymptomatic people without significant coronary disease. This phenomenon can be seen across most of the population but is most common in young, healthy people. Early repolarisation is best seen in the precordial leads. ST segments in these leads appear elevated, upwards and concave and are often associated with peaked and slightly asymmetrical T-waves with notch and slur on the R-wave. The other accompanying features are a shorter and depressed PR interval, abrupt transition, counterclockwise rotation, presence of U-waves and sinus bradycardia (Mehta et al. 1999).

ST depression may be described as 'upsloping', 'horizontal' or 'downsloping' (Figure 9.8), with downsloping ST depression being the most specific for myocardial ischaemia, and upsloping the least. Other causes of ST depression include RVH and LVH, RBBB and LBBB, and some drugs.

Non-specific ST depression is a common ECG finding and implies that the cause of the abnormality is not known, and that the ST segment change is minor. For ST-segment depression to be termed 'non-specific', the T-wave vector should be normal. If the T-wave vector is abnormal in the absence of other known causes of ST depression, it is suggestive of ischaemia. Significant ST depression has been defined as:

deviation from the J point of >1 mm (two small vertically ruled boxes)

deviation of >1 mm from 0.06 to 0.08 seconds after the J point (Scheidt 1986)

Key Point

You will note in some studies of ST-segment depression, significant ST depression is defined as >0.5 mm (one small square). Although this may be a more sensitive criteria for detecting ST-segment depression, in everyday clinical practice there is a lot of variability in ECG interpretation in terms of ST-segment amplitude; thus, setting the measurement criteria at this lower level may reduce diagnostic specificity.

Types of ST-segment depressions

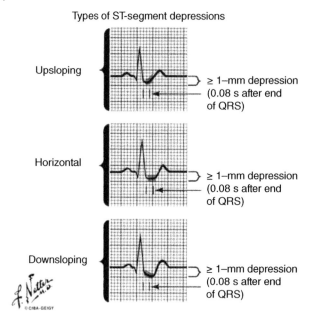

Figure 9.8 Types of ST-segment depression. *Source:* From Scheidt (1986). Courtesy of Novartis.

Transient ST-segment depression with inverted T-waves is usually a sign of reversible ischaemia affecting the sub-endocardial layers of myocardium (Scheidt 1986) and can occur as a result of acute reduction in coronary flow, or as a result of an acute increase in coronary demand, such as occurs with tachycardia (Sclarovsky 1999).

Downsloping ST-segment depression in the precordial leads, particularly in Leads V4 and V5 (Figure 10.5), are often due to extensive ischaemia as a result of stenosis of the left main coronary artery and/or triple vessel disease, and may produce lifethreatening haemodynamic disturbance, both systolic and diastolic (Sclarovsky et al. 1986a). This type of ST depression needs urgent investigation.

ST depression in the setting of non-ST-elevation myocardial infarction (NSTEMI) has been associated with poor outcomes (Patel et al. 2014) and therefore should not be dismissed without further investigation in the absence of an obvious cause, such as tachycardia.

T-Wave Abnormalities

The T-wave represents repolarisation of the ventricles. The wave of repolarisation moves predominantly from epicardium to endocardium (Hurst 1998). T-wave abnormalities often accompany abnormalities of the ST segment, but in some instances, occur in isolation. Although T-wave abnormalities are often associated with acute coronary syndromes, there are a number of other reasons why they may occur (Table 9.3) (Sclarovsky et al. 1986b).

Q-Waves

Pathological Q-waves (initial downward deflection of ≥40 ms in duration in any lead except III and aVR) are the most characteristic ECG finding of transmural MI of the left ventricle. Q-waves in V2 through V6 are considered abnormal if greater than 25% of R-wave amplitude. Q-waves appear when the infarcted muscle is electrically inert, and forces from other areas of the myocardium (such as the opposite

Table 9.3 T-wave abnormalities.

T-wave abnormality	Cause
'Flattened' T-waves	• Considered to be a non-specific abnormality with several potential causes such as ischaemia, cardiac scar, evolving infarction and electrolyte abnormality (Scheidt 1986)
Tall peaked T-wave ('hyperacute' T-wave)	• First ECG sign of a sudden narrowing or obstruction of an epicardial artery – caused by potassium leak through damaged membranes in the area of the infarct (Chesebro et al. 1991)
	• Hyperkalaemia
Inverted T-waves	• Normal finding in Lead III, aVR and V1
Deep symmetrical T-wave inversion	• May be a normal finding in V1–V3 for infants and children, and may persist into adolescence and young adulthood
	• No obvious cause, particularly in women
	• Chronic pericarditis, ventricular hypertrophy, intraventricular conduction defects
	• Hyperventilation
	• Mitral valve prolapse
	• Ventricular pre-excitation
	• Myocarditis
	• Electrolyte imbalance
	• Cardio-active drugs
	• Myocardial ischaemia
	• MI
	• Cerebral disease such as sub-arachnoid haemorrhage
	• Takotsubo Syndrome
Biphasic T-waves	• Myocardial ischaemia
	• Evolution of AMI
	• Takotsubo Syndrome
Pseudonormalisation of T-waves	• Where the T-wave has become inverted following an ischaemic event, a recurrent ischaemic event may result in the T-wave first becoming biphasic and then returning to what appears to be a normal configuration, which may then be followed by ST-segment elevation

wall) are reflected on the ECG. These forces may be represented by a vector directed away from the site of infarction and thus are seen as a negative wave (Q-wave) by electrodes overlying the infarcted region (Anderson et al. 2007).

Site of Infarction

Twelve-lead ECG leads that best detect changes in anatomically described locations of the myocardium according to the AHA (2007) are classified in Table 9.4.

Incremental ECG Leads

Right Ventricular Leads

Right ventricular myocardial infarction (RVMI) is usually associated with an inferior wall MI. Right ventricular involvement in inferior infarction is a strong, independent predictor of

Table 9.4 Anatomical region of the heart and associated ECG lead/s.

Anatomical region of the heart	ECG Lead
Inferior (or diaphragmatic) wall	II, II and aVF
Septal	V1 and V2
Anteroseptal	V1, V2, Vf3 and sometimes V4
Anterior	V3, V4 and sometimes V2
Apical	V3, V4 or both
Lateral	I, aVL, V5 and V6
Extensive anterior	I, aVL and V1 through V6
Posterior	V1 and V2[a]

[a] Posterior wall infarction does not produce Q-wave abnormalities in conventional leads and is diagnosed in the presence of tall R-waves in V1 and V2.

major complications and in-hospital mortality. The standard 12-lead ECG is mainly used to assess the left ventricle. ST segment elevation that is disproportionately greater in lead III than in lead II is pathognomonic for RVMI. If RVMI is suspected, right-sided precordial leads should be used to assess for RVMI. The V leads 4–6 are placed on the right side of the chest in the same anatomical position as left sided leads and are known as V4r, V5r and V6r. ST-segment elevation greater than 1 mm in Lead V4r, a lead placed in the right midclavicular line and 5th intercostal space, has been shown to be highly predictive of right ventricular infarction (Ondrus et al. 2013).

Posterior Leads

Posterior MI is usually associated with inferior and/or lateral MI but may occur in isolation. As typical ST-segment elevation is not seen on the standard 12-lead ECG, there is a risk of delayed diagnosis and management. Additional leads can be obtained to detect changes due to posterior MI. ST-segment elevation in Leads V7–V9 (precordial leads v4-6 are placed from the posterior axillary line.

A tall R-wave in V1 (in the absence of RVH, RBBB or Wolff–Parkinson–White syndrome) was thought to be a sign of posterior myocardial infarction, but new evidence suggests that it may more likely be associated with extensive lateral MI (Bayés de Luna et al. 2015). Posterior MI is suggested by the following changes in V1-3:

- Horizontal ST depression
- Tall, broad R-waves (>30 ms)
- Upright T-waves
- Dominant R-wave (R/S ratio > 1) in V2 (Burns 2021).

Obtaining a 12-Lead ECG

Suggested Resource

12 lead ECG placement of electrodes
RegisteredNurseRN (2017)
https://youtu.be/Rt4kjD4z8vM

Equipment Preparation

A 12-lead ECG may be obtained using an ECG machine (that is usually located on a mobile trolley) or from a bedside monitor that has 12-lead capability.

- Check that the equipment has no broken cables/wires and no damage to the housing.
- Inspect the cables/wires for cleanliness. They should be cleaned between uses.
- If the machine requires an external power source, plug the machine into a grounded alternating current wall outlet. If battery operated, ensure that the machine has been charged.
- Ensure that the machine has the appropriate cable/lead configuration attached.

- Ensure that there are sufficient consumables to undertake the procedure (ECG paper, 10 adhesive electrodes).
- Turn the machine on and ensure it is functional.
- Turn the ECG machine on and input patient information details if that is the unit practice (name, age, date and any other relevant details).
- Check that paper speed is set at 25 mm/s; sensitivity is set at 1 or 10 mm/s and baseline at centre.

Patient Preparation

Information and Consent

Although having an ECG is not a new procedure for many patients, others may be unaware of what is involved, and the appearance of the ECG machine may be frightening.

- Explain to the patient that an ECG is not an invasive test and should not cause pain, although removal of adhesive electrodes can cause some discomfort.
- In most settings, an ECG will only require a verbal consent from the patient, but as with any procedure, this should be obtained prior to the procedure, after explaining the reason for obtaining the ECG and what is involved.

Positioning

If you want to get a good ECG trace on the first attempt, ensure that the patient is comfortable. If the patient is not comfortable, you will find that they will hold themselves rigidly or wriggle to try and get comfortable, resulting in muscle tremor and a poor ECG tracing. Lying completely flat is uncomfortable for many patients, particularly those with heart failure.

- Position the patient in a supine position but lift the head of the bed slightly (around 15°). Ensure that the pillow is comfortably placed

and not causing the patient to 'hunch' their shoulders or neck forward. For patients with heart failure and other acute respiratory conditions, the ECG will have to be taken in a position tolerated by the patient.
- Ensure that the patient's extremities are not in contact with bedrails or footboards. This may result in reduced quality of the ECG tracing.

Patient Privacy

The procedure for obtaining a 12-lead ECG involves uncovering and exposing parts of the patient's body that are not normally exposed publicly. This may cause some embarrassment and anxiety for the patient, particularly if there is a likelihood of being observed by others who are not involved in the procedure of obtaining an ECG.

- Ensure that privacy is maintained and that unwelcome visitors during the procedure are discouraged.
- Demonstrate consideration of the patient's dignity by not exposing any more of the patient than needed to complete the ECG procedure.
- Cover the patient where possible during the procedure. Keeping them covered as much as possible and maintaining warmth will also prevent shivering, which could result in a poor ECG tracing.

Skin Preparation

Taking time to prepare the patient's skin for electrode adhesion will save time in the long run and contribute to obtaining a quality ECG trace.

- Ask the patient to remove jewellery from any area that may impede electrode placement.
- If the patient is diaphoretic, has excess oils or any material on the skin that may result in poor attachment of the electrodes, clean the skin with a cloth and warm water (soap can be

used if it does not irritate the patient's skin) and dry thoroughly.

- If the patient has excess body hair, remove the hair in the areas where electrodes will be placed, taking care not to cause any abrasions (with clippers if available, rather than shaving devices). Explain the rationale prior to removing body hair and get the patient's verbal permission to proceed. Excess body hair will result in poor attachment of the electrodes and a poor ECG trace. Furthermore, removal of the electrodes after the procedure will also result in a painful removal of the attached body hair.

Attaching the Electrodes

Correct lead placement is an important aspect of obtaining a 12-lead ECG, particularly when sequential ECGs are expected to be performed.

Limb Leads

Limb leads (using extremities) should be placed on the fleshy, lower aspects of the limbs, taking care to avoid bony prominences and muscle mass.

Key Point

ECGs recorded with torso placement of the extremity electrodes cannot be considered equivalent to standard ECGs and thus should not be used interchangeably with standard ECGs for serial comparison. Serial ECGs should use the same lead placement.

Precordial Leads

The 'angle of Louis', also known as the 'sternal notch', is the point where the clavicle joins the sternum. Run you finger from the top of the sternum and over the bony prominence of the sternal notch. Directly under this notch and to the side, you will palpate the second intercostal space. Slide your finger over the third and fourth ribs until you palpate the fourth intercostal space. Chest lead placement is as follows.

Lead V1 is placed in the fourth intercostal space to the right of the sternum.

Lead V2 is placed in the fourth intercostal space to the left of the sternum.

Lead V3 is placed directly between Leads V2 and V4.

Lead V4 is placed in the fifth intercostal space in the midclavicular line.

Lead V5 is placed horizontally with V4 in the anterior axillary line.

Lead V6 is placed horizontally with V4 and V5 in the midaxillary line.

- Precordial electrodes should be placed under the breast in women as breast tissue may impede conduction.
- If using pre-gelled electrodes, remove the backing and attach them firmly.
- Attach the lead wires to the electrodes.

Obtain the ECG

Ask the patient to relax and refrain from movement whilst obtaining the ECG. Obtain the 12-lead ECG by pressing the appropriate acquisition selector.

Check the Quality of the ECG

The ECG quality should be reviewed prior to disconnecting the patient.

- The ECG should have a straight baseline. If there is a wandering baseline, check that the leads are connected properly. Request that the patient does not move during the procedure and repeat the ECG.
- The ECG should have clearly defined waveforms and intervals. If there is artefact, this may be due to electrical interference or skeletal muscle tremor. Unplug or move any unnecessary electrical equipment away from the patient. Ensure that the patient is warm (reduce potential for shivering). Repeat the ECG.

Interpret the ECG

The ECG should be interpreted by someone with the knowledge and skills to do so. In the case of a patient who is symptomatic, if the nurse/technician performing the ECG does not have ECG interpretation skills, a senior nurse or doctor who is able to interpret the ECG should be promptly notified to do so. If no further ECG is required, the equipment should be disconnected and the patient made comfortable. The ECG leads should be cleaned prior to re-use on another patient.

Learning Activity 9.5

Most ECG machines include a printout of ECG measurements and offer an automated interpretation. Should we rely on the automated interpretation?

Suggested Resources

Intro to EKG interpretation – A systematic approach
Strong Medicine (2014)
https://youtu.be/ENyBhCJ2llY
ECG: a methodological approach.
Patient UK (2016)
https://patient.info/doctor/ecg-a-methodical-approach

Documentation

Interpretation of the ECG should be documented in the patient's case notes or file. If the ECG is part of an assessment for chest pain, the level of pain at the time the ECG is obtained (according to a pain scale) and should be documented on the ECG and in the case notes/file.

Learning Activity 9.6

Why is the ECG called a '12-lead ECG' when you only have 10 electrodes and 10 ECG leads?

Conclusion

The 12-lead ECG has for some years been used in cardiac assessment. Nurses working in a cardiac environment require advanced skills in ECG interpretation to recognise abnormalities that may indicate rhythm disturbance, ischaemia and infarction and other conditions with associated ECG abnormalities.

Learning Activity Answers

Learning Activity 9.1

Answer: Atrial repolarisation happens around the time of ventricular depolarisation, and as the atria only have a small muscle mass compared to the ventricles, the repolarisation wave of the atria is obscured by the relatively massive electrical depolarisation of the ventricles (the QRS complex).

Learning Activity 9.4

Answer: Conduction in a paced rhythm starts in the ventricles rather than normal conduction, thus depolarisation is prolonged. The QRS complexes are similar to those of ventricular rhythms, but a pacing spike should be visible before the QRS complex. If the lead is in the right ventricle (RV), it will produce a left bundle branch block (LBBB) pattern as the impulse moves across the myocardium from right to left. If the lead is in the left ventricle, it will produce a right bundle branch block (RBBB) pattern as the impulse moves across the myocardium from left to right. A single pacemaker lead device is placed in the right ventricle; an atrioventricular (AV) sequential pacemaker will have two leads: 1 in the right atria and one in the right ventricle; and cardiac resynchronisation therapy (CRT) device has a lead in the right atrium, right ventricle, and left ventricle via the coronary sinus vein. The QRS in CRT pacing has a BBB pattern but is a more complex ECG pattern due to the merging wave fronts of the impulse (Stipdonk et al. 2015). For further reading, the link to this article is provided in the reference list.

Learning Activity 9.5

Answer: Computerised ECG interpretation (CEI) should only be used as an adjunct to ECG interpretation by a health professional (HP) who has expertise in ECG interpretation. Automated interpretation may (rightly or wrongly) influence the HP interpretation of the ECG, particularly if there are time constraints, fatigue, or low level of expertise in ECG interpretation (Schläpfer and & Wellens, 2017). For further reading, the link to this article is provided in the reference list.

Learning Activity 9.6

Answer: Unipolar leads (use one electrode each) are the six precordial leads (V1–V6). The three augmented unipolar limb leads that are termed unipolar leads because there is a single positive electrode that is referenced against a combination of the other limb electrodes. The positive electrodes for these augmented leads are located on the left arm (aV_L), the right arm (aV_R), and the left leg (aV_F). In practice, these same electrodes are used for the bipolar leads I, II and III. Thus, nine electrodes are used to produce 12 views of the heart. The 10th electrode on the right lower limb is a ground electrode, which serves to reduce electrical interference.

References

Anderson, J.L., Adams, C.D., Antman, E.M. et al. (2007). ACC/AHA 2007 guidelines for the management of patients with unstable angina/non ST-elevation myocardial infarction: a report of the American College of Cardiology/American Heart Association Task Force on Practice Guidelines (Writing Committee to Revise the 2002 Guidelines for the Management of Patients With Unstable Angina/Non ST-Elevation Myocardial Infarction): developed in collaboration with the American College of Emergency Physicians, the Society for Cardiovascular Angiography and Interventions, and the Society of Thoracic Surgeons: endorsed by the American Association of Cardiovascular and Pulmonary Rehabilitation and the Society for Academic Emergency Medicine. *Circulation* **116** (7): e148–e304. doi: 10.1161/ CIRCULATIONAHA.107.181940. Epub 2007 Aug 6. Erratum in: Circulation. 2008 Mar 4;**117** (9): e180. PMID: 17679616.

Bayés de Luna, A., Rovai, D., Pons Llado, G. et al. (2015). The end of an electrocardiographic dogma: a prominent R wave in V1 is caused by a lateral not posterior myocardial infarction – new evidence based on contrast-enhanced cardiac magnetic resonance – electrocardiogram correlations. *European Heart Journal* **36** (16): 959–964.

Burns (2021). Posterior myocardial infarction. LITFL. https://litfl.com/posterior-myocardial-infarction-ecg-library (accessed 20 July 2021).

Casale, P.N., Deveroux, R.B., Alonso, D.R. et al. (1987). Improved sex-specific criteria of left ventricular hypertrophy for clinical and computer interpretation of electrocardiograms: validation with autopsy findings. *Circulation* **75**: 565–572.

Chabbra, L. and Spodick, D.H. (2012). Ideal isoelectric reference segment in pericarditis: a suggested approach to a commonly prevailing clinical misconception. *Cardiology* **122** (4): 210–212.

Chesebro, J.H., Zolhelyi, P., and Fuster, V. (1991). Pathogenesis of thrombosis in unstable angina. *American Journal of Cardiology* **68**: B2–B10.

Larkin, J. and Buttner, R. (2021). Trifascicular Block. *LITFL*. https://litfl.com/trifascicular-block-ecg-library (accessed 20 July 2021).

Meek, S. and Morris, F. (2002). ABC of clinical electrocardiography: Introduction I – Leads, rate, rhythm, and cardiac axis. *British Medical Journal* **324**: 415–418.

Mehta, M., Jain, A.C., and Mehta, A. (1999). Early repolarization. *Clinical Cardiology* **22**: 59–65.

Ondrus, T., Kanovsky, J., Novotny, T. et al. (2013). Right ventricular myocardial infarction: from pathophysiology to prognosis. *Experimental and Clinical Cardiology* **18** (1): 27.

Patel, J.H., Gupta, R., Roe, M.T. et al. (2014). Influence of presenting electrocardiographic findings on the treatment and outcomes of patients with non–ST-segment elevation myocardial infarction. *The American Journal of Cardiology* **113** (2): 256–261.

Scheidt, S. (1986). *Diagnosis of Cardiac Rhythm in Basic Electrocardiography*, 20–38. West Caldwell, NJ: CIBA-GEIGY Pharmaceuticals. *Medical Education Division*.

Sclarovsky, S. (ed.) (1999). *Electrocardiography of Acute Myocardial Ischaemic Syndromes*. London: Martin Dunitz Ltd.

Sclarovsky, S., Davidson, E., Strasberg, B. et al. (1986a). Unstable angina pectoris evolving to acute myocardial infarction: significance of ECG changes during chest pain. *American Heart Journal* **112**: 462.

Sclarovsky, S., Davidson, E., Strasberg, B. et al. (1986b). Unstable angina: the significance of ST segment elevation or depression in patients without evidence of increased myocardial oxygen demand. *American Heart Journal* **112**: 463–467.

The Global Use of Strategies to Open Occluded Coronary Arteries in Acute Coronary Syndromes (GUSTO) Investigators (1993). An international randomized trial comparing 4 thrombolytic strategies for acute myocardial infarction. *New England Journal of Medicine* **329**: 673–682.

10

Cardiac Monitoring in the Clinical Setting

Angela M. Kucia and Carol Oldroyd

Overview

Continuous electrocardiographic (ECG) monitoring may be initiated for a variety of reasons in clinical settings. The choice of monitoring system will depend upon the clinical indication for monitoring the patient, the types of monitoring system available, the available evidence-based guidelines and institutional policies and practices.

When ECG monitoring is initiated in the clinical setting, the nurse has a responsibility to ensure that it is maintained, continuously observed and that any abnormalities are promptly detected and acted upon. Nurses who are caring for patients with ECG monitoring should have appropriate skills to undertake these aspects of management. In a practical sense, there is a lot more to ECG monitoring than interpreting information and acting upon it. Nurses who are responsible for the delivery of care to patients with continuous ECG monitoring should be aware of specific issues related to electrical safety for patients and staff, the dignity and comfort of patients and the maintenance of skin integrity. This chapter will address a range of issues related to care of the monitored patient.

Learning Objectives

After reading this chapter, you should be able to:

- Describe the types of ECG monitoring systems currently available and the indications for their use.
- List the indications for undertaking ECG monitoring.
- Describe the types of settings where cardiac monitoring may be used.
- Discuss the elements of equipment and patient preparation for ECG monitoring.
- Discuss nursing responsibilities in the delivery of care to patients with cardiac monitoring
- Explain the concept of 'alarm' fatigue and strategies for avoidance.

Key Concepts

Arrhythmia monitoring; ischaemia monitoring; monitoring systems; electrical safety; telemetry; alarm fatigue

---

Cardiac Care: A Practical Guide for Nurses, Second Edition. Edited by Angela M. Kucia and Ian D. Jones.
© 2022 John Wiley & Sons Ltd. Published 2022 by John Wiley & Sons Ltd.

ECG Monitoring Systems and Lead Formats

The basic elements of ECG monitoring systems include a display screen, an amplifier to amplify the signal voltage, and leads and electrodes for connection to the patient. Hardwire monitors are usually located at the bedside and transmit information to a central monitor where it can be printed, stored and analysed. Contemporary monitoring systems are capable of monitoring and displaying multiple leads simultaneously, with advanced arrhythmia and ischaemia detection and calculation of ECG intervals. ECG monitoring is also used in conjunction with equipment such as a defibrillator, pacemaker and diathermy apparatus.

Monitoring systems have become increasingly complex and, in addition to arrhythmia monitoring and detection, are designed to monitor, collect and process data for a range of clinical parameters. Most basic ECG monitors include additional software and equipment to monitor non-invasive blood pressure, SpO_2, respirations, invasive haemodynamics, and temperature and allow acquisition and printout of a 12-lead ECG from the bedside. Many systems also offer continuous 12-lead ST-segment analysis. Other options can be added in areas such as intensive care, neonatal intensive care, paediatrics and anaesthetics.

Despite the advanced technology that is now available in cardiac monitoring systems, it is still necessary for experienced health care professionals to evaluate the information obtained from ECG monitoring, including the detection of false alarms, and to make decisions on a course of action in response to the information obtained. The type of monitoring selected for use in each clinical situation should be selected by health professionals who have expertise in the management of conditions in which ECG monitoring is indicated.

Key Point

Accurate electrode placement and selection of the appropriate leads to monitor are important when implementing continuous arrhythmia monitoring. For arrhythmia monitoring, V1 is commonly selected in adults because it is useful in distinguishing between ventricular tachycardia and aberrancy (Sandau et al. 2017).

Three-Electrode Monitoring Systems

Conventional cardiac monitoring using a three- or four-electrode configuration is the simplest form of cardiac monitoring. The ECG leads normally monitored using this configuration are the modified limb leads I, II and III. Lead II is the usual choice for monitoring since it normally provides the best amplitude for both the P waves and the QRS complexes; however, leads I or III can be used if they provide a better signal.

The normal format of electrode placement is for the right arm (RA) electrode to be placed in the infraclavicular fossa close to the right shoulder; the left arm (LA) electrode to be placed in the infraclavicular fossa close to the left arm and the left leg (LL) electrode usually placed on the abdomen or lower left chest wall. If a fourth electrode (RL) is present, this is a ground or reference electrode and can be placed anywhere but is usually placed on the right side of the abdomen (see Figure 10.1). Electrode positions can be changed if circumstances (such as trauma or surgery) dictate. This system can also be used to monitor a modified chest lead (MCL) such as MCL1. As the name suggests, this lead provides a substitute for V1.

Five-Electrode Monitoring Systems

In five-electrode monitoring systems, in addition to the electrodes previously described, a fifth electrode is used that can be placed in any of the pre-cordial chest lead positions, although V1 is the most common. Unlike MCL1, this system provides a true recording of V1, but it is not possible to record more than one chest lead at a time. It is helpful in determining the origin of broad complex rhythms but is not sensitive enough for use in monitoring for myocardial ischaemia. The anatomical placement of the RA, LA, RL, LL and V electrodes are the same as described in the Mason–Likar configuration described in Figure 10.1. Typically, cardiac monitors used with this electrode configuration have a 2-channel ECG display so that a limb lead and a V lead can be visualised simultaneously.

Twelve-Lead (10 Electrode) Monitoring Systems

Continuous 12-lead ST-segment monitoring utilises 10 electrodes that are attached in a configuration like that of the standard ECG. In order to avoid artefact due to movement and for patient comfort, the limb leads are placed in the Mason–Likar configuration (Figure 10.1), with the RA electrode placed at the right infraclavicular fossa medial to the border of the deltoid muscle; the LA electrode placed in a corresponding position on the left; the LL electrode placed at the left iliac fossa and the RL electrode usually placed at the right iliac fossa, although it can be placed in any position. When

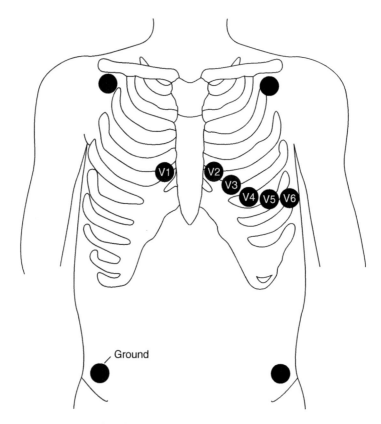

Figure 10.1 Mason–Likar configuration. *Source:* Reprinted from Sejersten et al. (2006). Copyright 2006, with permission from Elsevier.

making serial comparisons between ECGs, it is important to note that an ECG taken in a Mason–Likar configuration will differ from a standard 12-lead ECG with limb electrodes at the limb extremities, in that the limb lead QRS complexes may vary somewhat in amplitude and axis between the two configurations.

As standard ECGs are captured only at periodic intervals, transient episodes of ischaemia may go undetected, resulting in lost diagnostic and therapeutic opportunities. Continuous 12-lead ST-segment monitoring is useful for detecting ischaemia, particularly in patients who are unable to perceive angina symptoms, including those with diabetes mellitus and patients with impaired communication for reasons such as intubation, sedation or impaired mental status. Despite its clinical utility, ST-segment monitoring is underutilised.

Telemetry Monitoring Systems

Telemetry literally means 'the measurement or recording of signals at a distance' and in the context of ECG monitoring, telemetry is used for the radio transmission of ECG signals to remove the need for connecting wires to the patient. Telemetry systems may use the simple three-electrode system described above for arrhythmia monitoring only; or they may take the form of more complex systems that are also capable of ischaemia monitoring and have adjuncts such as non-invasive blood pressure monitoring and pulse oximetry.

The telemetry transmitter is a small box, which is attached to the patient by leads and electrodes (Figure 10.2). The transmitter sends a signal to a central monitoring system. This system is useful in that it allows the patient to mobilise within an area that is equipped to pick up the signal. This may be confined to patients in the coronary care unit, but often is extended to cardiac stepdown and other wards. The central monitoring system and staff who are responsible for monitoring may be in a different ward or area from the patient. One of the problems with this 'remote' transmission is that the responsibility for the maintenance of continued monitoring seems to fall somewhere between the nurses in the remote ward and those in the CCU. Patients often become disconnected from the monitoring system, either accidentally such as when an electrode becomes dislodged, or purposefully such as when the unit is removed for the patient to have a shower. This also happens when the patient wanders beyond the area where the signal can be picked up, or the patient may be sent to other departments for tests or procedures. Notifying a

Figure 10.2 Telemetry monitor.

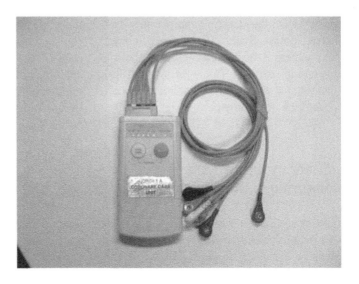

remote unit of telemetry disconnections can be time-consuming and burdensome.

Learning Activity 10.1

You are working on a general medical ward and you have two patients who are on telemetry monitoring. The cardiac rhythm is transmitted directly to the CCU monitor and you have no visual display of the cardiac rhythm in the medical ward. What are your responsibilities in caring for these patients?

Other problems that occur are that nurses in remote areas caring for the patient are not informed of the occurrence of arrhythmias and thus arrhythmias may not get noted or documented. This may result in the assumption that the patient is not at increased risk of an arrhythmia when in fact this is not the case. Moreover, when a potentially lethal arrhythmia occurs, it may be difficult to locate patients if they are not at their bed space or have not informed the staff caring for them of their whereabouts. The telemetry receiver is an expensive piece of equipment and can be easily lost if there is not a system in place for recording where it is being used and when it is returned.

Key Point

Demand for telemetry receivers is usually greater than the supply. Inappropriate use of telemetry affects clinician efficiency and increases health care costs without benefiting patients (Yeow et al. 2018). Institutional policies and guidelines should govern the use of telemetry systems.

Indications for Arrhythmia Monitoring in the Clinical Setting

Continuous ECG monitoring is commonly used in selected acute care settings such as intensive care units, CCUs, high dependency units, emergency departments, operating theatres and post-anaesthesia recovery rooms. The decision to undertake ECG monitoring in a patient will be influenced by local policies and guidelines and availability of monitored beds and equipment.

Four broad rationales for arrhythmia monitoring have been identified in the American Heart Association's 2017 Update to Practice Standards for Electrocardiographic Monitoring in Hospital Settings. They are:

1) Immediate recognition of sudden cardiac arrest to improve time to defibrillation.
2) Recognition of deteriorating conditions (such as development of non-sustained arrhythmias or prolonged QT-interval) that may lead to a life-threatening, sustained arrhythmia.
3) Facilitate or guide arrhythmia management.
4) Facilitate diagnosis of arrhythmia or cause of symptoms.

Indications for cardiac monitoring are outlined in Table 10.1.

Other conditions that are not specifically cardiac in nature but may require ECG monitoring include trauma, sepsis, acute respiratory failure, acute pulmonary embolus, major surgery, renal failure, electrolyte disturbance and ingestion of toxic substances. Although there are some suggested time intervals for continuation of ECG monitoring indicated in each of the clinical situations above, there are no definitive rules as to when cardiac monitoring should be discontinued. Given that resources such as monitored beds and portable telemetry units are often in short supply, discontinuation of cardiac monitoring can often pose some difficulties and may have medico-legal and ethical implications, particularly where monitoring must be discontinued for one patient to enable it to be used on another. Institutional guidelines can be a helpful support in making these decisions.

Table 10.1   Indications for arrhythmia monitoring in adults.

Indication	Timeframe
Resuscitation from cardiac arrest	Until the cause of the arrest is detected and treated
Targeted temperature management	Decision must be made on presumed cause of arrest
Suspected/known acute coronary syndromes	Presentation until acute coronary syndrome is ruled out; ischaemia is resolved or for at least 24 h after acute myocardial infarction and revascularization
Vasospastic angina	Until symptoms resolve
Takotsubo syndrome	Until symptoms resolve; QTc returns to normal limits; arrhythmias resolve (if present).
Cardiac surgery	Minimum of 48–72 h following cardiac surgery; or until discharge if there is a risk of atrial fibrillation
Newly diagnosed left main disease (or equivalent) requiring urgent bypass surgery	Diagnosis until 24–72 h following cardiac surgery or until discharge if there is a risk of atrial fibrillation
Non-urgent percutaneous intervention with complications such as vessel dissection, abrupt closure or no reflow	Minimum of 24 h or until complications resolve
Transcatheter structural interventions	≥3 d after procedure depending on procedure, device and patient factors
Temporary transvenous or transcutaneous pacing or permanent pacemaker lead implantation where the patient is pacemaker dependent	Until the cause of bradyarrhythmia is corrected or permanent pacemaker function is established
Severe bradyarrhythmias and/or advanced AV block including Mobitz Type II, complete heart block or new-onset bundle branch block in the setting of myocardial infarction (particularly anterior myocardial infarction)	Until the cause of bradyarrhythmia is corrected or definitive therapy (such as permanent pacing) is instituted
Re-entrant tachyarrhythmias such as Wolff–Parkinson–White (WPW) with rapid anterograde conduction	Until a definitive therapy is established, or a successful ablation procedure is undertaken
Ventricular arrhythmias such as ventricular tachycardia, ventricular fibrillation, Torsades de Pointes or potential for ventricular arrhythmias due to prolonged QT syndrome	Until the cause of the arrhythmia is corrected or a definitive therapy, such as implantation of a cardioverter defibrillator, has been established
Intra-aortic balloon counterpulsation (IABP)	Until IABP therapy is ceased (no further need to track rhythm for IABP function) and the patient is haemodynamically stable
Acute heart failure/pulmonary oedema	Until the signs and symptoms of heart failure are resolved; therapies that may contribute to arrhythmias (positive inotropic drugs) are discontinued; causative mechanisms such as ischaemia or tachyarrhythmias such as atrial fibrillation are resolved or controlled
Anaesthesia or conscious sedation	Until the patient is properly awake and alert

(Continued)

Table 10.1 (Continued)

Indication	Timeframe
Haemodynamic instability whatever the course	Until the cause of haemodynamic instability is corrected and the patient is clinically stable
	$\geq$24h until cause and treatment identified
Syncope with suspected cardiac cause	
During clinical exercise stress testing	During the exercise stress test and $\geq$5m of recovery following the test

Alarm Fatigue

Research suggests that 72–99% of clinical alarms are false alarms (Sendelbach and Funk 2013; Bach et al. 2018). Alarm fatigue refers to a state of sensory overload when clinicians are exposed to an excessive number of alarms, especially when a high number of these are false alarms. Alarm fatigue is dangerous as it can cause desensitisation to alarms resulting in alarms being missed or ignored. Patient deaths have been attributed to alarm fatigue. Various strategies have been proposed to reduce alarm fatigue without compromising patient safety (Winters et al. 2018). Table 10.2 outlines nursing considerations in the care of a patient with continuous cardiac monitoring.

Suggested Resource

Bach, T. A., Berglund, L. M., & Turk, E. (2018). Managing alarm systems for quality and safety in the hospital setting. BMJ open quality, 7(3), e000202. https://bmjopenquality.bmj.com/content/7/3/e000202.full

Learning Activity 10.2

After reading the article above, consider strategies that may be used to combat alarm fatigue in your unit. What might these be? How would you implement them?

Table 10.2 Nursing considerations in the care of the patient with continuous ECG monitoring.

Assemble the equipment that you will require

Monitor/transmitter	When using electrical equipment, such as a cardiac monitor, nurses should ensure that it has had a safety check as per the manufacturer's recommendations (usually annual). Nurses should be trained in the use of such equipment. Cables and leads should be intact and not frayed
	Patients who have cardiac monitoring in place are often attached to other electrical devices such as infusion pumps and have breaks in the skin for intravenous cannulation, which put them at increased risk of electrical shock. For this reason, cardiac monitoring areas should be cardiac protected according to national standards
	If a telemetry transmitter is to be used, it will require fresh batteries appropriately inserted. A telemetry pouch or pocket will be needed to hold the device

Table 10.2 (Continued)

Disposable electrodes	Standard adhesive electrodes are usually the least costly option and for this reason most institutions would prefer that these are used in the first instance
	For the diaphoretic patient, there are diaphoretic electrodes that are more expensive than the standard electrode, but they will not have to be replaced as often on a diaphoretic patient and thus are likely to be more cost-effective in this situation
	Some patients are sensitive to the adhesive and/or the gel in electrodes and hypoallergenic electrodes may be required
	The electrodes should be adhered in a way that ensures that there are no air bubbles beneath the electrode. It must be ensured that all backing material is removed from the electrode – any residual backing can cause irritation to the patient
	Correct placement of the electrodes is required to ensure a tracing that can be correctly interpreted. Cables are usually colour coded, but it is important to realise that there may be international differences in the colour code
Patient preparation	
Patient education	The application of a cardiac monitor can cause anxiety in patients and their families, especially when there are irregularities with the cardiac trace (which may in fact be due to artefact) or when the heart rate changes. A little time spent in reassuring patients and families about the function of the monitor and letting them know that irregularities in rate and rhythm will trigger alarms in the central monitor that will alert nurses if there are any problems with heart rhythm of may allay their fears
	When a patient is placed on telemetry, he or she needs to be educated about the area that they can mobilise within; to inform the nurse if an electrode becomes detached and not to shower or bath with the unit attached
Skin preparation	Gauze swabs or a cloth to clean the skin may be required, particularly in diaphoretic patients. The skin should be clean and dry prior to attachment of the adhesive electrodes
	If the patient has chest hair, it may need to be clipped. Shaving with a razor is not advised as it often results in grazing or small cuts which increases the risk of infection. If electrodes are placed directly over excess chest hair, impedance is increased, resulting in a poor trace and the electrode lifts, pulling at the chest hair, resulting in patient discomfort and a poor trace, electrodes have to be repeatedly replaced, resulting in discomfort to the patient each time the electrode is removed, increased cost in terms of electrode usage and the time taken to replace them frequently, and periods where the patient may be unmonitored due to 'loose lead'. A little time taken to attach electrodes properly when initiating monitoring will save time and resources and make the patient more comfortable. Regular checks of the skin are needed to detect allergy or irritation to the electrodes. Electrodes should be replaced if they roll up, lift, or become soiled or wet. When monitoring is discontinued, the electrodes and any residual adhesive should be removed. Patients are often unaware that electrodes are still attached (particularly underneath a woman's breast)
Comfort and dignity	Exposure of the torso for the purpose of attaching electrodes is often embarrassing for the patient. Privacy must be ensured, and the patient is covered as much as possible
	It is often not practical for the patient to wear his or her own clothing when attached to cardiac monitoring and other devices such as infusion pumps. Hospital gowns can be less than discreet in covering the patient. When attaching electrodes and leads, it should be borne in mind how this will impact on the patient's clothing cover; do not attach the leads over the top of a gown as this will make the gown sag at the top and lift at the bottom, exposing the patient

(Continued)

Table 10.2 (Continued)

	The leads should be looped so that there is no tension on them. Tension may cause them to become disconnected or cause discomfort to the patient
Hygiene needs	The patient with cardiac monitoring in place will need advice on how best to meet hygiene needs. The electrodes should not come into contact with water, and the patient may need some assistance in attending to hygiene
Management of monitoring	
Obtain a good-quality trace on the cardiac monitor	It must be ensured that the rhythm displayed on the monitor can be clearly seen and is free of artefact
Obtain a rhythm strip, diagnose the rhythm and	If any artefact is present, the cause must be rectified. It may be that an electrode has become detached or has poor contact with the skin
document	The electrode may be placed over the skeletal muscle or the patient's movement may result in artefact. Alternately, there may be electrical interference from another piece of electrical equipment such as an infusion pump or an electric bed
Ensure that appropriate alarm limits are set	Most systems will impose generic alarm settings, but this may need to be altered according to a patient's rhythm and condition. For example, a patient may normally be bradycardic due to beta-blocker use: thus, the low-rate alarm may need to be set lower to prevent continuous bradycardia alarms
Ensure appropriate supervision	It must be ensured that the monitored patient is under the direct care of a nurse who has had training in arrhythmia interpretation and management of arrhythmias

---

Learning Activity 10.3

Observe the trace in Figure 10.3. What are the likely causes of the poor trace and how may this be rectified?

Learning Activity 10.4

Multiple Choice Questions

1 Which of the following leads is the usual choice of monitoring when using a three-lead monitoring system?
   A Lead I
   B Lead II
   C Lead III
   D Lead aVr

2 When using telemetry to monitor patients, which of the following would be the main advantage in patient care?
   A It allows the patient to mobilise
   B The patient can maintain a normal diet
   C The patient can shower and bathe
   D The leads don't become entangled

3 Which of the following is not a consideration when choosing adhesive electrodes?
   A Cost
   B Colour
   C Diaphoresis
   D Patient's skin sensitivity/allergy

4 Which of the following is not an indication for continuous cardiac monitoring?
   A Exercise stress testing
   B Suspected acute coronary syndrome
   C Syncope due to dehydration
   D Syncope of suspected cardiac origin

5 Which is the preferred lead for monitoring in suspected ventricular tachycardia?
   A 1
   B II
   C III
   D V1

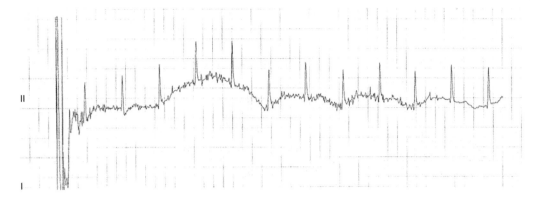

Figure 10.3 Cardiac trace with artefact.

Learning Activity Answers

Learning Activity 10.1

Answer: Your responsibility would be (i) to know the reason for monitoring, (ii) know who to contact to obtain information about cardiac rhythm if arrhythmia is suspected from a change in the patient's condition or observations, (iii) obtain printed records of arrhythmias to be documented in the patient's case notes; (iv) inform the CCU if the patient is purposely detached from the monitor for any reason or if the patient no longer requires monitoring, (v) ensure that the patient has regular checks to ensure that the monitor is still attached; (vi) ensure that adhesive electrodes are changed as needed and are not causing skin irritation), (ensure that the patient understands the reason for monitoring, care of the monitor and the range that the patient can ambulate without losing the monitoring trace. There should be agreement about who will review the patient's ECG activity on a daily basis (usually the home medical team). You may have identified more responsibilities based upon your institutional guidelines.

Learning activity 10.3

Answer: Artefact on an ECG trace is anything seen on the ECG that is not caused by the electrical currents generated by the heart. Sources of ECG artefact include electrical interference from power to electrical wall outlets, or from a remote device such as a mobile phone. Muscle tremor, patient movement, or loss of electrode contact can also cause ECG artefact.

To reduce artefact on the ECG, the following options can be tried:
- Obtain the ECG away from other equipment where possible.
- Switch off unnecessary equipment (for example electric bed) during ECG recording where possible.
- Ensure that cable and lead wires do not cross the power cables of other equipment or ventilator tubing.
- To reduce muscle tremor, provide a warm blanket to a shivering patient.
- To reduce patient movement, ensure that the patient is comfortable and relaxed prior to obtain the ECG.

- Check the lead wire-to-electrode connection and electrode-to-patient's skin adhesion.
- Adjust the ECG filter setting if nothing else works.

(Phillips 2008)

Learning activity 10.4

Answers: 1 (b); 2 (a); 3 (b); 4 (c); 5 (d)

References

Bach, T.A., Berglund, L.M., and Turk, E. (2018). Managing alarm systems for quality and safety in the hospital setting. *BMJ Open Quality* **7** (3): e000202.

Sandau, K.E., Funk, M., Auerbach, A. et al. (2017). Update to practice standards for electrocardiographic monitoring in hospital settings: a scientific statement from the American Heart Association. *Circulation* **136** (19): e273–e344. https://www.ahajournals.org/doi/pdf/10.1161/CIR.0000000000000527.

Sejersten, M., Pahlm, O., Pettersson, J. et al. (2006). Comparison of EASI-derived 12-lead electrocardiograms versus paramedic-acquired 12-lead electrocardiograms using Mason-Likar limb lead configuration in patients with chest pain. *Journal of Electrocardiology* **39** (1): 13–21.

Sendelbach, S. and Funk, M. (2013). Alarm fatigue: a patient safety concern. *AACN Advanced Critical Care* **24** (4): 378–386.

Winters, B.D., Cvach, M.M., Bonafide, C.P., Hu, X., Konkani, A., O'Connor, M.F., ... and Kane-Gill, S.L. (2018). Technological distractions (part 2): a summary of approaches to manage clinical alarms with intent to reduce alarm fatigue. *Critical Care Medicine*, **46** (1), 130-137. doi: https://doi.org/10.1097/CCM.0000000000002803.

Yeow, R.Y., Strohbehn, G.W., Kagan, C.M., Petrilli, C.M., Krishnan, J.K., Edholm, K., ... and Pahwa, A.K. (2018). Eliminating inappropriate telemetry monitoring: an evidence-based implementation guide. *JAMA Internal Medicine*, **178** (7), 971-978. doi: https://doi.org/10.1001/jamainternmed.2018.2409.

11

Arrhythmias

Angela M. Kucia

Overview

Arrhythmia is a generalised term used to indicate a disturbance in heart rhythm. Arrhythmias may be associated with coronary heart disease (CHD), congenital abnormalities and cardiomyopathies and can be induced by non-cardiac factors such as electrolyte imbalance and some drugs. The interpretation of cardiac arrhythmias plays an important role in the diagnosis of some cardiac disorders.

In some cases, an arrhythmia may go unnoticed by the patient, while in other cases there may be associated symptoms including palpitations, breathlessness, chest pain, heart failure or syncope. Symptoms produced by arrhythmias are usually those that are abnormally fast or slow. Importantly, arrhythmias are believed to be the underlying cause of sudden cardiac death syndrome. Arrhythmias producing circulatory impairment, myocardial ischaemia or an increased risk of sudden cardiac death require prompt and effective identification and treatment. This chapter describes the process of cardiac rhythm interpretation, the characteristics of normal sinus rhythm (SR), and common arrhythmias. You may wish to revisit Chapter 3 to review Cardiac Electrophysiology. The management of rhythm disturbances is discussed in Chapter 14.

Learning Objectives

After reading this chapter, you will be able to:

- Understand the significance of common cardiac arrhythmias.
- Use a systematic approach in arrhythmia interpretation.
- Define and identify common arrhythmias and understand the principles of treatment.
- Define and identify tachyarrhythmias and understand the principles of treatment.
- Identify circumstances in arrhythmia management that require expert help.

Key Concepts

Arrhythmia; disorders of conduction; tachycardia; bradycardia; rhythm interpretation

Mechanisms of Arrhythmia Generation

Any rhythm that does not meet the criteria of normal sinus rhythm (SR) is termed an arrhythmia.

Although automaticity is an intrinsic property of all myocardial cells, the sinoatrial (SA) node normally displays the highest intrinsic rate and in normal conditions is the normal pacemaker of the heart. All other pacemakers are referred to as subsidiary or latent pacemakers because they take over the function of initiating excitation of the heart only when the SA node is unable to generate impulses or when these impulses fail to propagate. These subsidiary pacemakers are located within the atria or ventricles and have intrinsically slower rates than the sinus node. Conditions that may cause the sinus node rate to drop below that of subsidiary pacemakers include increased vagal tone, drug effects, electrolyte abnormalities and sinus node disease. Conditions that may cause subsidiary pacemakers to be faster than the sinus node rate include increased sympathetic tone, some disease states and effects of drugs such as digitalis and sympathomimetics.

The mechanisms that cause cardiac arrhythmias generally fall into two categories: (1) focal activity or (2) reentry. Focal activity can arise from enhanced automaticity or triggered activity.

Automaticity

Automaticity is the property of cardiac cells to generate spontaneous action potentials (see Chapter 3) . Abnormal automaticity includes both reduced or increased automaticity (Antzelevitch & Burashnikov 2011).

Afterdepolarisations

Triggered activity results from the premature activation of cardiac tissues by afterdepolarisations (depolarisations that are triggered by one or more preceding action potentials) (Antzelevitch & Burashnikov 2011; Tse 2016). Early afterdepolarisations (EADs) can develop before full repolarisation, corresponding to phase 2 or phase 3 of the cardiac action potential and are thought to be associated with arrhythmias seen in heart failure and long QT syndromes. Delayed afterdepolarisations (DADs) can develop after full repolarisation, corresponding to phase 4 of the cardiac action potential. DADs occur with intracellular calcium overload such as can occur with exposure to digoxin or catecholamines, or in the setting of hypokalaemia, and hypercalcaemia, hypertrophy and heart failure (Tse 2016).

Key Point

Class IA and III antiarrhythmics can have a proarrhythmic effect because of their action in prolonging repolarisation in cardiac cells that may encourage afterdepolarisations (see Chapter 12).

Reentry

Re-entry occurs when an action potential fails to extinguish itself and reactivates a region that has recovered from refractoriness (Tse 2016). Re-entrant conduction abnormalities may lead to premature beats or sustained tachycardias in any part of the heart where conduction velocity is abnormally slow. The impulse can travel through an area of myocardium, depolarise it and then re-enter that same area to depolarise it again. Ischaemia, electrolyte abnormalities, some drugs and disease processes can facilitate this type of conduction abnormality (Jacobsen 2010).

Key Point

When an impulse travels the re-entry loop only once, a single premature beat results. If conduction velocity is slow enough and the refractory period of normal tissue is short enough, a single impulse could travel the loop numerous times, resulting in a run of premature beats or in a sustained tachycardia (Jacobsen 2010).

Arrhythmia interpretation

Cardiac monitoring is suitable for rhythm recognition but insufficient for diagnosis of myocardial infarction (MI) or more sophisticated ECG interpretation (see Chapter 10). Wherever possible, a 12-lead ECG should be recorded, since this provides additional information that is not present on a single rhythm strip. However, a 12-lead ECG recording is not always possible, and a cardiac monitor may be the only aid to identifying the patient's rhythm. Precise identification of many rhythm abnormalities requires experience and expertise, but in most cases an accurate description of the rhythm is sufficient to allow effective management (see Chapter 12).

The clinical significance of a rhythm that deviates from normal SR is dependent on various factors including the ventricular rate, myocardial conduction, and the patient's physiological and psychological response. Arrhythmia identification can be approached in a variety of ways, but a systematic approach to interpretation of the electrocardiographic waveforms and intervals gives the best result. Having first ensured that the ECG rhythm recording/monitor is clearly identified for a particular patient (to ensure safety), follow the steps, and answer the questions in Table 11.1.

1. Is the Rhythm Regular or Irregular?

This is not always as easy to determine as it seems. In most cases, it is possible to see if a rhythm is regular or not merely by looking at it on the monitor screen, but as the heart rate increases, beat-to-beat variation becomes more difficult to detect. In cases of doubt, placing a piece of paper along a rhythm strip printout and marking three consecutive R waves will provide additional information: where the rhythm is regular the marks should correspond to R waves anywhere along the strip; if not, then the rhythm is irregular.

Table 11.1 Systematic interpretation of rhythm.

Is the *rhythm* regular or irregular?

Normal sinus rhythm is regular

What is the *heart rate*?

The normal heart rate is between 60 and 100 bpm

- A heart rate < 60 bpm is termed 'bradycardia'
- A heart rate > 100 bpm is termed 'tachycardia'

To calculate heart rate:

One large box represents 0.2 s; thus, there are five large boxes in a second

Count how many complexes there are in a second and multiply by 60 to obtain the heart rate

This method is only reliable for regular heart rates, whereas, a full 60 seconds is required for irregular heart rates

Is the *P-wave* normal?

Does a normal P-wave precede each QRS complex?

- Normal sinus rhythm should have an upright P-wave in Lead II
- Normal P-wave width is <0.11 s (<3 small squares)

Is the *PR interval* normal?

Is the PR interval (measured from the beginning of P to the beginning of QRS complex) the same in each complex?

- The normal PR interval is 0.12–0.20 s (3–5 small squares)

Is the *QRS* normal?

Is the QRS narrow or wide?

- The QRS is measured from the first upward/downward deflection from baseline until return to baseline
- Normal QRS width is 0.06–0.10 s (1.5–2.5 small squares)

The most common reasons for irregular heart rhythms are atrial fibrillation (AF), ectopic beats and heart block. In AF, the rhythm is often described as 'irregularly irregular', meaning that it does not follow any discernable pattern. AF is very common, particularly in the older people, and the effect on the patient is often related to the ventricular rate. Heart blocks may follow a cyclical pattern, and careful analysis of the relationship between the P wave and QRS complex is required. Both atrial ectopic (atrial premature contraction) and ventricular ectopic (ventricular premature contraction) beats can make an essentially regular rhythm appear irregular. Ectopic beats are often benign, but investigation of possible underlying causes should be considered.

2. What Is the Ventricular Rate?

Provided that discernable QRS complexes are present, the next step is to determine the ventricular rate or bpm. There are several different ways of doing this – the simplest being to read the rate shown on most modern cardiac monitors. However, this may not always be accurate, particularly in the presence of peaked T-waves or an irregular rhythm such as AF, and caution is required if relying on this method. Other approaches include printing a rhythm strip and measuring the number of large squares between adjacent R-waves and dividing this number into 300. For example, if there are four large squares between the R-waves, then the rate is 300/4 giving a rate of 75 bpm. An alternative method involves counting the number of R-waves in 30 large squares and multiplying by 10. Both these methods give a reasonable approximation allowing the rhythm to be classified as regular (60–100 bpm), a bradycardia (less than 60 bpm) or a tachycardia (>100 bpm).

3. Are there P-Waves Present?

P-waves denote atrial depolarisation and appear before the QRS complex in SR. A normal P-wave is seen as an upright, rounded deflection in Lead II on the ECG, indicating that the impulse has originated in or near the sinoatrial (SA) node. Sometimes inverted P-waves are seen, indicating the impulse has originated closer to the AV node. Intermittent P-waves may indicate a type of heart block, and other forms of atrial activity exist, including flutter and fibrillation waves.

4. What Is the Relationship Between the P-Waves and the QRS Complexes?

Having examined both atrial and ventricular activities, the final step involves analysing the relationship between them. In SR, the P-wave should always be followed by a QRS complex, with a normal PR interval of 0.12–0.2 s (or three to five small squares). The PR interval is measured from the beginning of the P-wave to the beginning of the QRS. A distance greater than five small squares indicates some type of heart block is present. The significance of a shortened PR interval is often overlooked but may well indicate a pre-excitation syndrome and is particularly important in patients presenting with paroxysmal tachycardias.

5. Is the QRS Width Broad or Narrow?

Normal QRS duration is between 0.08 and 0.12 seconds (less than three small squares on the ECG paper, using standard paper speed of 25 mm/s). This interval represents the length of time the electrical impulse takes to depolarise the ventricles. A measurement of longer than three small squares indicates that there is a delay in the conduction of the impulse. This can be due to either a blockage in the conduction system (e.g. bundle branch block) or a result of the impulse being initiated from the ventricular myocardium. Widening of the QRS complex can also occur in electrolyte disturbances (e.g. hyperkalaemia) or with some drugs such as tricyclic antidepressants and some antiarrhythmic drugs.

Having systematically used the approach described above, it should now be possible to determine the cardiac rhythm. Although it is not always possible to precisely name the rhythm, this approach should at least allow for an accurate description, which in turn will direct appropriate management, and may prove particularly useful when communicating with colleagues who do not have access to the patient or actual rhythm strip (such as in telephone consultations with off-site medical staff).

Sinus Rhythm

Rhythms that originate in the sinus node and their characteristics are shown in Figure 11.1. Sinus rhythms include normal sinus rhythm (Figure 11.1a), sinus bradycardia (Figure 11.1b), sinus tachycardia (Figure 11.1c), and sinus arrhythmia (Figure 11.1d). Sinus rhythms are included in the group of supraventricular rhythms because the initial impulse for conduction occurs above the ventricles. The sinoatrial (or sinus) node is the normal pacemaker of the heart. The sinus node is in the wall of the right atrium and transmits impulses to the atria and the ventricles (see Chapter 3). Rhythms that originate from the sinus node have a P-wave preceding each QRS complex. The P-wave in a sinus rhythm is of consistent morphology that is upright in ECG leads I and II and inverted in aVR. Sinus P-waves are most prominently seen in leads II and V1.

Key Point

Although cells in several areas of the atria, coronary sinus, pulmonary veins, atrioventricular (AV) junction, AV valves and Purkinje system have the property of automaticity, under normal conditions, they have slower rates than the sinus node so that under normal conditions, they do not compete with the sinus node.

Normal Sinus Rhythm

The heart's usual rhythm is normal sinus rhythm (SR) (Figure 11.1a). SR is regular with a rate between 60 and 100 beats per minute (bpm) in adults.

The P-R interval is regular and between 0.12 and 0.20 seconds (3–5 small squares). The components of the normal cardiac cycle with normal waveforms and intervals can be seen in Chapter 9 (Figure 9.1).

Bradyarrhythmias

A bradyarrhythmia exists when the ventricular rate is less than 60 bpm. In some cases, the patient is asymptomatic, and no treatment is required. However, the bradycardia may be due to malfunction of the SA node, or a delay or blockage of AV conduction, in which case intervention may be required.

Tachyarrhythmias

Tachycardias are defined as a heart rate greater than 100 bpm and can be supraventricular or ventricular in origin. Tachycardias can result in hypotension and reduced tissue perfusion. Because the heart is beating faster, the amount of time between cardiac contractions is reduced, thus the ventricles do not have time to fill adequately before contraction and cardiac output decreases. Heart rate is a major determinant of oxygen requirement: the harder the heart must work, the greater its demand for oxygen. Persistent or prolonged tachycardia will, therefore, increase the amount of oxygen required by the myocardium, resulting in increased ischaemia in patients who cannot meet the increased demand.

Differentiating Between Supraventricular Tachycardia and Ventricular Tachycardia

Supraventricular tachycardia (SVT) is a term that is used to group together those tachyarrhythmias that originate above the ventricles and appear as a narrow QRS complex on the ECG and are more than 100 bpm at rest. Although the impulse is not originating from the SA node, ventricular depolarisation

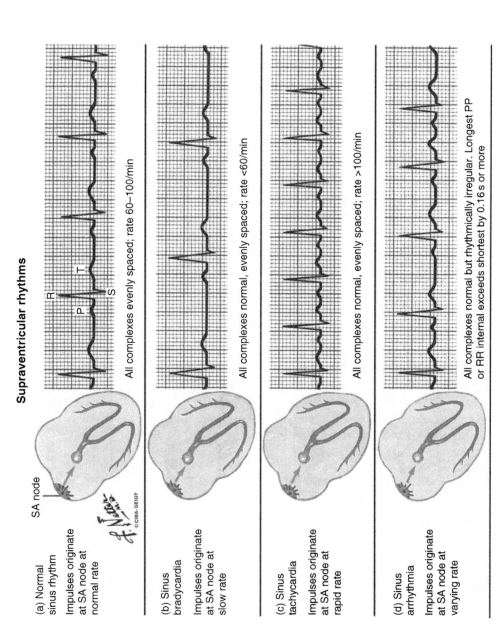

Supraventricular rhythms

SA node

(a) Normal sinus rhythm

Impulses originate at SA node at normal rate

All complexes evenly spaced; rate 60–100/min

(b) Sinus bradycardia

Impulses originate at SA node at slow rate

All complexes normal, evenly spaced; rate <60/min

(c) Sinus tachycardia

Impulses originate at SA node at rapid rate

All complexes normal, evenly spaced; rate >100/min

(d) Sinus arrhythmia

Impulses originate at SA node at varying rate

All complexes normal but rhythmically irregular. Longest PP or RR internal exceeds shortest by 0.16 s or more

Figure 11.1 Sinus rhythms. *Source:* Scheidt (1986). Basic Electrocardiography. Novartis Medical Education. U.S.A. Copyright Novartis A.G. Used with permission.

occurs normally and results in a narrow QRS complex. The rhythm is often regular but may be irregular in the presence of AF or variably conducted atrial flutter. SVT is sometimes referred to as a narrow complex tachycardia, but may present with a wide QRS due to

- pre-existing bundle branch block (BBB) or intraventricular conduction defect;
- aberrant conduction due to tachycardia (patient has normal QRS when in SR);
- electrolyte or metabolic disorder;
- conduction over an accessory pathway (pre-excitation) (Page et al. 2016).

> **Key Point**
>
> A broad complex tachycardia may be due to ventricular tachycardia, paced rhythm, artefact or SVT with a conduction abnormality (see Figure 11.2)

Ectopy, Aberrancy and Escape Beats

Unusual beats may be seen on the ECG that do not match the dominant rhythm (see Figure 11.3). These are usually classified as ectopic beats, aberrant beats or escape beats.

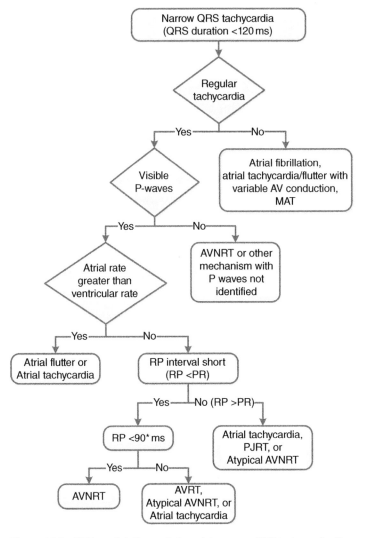

Figure 11.2 Differential diagnosis for adult narrow QRS tachycardia. *Source:* Page et al. (2016).

Unusual beats

(a) Premature contractions (occur early, before next sinus beat is expected)

1. Atrial

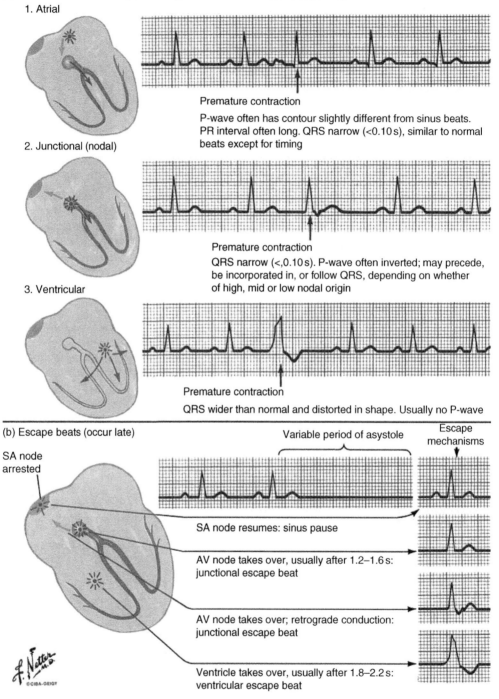

Premature contraction

P-wave often has contour slightly different from sinus beats. PR interval often long. QRS narrow (<0.10 s), similar to normal beats except for timing

2. Junctional (nodal)

Premature contraction

QRS narrow (<,0.10 s). P-wave often inverted; may precede, be incorporated in, or follow QRS, depending on whether of high, mid or low nodal origin

3. Ventricular

Premature contraction

QRS wider than normal and distorted in shape. Usually no P-wave

(b) Escape beats (occur late)

Variable period of asystole

Escape mechanisms

SA node arrested

SA node resumes: sinus pause

AV node takes over, usually after 1.2–1.6 s: junctional escape beat

AV node takes over; retrograde conduction: junctional escape beat

Ventricle takes over, usually after 1.8–2.2 s: ventricular escape beat

Figure 11.3 Ectopic and escape beats. *Source:* Scheidt (1986). Basic Electrocardiography. Novartis Medical Education. U.S.A. Copyright Novartis A.G. Used with permission.

Ectopy

An ectopic beat arises from a region of the heart muscle that is not normally responsible for impulse formation (i.e. the SA node). Infrequent atrial, junctional and ventricular ectopic beats (Figure 11.3a) are usually harmless but may cause palpitations and light-headedness if frequent, may be associated with an underlying disease state, or may indicate an increased risk of other arrhythmias.

Aberrancy

Aberrant ventricular conduction occurs when the supraventricular electrical impulse is conducted abnormally through the ventricular conducting system, such as in bundle branch block, resulting in a wide QRS complex that may be confused with a ventricular ectopic beat.

Escape Beats

Should the SA node fail, an automatic cell must take over to maintain beating of the heart. This is known as an escape beat (Figure 11.3b). Escape beats may be asymptomatic or associated with underlying pathology eventually leading to symptomatic bradycardia requiring treatment.

Suggested Resource

The ECG course – Ectopy and aberrancy (includes escape beats)
The Resuscitationist (2014)
https://youtu.be/O8lEDgPWdpY

Sinus Dysrhythmias

Sinus Bradycardia

Sinus bradycardia (SB) occurs when the heart rate is slower than 60 bpm. This rhythm is like normal SR, except that the RR interval is longer. Each P-wave is followed by a QRS complex in a ratio of 1:1 (see Figure 11.1b).

SB can occur naturally during sleep and be a normal finding in athletes, or a side effect of treatment such as beta-blockers, calcium-channel blockers, amiodarone and other antiarrhythmic drugs. Other causes include hypothermia, hypothyroidism, increased intracranial pressure, obstructive sleep apnoea, some infectious diseases and hypoxia. SB may be associated with inferior MI, where the right coronary artery supplies the inferior territory of the heart, including the sinus and AV nodes in many patients. SB is common in elderly patients but may be an early manifestation of sinus node dysfunction (Homoud 2019a).

Key Point

Vasovagal responses due to heightened parasympathetic activity and sympathetic withdrawal on the SA node may produce profound bradycardia and syncope. Vasovagal stimuli including coughing, vomiting, carotid sinus stimulation and Valsalva manoeuvres (Homoud 2019a).

Slow heart rates may be well tolerated, and intervention is not required in asymptomatic patients. Some patients may exhibit symptoms such as dyspnoea, dizziness, chest pain, syncope and hypotension. In symptomatic bradycardia, atropine is usually the first drug of choice if not contraindicated. If atropine is not successful in restoring in alleviating symptoms and haemodynamic stability, temporary pacing should be initiated if available. If pacing is not readily available, a dopamine or adrenaline infusion may be required (Homoud 2019a).

Sinus Tachycardia

Sinus tachycardia is classified as a sinus rhythm greater than 100 bpm. All the other

ECG characteristics are the same as for sinus rhythm (Figure 11.1c).

Physiological sinus tachycardia is not a 'true' arrhythmia but represents a response to some other physiological or pathological state. It is a normal response to stressors such as fever, pain, anxiety, exercise, hypovolaemia, shock and cardiac failure. It can also be caused by stimulants such as caffeine and alcohol, or drugs that cause sympathetic stimulation.

Inappropriate sinus tachycardia (IST) is unexplained by physiological demands and may occur at rest, with minimal exertion, or during recovery from exercise. IST may be associated with debilitating symptoms that include weakness, fatigue, lightheadedness and uncomfortable sensations, such as heart racing. Patients with IST often have resting heart rates >100 bpm and average rates that are >90 bpm in a 24 hours period. The cause of IST is unclear, but mechanisms related to dysautonomia, neurohormonal dysregulation and intrinsic sinus node hyperactivity have been proposed (Page et al. 2016).

The cause of the tachycardia and underlying condition of the myocardium will determine the prognosis. Management focuses on detecting and correcting any underlying causes.

Sinus Node Dysfunction

The sinoatrial (SA) node is normally the dominant pacemaker in the human heart. Sinus node dysfunction (SND), also referred to as 'sick sinus syndrome', is the term used to describe the inability of the SA node to generate a heart rate that meets the physiologic needs of an individual (Homoud 2019b). Patients with SND may be asymptomatic or highly symptomatic. Atrial myocytes found in the sinoatrial (SA) node are specialised into two different functional cells: pacemaker (P) cells that are responsible for pacemaker function, and transitional (T) cells that are responsible for propagating the impulse into the right atrium. Disruption in the pacemaker function of the SA node may result in inappropriate sinus bradycardia, or sinus pause/arrest where there are pauses of three seconds or more without atrial activity, usually due to a failure of P cells to generate the action potential. Disruption in the transitional function of the SA node may result in sinoatrial (SA) exit block, which is caused by the failure of the T cells to transmit the impulse (Dakkak and Doukky 2019). The most common cause of SND is replacement of SND tissue by fibrous tissue, which can also happen in other parts of the conducting system. Medications commonly associated with SND are beta-blockers, calcium-channel blockers, digoxin and antiarrhythmic drugs. SND is associated with various abnormalities of rhythm.

Sinus Pause/Sinus Arrest

A sinus pause or arrest refers to the transient absence of sinus P-waves on the electrocardiogram (ECG) that may last from 2 seconds to several minutes. The duration of the pause has no relationship to the cycle length of the base rhythm (i.e. the next P-wave does not necessarily occur at the expected time interval). An escape beat or rhythm may occur (See Figure 11.2b). A pause of 2 seconds or so may occur in normal hearts, but longer episodes of sinus arrest can produce symptoms of dizziness, syncope, and in rare circumstances, death (Homoud 2019c).

Sino-Atrial Exit Block

SA exit block manifests as the absence of a P-wave on the surface ECG. Sinus node depolarisation is normal, but in SA exit block, but the impulse fails to conduct surrounding atrial tissues. SA nodal exit block has sub-types that mirror those of AV block (first degree, second-degree types I and II, and third degree), but the abnormalities refer to conduction between the SA node and atria rather than between atria and ventricles. First- and third-degree SA exit blocks cannot be seen on the surface ECG and an electrophysiological study is required for diagnosis. Type 1 second-degree SA exit block manifests as progressive shortening of the PP interval before a P-QRS-T complex is dropped. The shortening PP interval may be helpful in discriminating between Type 1 second-degree SA

exit block and sinus pause. Type 2 second-degree SA exit block manifests as PP intervals surrounding the dropped complexes being two or more times that of the baseline PP interval. This point can distinguish Type 2 second-degree SA exit block from sinus pause (Haghjoo 2017).

Patients with SND are rarely haemodynamically unstable for a prolonged period but atropine, dopamine or adrenalin, as well as temporary cardiac pacing, may be required if unstable. Symptomatic patients with SND may be treated by discontinuing possible offending drugs and/or permanent pacemaker insertion if required (Homoud 2019c).

Key Point

Tachy-brady syndrome (see Figure 11.4) results from abnormal automaticity and conduction within the atrial tissue and commonly affects patients with SND. It is identified by bradycardia alternating with paroxysmal supraventricular arrhythmias, the most frequent being AF or atrial flutter (Dakkak and Doukky 2019). With abrupt cessation of the tachycardia, prolonged bradycardia or asystole occurs because of exaggerated overdrive suppression of abnormal pacemakers (Haghjoo 2017).

Suggested Resource

The following video gives a good explanation of types of SND and shows ECG examples:
Advanced EKGs – Sinus node dysfunction
Strong Medicine (2015)
https://youtu.be/H6yTQm2h8dc

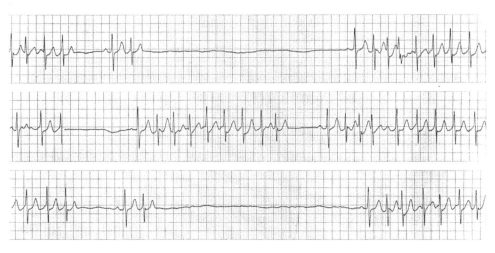

Figure 11.4 Tachy-brady syndrome. *Source:* Burns (2019).

Atrial Dysrhythmias

Non-sinus Supraventricular Rhythms

Non-sinus supraventricular rhythms are those that arise in the atria or the atrioventricular junction and adjacent tissue. These are shown in Figure 11.5 and discussed below.

Ectopic Atrial Rhythms

An ectopic atrial rhythm may occur when an ectopic focus in the atrium becomes the dominant pacemaker. The cause may be sinus node failure with development of an atrial escape rhythm that usually operates at 30–60 bpm or an ectopic focus that generates impulses faster that the SA node and therefore suppresses SA node impulse generation. As the ectopic focus is outside of the sinus node, the direction of atrial activation may be different and the P-wave morphology, axis and duration will depend on the site of the ectopic focus in the atrium (Prutkin 2019). The QRS complex will still be the same as the impulse follows the same pathway through the ventricles.

Atrial Tachycardia

Non-sinus atrial tachycardia (AT) refers to a rhythm above 100 bpm where there is a single (unifocal) ectopic focus within the atria that has a consistent P-wave of abnormal shape and/or size that falls before a narrow, regular QRS complex (Banchs 2018). Heart rates are highly variable in atrial tachycardia producing a rate usually between 100 and 250 (Kaplan and Lala 2019). AT is the least common of the SVTs and does not require the AV node, accessory pathways or ventricular tissue for initiation and maintenance (Budzikowski 2017). ATs can be classified as focal or macro-re-entrant. Focal ATs are thought to be due to automaticity although micro-re-entry and triggered activity (often found in digoxin toxicity), whereas macro-re-entrant atrial tachycardias involve a re-entry circuit within the atria itself. Paroxysmal atrial tachycardia (PAT) refers to episodic AT with an abrupt onset and termination.

Adenosine can be helpful in the diagnosis of AT and is usually effective in terminating focal AT, but not likely to be effective in re-entrant

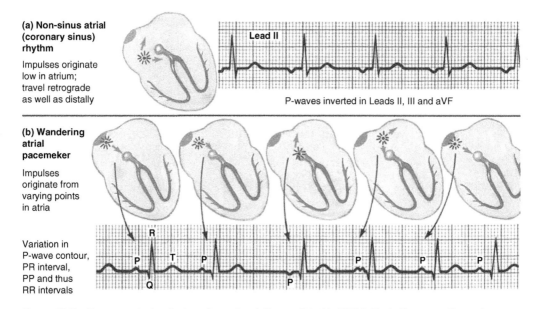

Figure 11.5 Supraventricular rhythms (non-sinus). *Source:* Scheidt (1986). Basic Electrocardiography. Novartis Medical Education. U.S.A. Copyright Novartis A.G. Used with permission.

Supraventricular rhythms

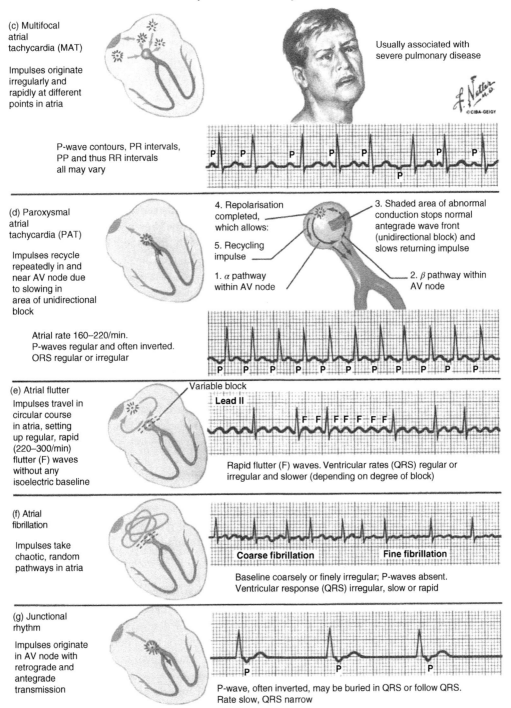

(c) Multifocal atrial tachycardia (MAT)

Impulses originate irregularly and rapidly at different points in atria

Usually associated with severe pulmonary disease

P-wave contours, PR intervals, PP and thus RR intervals all may vary

P P P P P P P
P

(d) Paroxysmal atrial tachycardia (PAT)

Impulses recycle repeatedly in and near AV node due to slowing in area of unidirectional block

4. Repolarisation completed, which allows:

5. Recycling impulse

1. α pathway within AV node

3. Shaded area of abnormal conduction stops normal antegrade wave front (unidirectional block) and slows returning impulse

2. β pathway within AV node

Atrial rate 160–220/min. P-waves regular and often inverted. ORS regular or irregular

P P P P P P P P P P P

(e) Atrial flutter

Impulses travel in circular course in atria, setting up regular, rapid (220–300/min) flutter (F) waves without any isoelectric baseline

Variable block

Lead II

F F F F F F F F

Rapid flutter (F) waves. Ventricular rates (QRS) regular or irregular and slower (depending on degree of block)

(f) Atrial fibrillation

Impulses take chaotic, random pathways in atria

Coarse fibrillation   **Fine fibrillation**

Baseline coarsely or finely irregular; P-waves absent. Ventricular response (QRS) irregular, slow or rapid

(g) Junctional rhythm

Impulses originate in AV node with retrograde and antegrade transmission

P   P   P

P-wave, often inverted, may be buried in QRS or follow QRS. Rate slow, QRS narrow

Figure 11.5   (Continued)

AT. If the diagnosis of AT is established, intravenous beta-blockers, diltiazem or verapamil are recommended to treat haemodynamically stable patients. If these are not effective, amiodarone may be helpful in slowing the ventricular rate. In unstable patients with focal AT, synchronised DCCV is recommended (Page et al. 2016). Non-pharmacological treatments are cardioversion, catheter ablation or surgical ablation in patients with complex congenital heart disease. Atrial tachycardia (AT) is associated with increased morbidity and mortality in adults with congenital heart disease, particularly after surgery for correction of congenital or valvular heart disease. In patients with structurally normal hearts, atrial tachycardia is associated with a low mortality rate (Budzikowski 2017).

Key Point

Atrial tachyarrhythmias with aberration may also present with a broad complex. Table 11.2 shows ECG criteria to differentiate VT from SVT in broad complex tachycardias.

Wandering Atrial Pacemaker

Wandering atrial pacemaker (WAP) is present when there are three or more P-waves that differ in morphology (Figure 11.5b). WAP is due to ectopic foci within the atrial myocardium that serve as dominant pacemakers that discharge in random fashion at a rate of less than 100 bpm. If the rate is above 100 bpm, the rhythm is called multifocal atrial tachycardia. As the rhythm is irregular, it may be mistaken for atrial fibrillation. It may also be confused with sinus rhythm with multifocal premature atrial contractions (Prutkin 2019).

Multifocal Atrial Tachycardia

Multifocal atrial tachycardia (MAT) is characterised by a rate above 100 bpm, at least three morphologically distinct P-waves, irregular PP intervals and an isoelectric baseline between the P-waves (Figure 11.5c) (Tandon et al. 2015). If the rate is less than 100 bpm, this rhythm is

referred to as wandering atrial pacemaker. MAT may be asymptomatic, or presentation symptoms may include palpitations, breathlessness, chest pain, lightheadedness and syncope. Symptoms usually improve when the underlying condition is treated, and MAT controlled. Morbidity is difficult to quantify because the underlying disease is the primary determinant of complications. Diltiazem or verapamil decrease the atrial activity and slow atrioventricular (AV) nodal conduction, thereby decreasing ventricular rate, but they do not return all patients to normal sinus rhythm. Beta-blockers are usually contraindicated due to the presence of chronic pulmonary disease in this patient cohort. Due to the multiple atrial foci, direct current (DC) cardioversion is not effective in restoring normal sinus rhythm and can precipitate more dangerous arrhythmias and thus contraindicated in MAT. AV-nodal ablation and permanent pacemaker implantation can be considered for people with persistent MAT (Tandon et al. 2015).

Atrial Fibrillation

AF is the most common sustained cardiac arrhythmia in clinical practice and is associated with an increased risk for death, heart failure, hospitalisation and thromboembolic events. AF is associated with several chronic diseases, including coronary disease, valvular heart disease, heart failure, hypertrophic cardiomyopathy, congenital heart disease, venous thromboembolic disease, chronic obstructive pulmonary disease and chronic kidney disease. AF is also associated with several risk factors for coronary disease including hypertension, obesity and diabetes (Ganz 2019). Sedentary lifestyle is a risk for AF, and conversely, athletes who undertake long-term endurance training are also at increased risk for AF. Obstructive sleep apnoea is common among patients with AF and may be a contributor to the initiation and progression of AF (Calkins et al. 2017). There also appears to be a genetic component: having a family member with AF is associated with a 40% increased risk for the arrhythmia (Lubitz et al. 2010). Potentially reversible causes of AF include surgery (particularly cardiac surgery); hyperthyroidism, inflammation and infection. Modest amounts of alcohol can trigger AF in some patients and AF commonly occurs in binge drinkers. Most cases occur during and following weekends or holidays when alcohol intake is increased and thus termed the 'the holiday heart syndrome' (Ganz 2019).

AF may be paroxysmal (self-terminating or intermittent); persistent (fails to self-terminate in 7 days); long-standing persistent (lasted more than 12 months) or permanent (a decision has been made to not pursue a rhythm control strategy). Paroxysmal AF commonly precedes chronic AF. Both symptomatic and asymptomatic episodes of AF are common.

The diagnosis of AF requires an ECG showing the typical pattern of AF with irregular RR intervals and no discernible distinct P-waves. AF occurs when multiple ectopic foci in the atria discharge at up to 600 times/min. There are no discernable P-waves, but small undulating waves (known as fibrillation or fibrillatory waves) appear on the ECG. The AV node is bombarded by electrical impulses from the atria and becomes relatively refractive to conduction, resulting in erratic transmission of impulses through the AV node, and subsequently, an irregular ventricular rhythm. This rhythm is frequently referred to as an 'irregularly irregular' rhythm, meaning there is no discernable pattern to its irregularity (Figure 11.5f).

AF reduces cardiac output due to loss of atrial kick (synchronised atrial mechanical activity), irregularity of ventricular response and an inappropriately rapid heart rate. The rapid rate at which the atria depolarise causes a quivering motion rather than effective contraction. This in turn leads to inadequate filling of the ventricles, which results in a fall in cardiac output. See Box 11.1 for a summary of AF management.

Box 11.1   Atrial fibrillation management.

Management guidelines for AF are continually evolving. Most guidelines include management algorithms for acute and chronic AF and the most recently available guidelines should be consulted. Management of AF may be based upon either a rhythm or rate control strategy. A rate control strategy is favoured in patients with minimal symptoms or in those in whom attempts at maintaining sinus rhythm are likely to be or are futile.

Most patients with new onset AF present with symptoms relating to the arrhythmia. Management issues include prevention of systemic embolisation and rhythm or rate control to reduce symptoms (Kumar 2019). The use of DCCV or pharmacological cardioversion from AF will depend upon individual circumstances, and in acute cases on haemodynamic stability or failure of pharmacological cardioversion. Most recently, AF management guidelines suggest a more integrated approach using the "ABC method": A Anticoagulation, Avoid stroke; B Better symptom control; C Comorbidities, Cardiovascular risk factors (Hindricks et al. 2021).

Pharmacotherapy

See Chapter 12 to review antiarrhythmic drugs used in AF and refer to current professional guidelines.

Anticoagulation

Warfarin and novel oral anticoagulants (NOACs) dabigatran, rivaroxaban, apixaban or edoxaban are commonly used to reduce the risk of ischaemic stroke and other embolic events in paroxysmal and permanent AF but use of anticoagulants must be balanced against the risk of bleeding. Tools to calculate risk scores for assessing the benefit from stroke reduction or the increase in bleeding risk with anticoagulation are available to guide clinicians, but do not have a high predictive ability. The CHA_2DS_2-VASc score is the most frequently used model worldwide. The risk of ischaemic stroke or peripheral embolisation (without antithrombotic therapy) increases as the number of risk factors in the risk score increase (Manning et al. 2017). Anticoagulation is not recommended for a score of 0 and is recommended for a score of 1 or greater in men and 2 or greater in women (Hindricks et al. 2021). If anticoagulation is indicated, novel oral anticoagulants are recommended in preference to warfarin (Brieger et al. 2018), but the choice of anticoagulant should be based on individual patient characteristics and patient choice.

Cardioversion

In the case of rapid AF and haemodynamic instability, electrical (DC) cardioversion may be required. Electrical cardioversion may also be used if pharmacological cardioversion fails or in haemodynamically stable patients at low thromboembolic risk (Brieger et al. 2018). In stable patients, DCCV may be indicated in new onset AF, AF that is rate controlled but with persistent symptoms, and where previous cardioversion has resulted in sinus rhythm being maintained for a reasonable length of time between procedures (Page et al. 2016).

Cardiac ablation

Catheter ablation is an effective treatment for AF and may be indicated in symptomatic, drug-refractory atrial fibrillation. The major benefits of AF ablation are improvement in survival and quality of life and decreased risk of stroke and heart failure. The procedure does, however, does

carry a significant risk of complications, some of which might result in life-long disability and/or death. Potential complications include cardiac tamponade, aortic puncture or tear, pericarditis or pericardial effusion, trans-ischaemic attack, or stroke, myocardial ischaemia or infarction, pulmonary vein stenosis, pharyngeal trauma, aspiration pneumonia, oesophageal perforation or haematoma, atrio-oesophageal fistula, gastroparesis (vagal nerve injury), gastric tear, phrenic nerve palsy, urethral stricture and atonic bladder (Voskoboinik et al. 2018). A decision to perform catheter or surgical AF ablation should only be made after a patient carefully considers the risks, benefits and alternatives to the procedure (Calkins et al. 2017).

Anticoagulation

Anticoagulants should not be interrupted during the procedure. Warfarin discontinuation with low-molecular-weight heparin bridging and short NOAC interruption are associated with an increased risk of cerebral thromboembolic complications. In studies of patients undergoing cardiac ablation, the risk of major bleed is double that in patients treated with uninterrupted warfarin compared with uninterrupted NOACs (Cardoso et al. 2018).

Follow-up

An integrated care approach should be adopted, delivered by multidisciplinary teams, including patient education and the use of eHealth tools and resources where available (Brieger et al. 2018). Traditional risk factors for CVD (see Chapter 5) should be managed to reduce AF burden and improve quality of life for people with AF (Brieger et al. 2018). Regular monitoring and feedback of risk factor control, treatment adherence and AF persistence should occur. Anticoagulation requirements should be reviewed at every follow-up appointment.

Atrial Flutter

Atrial flutter is a macro-re-entrant arrhythmia characterised by atrial rates between 240 and 400 bpm. It is best defined by the presence of uniform atrial activation known as 'flutter waves' that appear in a characteristic 'saw-tooth' pattern on the ECG (Figure 11.5e), with P-waves best visualised in Leads II, III, aVF or V1. The atrial rate is faster than the ventricular rate. Commonly, there is a 2:1 conduction ratio, although the block can be 4:1, or less commonly 3:1 or 5:1. The conduction rate may vary, known as 'variable block'.

Atrial flutter is divided into two types:

- Typical atrial flutter has a rate between 240 and 340 bpm and involves a single counter-clockwise re-entrant circuit that encircles the tricuspid valve annulus in the right atrium. A clockwise re-entrant pathway is less commonly seen.
- Atypical atrial flutter follows a different circuit that may involve the right or the left atrium.

Key Point

Flutter waves for typical atrial flutter are inverted (negative) in Leads II, III, aVF and V1 because of a counterclockwise re-entrant pathway, but may be upright (positive) when the re-entrant loop is clockwise.

Atrial flutter can occur in clinical settings like those associated with AF, and it is common for AF and atrial flutter to coexist in the same patient. Atrial flutter can be triggered by AT or AF. Patients with atrial flutter are thought to have the same risk of thromboembolism as patients with AF; thus, the recommendations for anticoagulation associated with pharmacological or electrical cardioversion are the same as for patients with AF. Synchronised DCCV is recommended for acute treatment of patients with atrial flutter who are haemodynamically unstable and unresponsive to pharmacological treatment.

Key Point

When using DCCV in rate-controlled patients with atrial flutter, be prepared for potential bradycardia and hypotension following reversion to sinus rhythm.

A rhythm control strategy is often chosen in the longer term as rate control is difficult in atrial flutter. Catheter ablation is often preferred to long-term pharmacological therapy (Page et al. 2016).

Key Point

As many patients with atrial flutter have periods of AF, risk assessment of atrial flutter patients should use current atrial AF risk scores for anticoagulation (Manning et al. 2017). Follow the AF guidelines for anticoagulation (pre- and post-procedure) when undertaking DCCV or cardiac ablation in patients with atrial flutter.

Junctional Dysrhythmias

Junctional Escape Rhythm

If the SA node fails, automatic cells in the AV node may take over the function of maintaining the heart's rhythm. This is known as a junctional rhythm. Rhythms originating in the junction have both retrograde (back to the atria) and antegrade (continuing down the bundle branches) conduction. Inverted P-waves may be seen immediately after the QRS or may be obscured by the QRS complex (Figure 11.5g). The intrinsic rate of the junction is about 50 bpm, and this rate will signify that the rhythm is an escape rhythm.

Accelerated Junctional Rhythm and Junctional Tachycardia

Junctional rhythms originate in the AV node and have both retrograde and antegrade conduction. The P-wave is often inverted and may be obscured by the QRS or follow the QRS (Figure 11.5g). Junctional tachycardia (JT), also known as junctional ectopic tachycardia (JET), is a narrow-complex tachycardia with typical rates of 120–220 bpm that is often mistaken for other rhythms. Occasionally, it may be irregular. The mechanism for JT is enhanced automaticity. Non-paroxysmal JT (accelerated AV junctional rhythm) occurs at a rate of 70–130 bpm and is more common in adults than paroxysmal junctional tachycardia. It is often due to digoxin toxicity or MI (Page et al. 2016). It is difficult to distinguish between JT and atrioventricular nodal re-entry tachycardia (AVNRT) as they share many common characteristics, but they have different mechanisms: AVNRT is due to re-entry and JT is usually due to enhanced automaticity from an ectopic focus in the AV junction (Chen et al. 2015).

> **Key Point**
>
> Junctional tachycardia is uncommon in adults and is usually benign. It is typically seen in infants after cardiac surgery for congenital heart disease children with a high rate of death due to heart failure or an uncontrollable, incessant tachyarrhythmia (Page et al. 2016).

Beta-blockers may be used for the treatment of JT, and diltiazem, verapamil or procainamide if beta-blockers are ineffective (Page et al. 2016).

> **Suggested Resource**
>
> Basic electrophysiology, part 8 – Junctional rhythms
> 32bravo711 (2016)
> https://youtu.be/NbeGjPE8qd0

Ventricular Rhythms and Tachyarrhythmias

Mechanisms of VAs include enhanced normal automaticity, abnormal automaticity, triggered activity induced by early or late afterdepolarisations, and re-entry (Al-Khatib et al. 2018). Ventricular rhythms have been described in Table 11.2.

Common causes of VAs include ischaemic heart disease, structural heart disease (including cardiomyopathies), congenital structural cardiac disorders, acquired and inherited channelopathies, electrolyte imbalances (hypokalaemia, hypomagnesaemia, hypocalcaemia), some antiarrhythmic medications, sympathomimetic agents, including intravenous inotropes and illicit drugs such as methamphetamine or cocaine (Compton 2017). Ventricular tachycardia (VT) and ventricular fibrillation (VF) are the most common cause of sudden death. VAs can be seen as a spectrum of arrhythmias that range from a ventricular premature beat (VPB) to ventricular fibrillation (VF) (see Table 11.2).

Ventricular Premature Beats (VPBs)

Sporadic occurrence of VPBs is not uncommon in the general population and occurs increasingly with age. Conditions in which VBPs are commonly seen include ischaemic heart

Table 11.2 The spectrum of ventricular arrhythmias.

Ventricular premature beats

VPB, also called premature ventricular complex (PVC) (see Figure 11.6).	A VBP is an ectopic firing of a focus within the ventricles that bypasses the His-Purkinje system and depolarises the ventricles directly. A VPB occurs earlier than would be expected for the next sinus impulse. The QRS complex is abnormally wide ($\geq 120\,ms$) and morphologically bizarre due to abnormal and delayed conduction. VPBs arising from the right ventricle have LBBB; those arising from the left ventricle have RBBB and there is discordance between the ST-segment and T-wave (see Figure 11.6). Discordance, a pattern of repolarisation abnormality in which the direction of the ST-segment and T-wave are opposite to the main vector of the QRS complex, is seen. An inverted P-wave may be seen after the QRS if there is atrial capture due to retrograde conduction. VPBs may be unifocal (same QRS morphology originating from the same ventricular focus) or multifocal (different QRS morphology originating from different foci in the ventricle) if more than one VPB is seen. The VPB is usually followed by a full compensatory pause (the next normal beat arrives after an interval that is equal to double the preceding RR interval
Couplets	Two consecutive VPBs. These may be unifocal or multifocal.
Salvos	Three or more consecutive VPBs. Technically this fits the definition of non-sustained VT (below) but in practice usually describes five beats or less
Ventricular bigeminy/trigeminy/ quadrigeminy	Used to describe a pattern of regularly recurring VPBs (every second beat a VPB = bigeminy; every third beat = trigeminy; every fourth beat = quadrigeminy). VPBs may reoccur regularly but with less frequency (every fifth beat etc.)
R on T phenomenon	The R-wave of the VPB falls on the T-wave of the preceding complex (the vulnerable part of the cardiac cycle) that may trigger VF

Ventricular rhythms (other than tachycardias)

Idioventricular rhythm (IVR)	When the SA node is blocked or depressed, latent pacemakers (can be atrial, junctional or ventricular) can generate escape beats or an 'escape' rhythm. When the ventricle generates the rhythm, it is known as 'IVR' or 'ventricular escape rhythm' (Figure 11.7a). IVR is a slow and regular rhythm and has a rate of less than 50 bpm. P-waves are absent, and the QRS interval is prolonged (Gangwani and Nagalli 2021)
Accelerated ventricular rhythm	Usually presents at a rate between 50 and 100 bpm and typically occurs with underlying ischaemic or structural heart disease (Figure 11.7b). Often seen as a 'reperfusion arrhythmia'. Treatment is not usually required unless the AVR is prolonged with haemodynamic compromise

(Continued)

Table 11.2 (Continued)

Ventricular tachycardias	
Non-sustained VT	More than three beats that terminate spontaneously
Sustained VT	Lasts more than 30 s or requires termination due to haemodynamic compromise in less than 30 s (Al-Khatib et al. 2018)
Monomorphic VT	The QRS originates from a single ventricular focus and the rhythm has identical QRS complexes (see Figure 11.7c)
Bidirectional VT	The QRS has an alternating frontal plane axis from beat to beat (alternating positive and negative complexes). Bidirectional VT is most often seen in the setting of digitalis toxicity or catecholaminergic polymorphic VT
Polymorphic VT	The QRS originates from multiple ventricular foci and change shape or have multiple forms
Torsades de Pointes (TdP)	A type of polymorphic VT that occurs with QT prolongation. The name is derived from the appearance of the QRS complexes that appear to twist around the isoelectric line (see Figure 11.8). Both QT-prolongation and polymorphic VT must be present for a diagnosis of TdP.
Catecholaminergic polymorphic VT (CPVT)	This is a polymorphic VT that can be triggered by stress, exercise, strong emotional states and catecholamine administration. Patients may present with syncope or with sudden cardiac death if CPVT degrades into VF (Compton 2017).
VT (electrical) storm	VT storm (also referred to as electric or arrhythmic storm) can be defined as 'a state of cardiac electrical instability that is defined by ≥3 episodes of sustained VT, VF or appropriate shocks from an ICD within 24 h' (Al-Khatib et al. 2018).
Ventricular flutter	A regular ventricular arrhythmia with around 300 complexes/minute. Complexes have a monomorphic sine wave appearance and no isoelectric interval between successive QRS complexes (Al-Khatib et al. 2018).
Ventricular fibrillation	Rapid, grossly irregular electrical activity with marked variability in electrocardiographic waveform, ventricular rate usually >300 bpm (cycle length: <200 ms) (Al-Khatib et al. 2018).

disease, structural heart disease, congenital heart disease, pulmonary diseases, sleep apnoea and endocrine disorders. Stimulants including nicotine, alcohol, sympathomimetic agents or illicit drugs (cocaine, amphetamines) can trigger VPBs (Manolis 2019). VPBs produce few or no symptoms and rarely cause haemodynamic compromise unless they occur frequently in a patient with severely depressed LV function or when associated with an underlying bradycardia. Frequent VPBs can, however, cause a reversible cardiomyopathy and increase the risk of developing systolic heart failure (Manolis 2019).

Palpitations is the most common symptom. Patients often report 'missing a beat' due to the post-VPB pause or intermittently 'feeling a thud', which occurs because of the hypercontractility of the post-VPB beat. The sensation produced by ectopic beats often causes anxiety and in turn, a

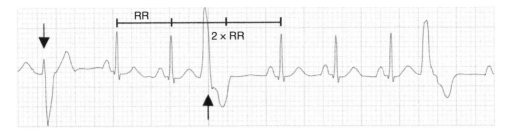

Figure 11.6 Ventricular premature beat. *Source:* Burns (2019). #FOAMed Medical Education Resources by LITFL. https://litfl.com/wp-content/uploads/2018/08/multifocal-PVC.jpg. Accessed under the Creative Commons Attribution-Share Alike 4.0 Unported license. https://creativecommons.org/licenses/by-nc-sa/4.0/.

Ventricular rhythms

QRS >0.10 s: No P-waves (ventricular impulse origin)

(a) Rate <40/min: idioventricular rhythm

(b) Rate 40–120: accelerated idioventricular rhythm (AIVR)

Short bursts (usually <20 s) of AIVR, often a few days after MI. Usually asymptomatic with no progression to ventricular tachycardia or ventricular fibrillation

(c) Rate >120: ventricular tachycardia

Infarct

Slowed conduction in margin of ischaemic area permits circular course of impulse and re-entry with rapid repetitive depolarisation

Rapid, bizarre, wide QRS complexes

(d) Ventricular fibrillation

Chaotic ventricular depolarisation

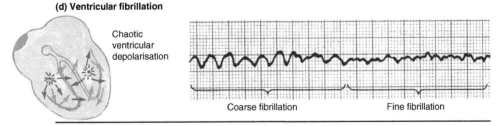

Coarse fibrillation   Fine fibrillation

Figure 11.7 Ventricular rhythms. *Source:* Scheidt (1986). Basic Electrocardiography. Novartis Medical Education. U.S.A. Copyright Novartis A.G. Used with permission.

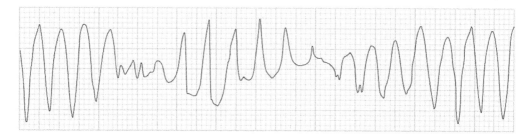

Figure 11.8 Torsades de Pointes. *Source:* #FOAMed Medical Education Resources by LITFL. https://litfl.com/wp-content/uploads/2018/08/ECG-strip-Torsades-de-pointes-TDP.jpg. Accessed under the Creative Commons Attribution-Share Alike 4.0 Unported license. https://creativecommons.org/licenses/by-nc-sa/4.0/.

catecholamine surge provoked by anxiety may cause additional ectopy and palpitations. Awareness of ectopic beats often is increased during periods of rest and patients often report that they are worse when lying on their left side as this brings the heart closer to the chest wall.

Correctable causes of VPBs should be identified and addressed. A twelve-lead ECG forms part of the standard evaluation of VPBs, but they may not always be present at the time the ECG is undertaken. Unexplained VPBs should be investigated using Holter monitoring (see Chapter 8) to quantify frequency and characterises of the ectopic beats. Echocardiography should be undertaken to detect any abnormalities in cardiac structure and function. An exercise stress test (EST) should be used to evaluate the response of VPBs to exercise, whether VT can be induced with exercise, and screen for underlying myocardial ischaemia (see Chapter 8).

Management of VBPs depends upon underlying causes and patient symptoms. For patients who are symptomatic despite avoidance of known triggers, therapeutic options include antiarrhythmic medications or radiofrequency catheter ablation (see Chapter 12). Beta-blockers are usually the first line of treatment unless contraindicated (Manolis 2019).

Idioventricular Rhythm

Idioventricular rhythm (IVR) (see Figure 11.7a) is an escape rhythm originating in the ventricles that occurs in response to a failure of SA node and AV nodal pacemakers to function.

The rate is usually less than 40bpm and the rhythm is usually transient. If IVR persists, symptomatic hypotension may occur. As with escape beats, the underlying pathology and symptoms will dictate whether treatment is required.

Accelerated IVR (AIVR) (Figure 11.7b) results when the rate of an ectopic ventricular pacemaker exceeds that of the sinus node. AIVR is often seen in the setting of acute myocardial infarction during reperfusion.

Ventricular Tachycardia

VT is present when three or more consecutive complexes originating in the ventricles occur in rapid succession at a rate that is greater than 100bpm (see Figure 11.7c). VT is often preceded by ectopic beats. The causes of VT include those of VBPs. Additionally, scarring due to MI or cardiac surgery can predispose to VT. Inherited channelopathies (long QT Syndrome, short QT syndrome, Brugada syndrome and CPVT) predispose to VT and VF. Acquired channelopathies commonly resulting from drugs that prolong the QT interval and those that slow myocardial conduction (see Chapter 12) may also promote re-entrant VT. Hypokalaemia and hypomagnesaemia may also predispose patients to VT and VF, particularly those with pre-existing structural heart disease (Compton 2017).

Monomorphic VT

Ventricular tachycardia is always serious, and the rate may be so fast that adequate ventricular filling is not possible. Because coronary blood flow occurs predominantly during diastole, high heart rates reduce filling time, resulting in poor coronary blood flow and myocardial ischaemia. VT can lead to heart failure and shock with pulmonary oedema and requires urgent treatment. There is a high risk of VT deteriorating to ventricular fibrillation (VF) and cardiac arrest. Initial management of a patient with VT will depend upon haemodynamic stability.

Haemodynamically Stable Monomorphic VT

Occasionally, VT will occur for periods where there is no haemodynamic decompensation, but VT may deteriorate into unstable states and more malignant arrhythmias without warning. Initial treatment is cardioversion with antiarrhythmic therapy (amiodarone, lignocaine or procainamide) or DCCV (Ganz and Buxton 2018).

Haemodynamically Unstable but Responsive Monomorphic VT

Patients with VT who are haemodynamically unstable but still responsive with a discernible blood pressure and pulse should have urgent cardioversion following administration of sedation. Patients should initially be treated with a synchronised 100-joule shock from a biphasic defibrillator (200-joules if using a monophasic defibrillator), with escalating energy levels for subsequent shocks if required (Ganz and Buxton 2018).

Haemodynamically Unstable Pulseless Monomorphic VT

A patient with VT who is haemodynamically unstable and pulseless should be managed with a synchronised shock at maximal energy and cardiopulmonary resuscitation (CPR). Subsequent shocks, if required, should be at the highest output available on the defibrillator (Ganz and Buxton 2018). Advanced cardiac life support (ACLS) resuscitation algorithms should be followed (see Chapter 20).

Polymorphic VT

Some episodes of polymorphic VT cause haemodynamic collapse and degenerate into VF, but many episodes terminate spontaneously. Patients with haemodynamically unstable or pulseless polymorphic VT require defibrillation.

Long-term treatment for VT depends on the reversibility or trigger/s or susceptibility to further ventricular arrhythmias. Pharmacological management may be adequate for some patients, whereas others may choose or require VT ablation. Patients without a reversible cause of sustained VT will likely need an implantable cardioverter defibrillator (ICD) (see Chapter 12).

Key Point

It is sometimes difficult to distinguish between VT and a broad complex SVT. Although VT is more likely than SVT to cause hypotension and haemodynamic instability, the haemodynamic stability of a patient isn't necessarily helpful in distinguishing between VT and SVT (Vereckei 2014). Many patients tolerate VT and SVT, whilst patients with underlying disease processes may be unstable with VT or SVT. Table 11.3 displays ECG criteria to help distinguish between the VT and SVT.

Ventricular Fibrillation

Ventricular fibrillation results in cardiac arrest and if left untreated is rapidly fatal. Usually simple to recognise, VF (Figure 11.7d) occurs when portions of the ventricular myocardium depolarise independently of each other, at a fast, irregular rate. Co-ordinated ventricular activity and muscular contraction is replaced by a quivering motion, thus cardiac output is critically compromised. Irregular, chaotic and abnormal deflections of varying height and width are evident on the ECG, with no identifiable QRS complexes. VF is most seen in the early phase of MI, often occurring following a ventricular ectopic beat that interferes with repolarisation (R on T ectopic). As discussed above, VF can be precipitated by an episode of VT, which can degenerate into VF.

> **Key Point**
>
> Multiple recurrences of ventricular arrhythmias over a short period of time (typically 24 h) are referred to as 'electrical storm' or 'arrhythmic storm'. In most instances, the arrhythmia is ventricular tachycardia (VT), but polymorphic VT and ventricular fibrillation (VF) can also result in electrical storm. The arrhythmias can be self-terminating but frequently are terminated using antiarrhythmic drugs or device-related therapies (defibrillation or anti-tachycardia pacing).
>
> 'Incessant VT' is defined as haemodynamically stable VT which persists for longer than 1 h (Passman 2019).

> **Learning activity 11.1**
>
> Find an ECG with a broad complex tachycardia. Visit the website below and work through the various criteria provided for differentiating between VT and SVT.

> **Suggested resource**
>
> Life in the Fastlane (LIFL)
> https://litfl.com/vt-versus-svt-ecg-library/

Asystole

Asystole refers to the absence of cardiac output and ventricular depolarisation and it eventually occurs in all dying patients. It may occur as a primary condition as a result of the failure of the heart's electrical system to generate a ventricular depolarisation due to conditions such as ischaemia or degeneration of the conducting system. Primary asystole is usually preceded by a bradyarrhythmia due to sinus node block-arrest, complete heart block or both. Secondary asystole is due to factors other than the failure

of the heart's conducting system to generate an impulse. Severe tissue hypoxia with metabolic acidosis is usually the common pathway and the outcome is generally poor. Asystole is the terminal rhythm following unresolved VF (Shah 2020). The management of cardiac arrest due to asystole is covered in Chapter 20.

> **Suggested Resource**
>
> The ECG course – Ventricular rhythms
> The Resuscitationist (2014)
> https://youtu.be/L83yVPXiLSk

Heart Block Related to Atrioventricular Nodal Conduction

Atrioventricular block occurs when there is a delay or failure in impulse conduction from the atria to the ventricles. It may be transient or permanent and can be classified as first, second or third degree (see Figure 11.9).

First-degree AV Block

Atrial conduction is prolonged in first-degree block (Figure 11.9d). The rate is usually within normal limits, so technically first-degree block is not a bradycardia, but it is practical to consider along with other AV blocks. The impulse is delayed passing through the AV node to the ventricles, resulting in prolongation of the PR interval on the ECG. A QRS complex follows every P-wave, and the rhythm is regular. A prolonged conduction time is frequently found in athletes and older people. First-degree block can also present in patients on beta-blocker therapy, with digoxin toxicity and electrolyte disturbance, such as hyperkalaemia. It is also associated with myocardial ischaemia, myocardial infarction (MI), myocarditis and hypoxia.

If the heart rate is normal and the patient is unaffected, there is no need for treatment. If, however, the block is associated with organic heart disease, such as MI, the patient might be

Atrioventricular conduction variations

(a) Fixed normal PR interval
    Sinus rhythm

(b) Fixed but short PR interval
    1. Junctional or coronary sinus rhythm
    2. Wolff–Parkinson–White syndrome

(c) P wave related to each QRS complex, but variable PR interval
    1. Wandering atrial pacemaker
    2. Multifocal atrial tachycardia

(d) Fixed but prolonged PR interval
    First-degree AV block

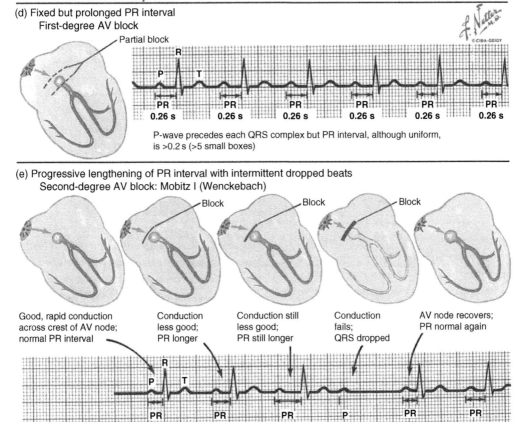

(e) Progressive lengthening of PR interval with intermittent dropped beats
    Second-degree AV block: Mobitz I (Wenckebach)

(f) Sudden dropped QRS without prior PR lengthening
    Second-degree AV block: Mobitz II (non-Wenckebach)

Figure 11.9 Atrioventricular conduction variations. *Source:* Scheidt (1986). Basic Electrocardiography. Novartis Medical Education. U.S.A. Copyright Novartis A.G. Used with permission.

at risk of progressing to second- or third-degree block and should be observed accordingly.

Second-degree AV Block

There are two types of second-degree AV heart block: Mobitz type I (Wenckebach) and Mobitz Type II.

Mobitz Type I (Wenckebach)

In Mobitz type 1 AV block, commonly referred to as Wenckebach, there is a progressive prolongation of the PR interval over several heart beats (Figure 11.9e). The phenomenon repeats itself with a gradual lengthening of the PR interval over three to six beats until an impulse is totally blocked, and the P wave occurs without a corresponding QRS complex, and a pause ensues. The resulting ventricular rhythm is irregular, but follows a predictable, cyclical pattern. The rate can be normal but is often slow, varying from 75 down to 40 bpm. Second-degree heart block is usually localised to the AV node. It is characteristically periodic and of shorter duration than Mobitz type II block. It may be seen in acute or chronic ischaemia involving the conduction system, cardiomyopathy, myocarditis, endocarditis, hyperkalaemia, vagotonia and following cardiac surgery or cardiac ablation. It may also be associated with AV nodal blocking medications and is commonly seen in digoxin overdose. Treatment involves reversal of underlying causes, such as avoidance of AV nodal blocking drugs or treatment of ischaemia. Mobitz type I AV block does not usually cause haemodynamic compromise, but if haemodynamic compromise does occur, atropine may be used, followed by transcutaneous pacing if required. It does not usually require pacing unless there is evidence of haemodynamic instability. Atropine may also be used followed by transcutaneous pacing if required. If the patient remains unstable, transvenous pacing may be required. Hypotension may need treatment with dopamine or dobutamine. If no reversible cause of the arrhythmia is found, or if symptoms persist despite treatment of reversible causes, permanent pacing may be required (Sauer 2019a).

Mobitz Type II

Mobitz type II heart block is characterised by occasional non-conducted P-waves without a preceding lengthening of the PR interval (Figure 11.9f). The 'dropped' beat can occur irregularly or regularly every second, third or fourth beat and in this case is referred to as 2:1, 3:1, 4:1 AV block, respectively. The block in conduction occurs beneath the AV node in the bundle of His or bilaterally in the bundle branches. It is less common than Mobitz type I but is frequently associated with haemodynamic compromise when it occurs and often progresses to complete heart block.

Causes and treatment of Mobitz type II AV block are like those for Mobitz type I (Sauer 2019b). In the setting of MI, Mobitz type II block is often associated with irreversible myocardial damage, and deterioration to complete AV block is common. Prophylactic temporary pacing is used to avert the need for pacemaker insertion in a compromised patient in case complete heart block develop suddenly.

Third-degree (Complete) AV Block

In third-degree or 'complete' heart block (CHB) (Figure 11.10a), there is no conduction from the atria to the ventricles. In most cases, the pacemaker function is taken over by a focus below the block acting as a 'safety net', with the heartbeat sustained by impulses from the area around the AV node, or the ventricles. The QRS complex can be either broad or narrow depending on the site where the impulses are being generated. A nodal rhythm gives a rate of around 40–60 beats with a narrow complex, whereas a ventricular rhythm gives a rate of 15–40 bpm with broad complexes (Figure 11.10a). If an 'escape' rhythm fails to develop, ventricular standstill will occur, and the patient will require immediate resuscitation.

The atrial rate may be normal and regular, and the ventricular rate is also regular, but impulse transmission between the atria and ventricles is absent. The P-wave does not precede a QRS complex on the ECG. The lower down the conduction pathway an escape rhythm is generated, the slower the ventricular rate will be and less well tolerated by the patient.

Causes for third-degree (complete) AV block are like those of second-degree AV block. Many antihypertensive, antianginal, antiarrhythmic, and heart failure medications can cause AV block. Potentially aggravating or causative medications should be withdrawn (Agrawal and Guzman 2018). When associated with inferior MI, drug toxicity, acute pericarditis or myocarditis, total AV block is usually a transient phenomenon, although temporary pacing may be required if the patient is symptomatic or haemodynamically compromised (see Chapter 12). The clinical presentation of CHB is variable depending upon the rate of the underlying escape rhythm and the presence of comorbid conditions (Sauer 2019c), but few patients who acutely develop third degree AV block are asymptomatic. Most are haemodynamically unstable and cardiovascular collapse and death may result. In acute anterior MI, the development of complete heart block usually indicates extensive myocardial damage, and there is immediate danger of impending asystole and requires immediate preparation for temporary pacing (Agrawal and Guzman 2018).

Atropine may be used in haemodynamically patients with caution. If the site of block is in the AV node, atropine may be useful, but if the block is in the His bundle, atropine may lead to an increased atrial rate, and a greater degree of block can occur with a slower ventricular rate. Atropine is unlikely to be successful in wide-complex bradyarrhythmias. In patients with suspected acute MI, atropine can cause increased ventricular irritability and potentially dangerous ventricular arrhythmias (Agrawal and Guzman 2018).

Isoproterenol is more likely to facilitate conduction with a distal level of block compared with atropine, but patients with a distal block are more likely to have a contraindication, such as myocardial ischaemia/infarction. Isoproterenol should only be used as a temporary measure until pacing (preferably transvenous) is initiated (Agrawal and Guzman 2018). Permanent pacing may be required if the arrhythmia is not resolved.

Atrioventricular Dissociation

Atrioventricular dissociation may occur when P-waves and QRS complexes occur independently, with the ventricular rate being higher than the atrial rate (Figure 11.10b). AV dissociation is usually a benign phenomenon that can result from (i) slowing of the dominant pacemaker (sinus node), which allows an escape junctional or ventricular rhythm or (ii) acceleration of a normally slower (subsidiary) pacemaker, such as a junctional site or a ventricular site that activates the ventricles without retrograde atrial capture.

Key Point

Complete heart block may be described as a type of AV dissociation as the atria and ventricles operate independently, but a rhythm is usually labelled AV dissociation when the ventricular rate is faster than the atrial rate.

Suggested Resource

Intro to EKG interpretation – AV block-Strong Medicine (2014) https://youtu.be/iiinZvwBSuE

Suggested Resource

Kusumoto, F.M., Schoenfeld, M. H., Barrett, C. et al. (2019). 2018 ACC/AHA/HRS guideline on the evaluation and management of patients with bradycardia and cardiac conduction delay: a report of the American College of Cardiology/American Heart Association Task Force on Clinical Practice Guidelines and the Heart Rhythm Society. *Circulation* 140 (8): e382–e482. https://doi.org/10.1161/CIR.0000000000000627

Atrioventricular conduction variations

(a) No relationship between P-waves and QRS complexes: QRS rate *slower* than P rate

Third–degree (complete) AV block

1. Impulses originate at both SA node (P-waves) and below site of block in AV node (junctional rhythm) conducting to ventricles

Block

Atria and ventricles depolarize independently. QRS complexes less frequent; regular at 40–55/min but normal in shape

2. Impulses originate at SA node (P-waves) and also below site of block in ventricles (idioventricular rhythm)

Block

Atria and ventricles depolarize independently. QRS complexes less frequent; regular at 20–40/min but wide and abnormal in shape

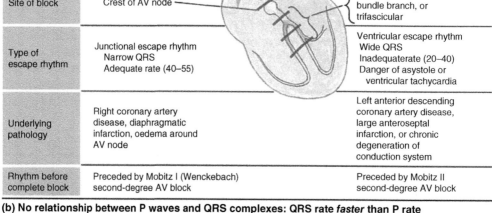

Features of two types of atrioventricular block

	'High'	'Low'
Site of block	Crest of AV node	Bundle of His, bilateral bundle branch, or trifascicular
Type of escape rhythm	Junctional escape rhythm Narrow QRS Adequate rate (40–55)	Ventricular escape rhythm Wide QRS Inadequate rate (20–40) Danger of asystole or ventricular tachycardia
Underlying pathology	Right coronary artery disease, diaphragmatic infarction, oedema around AV node	Left anterior descending coronary artery disease, large anteroseptal infarction, or chronic degeneration of conduction system
Rhythm before complete block	Preceded by Mobitz I (Wenckebach) second-degree AV block	Preceded by Mobitz II second-degree AV block

(b) No relationship between P waves and QRS complexes: QRS rate *faster* than P rate

AV dissociation

Slower supraventricular rhythm

Rapid ventricular rhythm, which does not conduct retrograde to atria or shut off sinus

P-waves less frequent than QRS complexes and totally unrelated to them

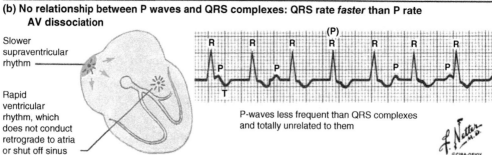

Figure 11.10 Atrioventricular conduction variations: Complete heart block and AV dissociation. *Source:* Scheidt (1986). Basic Electrocardiography. Novartis Medical Education. U.S.A. Copyright Novartis A.G. Used with permission.

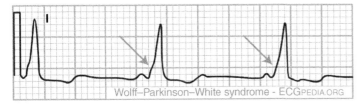

Figure 11.11 Wolff Parkinson White pattern. *Source:* CardioNetworks: De-Rhythm_WPW.png. Accessed under the Creative Commons Attribution-Share Alike 3.0 Unported license. https://creativecommons.org/licenses/by-sa/3.0/deed.en.

Re-entrant Tachycardias

When an accessory pathway is present, conduction from the atria to the ventricles may occur exclusively via the AV node, exclusively via the accessory pathway, or a combination of both (DiBiase and Walsh 2018).

Atrioventricular Re-entrant Tachycardia

Atrioventricular re-entrant (or reciprocating) tachycardia (AVRT) has an anatomically defined circuit that consists of two pathways: the normal AV conduction system and an AV accessory pathway that is necessary for initiation and maintenance of the tachycardia. Differences in conduction time and refractoriness between the normal conduction system and the accessory pathway, and a properly timed premature impulse of atrial, junctional or ventricular origin can initiate re-entry (DiBiase and Walsh 2018). AVRT has two types of accessory pathways: orthodromic or antidromic. If the impulse is conducted down the AV node and up the accessory pathway, the QRS will be narrow (orthodromic AVRT). This accounts for around 95% of cases of AVRT. Rarely, the impulse is conducted down the accessory and up the AV node resulting in a wide QRS (antidromic AVRT) (Goldberger et al. 2018).

Key Point

In narrow QRS orthodromic AVRT, any delta wave that may be seen in sinus rhythm is lost since antegrade conduction is not occurring via the accessory pathway and the ventricle is not pre-excited (DiBiase and Walsh 2018).

Wolff–Parkinson–White (WPW) Syndrome

WPW syndrome is a rare condition most found among those with a first-degree relative with a pre-excitation syndrome. Presentation symptoms for WPW syndrome include palpitations, lightheadedness, dizziness, syncope, chest pain and cardiac arrest (DiBiase and Walsh 2019).

In sinus rhythm, WPW syndrome is associated with a classic ECG pattern of pre-excitation with two major features:

- A short PR interval (less than 0.12 seconds)
- A delta wave (initial slurring of the QRS complex) (see Figure 11.11)

Key Point

A WPW pattern (ECG abnormalities in asymptomatic patients) is more commonly seen than symptomatic WPW syndrome. A WPW pattern may appear intermittently on an ECG and can disappear permanently over time. Identification of a short PR interval and a delta wave confirms the diagnosis of the WPW pattern (DiBiase and Walsh 2019).

Diagnosis of WPW Syndrome

WPW syndrome is typically diagnosed in a patient with a pre-existing WPW pattern on an ECG, who develops an arrhythmia that involves the accessory pathway, though some patients may present with arrhythmia and no known history of the WPW pattern. AVRT is the most frequently occurring re-entrant tachycardia associated with WPW syndrome. AF and atrial flutter are less commonly seen. Ventricular fibrillation (VF) and sudden death can result from a rapid ventricular response during AF or atrial flutter if it persists and deteriorates into VF, but this appears to be a rare occurrence (DiBiase and Walsh 2019).

Key Point

Some medications, primarily AV nodal blockers (verapamil, adenosine, digoxin), have been associated with an increased risk of VF for patients with pre-excitation and AF, due to preferential conduction via the accessory pathway (DiBiase and Walsh 2019).

An electrophysiological study can be used to risk stratify asymptomatic patients with a WPW pattern and ablation (see Chapter 12)

may be used to treat symptomatic WPW or asymptomatic WPW in persons with high-risk features or high-risk occupations.

Suggested Resource

Advanced EKGs – Wolff–Parkinson–White (WPW) syndrome
Strong Medicine (2016)
https://youtu.be/edf3Hq7XhKM

Atrioventricular Nodal Re-entry Tachycardia (AVNRT)

AVNRT is the most common type of re-entrant supraventricular tachycardia (SVT). The substrate for AVNRT is the presence of dual AV nodal pathways. Patients with AVNRT have two pathways connecting into the AV node that form part of a re-entrant circuit (Figure 11.12).

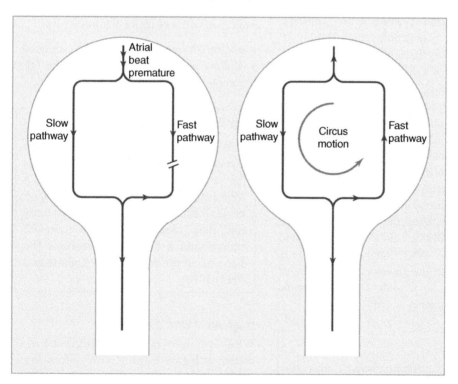

Figure 11.12 AVRNT Pathways. A premature atrial impulse finds the fast pathway refractory, allowing conduction only down the slow pathway (left). By the time the impulse reaches the His bundle, the fast pathway may have recovered, allowing retrograde conduction back up to the atria—the resultant "circus movement" gives rise to slow-fast atrioventricular nodal re-entrant tachycardia (right). *Source:* Esberger et al. (2002). Copyright 2019 BMJ Publishing Group Ltd. Reprinted with permission.

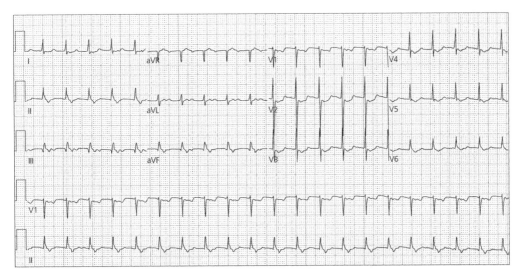

Figure 11.13 Twelve-lead ECG from a patient with AVNRT. There are inverted P waves at the terminal portion of the QRS complexes most prominent in the inferior leads, consistent with retrograde atrial activity. *Source:* Chan and Harrigan (2009)

AVRNT typically has an abrupt onset and termination. Episodes may last from seconds or minutes to days, and in the absence of structural heart disease, is usually well tolerated. Symptoms include palpitations, anxiety, light-headedness, chest discomfort, nervousness and dyspnoea. Polyuria sometimes occurs after termination of an episode due to the release of atrial natriuretic factor. Patients with coronary artery disease may experience angina or MI and patients who have heart failure may experience a worsening of their symptoms if AVNRT develops. Asystole can transiently occur at the termination of AVNRT due to tachycardia-induced depression of the sinus node (Olshansky and Sullivan 2017). A twelve-lead ECG from a patient with AVRNT is shown in Figure 11.13.

Suggested Resource

Atrioventricular re-entrant tachycardia (AVRT) and AV nodal re-entrant tachycardia (AVNRT)
khanacademymedicine (2014)
https://youtu.be/tRuvXP-H164

Learning Activity 11.1

Undertake the rhythm challenge via the link below:
Rhythm Challenge
The Resuscitationist (2014)
https://youtu.be/PR9tnDxCBag

Conclusion

Cardiac arrhythmias are one of the main complications in the acute cardiac patient. Effective patient care and intervention depend on accurate assessment, observation and recognition of relevant signs and symptoms. Identification of the arrhythmia can be achieved using a systematic approach, classifying the arrhythmia as either a bradycardia or a tachycardia. Management is determined by the haemodynamic status of the patient. A haemodynamically unstable patient requires prompt intervention, whilst the stable patient allows more time for rhythm analysis. Management of arrhythmias aims to restore sinus rhythm or, if this is not possible, to control the ventricular rate and maximise cardiac output using either drugs or electrical intervention. Patients' haemodynamic tolerance varies, and the focus of any intervention should always be the condition of the patient.

References

Agrawal, A. and Guzman, D.B. (2018). Third-Degree Atrioventricular Block (Complete Heart Block) Treatment and Management. In: (ed. F. Talavera, B. Oshansky, and J.N. Rottman). *Medscape*. https://emedicine.medscape.com/article/162007-treatment#d8.

Al-Khatib, S.M., Stevenson, W.G., Ackerman, M.J. et al. (2018). 2017 AHA/ACC/HRS guideline for management of patients with ventricular arrhythmias and the prevention of sudden cardiac death: a report of the American College of Cardiology/American Heart Association Task Force on Clinical Practice Guidelines and the Heart Rhythm Society. *Journal of the American College of Cardiology* **72** (14): e91–e220.

Antzelevitch, C., & Burashnikov, A. (2011). Overview of basic mechanisms of cardiac arrhythmia. Cardiac electrophysiology clinics, **3** (1), 23–45.

Banchs, J.V. (2018). Atrial tachycardia: diagnosis and treatment. *Cardiology Advisor*. https://www.thecardiologyadvisor.com/home/decision-support-in-medicine/cardiology/atrial-tachycardia-diagnosis-and-treatment.

Brieger, D., Amerena, J., Attia, J.R., Bajorek, B., Chan, K.H., Connell, C., . . . & Hendriks, J. (2018). National Heart Foundation of Australia and Cardiac Society of Australia and New Zealand: Australian clinical guidelines for the diagnosis and management of atrial fibrillation 2018. *Medical Journal of Australia*, **209** (8), 356–362. https://doi.org/10.5694/mja18.00646.

Brugada, P., Brugada, J., Mont, L. et al. (1991). A new approach to the differential diagnosis of a regular tachycardia with a wide QRS complex. *Circulation* **83** (5): 1649–1659.

Budzikowski, A.S. (2017). Atrial tachycardia. In: (ed. C.S. Cho and J.N. Rottman). Medscape. https://emedicine.medscape.com/article/151456-overview.

Burns, E. (2019). Tachy-brady syndrome. #FOAMed Medical Education Resources by LITFL. https://litfl.com/wp-content/uploads/2018/08/Brady-Tachy-Brady-Syndrome.jpg.

Calkins, H., Hindricks, G., Cappato, R. et al. (2017). 2017 HRS/EHRA/ECAS/APHRS/SOLAECE expert consensus statement on catheter and surgical ablation of atrial fibrillation. *EP Europace* **20** (1): e1–e160. https://doi.org/10.1093/europace/eux274.

Cardoso, R., Knijnik, L., Bhonsale, A., Miller, J., Nasi, G., Rivera, M., . . . & Calkins, H. (2018). An updated meta-analysis of novel oral anticoagulants versus vitamin K antagonists for uninterrupted anticoagulation in atrial fibrillation catheter ablation. *Heart Rhythm*, **15** (1), 107–115. DOI: https://doi.org/10.1016/j.hrthm.2017.09.011.

Chan, T.C. and Harrigan, R.A. (2009). What is the ECG differential diagnosis of narrow complex tachycardia? In: *Critical Decisions in Emergency and Acute Care Electrocardiography* (ed. W. Brady and J. Trewitt), 444–451. Oxford, UK: Wiley-Blackwell.

Chen, H., Shehata, M., Cingolani, E., Chugh, S.S., Chen, M., & Wang, X. (2015). Differentiating atrioventricular nodal re-entrant tachycardia from junctional tachycardia: conflicting reponses?. *Circulation: Arrhythmia and Electrophysiology*, **8** (1), 232–235. https://doi.org/10.1161/CIRCEP.114.002169.

Compton, S.J. (2017). Ventricular tachycardia. In: (ed. J.N. Rottman). *Medscape*. https://emedicine.medscape.com/article/159075-overview#a5.

Dakkak, W. and Doukky, R. (2019). *Sick Sinus Syndrome: Stat Pearls*. Treasure Island (FL): StatPearls Publishing https://www.ncbi.nlm.nih.gov/books/NBK470599.

DiBiase, L. and Walsh, E.P. (2018). Atrioventricular reentrant tachycardia (AVRT) associated with an accessory pathway. In: (ed. S.L. Levy, B.P. Knight, and B.C. Downey). *UpToDate.* http://www.uptodate.com/home/index.html.

DiBiase, L. & Walsh, E.P. (2019). Wolff-Parkinson-White syndrome: Anatomy, epidemiology, clinical manifestations, and diagnosis. In: (ed. S.L. Levy, B.P. Knight and B.C. Downey). *UpToDate.* http://www.uptodate.com/home/index.html.

Esberger, D., Jones, S., & Morris, F. (2002). Junctional tachycardias. *BMJ*, **324** (7338), 662–665. doi: https://doi.org/10.1136/bmj.324.7338.662.

Gangwani, M.K. and Nagalli, S. (2021). Idioventricular Rhythm. [Updated 2021 Apr 7]. In: StatPearls [Internet]. Treasure Island (FL): StatPearls Publishing; 2021 January-. https://www.ncbi.nlm.nih.gov/books/NBK554520.

Ganz, L.I. (2019). Epidemiology of and risk factors for atrial fibrillation. In: (ed. P.J. Zimetbaum and G.M. Saperia). *UpToDate.* http://www.uptodate.com/home/index.html.

Goldberger, A.L., Goldberger, Z.D., and Shvilkin, A. (2018). *Clinical Electrocardiography: A Simplified Approach E-Book: A Simplified Approach*, 9e, 184. Elsevier Health Sciences.

Ganz, L. and Buxton, A. (2018). Sustained monomorphic ventricular tachycardia in patients with structural heart disease: treatment and prognosis *UpToDate.* Waltham, MA: UpToDate Inc. https://www.uptodate.com/contents/sustained-monomorphic-ventricular-tachycardia-in-patients-with-structural-heart-disease-treatment-and-prognosis (accessed 10 February 2022).

Haghjoo, M. (2017). Bradyarrhythmias. In: *Practical Cardiology* (ed. M. Maleki, A. Alizadehasl and M. Haghjoo), 261–268. Elsevier Health Sciences https://doi.org/10.1016/B978-0-323-51149-0.00015-8.

Hindricks, G., Potpara, T., Dagres, N., Arbelo, E., Bax, J.J., Blomström-Lundqvist, C., ... & Watkins, C.L. (2021). 2020 ESC Guidelines for the diagnosis and management of atrial fibrillation developed in collaboration with the European Association for Cardio-Thoracic Surgery (EACTS) The Task Force for the diagnosis and management of atrial fibrillation of the European Society of Cardiology (ESC) Developed with the special contribution of the European Heart Rhythm Association (EHRA) of the ESC. European heart journal, **42** (5), 373–498. https://doi.org/10.1093/eurheartj/ehaa612

Homoud, M.K. (2019a). Sinus bradycardia. In: (ed. J. Piccini and B.C. Downey). UpToDate. http://www.uptodate.com/home/index.html.

Homoud, M.K. (2019b). Sinus node dysfunction: Epidemiology, etiology, and natural history. In: (ed. S. Levy and B.C. Downey). UpToDate. http://www.uptodate.com/home/index.html.

Homoud, M.K. (2019c). Sinoatrial nodal pause, arrest, and exit block. In: (ed. B. Olschansky and B.C. Downey). UpToDate. http://www.uptodate.com/home/index.html.

Jacobsen, C. (2010). Arrhythmias and conduction disturbances. In: *Cardiac Nursing*, 6e (ed. S.L. Woods, E.S. Sivarajan, M. Underhill and E.J. Bridges), 333–337. Philadelphia: Wolters Kluwer Health/Lippincott, Williams & Wilkins.

Kaplan, J. & Lala, V. (2019). Paroxysmal atrial tachycardia. *Stat Pearls*. Treasure Island (FL): StatPearls Publishing. https://www.ncbi.nlm.nih.gov/books/NBK538317.

Kumar, K. (2019). Overview of atrial fibrillation. In: (ed. P.J. Zimetbaum and G.M. Saperia). *UpToDate.* http://www.uptodate.com/home/index.html.

Lubitz, S.A., Yin, X., Fontes, J.D. et al. (2010). Association between familial atrial fibrillation and risk of new-onset atrial fibrillation. *JAMA 304* (20): 2263–2269. https://doi.org/10.1001/jama.2010.1690.

Manning, W.J., Singer, D.E., and Kasner, S.E. (2017). Atrial fibrillation: Risk of embolization. *UpToDate.* (accessed 23 May).

Manolis, A.S. (2019). Ventricular premature beats. In: (ed. H. Calkins and B.C. Downey). *UpToDate.* http://www.uptodate.com/home/index.html.

Olshansky, B. and Sullivan, R.M. (2017). Atrioventricular nodal reentry tachycardia. *Medscape.* https://emedicine.medscape.com/article/160215-overview (accessed 21 May 2019).

Page, R.L., Joglar, J.A., Caldwell, M.A. et al. (2016). 2015 ACC/AHA/HRS guideline for the management of adult patients with supraventricular tachycardia: a report of the American College of Cardiology/American Heart Association Task Force on Clinical Practice Guidelines and the Heart Rhythm Society. *Journal of the American College of Cardiology* **67** (13): e27–e115. https://doi.org/10.1016/j.jacc.2015.08.856.

Passman, R. (2019). Electrical storm and incessant ventricular tachycardia. In: (ed. M.S. Link and B.S. Downey). *UpToDate.* https://www.uptodate.com.

Pava, L.F., Perafán, P., Badiel, M. et al. (2010). R-wave peak time at DII: a new criterion for differentiating between wide complex QRS tachycardias. *Heart Rhythm* **7** (7): 922–926.

Prutkin, J.M. (2019). ECG tutorial: Atrial and atrioventricular nodal (supraventricular) arrhythmias. In: (ed. A.L. Goldberger and G.M. Saperia). *UpToDate.* https://www.uptodate.com.

Sauer, W.H. (2019a). Second degree atrioventricular block: Mobitz type I (Wenckebach block). In: (ed. L.I. Ganz and B.C. Downey). UpToDate. https://www.uptodate.com.

Sauer, W.H. (2019b). Second degree atrioventricular block: Mobitz type II. In: (ed. L.I. Ganz and B.C. Downey). UpToDate. https://www.uptodate.com.

Sauer, W.H. (2019c). Third degree (complete) atrioventricular block. In: (ed. L.I. Ganz and B.C. Downey). UpToDate. https://www.uptodate.com.

Scheidt, S. (1986). *Basic Electrocardiography.* New Jersey: Ciba-Geigy Pharmaceuticals.

Shah, S.N. (2020). Asystole. *eMedicine.* https://emedicine.medscape.com/article/757257-overview#a3 (accessed 23 July 2021).

Tandon, N., Hemphill, R.R., Huott, M.A., and Reddy, P.C. (2015). Multifocal atrial tachycardia. In: (ed. F. Talavera, P. Blackburn, and J.N. Rottman). *Medscape.* https://emedicine.medscape.com/article/155825-overview#a3.

Tse, G. (2016). Mechanisms of cardiac arrhythmias. Journal of arrhythmia, **32** (2), 75–81.

Vereckei, A. (2014). Current algorithms for the diagnosis of wide QRS complex tachycardias. *Current Cardiology Reviews, 10*(3), 262–276. doi: https://doi.org/10.2174/1573403X10666140514103309.

Vereckei, A., Duray, G., Szénási, G., Altemose, G.T., & Miller, J.M. (2008). New algorithm using only lead aVR for differential diagnosis of wide QRS complex tachycardia. *Heart Rhythm, 5*(1), 89–98. https://doi.org/10.1093/eurheartj/ehl473.

Voskoboinik, A., Sparks, P.B., Morton, J.B. et al. (2018). Low rates of major complications for radiofrequency ablation of atrial fibrillation maintained over 14 years: a single centre experience of 2750 consecutive cases. *Heart, Lung and Circulation* **27** (8): 976–983. https://doi.org/10.1016/j.hlc.2018.01.002.

12

Assessment and Management of Cardiac Rhythm Disturbances (Arrhythmias)

Carolyn E. Shepherd, Jenny Tagney, and Angela M. Kucia

Overview

A cardiac rhythm disturbance (arrhythmia or dysrhythmia) may refer to abnormalities in heart rate, regularity of rhythm, site of impulse origin or sequence of activation. Cardiac arrhythmias can occur at any age and range from harmless to life threatening. Timely, accurate diagnosis is essential in reducing the risk of associated complications of abnormal rhythm such as stroke, hypotension and heart failure. In the longer term, arrhythmias may impair left ventricular function. Nurses have a vital role in arrhythmia recognition and in providing support and information to people with arrhythmias.

This chapter outlines key points to include when taking a clinical history from a patient presenting with a cardiac arrhythmia or suspected cardiac arrhythmia, and the related diagnostic tests. It will provide an overview of treatment options including self-help strategies, pharmacological therapies, direct current cardioversion (DCCV) and catheter ablation. It will conclude with an overview of pacemakers and defibrillators, including the benefits and burdens of device therapy. For more detailed information about individual arrhythmias and their management, refer to Chapter 11.

Learning Objectives

After reading this chapter, you should be able to:

- Describe the steps in the assessment of a patient presenting with an arrhythmia or suspected arrhythmia.
- Describe the diagnostic tests used in patients presenting with an arrhythmia or suspected arrhythmia.
- Describe the basis of contemporary pharmacological therapies for arrhythmias
- Identify the role of direct current cardioversion in arrhythmia management
- Describe the rationale behind catheter ablation
- Explain the use of devices in the management of arrhythmias.

Key Concepts

Arrhythmia diagnosis, arrhythmia management, catheter ablation, device therapy.

Assessment

An accurate, structured and detailed clinical history from a patient presenting with an arrhythmia or a suspected arrhythmia is

Cardiac Care: A Practical Guide for Nurses, Second Edition. Edited by Angela M. Kucia and Ian D. Jones.
© 2022 John Wiley & Sons Ltd. Published 2022 by John Wiley & Sons Ltd.

essential. This not only provides clues as to the possible origin of the arrhythmia but guides physical examination and assists in determining the possible clinical severity of the condition and whether urgent investigation or action is required. Arrhythmia can present with a variety of different symptoms. The most common complaint for patients presenting with arrhythmia is palpitations. Palpitations, defined as subjective awareness of an abnormal heartbeat, are amongst the most common symptoms that prompt patients to see their general practitioner (GP). Palpitations are often frightening for the patient, but most are due to benign atrial or ventricular extrasystoles (Gale and Camm 2016). It is important to bear in mind that some patients with an arrhythmia may present with other symptoms such as unexplained fatigue, dyspnoea, dizziness, reduced exercise tolerance, pre-syncope/syncope or angina. A symptomatic patient with suspected arrhythmia will require prompt assessment to ascertain haemodynamic status; cardiac rhythm; evidence of structural or coronary heart disease, pre-excitation or channelopathy; and systematic factors that may have triggered or exacerbated the patient's symptoms. 'Red-flag' features that should trigger an in-patient cardiology review include:

- associated syncope
- palpitations triggered by exercise
- symptoms/evidence of ischaemic or structural heart disease
- accessory pathway or channelopathy
- family history of cardiomyopathy or sudden death (Hothi and Sprigings 2017).

Some arrhythmias have no symptoms and may be found during a routine health check. Random pulse checks are recommended in patients over 65 years old to facilitate diagnosis of arrhythmia, particularly atrial fibrillation (Cole et al. 2018). For information about different types of arrythmias, refer to Chapter 11.

Taking a Clinical History

In obtaining the clinical history, it is important to use a systematic and structured approach using targeted questions that will assist in identifying the key features of the complaint (see Table 12.1). For patients presenting with palpitations, the prognostic implications are dependent on the underlying aetiology, as well as clinical characteristics of the patient (Raviele et al. 2011).

Key Point

Some arrhythmic conditions, particularly those related to syncope or cardiac arrest, may lead to driving restrictions. Driving regulations relating to specific medical restrictions vary from country to country and state to state. Patients should be advised about driving restrictions that may apply whilst awaiting a diagnosis or following a diagnosis that necessitates driving restrictions. Arrhythmias may have an impact on employment and life or travel insurance.

Physical Examination

An examination of the patient will be guided by points ascertained within the clinical history and should include looking for evidence of any organic diseases that could explain the symptoms, such as thyroid dysfunction, or any structural heart disease such as valvular disorders. Arrhythmias may occur in structurally normal hearts and in the absence of a known cause. Examination should include cardiac auscultation, peripheral vascular assessment including carotid artery auscultation and signs of peripheral oedema, examination of the neck for signs of swelling/goitre, eyes for exophthalmos (thyrotoxic) or pallor (anaemia), breath sounds, nail beds for colour (pallor may

Table 12.1 Patient history.

Relevant medical history	Rationale
Previous history cardiac disease	Ischaemic heart disease, cardiomyopathies, valvular disease, rheumatic fever, congenital heart disease, hypertension, Takotsubo syndrome and heart failure may be associated with atrial and ventricular arrhythmias and disturbances. Mitral valve disease can predispose to atrial fibrillation
Co-existing medical conditions	Co-existing medical conditions that may trigger or exacerbate arrhythmias include chronic obstructive pulmonary disease, sleep apnoea, neurological conditions including stroke and epilepsy, and thyrotoxicosis, diabetes, anaemia, pheochromocytoma, and pregnancy, excessive fatigue, infection and sepsis, cancer and chemotherapy, general anaesthesia, pulmonary embolus
Psychosomatic disorders	Psychological factors such as stress, anxiety or panic disorder, and anger (Lampert 2016) are more likely to cause sinus tachycardia but may trigger supraventricular tachycardia (SVT) or ventricular tachycardia (VT) (Hothi and Sprigings 2017).
Family history of cardiac disease, tachycardia or sudden cardiac death	Ischaemic heart disease, early-onset atrial fibrillation, channelopathies and cardiomyopathies have a genetic component (Hothi and Sprigings, 2017). Around 50% of inherited arrhythmia disorders associated with a structurally normal heart (long and short QT syndrome, Brugada syndrome, catecholaminergic polymorphic ventricular tachycardia, early repolarisation syndrome and idiopathic ventricular fibrillation) are diagnosed during a health check-up or during screening as a family member of a deceased person (Hocini et al. 2014).
Medications at the time of palpitations	Prescribed medications, including some antiarrhythmics, antianginals, antiemetics, gastrointestinal stimulants, antibacterials, narcotics, antipsychotics, inotropes, digoxin, anaesthetic agents, bronchodilators, and drugs that cause electrolyte imbalances, can cause arrhythmias (Barnes and Hollands 2010). Some herbal substances and dietary supplements may trigger arrhythmias
	Check if the patient is on an anticoagulant or antiplatelet medication, which may indicate a prior diagnosis of atrial fibrillation
	Check for a history of allergies or previous adverse reactions to medications
Drugs and other substances	Caffeine, illicit drugs (e.g. cocaine, amphetamines, 'ecstasy'), alcohol and smoking can trigger arrhythmias (Hothi and Sprigings 2017).
Electrolyte imbalance	Hypo- or hyperkalaemia, hypo- or hypercalcaemia and hypomagnesaemia may trigger arrhythmias (Hothi and Sprigings 2017).

(Continued)

Table 12.1 (Continued)

Relevant medical history	Rationale
Prior history of palpitations/arrhythmia • Age at the first episode • Number of previous episodes • Frequency of episodes	Congenital long QT syndrome, Brugada syndrome and catecholaminergic polymorphic ventricular tachycardia are responsible for sudden cardiac death (SCD) in young and apparently healthy individuals. AVNRT is reported more frequently in women, with the age of onset being >30; AVRT is often reported in a younger age group (Page et al. 2016). Ageing of the heart is associated with an increasing incidence of arrhythmias and disorders of the SA node and conduction system
Onset of palpitations • Activity (during sport or normal exercise) • During rest or sleep • Position (supine, standing, squatting or bending) • Abrupt or slowly arising	Sustained supraventricular and ventricular tachyarrhythmias may be provoked by sympathetic stimulation and catecholamine excess, as occurs during exercise or at times of stress (Zimetbaum 2018). Extrasystoles may be felt on lying down in the left lateral decubitus or supine positions where the apex of the heart is closer to the chest wall. AV nodal re-entrant tachycardia may be precipitated by bending over and then standing up and may terminate on lying down (Zimetbaum 2018).
Symptoms • Onset of symptoms preceding arrhythmia or during arrhythmia	• Chest pain, syncope or near syncope, sweating, pulmonary oedema, anxiety, nausea or vomiting • An irregular pounding feeling in the neck may be felt due to atrioventricular dissociation with occasional atrial contraction against a closed tricuspid and mitral valve (Zimetbaum 2018)
Type of palpitations • Regular/irregular • Slow/fast • Permanent/intermittent • 'Missed' beats • Stop/start abruptly or build up slowly	• An irregular rhythm may indicate atrial fibrillation (AF) • Slow heart rate may indicate sinus bradycardia or heart block • Permanent may indicate atrial arrhythmias. Intermittent may indicate paroxysmal atrial arrhythmias, atrio-ventricular (AV) nodal re-entrant tachycardias, ventricular tachycardia or heart block
End of the episode • Spontaneous • Vagal manoeuvres • Drug administration • Decreasing abruptly or slowly	

Suggested Resource

An approach to palpitations
Strong Medicine (2018)
https://youtu.be/ep7nkE4KvLk

indicate anaemia) and splinter haemorrhage (one of the signs of endocarditis). Baseline observations of pulse, blood pressure, respiratory rate and oxygen saturations should be taken. Further investigations, including laboratory tests, may be required to confirm a suspected diagnosis. See Chapter 6 for further details about cardiovascular assessment.

Screening for Atrial Fibrillation

Opportunistic screening in the clinic or community is recommended for persons over 65 years of age, preferably by ECG rather than pulse check or pulse-based devices. In patients with implanted pacemakers and defibrillators, the device should be regularly interrogated for occurrence of AF. A transthoracic echocardiogram should be performed in all patients with newly diagnosed AF to identify valvular heart disease and quantify left ventricular function and atrial size. Transthoracic echo can be considered prior to electrical or pharmacological cardioversion if intracardiac thrombus is a consideration (Brieger et al. 2018).

Suggested Resource

Giskes, K., Lowres, N., and Li, J. et al. (2021). Atrial fibrillation self-screening, management and guideline recommended therapy (AF SELF SMART): a protocol for atrial fibrillation self-screening in general practice. *IJC Heart and Vasculature* 32: 100683. https://doi.org/10.1016/j.ijcha.2020.100683

Diagnostic Investigations

Laboratory Investigations

There are no evidence-based guidelines for laboratory work-up of patients with palpitations. Ruling out anaemia, hyperthyroidism and electrolyte disturbance is reasonable, in addition to testing for specific disorders that may be suggested by the history and physical examination (Zimetbaum 2018). For further information about common laboratory investigations used in cardiac disorders, see Chapter 7.

Electrocardiographic Investigations

Refer to Chapter 3 to review cardiac electrophysiology and Chapter 9 for review of electrocardiography.

12-Lead ECG

In assessment of the patient with suspected arrhythmia, a baseline 12-lead ECG is used to ascertain rate, rhythm and conduction, and to look for any abnormal patterns to distinguish the potential mechanism of the arrhythmia. Table 12.2 provides some examples of Common key ECG patterns for syndromes associated with increased risk of arrhythmia. If the patient is experiencing symptoms at the time of the ECG, a systematic analysis of the ECG should be undertaken to define the arrhythmia. It is important to identify any patterns on the otherwise normal ECG that could lead to an arrhythmia causing sudden cardiac death (SCD). The 12-lead ECG can be used to detect prognostic markers for SCD by identifying specific patters of electrical disturbance that can predispose to malignant arrhythmia (Rizzo et al. 2016).

Holter Monitoring

The Holter monitor is like standard electrocardiography, but with fewer leads and electrodes. Indications for Holter monitoring are similar to those of a 12-lead ECG, but a Holter monitor can be used for 24–48 hour periods whilst the patient undertakes normal activities to increase the chance of detecting an abnormality. As patients are expected to engage in normal daily activities, electrodes are placed over bones to minimise artefact from muscular activity and movement. The electrodes are connected to a small recorder that is attached to a belt or hung around the patient's neck, keeping a log of the heart's electrical activity throughout the recording period. The main limitation of Holter

Table 12.2 Common key ECG patterns for syndromes associated with increased risk of arrhythmia.

Syndrome	Characteristics of ECG in the absence of arrhythmia
Wolff–Parkinson–White (WPW) syndrome	• Short PR interval (<0.12 s) • Delta wave (slurred and broad upstroke of the QRS complex) • QRS complex is wide (>0.12 s) and bizarre in appearance • Increases risk of AVRT, atrial fibrillation or flutter.
Long QT syndrome (LQTS) – congenital or acquired	• Prolonged QT interval • Disorder of myocardial repolarisation • QT interval varies with heart rate and is adjusted for heart rate (QTc) • QTc of >450 ms for men and > 460 ms for women is considered abnormal and a QTc >500 ms is highly abnormal for men and women (Giudicessi et al. 2019) • Increases risk of torsade de pointes (polymorphic ventricular tachycardia), which may be lethal
Short QT syndrome	• Rare inherited channelopathy • The lower limit of the normal QT interval and the value below, which it could be considered arrhythmogenic, are unclear, but in most cases of arrhythmia is less than 360 ms (Antzelevitch 2019)
Brugada syndrome (BrS) (referred to as 'Brugada pattern' in asymptomatic people with typical ECG features)	• Pseudo-right bundle branch block • Persistent ST-segment elevation in leads V1 and V2 • Associated with ventricular arrhythmias and SCD ECG patterns diagnostic for BrS (Type 1) or suggestive of BrS (Types 2 and 3) *Type 1 (coved) (Figure 12.1)* • diagnostic for Brugada • characteristic ECG pattern (coved type ST-segment elevation ≥2 mm followed by a negative T-wave in ≥1 of the right precordial leads V1 to V2) • observed spontaneously or during a sodium-channel blocker test. *Type 2 and 3 ("saddle-back type") (Figure 12.1)* • only suggestive of BrS • characterised by an ST-segment elevation in ≥1 right precordial lead (V1 to V3), followed by a convex ST • the r′-wave may or may not overlap the J point, but it has a slow downward slope • the ST segment is followed by a positive T-wave in V2 and is of variable morphology in V1 (Brugada et al. 2018)
Early repolarisation (ER) syndrome (J-waves or J-point elevation)	• ER syndrome is associated with an increased risk for arrhythmic death and idiopathic ventricular fibrillation (VF) • J-point elevation ≥1 mm in ≥2 contiguous inferior and/or lateral leads with a 'notching' appearance (positive J-deflection inscribed in the S wave) or 'slurring' (a gradual transition of the QRS to the ST-segment) in two inferior, lateral or infero-lateral leads. The simultaneous presence of ST-segment elevation is not necessary for diagnosis (Haïssaguerre et al. 2008)

Table 12.2   (Continued)

Syndrome	Characteristics of ECG in the absence of arrhythmia
Left ventricular hypertrophy (LVH)	• Sokolow–Lyon and Cornell ECG criteria for LVH are associated with an increased risk of SCD (Porthan et al. 2019)
Short coupled premature ventricular contractions (PVCs)	• Variability in premature ventricular contraction (PVC) coupling interval increases the risk of cardiomyopathy and sudden death (Hamon et al. 2017)
ECG abnormalities associated with myocardial ischaemia/infarction or drug toxicity	• ST-segment elevation or depression and T-wave abnormalities due to myocardial ischaemia or infarction are associated with increased risk of arrhythmia • ST-segment and T-wave abnormalities and QRS complex width changes due to drug toxicity are associated with increased risk of arrhythmia
Bundle branch block	Conduction disorders become more common with age, and may either be asymptomatic, or cause haemodynamic changes requiring treatment, particularly if occurring in the setting of myocardial ischaemia or infarction

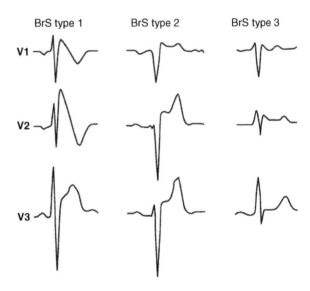

Figure 12.1   ECG patterns associated with Brugada Syndrome. The 3 BrS ECG types. Type 1 (left) is the typical BrS type ECG and diagnostic for BrS. BrS types 2 (middle) and BrS type 3 (right) are not specific BrS patterns, but raise suspicion of BrS and may be observed in subjects with intermittent BrS type 1 ECG. *Source:* Reproduced with permission. Delise and Zeppilli (2021).

monitoring is that it is only worn for a relatively short period, and symptoms or arrhythmia events may not occur during the time that the patient is wearing the monitor.

Implantable Loop Recorder

An implantable loop recorder (ILR) is a single-lead ECG monitoring device that can store ECG data automatically in response to a significant bradyarrhythmia or tachyarrhythmia, or in response to patient activation. ILRs are subcutaneously implanted, usually in the left parasternal region. An ILR is useful when symptoms are infrequent or when aggregate long-term data, such as burden of AF, are required. Disadvantages include the need for a minor surgical procedure and the cost of the device. Moreover, the ILR may not always be able to differentiate between supraventricular and ventricular arrhythmias, and oversensing may exhaust the memory (Mittal et al. 2015).

Indications for insertion of an ILR are

- diagnosis in patients with recurrent unexplained episodes of palpitations or syncope
- long-term monitoring in patients at risk for or with documented atrial fibrillation (AF)
- risk stratification in patients with previous myocardial infarction
- risk stratification in certain genetic disorders

Contraindications to the insertion of an ILR includes the presence of active bleeding or infection.

Patch Device

Patch devices are an alternative to loop recorders and Holter monitors. They attach externally through adhesive to the chest wall or sternum and record and store rhythm data in a single lead. They are leadless and can be self-applied and have patient-trigger capability to allow for symptom–rhythm correlation (Kusumoto et al. 2019).

Smartphone Technology

Rapid progress is being made in the use of smartphone technology for cardiac monitoring and arrhythmia detection. This technology generally relies upon an external device with metal sensors to be connected to the mobile phone to create a rhythm strip that can be transmitted to their physician using a smartphone app and Wi-Fi connectivity or a data enabled cellular network plan (Nguyen and Silva 2016). Other smartphone products use photoplethysmography through a phone camera and light to detect atrial fibrillation (Garabelli et al. 2017).

> **Key Points**
>
> Holter monitors should only be used for symptoms that occur frequently (daily to weekly). If symptoms occur less frequently, an ILR should be considered.
>
> Single-lead ECG devices do not always allow for a precise diagnosis of the type of arrhythmia recorded. A 12-lead ECG may be more accurate.

Electrophysiology (EP) Studies

An electrophysiology study (EPS) is a minimally invasive procedure that is typically performed in a cardiac catheter or EPS laboratory to assess cardiac electrical activity and conduction. Common indications and contraindications for EPS are shown in Box 12.1.

Multipolar electrode catheters are positioned in the heart via multiple venous accesses (usually femoral, but subclavian, internal jugular or brachial approach may be used). The catheters are positioned at various intra-cardiac sites to record electrical activity. Programmed electrical stimulation can be used to induce arrhythmias in the atria and the ventricles (Homoud 2019). Complications associated with EPS study occur in around 2% of people and are mostly associated with cardiac catheterisation and are like those listed in Table 8.3. Serious ventricular tachyarrhythmias are frequently induced during diagnostic electrophysiology testing. Whilst these arrhythmias can usually be terminated promptly by using overdrive pacing or external defibrillation, there is a risk of prolonged hypotension and, rarely, sudden death resulting from arrhythmias that are difficult to terminate (Homoud 2019). Box 12.2 outlines preparation for patients undergoing EPS.

Imaging

This standard investigation provides information on heart size, position and allows review of the lung fields. Following device implants, a

---

Box 12.1   Indications and contraindications for EPS Indications.

Indications

Identify cause, define prognosis, and determine therapy

- Sinus node dysfunction (SND) to assess the relation between clinical symptoms and SND in symptomatic patients with documented sinus bradyarrhythmias where diagnosis cannot be established by non-invasive means (Muresan et al. 2019).
- Abnormal atrioventricular conduction blocks that cannot be localised by non-invasive means (Muresan et al. 2019).
- Narrow QRS complex tachycardia and (a) frequent or poorly tolerated episodes of tachycardia that do not adequately respond to drug therapy; (b) to identify the site of origin, mechanism, and electrophysiological properties of the pathways of the tachycardia to choose appropriate therapy (c) in patients who prefer ablative therapy compared to pharmacological treatment; (d) there is a concern about the pro-arrhythmic properties of an antiarrhythmic or they are not candidates for anti-arrhythmic therapy (Muresan et al. 2019).
- Wide complex tachyarrhythmias where diagnosis cannot be established by non-invasive means.
- Ventricular pre-excitation in patients who have survived cardiac arrest (CA) or who

have unexplained syncope to explore options for ablation.
- Symptomatic patients with ECG suggestive of pre-excitation who may be at high risk of SCD due to AF progressing to VF (Muresan et al. 2019).
- Congenital heart disease to determine the nature of the arrhythmia in patients where there is clinical suspicion of arrhythmia disorders, including syncope (Muresan et al. 2019).
- Unexplained syncope, where initial evaluation suggests an arrhythmic cause (Brignole et al. 2018).

Risk stratification

- Symptomatic young (8–21 years) patients with ECG suggestive of pre-excitation who may be at high risk of SCD due to AF progressing to ventricular fibrillation (Homoud et al. 2019).
- Coronary artery disease to assess the inducibility of VT in high-risk patients for ventricular arrhythmia occurrence (Muresan et al. 2019).

Contraindications

Absolute contraindications to EPS include unstable angina, infection, active bleeding, and congestive heart failure (not caused by the arrhythmia) (Homoud et al. 2019).

---

chest X-ray (CXR) shows the position of the device and the leads. The integrity of the leads can also be assessed. For further information about CXR, refer to Chapter 8.

Transthoracic Echocardiography

Echocardiography looks at the structure and function of the heart and may assist in finding

causal factors for an arrhythmia. Important findings that can help inform arrhythmia risk and guide management are:

- Valvular disease
- Chamber enlargement or irregularity
- Reduced left ventricular function
- Myocardial regional wall motion abnormalities (may relate to previous surgical scars or myocardial damage or dilatation)

Box 12.2   Patient preparation for electrophysiology (EP) study.

In addition to general preparation for cardiac diagnostic tests listed in Table 12.1, there are some activities to be undertaken to prepare patients for EP study:

- The patient should fast for 6–8 hours prior to the procedure except for oral medications with sips of water.
- Some cardiovascular medications (i.e. beta-blockers, dihydropyridine calcium-channel blockers, digoxin and antiarrhythmic medications) may need to be held for one or more days prior to the procedure (Homoud 2019) as ordered by the cardiologist.
- Hair should be removed from the groin area and possibly the area below the left collar bone where the catheters will be inserted.
- Premedication may be ordered to help the patient relax during the procedure.
- Continuous cardiac monitoring, blood pressure monitoring (noninvasively or via arterial monitoring) and pulse oximetry should be in place throughout the procedure.

- Defibrillation pads should be placed on the patient prior to beginning the procedure so as not to disrupt sterile field in the event electrical defibrillation is required.
- Intravenous access is required for administration of sedation and pharmacological management of any rhythm-related complications.
- Emergency trolley and equipment should be readily available in case of haemodynamic compromise resulting from arrhythmia.
- The patient should be informed that the EP study may take several hours and the test may be have negative or equivocal result.
- Sedation may be required if the study takes longer than normal or if the patient proceeds on to having an ablation. In this case, airway protection may be required until the patient has recovered from sedation.
- IV heparin is used if catheterisation of the left atrium (LA) is effected *via* transseptal puncture (Earley 2009).

- Structural abnormalities of the myocardium such as septal hypertrophy (hypertrophic cardiomyopathies) aneurysms or undiagnosed congenital abnormalities

More detailed information about echocardiography can be found in Chapter 8.

Cardiac Magnetic Resonance Imaging

CMR may be useful to detect and characterise underlying structural heart disease in patients with arrhythmia (Al-Khatib et al. 2018). See Chapter 8 for more information about CMR.

Coronary Angiography

A coronary angiogram may be used to detect an underlying ischaemic cause of arrhythmia.

More detailed information on coronary angiography is available in Chapter 8.

Diagnosis of Cardiac Channelopathies

Ion channel abnormalities in the myocardial cellular membrane that affect the cardiac action potential can predispose to life-threatening arrhythmias and sudden unexpected death. Long QT syndrome (LQTS), short QT syndrome (SQTS), Brugada syndrome (BS) and catecholaminergic polymorphic ventricular tachycardia (CPVT) are cardiac channelopathies caused by gene mutations (Behere and Weindling 2015). Provocative testing for diagnosis of channelopathies associated with potentially lethal ventricular arrhythmias can be undertaken using an exercise test or pharmacological agents. Testing should be undertaken in an area that has comprehensive monitoring and resuscitation equipment, including a defibrillator. The person undergoing testing should be continuously monitored by experienced personnel trained in advanced resuscitation and with an expert physician promptly available (Obeyesekere et al. 2011). More detailed information on exercise testing and contraindications is available in Chapter 8.

Drugs used in pharmacological testing for channelopathies associated with ventricular arrhythmias. Drugs commonly infused for pharmacological testing for channelopathies associated with ventricular arrhythmias are listed below:

- Brugada Syndrome: flecainide, ajmaline or procainamide
- LQTS: epinephrine (adrenalin) or adenosine
- CPVT: epinephrine

Genetic Testing Following Sudden Unexpected Death

In a patient with sudden unexpected death (SUD), a genetic assessment looking for underlying pathogenic mutations which may explain the SUD may be undertaken. Gene mutations cannot be identified in all cases, but it is probable that some mutations associated with arrhythmia and SUD have not yet been recognised. Clinical and/or genetic investigation of immediate relatives of the deceased person (cascade screening) may be undertaken to identify individuals at risk for potentially treatable life-threatening arrhythmias.

For further information about channelopathies, see Chapter 18.

Treatment Strategies for Arrhythmia

Vagal Stimulation Techniques

Haemodynamically stable episodic SVT can be effectively managed using vagal stimulation techniques to slow the heart. These include the Valsalva manoeuvre, ice to the face or carotid sinus massage (in cases with no audible bruit and no known carotid artery stenosis) (Page et al. 2016). Vagal manoeuvres can be performed in a variety of clinical settings for diagnostic and/or therapeutic purposes. Vagal manoeuvres increase vagus nerve activation to slow and terminate a tachycardia. Vagal manoeuvres are an effective first-line therapeutic intervention for patients with supraventricular tachycardia (SVT) and acute treatment of SVT of unknown mechanism, atrioventricular re-entrant tachycardia (AVRT), and atrioventricular nodal re-entrant tachycardia (AVNRT). In a standard Valsalva manoeuver, the patient is placed in a supine or semi-recumbent position, instructed to inhale normally and then to exhale forcefully against a closed glottis for 10–15 seconds. A modified Valsalva manoeuver begins with the standard manoeuver but is followed by supine positioning and passive leg raising (Frish and Zimetbaum 2018).

Learning Activity 12.1

Watch the video below to see how the modified Valsalva manoeuvre is performed.

Suggested Resource

Modified Valsalva manoeuvre for supraventricular tachycardia
The Lancet (2015)
https://youtu.be/8DIRiOA_OsA

Pharmacological Therapy

Pharmacological therapy may be required to treat arrhythmias. The aim of pharmacological treatment depends on the type of arrhythmia. Medication can be used to restore normal rhythm, control heart rate and/or symptoms and prevent life-threatening arrhythmias. Antiarrhythmic drugs are usually classified according to their general effects on the cardiac action potential. The Vaughan Williams antiarrhythmic drug classification scheme was devised in 1970 (Vaughan Williams 1970) and is still the most widely used classification scheme, though it has limitations due to better understanding of cardiac electrophysiology and mechanisms of cardiac arrhythmias, and newer antiarrhythmic drugs. Not all antiarrhythmic drugs fit into the Vaughan Williams classification, with many exerting effects from more than one class. Table 12.3 shows the class and actions of commonly used antiarrhythmic drugs. The physiology of the action potential can be reviewed in Chapter 3. Common safety considerations for antiarrhythmic medications are listed in Box 12.3.

Key Point

Some anti-arrhythmic drug therapies (for example flecainide) must be avoided if the heart is not structurally normal.

Table 12.3 Class and actions of commonly used antiarrhythmic drugs.

Vaughan Williams Class	Common drugs	Arrhythmia treated	Drug action/effect on the action potential
Class 1: Sodium (Na)-channel blockers Modulate or block the sodium channels. Subdivided into classes A, B and C according to their duration of action.	**Class Ia** Disopyramide, procainamide, quinidine	Effective in treating AF but not commonly used due to side-effects	Prolongs repolarisation Increases QT interval
	Class Ib Lignocaine (lidocaine), mexiletine	Lignocaine is used intravenously to treat VT and VF, but toxicity can occur at higher doses. Mexiletine is available orally to treat VT.	Shortens repolarisation
	Class Ic Flecainide, propafenone, moricizine	Atrial and ventricular arrhythmias. Flecainide can be used on an as-needed basis in the outpatient setting ('pill in pocket' approach) if indicated. Flecainide cannot be used in patients with structural heart disease (Ruskin 1989): In rare cases, flecainide may cause rapid 1:1 conduction (Colangelo et al. 2021)	No effect on repolarisation. Reduce conductivity
Class II: Beta-blockers	Acebutalol, atenolol, bisoprolol, carvedolol, esmolol, metoprolol, nadolol, propranolol	Atrial and ventricular arrhythmias, AV-nodal re-entrant tachycardia. Caution in patient with acute heart failure, bronchospasm, renal disease, pulmonary disease	β-adrenergic inhibition Sinus rate slowed AV nodal refractoriness increased (Al-Khatib et al. 2018)

Table 12.3 (Continued)

Vaughan Williams Class	Common drugs	Arrhythmia treated	Drug action/effect on the action potential
Class III: Potassium-channel blockers	Amiodarone	Atrial and ventricular arrhythmias. Long half-life Serious and wide-ranging side effects limit utility, particularly in younger people. Caution in renal disease and pulmonary disease	Beta-blocking properties. Prolongs repolarisation. Sinus rate slowed, QTc prolonged, AV nodal refractoriness increased (Al-Khatib et al. 2018)
	Dronedarone	Atrial arrhythmias only. Should not be used in patients with severe or decompensated heart failure or in permanent AF (King and McGuigan 2019).	Similar effects to amiodarone
	Sotalol	Atrial arrhythmias, treatment of life-threatening ventricular arrhythmias. Increased risk of ventricular tachycardia/torsades de pointes	Also has class II effects Prolongs phase 3 (Levine 2019) Decreases slope of phase 4 (Levine 2019)
Class IV: Calcium-channel blockers	Diltiazem Verapamil	SVT, AF and A flutter, AV-nodal re-entrant tachycardia, multifocal atrial tachycardia. Verapamil has been associated with an increased risk of VF in patients with pre-excitation and AF (Dibiase and Walsh 2018).	Sinus rate slowed, PR prolonged, AV nodal conduction slowed (Al-Khatib et al. 2018)
Class V: Work by other or unknown mechanisms (direct nodal inhibition)	Adenosine	SVT. Extreme caution in any patient with SVT involving an accessory pathway, including WPW syndrome. Should not be used in irregular or polymorphic broad-complex tachycardias (Singh and McKintosh 2019)	Interrupts re-entry pathways through the AV node and restores sinus rhythm
	Digoxin	AF, A Flutter. Caution in renal disease and hypokalaemia. Increased risk of VF in patients with pre-excitation and AF (DiBiase and Walsh 2018)	Enhances vagotonic responses and inhibits sympathetic activity (Campbell and MacDonald 2003)

(Continued)

Table 12.3 (Continued)

Vaughan Williams Class	Common drugs	Arrhythmia treated	Drug action/effect on the action potential
	Magnesium sulphate	AF, SVT, VF, TdP (Baker 2016)	Magnesium regulates the movement of ions through voltage-dependent Na^+, K^+ and Ca^{2+} channels in myocardial cells (Baker 2016)

Suggested Resource

Up to date information can be found about antiarrhythmic drugs, indications and side effects on the websites below:
- RxList www.rxlist.com
- NICE British National Formulary www.nice.org.uk/bnf (available in UK only)

Suggested Resources

Series on Antiarrhythmics
Strong Medicine (2017)

Lesson 1: Introducti on
https://youtu.be/H2O5Hhj0bos

Lesson 2: Sodium-channel blockers
https://youtu.be/CG2L9D2GXo4

Lesson 3: Beta-blockers
https://youtu.be/pK97Ni0fGJ8

Lesson 4: Potassium-channel blockers
https://youtu.be/jnZAmU-9wUY

Lesson 5: Calcium-channel blockers
https://youtu.be/Rmo1FzDwZ7E

Lesson 6: Digoxin, adenosine, atropine, iso-proterenol, and ivabradine
https://youtu.be/bbE5Kiq6hGI

Lesson 7: How to choose the right meds and classic pitfalls
https://youtu.be/5jMPVrgFk8U

Box 12.3 Safety considerations for antiarrhythmic medications.

Safety is of prime concern when prescribing antiarrhythmic medications. Consideration should be given to the following:

- Check for any potential interactions between the antiarrhythmic medication and the patient's other prescribed medications.
- Check for safety of antiarrhythmic medications if the patient is pregnant or lactating.
- Continuous cardiac monitoring may be required when starting some antiarrhythmic drugs.
- Anti-arrhythmic drugs can be pro-arrhythmic, especially those in Class 1a and 1c.
- Antiarrhythmic medication is contra-indicated in patients with heart block unless a cardiac pacemaker is in situ
- Elimination of antiarrhythmic drugs may be reduced and lead to toxicity in renal or hepatic impairment.
- Record baseline blood tests in order to detect any abnormalities caused by the drug over time.
- Hypokalaemia, hyperkalaemia, or hypo-magnesaemia may affect the actions of the antiarrhythmic drugs. Imbalances should be corrected as soon as possible.
- Some antiarrhythmic drugs can be tested for in the bloodstream in order to ensure therapeutic levels.
- The ECG and antiarrhythmic medication should be reviewed at all follow-up appointments.

Electrical (Direct Current) Synchronised Cardioversion

Direct current synchronised cardioversion (DCCV) may be used to restore sinus rhythm in patients with AF, atrial flutter, SVT (including AVNRT, AVRT, atrial tachycardia not responsive to vagal manoeuvres or pharmacotherapy) and conscious VT. DCCV involves delivering an electrical current from a defibrillator through the chest wall and the heart muscle using two electrode patches to restore sinus rhythm. The electrode patches (pads) are attached to the chest wall in an anteroposterior or antero-lateral position. Higher success rates and lower energy requirements for successful cardioversion have been found with the anterior–posterior configuration but an anterior-lateral pad configuration may be preferred for ease of application. The device manufacturer's guidelines should be followed regarding pad placement. If DCCV does not work in the first position, it may be repeated using an alternative position (Roberts 2018). The shock is automatically timed (synchronised) by the defibrillator to be delivered on the stroke of the R-wave. This avoids the vulnerable period of the electrical cycle (repolarisation) as a shock at this time could cause ventricular fibrillation. A button on the defibrillator enables this feature.

DCCV is performed under sedation, usually with midazolam or a general anaesthetic. The patient must be fasted and have a normal serum potassium concentration. Digoxin should be held on the day of the procedure to reduce the risk of VF (Roberts 2018).

Routine preparation and monitoring involved in electrical cardioversion includes the following:

- Standard cardiorespiratory monitoring including continuous ECG trace, blood pressure, oxygen saturation and end-tidal CO_2 monitoring.
- Intravenous access for administration of emergency drugs should complications occur.
- Supplemental oxygen, suction device and intubation equipment availability.
- Resuscitation equipment and medications should be readily available in case of an emergency (Knight 2019).

Key Point

Care should be taken to ensure that the patient's arms will not come into contact with hard bed surfaces as activation of the thoracic skeletal muscles during delivery of the shock may cause patients arms to jerk strongly (Knight 2019).

Key Point

Oxygen should be removed from the patient or turned off just prior to delivery of the shock and restarted after shock delivery as it is a fire hazard if electrical arcing occurs (Knight 2019).

Patients who cannot be converted to sinus rhythm or have an early recurrence of arrhythmia may be considered for a repeat procedure with pre-treatment with an antiarrhythmic drug such as sotalol or amiodarone (Roberts 2018).

Key Point

The defibrillator pads should be placed at a minimum of 15 cm apart from an implanted cardiac device and the device function should be checked following cardioversion.

When available, a biphasic defibrillator is preferred due to greater efficacy. The amount of energy selected for cardioversion may vary between different unit protocols or national guidelines. Knight (2019) suggests the following:

- Atrial fibrillation: 120–200 J for biphasic devices and 200 J for monophasic devices.
- Atrial flutter: 50–100 J for biphasic devices and 100 J for monophasic devices.
- Ventricular tachycardia with a pulse: 100 J for biphasic devices and 200 J for monophasic devices.

A higher initial energy may be considered in obese patients or in patients known to be difficult to cardiovert to increase the likelihood of early successful cardioversion and decrease the duration of sedation (Knight 2019).

Risks Associated with Electrical Cardioversion

Appropriate anticoagulation management at the time of the cardioversion is essential to reduce the risk of stroke (Page et al. 2016). With AF or atrial flutter for ≥48 h or unknown duration and no anticoagulation has been in place for the preceding 3 weeks, it is reasonable to perform a transoesophageal echo (TOE) first in order to exclude clot. Anticoagulation is required following the DCCV for at least 4 weeks, and possibly for longer in patients with a high risk of stroke.

- Thromboembolism
- Sedation-related complications
- Ventricular arrhythmias
- Bradyarrhythmias and conduction abnormalities
- Skin burn or irritation from electrodes
- Muscle soreness.
- Acute pulmonary oedema
- Hypotension
- Myocardial dysfunction (Knight 2019)

Suggested resource

The CHA$_2$DS$_2$-VASc Score for Atrial Fibrillation Stroke Risk medical calculation tool is commonly used in assessing stroke risk for patients with AF and is useful in guiding decisions about anticoagulation. The ORBIT Bleeding Risk Score for Atrial Fibrillation assesses bleeding risk with anticoagulation.

Calculators for these risk scores (and many other tools) can be found at https://www.mdcalc.com/

Key Point

If an R-wave is not present and sensed by the defibrillator (as in rhythms such as TdP or VF), synchronised cardioversion cannot be used because in synchronised mode, the defibrillator will not deliver a shock until an R-wave is sensed.

Ensure that the defibrillator is correctly sensing the R-wave and not some other ECG wave (such as a large T-wave).

Learning Activity 12.2

Read the full referenced articles included in this section for more comprehensive information about pharmacological and electrical cardioversion management for supraventricular arrhythmias.

Identify the professional organisational guidelines that direct practice for management of arrhythmias in your workplace. If you have unit guidelines, are these up to date and in line with current guidelines? Be aware that new guidelines, or focused updates to guidelines, are frequently released as new evidence becomes available.

Defibrillation

Defibrillation is non-synchronised random administration of a direct current (DC) shock during a cardiac cycle to terminate ventricular fibrillation, polymorphic ventricular tachycardia and pulseless ventricular tachycardia. The electrical current traverses the myocardium and causes all myocardial cells to contract simultaneously, thereby interrupting and terminating the abnormal electrical activity and allowing the sinus node to resume its function as the normal pacemaker. As with supraventricular tachycardia, guidelines for energy selection may vary. Knight (2019) suggests that for VF or pulseless VT, 120–200 J for biphasic devices and 360 J for monophasic devices. See Chapter 20 for management algorithms for cardiac arrest.

Cardiac Ablation

Catheter ablation is a surgical procedure that aims to provide a definitive solution for patients with various types of supraventricular and ventricular arrhythmias by applying energy to electrically cauterise the culprit tissue. The energy form used may be radiofrequency (heat), cryo (cold), or laser energy.

Supraventricular and Re-entrant Arrhythmias

Cardiac ablation may be used to treat AF (see indications, contraindications, and risk in Box 12.1); atrial flutter (similar indications, contraindications and risks as in AF ablation); paroxysmal SVT and WPW (indicated for symptomatic WPW or asymptomatic WPW in persons with high-risk features or high-risk occupations).

Atrial fibrillation ablation

Pulmonary veins are considered to be the main target for AF ablation in the majority of cases. The impulses thought to be the initiators of AF often arise from inside the pulmonary veins. In patients with paroxysmal AF there is no need to induce AF at the start of the procedure. A set of burn or freeze lines are drawn around the veins and once the procedure is complete, pacing manoeuvres are used to check that AF is not immediately inducible. These lines take around 3 months to heal and episodes of AF are to be expected during this period.

Surgical ablation of AF, although less widely available than catheter-based AF ablation, may be an option for patients at larger medical centres. For patients with a history of AF who are undergoing coronary artery bypass surgery or mitral valve replacement, surgical ablation to promote AV synchrony and sinus rhythm may be done at the same time (Calkin et al. 2017).

Ventricular Arrhythmias

Cardiac ablation may be used to treat PVCs in a structurally normal heart and PVC-induced cardiomyopathy (Ganz 2019a). Cardiac ablation may be suitable in the following circumstances:

- medication is not effective or suitable;
- scar-related heart disease presents with incessant VT (monomorphic) or an electrical storm (multiple episodes of ventricular arrhythmias over a short period of time);
- ischaemic heart disease with recurrent ICD shocks due to sustained VT (Breitenstein et al. 2019);
- arrhythmogenic right ventricular cardiomyopathy (Ganz 2019a).

In addition to the general potential complications of cardiac ablation, uncontrolled VT is a risk of the procedure (Cheung et al. 2018). Patients undergoing catheter ablation of myocardial infarct-associated VT have an increased risk of adverse outcomes compared with other forms of cardiac ablation due to significant comorbidities that can increase the risks of adverse outcomes such as congestive heart failure and pulmonary disease (Cheung et al. 2018).

Procedure

The procedure is initially like that of an electrophysiological (EP) study. The culprit tachycardia is induced with sequential pacing manoeuvres from the catheters, with or without the pharmacological assistance of certain intravenous drugs (isoprenaline and/or atropine). Once a precise diagnosis of the mechanism of the arrhythmia is made, applying radio-frequency (heat) or cryo energy (cold) to the culprit tissue, or to a defined area involved in the abnormal electrical circuit, successfully eradicates the arrhythmia in the vast majority of cases (Page et al. 2016). Short bursts of non-sustained arrhythmia can occur for a few days or weeks following the procedure but usually settle without intervention. The procedure can be repeated if required.

> **Key Point**
>
> Individuals undergoing ablation for SVT should be made aware that the procedure carries a small risk of damage to the AV node and consequently a requirement for a pacemaker.

> **Key Point**
>
> AV node ablation following pacemaker implantation may be used for people with AF who are unresponsive to rate and rhythm control therapies. This strategy allows for the discontinuation of rate-controlling medications, but as AF has not been eradicated, anticoagulation is still required.

> **Suggested Resource**
>
> Brugada, J., Katritsis, D.G., Arbelo, E., et al. (2020). 2019 ESC Guidelines for the management of patients with supraventricular tachycardia. *European Heart Journal* 41 (5): 655–720. https://academic.oup.com/eurheartj/article/41/5/655/5556821

Temporary Pacing

Temporary cardiac pacing is generally indicated for the acute management of serious bradyarrhythmias resulting from conditions that include primary abnormality of cardiac automaticity and/or conduction (idiopathic); conduction defect secondary to acute myocardial infarction; failure of previously implanted pacemaker device; unintended side effect, toxicity or overdose of cardioactive drugs; or severe electrolyte abnormalities (Sullivan et al. 2016). Several approaches to temporary pacing are available, including transvenous, transcutaneous, epicardial and transoesophageal (Alsheikh-Ali and Link 2017).

Temporary Transvenous Pacing

Transvenous pacing is the preferred form of temporary pacing if permanent pacing is not deemed necessary. It is more stable than transcutaneous pacing, more comfortable for the patient and can be used for a longer duration. The limitation of transvenous pacing in an emergency situation is that it requires expertise in both venous and cardiac anatomy in order to effectively access the vasculature and advance the electrode into the heart. A femoral vein approach is commonly used, particularly if the need for a pacemaker arises during percutaneous coronary interventions but has the disadvantages of risk of deep vein thrombosis, infection and patient immobility – consequently it is not used for long periods of time. The preferred access sites for temporary transvenous pacing leads are the left subclavian vein and the right internal jugular vein. The subclavian approach permits more freedom of patient motion (Hayes 2019a). Equipment for transvenous pacing includes an external pulse generator that attaches to the electrodes, allowing for the adjustment of pacing output, pacing rate, pacing mode and sensitivity to intrinsic activity. Most pacing systems support single or dual chamber pacing.

> **Suggested Resource**
>
> Medtronic Academy has a series of instructional videos and resources for preparation and maintenance of temporary transvenous pacing. Although the videos relate to Medtronic devices, the underlying principles are generally transferable to other pacing systems. You will need to register, but there is no charge.
> Medtronic Academy
> https://www.medtronicacademy.com

Transcutaneous Pacing

Transcutaneous pacing is generally used in an emergency until a perfusing rhythm is established, or until transvenous pacing or permanent pacing is available. It is not recommended for patients who present in asystole. Most external defibrillators have a pacing capability. Pacing is delivered via pads that can also be used for defibrillation and placed in the same position as for defibrillation. Transcutaneous pacing may cause a burning sensation of the skin and painful skeletal muscle contraction, especially with higher current use, and sedation is required. Many patients tolerate the pacing poorly, and the incidence of cardiac capture varies (Bunch et al. 2014).

Suggested Resources

The videos below will provide information and give a demonstration of transcutaneous pacing principles:
X Series Pacing
Zoll Medical (2016)
https://youtu.be/L43BOnTp_lQ
LIFEPAK 20/20E Defibrillator/Monitor
Noninvasive (Transcutaneous) Pacing
Physio Control (2014)
https://youtu.be/Nb0fDABC6UY

Other Forms of Temporary Pacing

Pacing via epicardial wires is used following cardiac surgery to maintain adequate heart rate should bradycardia occur or to override and reduce heart rate should tachyarrhythmias occur in the postoperative period. The wires are externalised and attached to an external pacing generator (Hayes 2019a).

Transoesophageal pacing can be used for atrial pacing, but it is uncomfortable to place, unreliable and painful, as it requires high current for capture and thus is rarely used (Hayes 2019a).

Implantable Cardiac Devices

Cardiac rhythm management devices include pacemakers and implantable cardioverter defibrillators (ICDs). The choice of device for an individual depends on the underlying pathophysiology, the individual's age, activity level and intrinsic heart rhythm.

A pacemaker is designed to treat abnormally slow heart rhythms, and an ICD to treat abnormally fast heart rhythms. An ICD also has pacing functionality. Pacemakers and ICDs detect and record abnormal rhythms and can be interrogated to provide current and historical information about any rhythm abnormalities experienced by the patient.

A loop recorder is another implantable device that detects and records abnormal rhythms to guide arrhythmia management but does not have a treatment function. Many loop recorders can also be interrogated using the same device as a pacemaker.

Implantable Pacemakers

Most contemporary pacemakers have two components: a pulse generator (the battery) that provides the electrical impulse for myocardial stimulation; and one or more electrodes, commonly referred to as leads, that deliver the electrical impulse from the pulse generator to the myocardium. Pulse generators are usually implanted in a pre-pectoral position in the infraclavicular region of the anterior chest wall though other sites may be used if needed. Impulses from the pulse generator are transmitted to the myocardium via transvenous leads. Transvenous leads are usually placed percutaneously or with a cephalic cutdown (Hayes 2019b). Epicardial cardiac pacemaker systems have a pulse generator and leads that are surgically attached directly to the epicardial surface of the heart and are occasionally used for patients with vascular access problems. Leadless cardiac pacing systems have recently been developed and approved for use for patients requiring single ventricle (right ventricular only) pacing. In the leadless system, the pulse generator and the electrode are in one self-contained unit, which is positioned via the femoral vein. It is anticipated that leadless systems will offer the advantage of long-term pacing capability without lead-associated complications. (Hayes 2019b).

The number of leads used and the chambers of the heart where pacing electrodes are placed vary:

- Single lead (single chamber): right atrium for atrial pacing or the right ventricle to pace the ventricle
- Two leads (dual chamber): right atrium and right ventricle
- Three leads for cardiac resynchronisation therapy (CRT): right atrium, right ventricle and left ventricle
- Leadless pacemaker: direct implant into the right ventricle (Stevenson and Voskoboinik 2018).

The functions of a pacemaker device are classified by the nature of their pacing mode, using a simple coding system expressed as a series of up to five letters (see Table 12.4). Pacemakers also detect and record abnormal rhythms, and these can be assessed by device interrogation.

Suggested Resource

Pacemaker codes and modes – Explained Understanding Pacemakers (2017)
https://youtu.be/L-lMhDQTq7w

Pacing for Bradycardia

Failure of impulse generation in the sinus node or propagation of the impulse via the atrioventricular (AV) node and/or the His–Purkinje network results in bradycardia. If the bradycardia is sufficiently slow or prolonged, it results in symptoms. You may wish to review normal cardiac conduction in Chapter 3.

Sinus Node Disease

Sinus node disease (SND), also known as sick sinus syndrome (SSS), can result in sinus bradycardia, chronotropic incompetence or sinus arrest and is the most common reason for pacemaker implantation (see Chapter 11). It is most often idiopathic and seen in elderly people (Nikolaidou et al. 2018).

Atrioventricular Node Disease

Acquired AV block is the second most common indication for permanent pacemaker insertion. AV block is usually idiopathic but can also result from myocardial ischaemia and infarction; medications including beta-blockers, calcium-channel blockers and digoxin; infection including brucellosis and Lyme disease; and cardiac surgery, most commonly involving the aortic valve. AV block is classified as follows:

- First-degree heart block is associated with a fixed but prolonged PR interval
- Second-degree heart block is sub-classified as (a) Mobitz Type I (Wenkebach) with cycles of progressive prolongation of PR interval until the P-wave fails to be conducted; and (b) Mobitz Type II in which the

Table 12.4 Commonly used pacemaker codes.

Position 1	Position II	Position III	Position IV	Position V
Chamber(s) paced	Chamber(s) sensed	Response to sensing	Rate modulation	Multisite pacing
0 = None	0 = None	0 = None	0 = None	0 = None
A = Atrium	A = Atrium	T = Triggered	R = Rate modulation	A = Atrium
V = Ventricle	V = Ventricle	I = Inhibited		V = Ventricle
D = Dual (A + V)	D = Dual (A + V)	D = Dual (T + I)		D = Dual (A + V)

Source: Adapted from Bernstein et al. (2002).

PR interval is constant but ventricular activation fails either intermittently or in a fixed ratio to the P-wave rate, usually 2:1. 3:1 or 4:1

- Third-degree heart block, also called complete heart block or AV dissociation, in which atrial and ventricular activity are independent of each other. The ventricular rhythm is an escape rhythm, with a rate that is usually around 30–40 beats/min (Nikolaidou et al., 2018).

The decision to implant a pacemaker is guided by symptoms associated with an arrhythmia, such as dizziness, light-headedness, syncope, fatigue, poor exercise tolerance and the location of the conduction abnormality. Disease below the AV node in the His–Purkinje system is generally considered to be less stable; thus, permanent pacemaker insertion is more likely to be recommended. Other indications for permanent pacemaker insertion include neurogenic syncope (in selected cases); unexplained syncope in a patient with sinus node dysfunction; bifascicular or trifascicular block associated with syncope attributed to transient complete heart block in the absence of other causes; and syncope without clear provocative events and with a hypersensitive cardio-inhibitory response of 3 seconds or longer (Nikolaidou et al., 2018). Some patients may be entirely dependent on their pacemakers and have no intrinsic (underlying) rhythm, while others may only pace intermittently, and the pacemaker is in place as a back-up in case of lapses in intrinsic activity.

Cardiac Resynchronisation/ Biventricular Pacing

Cardiac resynchronisation therapy (CRT) may be used in some patients with heart failure who have left ventricular (LV) dysfunction and poorly coordinated ventricular contraction that causes a reduction in LV stroke volume. Pacing both the left and the right ventricles of the heart simultaneously (biventricular pacing) can improve systolic function by resynchronising the heart contraction. CRT is not indicated in all patients with heart failure but can reduce symptoms and the number of hospitalisations and improve length of survival for many with heart failure (Atherton et al. 2018). CRT devices can be sub-divided into CRT P (cardiac resynchronisation-pacemaker) or CRT D (cardiac resynchronisation therapy with added defibrillator capacity).

Suggested Resource

Understanding pacemakers
Zero to Finals (2018)
https://youtu.be/53_jyoA47Fk

Implantable Cardioverter Defibrillators

Defibrillation

Indications for ICD implantation can be categorised as primary and secondary prophylaxis against sudden cardiac death (SCD). The greatest predictors of risk for SCD include poor LV systolic dysfunction (ejection fraction below 30–40%), Class II to IV heart failure symptoms using the New York Heart Association (NYHA) functional class classification system (Beyerbach 2019a). Other possible indications for ICD include VT in the setting of structural heart disease, syncope of undetermined origin, inducible VT or VF at EPS, hypertrophic cardiomyopathy, arrhythmogenic right ventricular dysplasia, LQTS, Brugada syndrome, CPVT, cardiac sarcoidosis, giant cell myocarditis and Chagas disease.

There is good evidence to support the use of an ICD for secondary prophylaxis. An ICD has been shown in several studies to be superior to antiarrhythmic drug therapy in patients with a history of life-threatening ventricular tachycardia VT and VF without a completely reversible cause (Beyerbach 2019a).

People with an ICD often describe delivery of a shock from the ICD as like being suddenly kicked or punched in the chest, though if the heart rate is very rapid, the person may have lost consciousness by this point. There may be some warning such as dizziness or light-headedness. Advice should be given to people with an ICD to sit or lie down if this occurs. The shock from the ICD does not harm anyone in contact with the person at the time of the shock. After the shock, the centre responsible for on-going care of the person with the ICD should be informed, and a check normally follows. If recovery is slow, or more than one shock occurs, then an ambulance should be called.

Key Point

Some ICDs can detect fluid build-up in the thoracic cavity in heart failure patients. The device has an audible alert that prompts the patient to contact their physician if this occurs. It is important to educate the patient about this alert as it is not uncommon for them to be alarmed if they do not know what it is.

Cardioversion

ICDs can be programmed to deliver synchronised shocks for ventricular tachycardia VT with relatively low energy.

Anti-tachycardia Pacing

Pacing faster than the rate of an arrhythmia can sometimes break the circuit and terminate it. Anti-tachycardia pacing (ATP), also known as overdrive pacing, may be useful in terminating atrial flutter or atrial tachycardia. Atrial fibrillation sometimes alternates with atrial flutter (Crossley et al. 2019). ICDs usually have an AT pacing function to terminate ventricular tachycardia with ventricular pacing and to terminate the arrhythmia and avoid the need for a shock to be delivered (Landolina et al. 2016).

Implantation Procedure for Cardiac Devices

Cardiac devices are implanted under sterile conditions in the cardiac catheter laboratory or operating theatre. The implantation procedure for pacemakers and ICDs is similar. Local anaesthesia is used at the site of the pulse generator insertion, with procedural sedation provided for patients in whom anxiety or pain control is needed. A pocket is made for the generator box subcutaneously in the chest wall below the clavicle. The leads are implanted via the subclavian or cephalic vein using fluoroscopy to guide them into place. Vital signs are monitored throughout the procedure and the device is checked at the end of the procedure to ensure correct functioning. The wound is closed either with glue, dissolvable or nondissolvable sutures. Following device implantation, a posteroanterior (PA) and lateral chest radiograph should be obtained to establish the position of the pulse generator and the associated lead(s) and to exclude complications such as pneumothorax. Patients should also have a 12-lead electrocardiogram (ECG) recorded post implant. This is particularly helpful in the case of cardiac resynchronisation therapy to verify biventricular capture (Ganz 2019a). Implantation takes around 60–90 minutes depending on the complexity of the device.

Subcutaneous Implantable Cardioverter Defibrillator

The subcutaneous implantable cardioverter defibrillator (S-ICD) was initially developed to avoid the complications of transvenous access in children and young adults with complicated congenital heart defects or in individuals who were unsuitable for a transvenous system due to problems with venous access. Rather than being placed within the right ventricle, the defibrillator lead is vertically positioned in the subcutaneous tissue of the chest, parallel to and slightly to the left of the sternal midline, followed by a horizontal segment at the level of the sixth rib. Here, it is connected to the generator box, which is positioned on the side of the chest, under the arm. This generator box is slightly larger than the traditional ICD. The S-ICD does not act as a pacemaker and programming choices are limited compared to traditional ICDs (Stiles 2019).

Post Procedure

> **Suggested Resource**
>
> Nursing care of patient with pacemaker
> Mometrix (2019)
> https://youtu.be/5JczIZiyZbQ

The patient may be suitable for same day discharge if there are no complications apparent within the initial 6 hours post-procedure. The patient should be advised to keep the wound dry for 5–7 days post-operatively. Any signs of infection should be reported immediately. If non-dissolvable sutures are used, they can be removed in 7–10 days after the procedure. Patients are usually followed up annually in dedicated pacing clinics to monitor functioning of the device (state of the battery, appropriateness of pacing, any increased resistance in the leads that may indicate damage or altered position) and review the device generator site.

Remote monitoring of devices is becoming more readily available.

> **Suggested Resource**
>
> There are many websites with advice for patients who have had a cardiac device implanted.
> See the example below:
> Pacemakers and implantable defibrillators
> Medline Plus
> https://medlineplus.gov/pacemakersand-implantabledefibrillators.html

> **Key Point**
>
> Patients are given a card with details of the make and model of the device implanted, a personal identity number and a 24 hours emergency phone number. The patient should be advised to always carry this.

Some manufacturers of implantable devices provide device interrogators that can be used in the home or in settings such as an emergency department (ED) (see Figure 12.2). The device has a small antenna that is placed over the pacemaker and the signals from the pacemaker are then transmitted to a remote site that reports the findings to the patient's

Figure 12.2 Medtronic Carelink monitor.

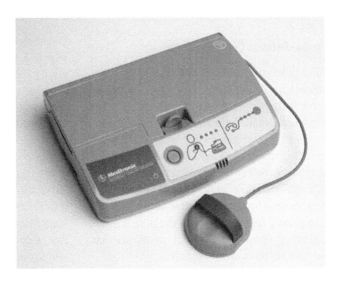

cardiologist and in the case of ED interrogation, to the treating physician). Remote monitoring reports are not as comprehensive as a complete device interrogation. Remote monitoring has been shown to improve survival in patients with an ICD or pacemaker.

Implantable Device Complications

Procedure-Related Complications

Complications associated with transvenous lead implantation includes bleeding (particularly for those on antiplatelet therapy), haematoma due to pocket bleed, pocket erosion (pulse generator or wires protrude through the device implantation site), infection, lead dislodgement, pneumothorax, haemothorax, air embolism, cardiac perforation, thrombosis of the implant vein, tricuspid valve regurgitation, and although rare, death may occur. Infection may occur at the time of implant or later and can be life-threatening. Complete removal of the pulse generator and all leads and treatment with antibiotic therapy is required unless there are exceptional circumstances in which this cannot be done. Extraction of leads carries a risk of vascular and/or cardiac injury due to the fibrous connections that develop between the leads and the vascular wall and endocardial surface (Weinstock 2019).

Device-Related Complications

Pulse generator problems are rare but are a significant problem for pacemaker-dependent patients if they occur. Lead malfunctions are rare and more likely to occur in ICD leads; presents with symptoms related to the failed lead including inappropriate ICD shocks, dizziness or syncope. Safety threshold values for pacing and defibrillation may change over time. Patients with implanted cardiac devices should be regularly followed up and the device interrogated to identify any device problems that may not yet be clinically apparent.

Suggested Resource

YouTube

Medmastery has produced a series of short videos that outline common pacemaker malfunctions, how to recognise them, why they occur and what needs to be done to fix the problem.
Common pacemaker problems
Medmastery (2015)
Part 1: Failure to capture https://youtu.be/xD1EqK0c46E
Part 2: Undersensing https://youtu.be/KRDkkrzw5iE
Part 3: Oversensing https://youtu.be/rj0qwxHgs_s

Key Point

Older implantable cardiac devices may not be MRI safe. Whilst most newer devices are MRI compatible, checks must be made to ensure that both the generator and the leads are MRI safe. Older leads may have been left *in situ* due to risk of removing them, and new leads inserted. The older leads may not be MRI safe. Checks must be made to see if the patient has older device leads *in situ*.

Other Complications

Pacemaker syndrome is a phenomenon in which a patient feels symptomatically worse after pacemaker placement and presents with progressively worsening symptoms of congestive heart failure. Pacemaker syndrome is most associated with single lead VVI pacemakers but has been reported in other pacing configurations. It can be caused by loss of synchrony between the atria and ventricles with loss of 'atrial kick' that contributes to cardiac output; retrograde ventriculo-atrial conduction; altered ventricular activation pattern; and absence of rate response to physiological need. Initial management is symptom support and longer term may involve optimizing pacemaker settings or replacing a single-chamber device with dual chamber or CRT (Beyerbach 2019b).

Phrenic nerve stimulation can occur due to inadvertent stimulation of the phrenic nerve, usually by a left ventricular lead. It can be continuous or paroxysmal and can cause dyspnoea, uncomfortable muscle twitching, hiccups and general malaise. It may not be apparent in the supine position and thus not detectable during the implantation procedure (Moubarak et al. 2014).

Phantom shock, a perception of having received a shock when no shock was delivered, occurs in around 9% of patients, usually those who have received an ICD shock previously (Berg et al. 2013).

Key Point

Some patients twist or rotate the device pulse generator within its pocket, known as 'Twiddler's syndrome', resulting in lead dislodgement and device malfunction (Ganz 2019b).

Key Point

Psychological distress, manifesting as anxiety and depression, is commonly found in people with an ICD. Contributing issues include fear of dying, fear of the device delivering a shock, limitations on normal life activities and changes in family dynamics, Moreover, partners of those with an ICD have been found to have equal or higher levels of anxiety, particularly in the first year following implantation (Rottmann et al. 2018).

Learning Activity 12.3

Undertake a literature search to identify studies of strategies to reduce symptoms of anxiety and depression in patients with an ICD. Have these strategies been successful or unsuccessful? Are there any strategies that you could use in your practice to support people with an ICD?

Practical Advice for Patients Following Device Implantation

Driving

Driving restrictions for patients with implantable devices are necessary when it poses a threat to others (Watanabe et al. 2017) but requires significant life adjustment and may be associated with decreased quality of life (Timmermans et al. 2018) and financial implications for those who are dependent on driving for their employment. Regulations vary around the world regarding fitness to drive following device implantation and are likely different for private versus commercial licences. The regulations for the country in which the patient resides (or drives) should be consulted.

Suggested Resources

Cardiovascular disorders: assessing fitness to drive
GOV.UK
https://www.gov.uk/guidance/cardiovascular-disorders-assessing-fitness-to-drive
Assessing Fitness to Drive for commercial and private vehicle drivers Austroads/National Transport Commission (Australia 2016)
https://austroads.com.au/drivers-and-vehicles/assessing-fitness-to-drive

---

Travel

Flying is generally safe 48 hours after an uncomplicated implant procedure if there is no pneumothorax, but restrictions of ipsilateral arm movement and avoidance of heavy lifting precludes the use of overhead lockers if travelling alone. The patient should always carry their Implant Identification Card for presentation at security checkpoints in airports or in emergency departments whilst traveling. X-ray security scanners are safe for device patients. The metal in the device may set off alarms when passing through airport security a hand search or use of a hand-held wand by security staff may result. Patients should be advised to place their hand vertically over the device to avoid the wand passing too close to the device. Airport security causes no harm to devices if the patient does not linger in the area (Stevenson and Voskoboinik 2018).

Exercise

Vigorous arm movements ipsilateral to the device should be avoided in the initial post-implantation period. Until recently, guidelines recommended against all moderate and high-intensity sports for people with ICDs as the risk profile was uncertain. Newer guidelines suggest that moderate leisure-time physical exercise is safe and clinically recommended for most individuals with ICDs (Kiuchi et al. 2019). Recently published long term results from the Multinational ICD Sports Registry showed that in young athletes, shocks related to competition/practice are not uncommon, but there were no serious adverse sequelae. The rates of lead malfunction in this cohort was similar to that reported for unselected paediatric populations (Saarel et al. 2018). Heidbuchel and colleagues (2019) found that participants in recreational sports had less frequent appropriate and inappropriate shocks during physical activity than participants in competitive sports. There does not appear to be consensus in current guidelines relating to participation in sports for people with an ICD. The decision to continue participating in sports should be shared between athletes and their physicians, taking into account the risk related to the underlying disease and the person's values and preferences (Lampert 2019).

Sexual Intimacy

For most people with an ICD sexual activity once the surgical site has healed, but avoidance of sexual activity is well documented in patients with ICDs (Rav Acha et al. 2017). Reasons for this include inadequate communication about sex between cardiovascular patients and their health providers as sex and intimacy are seen as topics not to be discussed with others; reduced interest in sex post ICD implant (possibly due to anxiety, depression, or change in body image); and fear of sex-induced ICD shock (Rav Acha et al. 2017). Intimate partners are also concerned for themselves and the person with an ICD if a shock is delivered during sexual activity. They need to be reassured that An ICD shock during sex is not a common occurrence, and that the shock will not be transmitted to a partner. It is essential that the person with the ICD and their partner receive counseling about sexual activity.

Suggested Resources (for patients)

After an implantable ICD
St. Vincent's Hospital Heart Health
https://www.svhhearthealth.com.au/rehabilitation/after-an-implantable-defibrillator-icd

Implantable cardioverter defibrillator (ICD)
British Heart Foundation
https://www.bhf.org.uk/informationsupport/treatments/implantable-cardioverter-defibrillator

---

Electromagnetic Interference

Electrical interference may cause devices to sense external signals as intrinsic cardiac signals, resulting in inhibition of pacing and possibly inappropriate defibrillation. Magnets flick a switch in pacemakers and defibrillators, which can result in asynchronous pacing or inactivation of defibrillation. This rarely happens with modern devices and normal household appliances, but it is recommended that mobile phones be kept 15 cm away from the device. Airport security is discussed under 'travel' above. Store antitheft devices are safe if the person with the device does not linger in the area. Some medical and dental procedures may require advice from a cardiologist and a device check post procedure. These include surgery using diathermy, medical radiation treatment, MRI, transcutaneous nerve stimulation and electroconvulsive therapy (Stevenson and Voskoboinik 2018).

End-of-Life Considerations for People with Implantable Cardiac Devices

People with ICDs, including CRT-D devices, who are approaching the end of their life should be given opportunities to discuss the option of deactivation of their device (Pitcher et al. 2016). Terminal illnesses, including end-stage heart failure, puts the person at risk of developing tachyarrhythmias that might lead to shock therapy. At this point shock therapy would be inappropriate, painful and distressing. Close collaboration between relevant health professionals, the patient and their family must happen to ensure timely deactivation, and it should be requested and appropriate.

Key Point

Cardiac devices need to be removed prior to cremation due to potential damage to the crematory chamber from flying metal. If there are no plans for cremation, a patient may be buried with their device in situ (Stevenson and Voskoboinik 2018).

Advanced Nursing Roles in Arrhythmia Management

Managing rhythm disturbances is now a highly specialised area within cardiology. It is developing rapidly as a speciality as new techniques, procedures and equipment become available. The emotional and economic distress associated with some arrhythmias is now well recognised. A holistic approach to arrhythmia management includes involving the patient in self-management strategies to complement medical management.

A major contribution to the improved management and support of patients with arrhythmias in the United Kingdom has been the appointment of specialist nurses as arrhythmia care co-ordinators who provide nurse-led arrhythmia clinics, DCCV clinics, procedure follow-up clinics and telephone support lines to provide advice and information to patients and general practitioners. This strategy was initially funded by the British Heart Foundation and has demonstrated reduced emergency department presentations, reduced re-admissions resultant cost savings (Ismail and Coulton 2016).

Suggested Resources

Pacemaker Codes and Modes – Explained Understanding Pacemakers (2017) https://youtu.be/L-lMhDQTq7w
Glikson, et al. (2021). 2021 ESC Guidelines on cardiac pacing and cardiac resynchronization therapy: Developed by the Task Force on cardiac pacing and cardiac resynchronization therapy of the European Society of Cardiology (ESC) With the special contribution of the European Heart Rhythm Association (EHRA). *European Heart Journal*, *42*(35), 3427-3520. https://doi.org/10.1093/eurheartj/ehab364

References

Al-Khatib, S.M., Stevenson, W.G., Ackerman, M.J. et al. (2018). 2017 AHA/ACC/HRS guideline for management of patients with ventricular arrhythmias and the prevention of sudden cardiac death: a report of the American College of Cardiology/American Heart Association Task Force on Clinical Practice Guidelines and the Heart Rhythm Society. *Journal of the American College of Cardiology* **72** (14): e91–e220. https://doi.org/10.1016/j.jacc.2017.10.054.

Alsheikh-Ali, A.A. and Link, M.S. (2017). Temporary transvenous pacing. In: *Cardiology Procedures*, 187–193. London: Springer https://doi.org/10.1007/978-1-4471-7290-1_22.

Antzelevitch, C. (2019). Short QT syndrome. In: (ed. M.S. Link and B.C. Downey). *UpToDate*, http://www.uptodate.com/home/index.html.

Atherton, J.J., Sindone, A., De Pasquale, C.G., Driscoll, A., MacDonald, P.S., Hopper, I., . . . & Thomas, L. (2018). National Heart Foundation of Australia and Cardiac Society of Australia and New Zealand: guidelines for the prevention, detection, and management of heart failure in Australia 2018. *Heart, Lung and Circulation*, **27** (10), 1123–1208. https://doi.org/10.1016/j.hlc.2018.06.1042

Baker, W.L. (2016). Treating arrhythmias with adjunctive magnesium: identifying future research directions. *European Heart Journal–Cardiovascular Pharmacotherapy*, **3** (2), 108-117. https://doi.org/10.1093/ehjcvp/pvw028.

Barnes, B.J., & Hollands, J.M. (2010). Drug-induced arrhythmias. *Critical Care Medicine*, **38**, S188-S197. http://dx.doi.org/https://doi.org/10.1097/CCM.0b013e3181de112a.

Behere, S.P. and Weindling, S.N. (2015). Inherited arrhythmias: the cardiac channelopathies. *Annals of Pediatric Cardiology* **8** (3): 210. https://dx.doi.org/10.410 3%2F0974-2069.164695.

Berg, S.K., Moons, P., Zwisler, A.D., Winkel, P., Pedersen, B.D., Pedersen, P.U., & Svendsen, J.H. (2013). Phantom shocks in patients with implantable cardioverter defibrillator: results from a randomized rehabilitation trial (COPE-ICD). *Europace*, **15** (10), 1463-1467. https://doi.org/10.1093/europace/eut087

Bernstein, A.D., Daubert, J.C., Fletcher, R.D. et al. (2002). The revised NASPE/BPEG generic code for antibradycardia, adaptive-rate, and multisite pacing. *Pacing and Clinical Electrophysiology* **25** (2): 260–264.

Beyerbach, D.M. (2019a). In: (ed. J.N. Rottman). Pacemakers and Implantable Cardioverter-Defibrillators. *Medscape*. https://emedicine.medscape.com/article/162245-overview.

Beyerbach, D.M. (2019b). What is pacemaker syndrome? In: (ed. J.N. Rottman), *Medscape*. https://www.medscape.com/answers/162245-111843/what-is-pacemaker-syndrome.

Bunch, T.J., Osborn, J.S., and Day, J.D. (2014). Temporary cardiac pacing. In: *Cardiac Pacing and ICDs* (ed. K.A. Ellenbogen and K. Kaszala), 134–149. https://doi.org/10.1002/9781118459553.

Breitenstein, A., Sawhney, V., Providencia, R. et al. (2019). Ventricular tachycardia ablation in structural heart disease: impact of ablation strategy and non-inducibility as an end-point on long term outcome. *International journal of cardiology* **277**: 110–117.

Brieger, D., Amerena, J., Attia, J.R., Bajorek, B., Chan, K.H., Connell, C., . . . & Hendriks, J. (2018). National Heart Foundation of Australia and Cardiac Society of Australia and New Zealand: Australian clinical guidelines for the diagnosis and management of atrial fibrillation 2018. *Medical Journal of Australia*, **209** (8), 356–362. https://doi.org/10.5694/mja18.00646.

Brignole, M., Moya, A., de Lange, F.J. et al. (2018). 2018 ESC Guidelines for the diagnosis and management of syncope. *European Heart Journal* **2001** (22): 1256–1306.

Brugada, J., Campuzano, O., Arbelo, E. et al. (2018). Present status of Brugada syndrome: JACC state-of-the-art review. *Journal of the American College of Cardiology* **72** (9): 1046–1059.

Calkins, H., Hindricks, G., Cappato, R., Kim, Y.H., Saad, E.B., Aguinaga, L., ... & Yamane, T. (2018). 2017 HRS/EHRA/ECAS/APHRS/SOLAECE expert consensus statement on catheter and surgical ablation of atrial fibrillation. *EP Europace*, **20** (1), e1–e160. https://academic.oup.com/europace/article-abstract/20/1/e1/4158475

Campbell, T.J. and MacDonald, P.S. (2003). Digoxin in heart failure and cardiac arrhythmias. *Medical Journal of Australia* **179** (2): 98–102. www.mja.com.au/system/files/issues/179_02_210703/cam10066_fm.pdf.

Cheung, J.W., Yeo, I., Ip, J.E., Thomas, G., Liu, C.F., Markowitz, S.M., . . . & Kim, L.K. (2018). Outcomes, costs, and 30-day readmissions after catheter ablation of myocardial infarct – associated ventricular tachycardia in the real world: nationwide readmissions database 2010–2015. *Circulation: Arrhythmia and Electrophysiology*, **11** (11), e006754. https://doi.org/10.1161/CIRCEP.118.006754.

Colangelo, T., Johnson, D., and Ho, R. (2021). Flecainide-induced atrial flutter with 1: 1 conduction complicated by ventricular fibrillation after electrical cardioversion. *Texas Heart Institute Journal* **48** (2): e197099.

Cole, J., Torabi, P., Dostal, I., Homer, K. and Robson, J., 2018. Opportunistic pulse checks in primary care to improve recognition of atrial fibrillation: a retrospective analysis of electronic patient records. *British Journal of General Practice*, **68** (671), pp.e388–e393. https://doi.org/10.3399/bjgp18X696605.

Crossley, G.H., Padeletti, L., Zweibel, S., Hudnall, J.H., Zhang, Y., & Boriani, G. (2019). Reactive atrial-based antitachycardia pacing therapy reduces atrial tachyarrhythmias. *Pacing and Clinical Electrophysiology*. https://doi.org/10.1111/pace.13696.

Delise, P. and Zeppilli, P. (ed.) (2021). Brugada ECG Pattern and Brugada Syndrome. In: *Sport-related Sudden Cardiac Death*, 151–158. Springer International Publishing https://doi.org/10.1007/978-3-030804473_11.

DiBiase, L. and Walsh, E.P. (2018). Treatment of symptomatic arrhythmias associated with the Wolff-Parkinson-White syndrome. In: (ed. S.L. Levy, B.P. Knight, and B.C. Downey), *UpToDate*. http://www.uptodate.com/home/index.html.

Earley, M.J. (2009). How to perform a transseptal puncture. *Heart* **95** (1): 85–92.

Frish, D.R. and Zimetbaum, P.J. (2018). Vagal maneuvers. In: (ed. B. Olshansky and B.C. Downey), *UpToDate*. https://www-uptodate-com.access.library.unisa.edu.au/contents/vagal-maneuvers?topicRef = 902&source = see_link (accessed 16 October 2019).

Gale, C.P. and Camm, A.J., 2016. Assessment of palpitations. *BMJ*, **352**, p.h5649. https://doi.org/10.1136/bmj.h5649.

Garabelli, P., Stavrakis, S. and Po, S., 2017. Smartphone-based arrhythmia monitoring. *Current Opinion in Cardiology*, **32** (1), pp.53-57. https://doi.org/10.1097/HCO.0000000000000350.

Ganz L.I. (2019a). Overview of catheter ablation of cardiac arrhythmias. In: (ed. S. Levy and B.C. Downey), *UpToDate*. http://www.uptodate.com/home/index.html.

Ganz L.I. (2019b). Cardiac implantable electronic devices: long-term complications. In: (ed. J. Piccini and B.C. Downey), *UpToDate*. http://www.uptodate.com/home/index.html.

Giudicessi, J.R., Noseworthy, P.A., & Ackerman, M.J. (2019). The QT interval: an emerging vital sign for the precision medicine era?. *Circulation*, **139** (24), 2711–2713.

Haïssaguerre, M., Derval, N., Sacher, F., Jesel, L., Deisenhofer, I., de Roy, L., . . . & De Chillou, C. (2008). Sudden cardiac arrest associated with early repolarization. *New England Journal of Medicine*, **358** (19), 2016-2023. https://doi.org/10.1056/NEJMoa071968.

Hamon, D., Rajendran, P.S., Chui, R.W., Ajijola, O.A., Irie, T., Talebi, R., . . . & Ardell, J.L. (2017). Premature ventricular contraction coupling interval variability destabilizes cardiac neuronal and electrophysiological control: insights from simultaneous cardioneural mapping. *Circulation: Arrhythmia and Electrophysiology*, **10** (4), e004937. https://doi.org/10.1161/CIRCEP.116.004937.

Hayes, D.L. (2019a). Temporary cardiac pacing. In: (ed. L.I. Ganz and B.C. Downey), *UpToDate*. http://www.uptodate.com/home/index.html.

Hayes, D.L. (2019b). Permanent cardiac pacing: Overview of devices and indications. In: (ed. M.S. Link & B.C. Downey), *UpToDate*. http://www.uptodate.com/home/index.html.

Heidbuchel, H., Willems, R., Jordaens, L., Olshansky, B., Carre, F., Lozano, I.F., ... & Lampert, R. (2019). Intensive recreational athletes in the prospective multinational ICD Sports Safety Registry: results from the European cohort. *European Journal of Preventive Cardiology*, **26** (7), 764–775.

Hocini, M., Pison, L., Proclemer, A., Larsen, T.B., Madrid, A., Blomström-Lundqvist, C. and Conducted by the Scientific Initiative Committee, European Heart Rhythm Association, 2014. Diagnosis and management of patients with inherited arrhythmia syndromes in Europe: results of the European Heart Rhythm Association Survey. *Europace*, **16** (4), pp.600-603. https://doi.org/10.1093/europace/euu074.

Homoud, M.K. (2019). Invasive cardiac electrophysiology studies. In: (ed. B.S. Knight and B.C. Downey), *UpToDate*. http://www.uptodate.com/home/index.html.

Hothi, S. and Sprigings, D. (2017). Palpitations. In: *Acute Medicine: A Practical Guide to the Management of Medical Emergencies*, 5e (ed. D. Sprigings and J.B. Chambers), 53–59.

Ismail, H., & Coulton, S. (2016). Arrhythmia care co-ordinators: their impact on anxiety and depression, readmissions and health service costs. *European Journal of Cardiovascular Nursing*, **15** (5), 355-362. https://doi.org/10.1177/1474515115584234.

King, G.S. and McGuigan, J.J. (2019). *Antiarrhythmics: Stat Pearls*. Treasure Island (FL): StatPearls Publishing https://www.ncbi.nlm.nih.gov/books/NBK482322.

Kiuchi, M.G., Schlaich, M., Ho, J., Carnagarin, R., & Villacorta, H. (2019). Lifestyle advice for patients with ICDs: physical activity–what is healthy and what is contraindicated. *E-journal of Cardiology Practice*, **17** (11).

Knight, B.P. (2019). Cardioversion for specific arrhythmias. In: (ed. R.L. Page and B.C. Downey), *UpToDate*. http://www.uptodate.com/home/index.html.

Kusumoto, F.M., Schoenfeld, M.H., Barrett, C., Edgerton, J.R., Ellenbogen, K.A., Gold, M.R., . . . & Lee, R. (2019). 2018 ACC/AHA/HRS guideline on the evaluation and management of patients with bradycardia and cardiac conduction delay: a report of the American College of Cardiology/American Heart Association Task Force on Clinical Practice Guidelines and the Heart Rhythm

Society. *Circulation*, **140** (8), e382-e482. DOI: https://doi.org/10.1161/CIR.0000000000000627.

Lampert, R. (2016). Behavioral influences on cardiac arrhythmias. *Trends in Cardiovascular Medicine*, **26** (1), 68–77. https://doi.org/10.1016/j.tcm.2015.04.008.

Lampert, R. (2019). Update on sports participation for athletes with implantable cardioverter defibrillators. *International Journal of Cardiovascular Sciences*, **32**, 391–395.

Landolina, M., Lunati, M., Boriani, G., Ricci, R.P., Proclemer, A., Facchin, D., . . . & Molon, G. (2016). Ventricular antitachycardia pacing therapy in patients with heart failure implanted with a cardiac resynchronization therapy defibrillator device: efficacy, safety, and impact on mortality. *Heart Rhythm*, **13** (2), 472-480. https://doi.org/10.1016/j.hrthm.2015.10.022.

Levine, E. (2019). Classifications of antiarrhythmic agents, *Medscape*. https://emedicine.medscape.com/article/2172024-overview (accessed 21 August 2019).

Mittal, S., Sanders, P., Pokushalov, E. et al. (2015). Safety profile of a miniaturized insertable cardiac monitor: results from two prospective trials. *Pacing and Clinical Electrophysiology* **38** (12): 1464–1469. https://doi-org.access.library.unisa.edu.au/10.1111/pace.12752.

Moubarak, G., Bouzeman, A., Ollitrault, J., Anselme, F., & Cazeau, S. (2014). Phrenic nerve stimulation in cardiac resynchronization therapy. *Journal of Interventional Cardiac Electrophysiology*, **41** (1), 15-21. https://doi.org/10.1007/s10840-014-9917-8.

Muresan, L., Cismaru, G., Martins, R.P. et al. (2019). Recommendations for the use of electrophysiological study: Update 2018. *Hellenic Journal of Cardiology* **60** (2): 82–100.

Obeyesekere, M.N., Klein, G.J., Modi, S., Leong-Sit, P., Gula, L.J., Yee, R., . . . & Krahn, A.D. (2011). How to perform and interpret provocative testing for the diagnosis of Brugada syndrome, long-QT syndrome, and catecholaminergic polymorphic ventricular tachycardia. *Circulation: Arrhythmia and Electrophysiology,* **4** (6), 958-964. https://doi.org/10.1161/CIRCEP.111.965947.

Nguyen, H.H., & Silva, J.N. (2016). Use of smartphone technology in cardiology. *Trends in Cardiovascular Medicine,* **26** (4), 376-386. https://doi.org/10.1016/j.tcm.2015.11.002.

Nikolaidou, T., Fox, D.J., & Brown, B.D. (2018). Bradycardia pacing. *Medicine,* **46** (10), 646-651. https://doi.org/10.1016/j.mpmed.2018.07.002.

Page, R.L., Joglar, J.A., Caldwell, M.A., Calkins, H., Conti, J.B., Deal, B.J., . . . & Indik, J.H. (2016). 2015 ACC/AHA/HRS guideline for the management of adult patients with supraventricular tachycardia: a report of the American College of Cardiology/American Heart Association Task Force on Clinical Practice Guidelines and the Heart Rhythm Society. *Journal of the American College of Cardiology,* **67** (13), e27-e115. https://doi.org/10.1016/j.jacc.2015.08.856.

Pitcher, D., Soar, J., Hogg, K., Linker, N., Chapman, S., Beattie, J.M., . . . & Patterson, G. (2016). Cardiovascular implanted electronic devices in people toward the end of life, during cardiopulmonary resuscitation and after death: guidance from the Resuscitation Council (UK), British Cardiovascular Society and National Council for Palliative Care. *Heart,* **102** (Suppl. 7), A1-A17. http://dx.doi.org/10.1136/heartjnl-2016-309 721.

Porthan, K., Kenttä, T., Niiranen, T.J., Nieminen, M.S., Oikarinen, L., Viitasalo, M., . . . & Albert, C.M. (2019). ECG left ventricular hypertrophy as a risk predictor of sudden cardiac death. *International Journal of Cardiology,* **276**, 125–129. https://doi.org/10.1016/j.ijcard.2018.09.104.

Rav Acha, M., Hasin, T. (2017). Sexual Function in Adults with Implantable Cardioverter-Defibrillators/Pacemaker Recipients. In: Proietti, R., Manzoni, G., Pietrabissa, G., Castelnuovo, G. (eds) Psychological, Emotional, Social and Cognitive Aspects of Implantable Cardiac Devices. Springer, Cham. https://doi.org/10.1007/978-3-319-55721-2_6

Raviele, A., Giada, F., Bergfeldt, L., Blanc, J.J., Blomstrom-Lundqvist, C., Mont, L., . . . & Document reviewers. (2011). Management of patients with palpitations: a position paper from the European Heart Rhythm Association. *Europace,* **13** (7), 920-934. https://doi.org/10.1093/europace/eur130.

Rizzo, C., Monitillo, F., & Iacoviello, M. (2016). 12-lead electrocardiogram features of arrhythmic risk: a focus on early repolarization. *World Journal of Cardiology,* **8** (8), 447. https://doi.org/10.4330/wjc.v8.i8.447.

Roberts, P.R. (2018). Direct current cardioversion. *Medicine* **46** (10): 663. https://doi-org.access.library.unisa.edu.au/10.1016/j.mpmed.2018.07.011.

Rottmann, N., Skov, O., Andersen, C.M. et al. (2018). Psychological distress in patients with an implantable cardioverter defibrillator and their partners. *Journal of Psychosomatic Research* **113**: 16–21. https://doi-org.access.library.unisa.edu.au/10.1016/j.jpsychores.2018.07.010.

Ruskin, J.N. (1989). The cardiac arrhythmia suppression trial (CAST). *New England Journal of Medicine* **321** (6): 386–388.

Saarel, E.V., Law, I., Berul, C.I., Ackerman, M.J., Kanter, R.J., Sanatani, S., ... & Lampert, R.J. (2018). Safety of sports for young patients with implantable cardioverter-defibrillators: long-term results of the Multinational ICD Sports Registry. *Circulation: Arrhythmia and Electrophysiology,* **11** (11), e006305.

Singh, S. and McKintosh, R. (2019). *Adenosine.* Treasure Island (FL): StatPearls Publishing https://www.ncbi.nlm.nih.gov/books/NBK519049.

Stevenson, I. and Voskoboinik, A. (2018). Cardiac rhythm management devices. *Australian Journal of General Practice* **47** (5): 264. www1.racgp.org.au/ajgp/2018/may/cardiac-rhythm-management-devices.

Stiles, M.K. (2019). Implantable cardioverter-defibrillators: Optimal programming. In: (ed. J. Piccini and B.C. Downey), *UpToDate.* http://www.uptodate.com/home/index.html.

Sullivan, B.L., Bartels, K., & Hamilton, N. (2016). Insertion and management of temporary pacemakers. *Seminars in Cardiothoracic and Vascular Anesthesia* (Vol. **20**, No. 1, pp. 52–62). Sage CA: Los Angeles, CA: SAGE Publications. https://doi-org. access.library.unisa.edu.au/10.1177/ 1089253215584923.

Timmermans, I., Jongejan, N., Meine, M., Doevendans, P., Tuinenburg, A., & Versteeg, H. (2018). Decreased quality of life due to driving restrictions after cardioverter defibrillator implantation. *Journal of Cardiovascular Nursing*, **33** (5), 474-480. https://doi.org https://doi.org/10.1097/ JCN.0000000000000474.

Watanabe, E., Abe, H., & Watanabe, S. (2017). Driving restrictions in patients with implantable cardioverter defibrillators and pacemakers. *Journal of Arrhythmia*, **33** (6), 594-601. https:// doi.org/10.1016/j.joa.2017.02.003.

Weinstock, J. (2019). Cardiac implantable electronic device lead removal. In: (ed. J. Piccini and B.C. Downey), *UpToDate*. http:// www.uptodate.com/home/index.html.

Vaughan Williams, E.M. (1970). Classification of antiarrhythmic drugs. *Symposium on Cardiac Arrhythmias, Sweden, Astra 1970*.

Zimetbaum, P.J. (2018). Overview of palpitations in adults. In: (ed. M.D. Aronson and J. Givens), *UpToDate*. http://www.uptodate. com/home/index.html.

Part IV

Detection and Management of Acute Coronary Syndromes

13

Pathogenesis of Acute Coronary Syndromes

Angela M. Kucia and John D. Horowitz

Overview

Cardiovascular atherosclerotic disease is the leading cause of death in Western industrialised nations, as well as in developing countries. The pathogenesis of acute coronary syndrome (ACS) usually involves atherosclerotic plaque rupture, platelet activation and thrombus formation. Mechanisms leading to adverse coronary events are complex and variable and are not predicted solely by the presence, severity and metabolic activity of atherosclerotic disease alone. Inflammatory activation and coronary artery spasm represent important components of the various acute coronary syndromes.

Key Concepts

Atherosclerosis; plaque rupture or erosion; endothelial dysfunction; thrombogenesis; vasoconstriction

---

Acute Coronary Syndrome

The term 'acute coronary syndrome' refers to a range of conditions generally associated with symptomatic coronary artery disease (CAD) including ST-segment elevation myocardial infarction (STEMI), non-ST-segment elevation myocardial infarction (non-STEMI), unstable angina (UA) that result in abrupt onset of myocardial ischaemia or infarction or possibly sudden cardiac death (SCD). The pathogenesis of ACS usually involves atherosclerotic plaque rupture, platelet activation and thrombus formation.

Although STEMI, non-STEMI and UA resulting from CAD generally share a common pathophysiological base, these conditions differ in severity and outcome, according to the nature and severity of contributing factors. Not all causes of STEMI, non-STEMI and UA have an atheromatous pathogenesis. This has led to the need for universal definitions of myocardial injury and myocardial infarction and subsequent modifications (see Chapter 14).

Learning Objectives

After reading this chapter, you should be able to:

- Describe the factors related to the process of atherosclerosis.
- Discuss the differences between stable and vulnerable plaques.
- Describe the process of thrombogenesis and the factors related to thrombus formation at the site of a plaque rupture.
- Demonstrate an understanding of the role of endothelium and the role of endothelial dysfunction in the development of ACS.

Cardiac Care: A Practical Guide for Nurses, Second Edition. Edited by Angela M. Kucia and Ian D. Jones.
© 2022 John Wiley & Sons Ltd. Published 2022 by John Wiley & Sons Ltd.

Key Point

Coronary artery spasm, coronary microvascular dysfunction, spontaneous coronary thrombosis/emboli, coronary artery dissection, myocarditis, takotsubo syndrome, various cardiomyopathies and many non-cardiac conditions may cause troponin elevation (Pasupathy et al. 2017). Some of these may be associated with typical signs and symptoms of myocardial ischaemia or infarction in the absence of obstructive coronary disease.

Suggested Resource

Pathogenesis of atherosclerosis
PhysioPathoPharmaco (2017)
https://youtu.be/N33JsBeziEY

Atherosclerosis

Acute coronary syndromes generally result from atherosclerosis, which causes plaque formation in the inside lumen of medium- and large-sized coronary arteries. Plaque may cause partial obstruction of the coronary artery, a process which is usually asymptomatic, or, in the setting of plaque rupture and associated thrombosis, can progress rapidly to total coronary occlusion. Atherosclerosis is a progressive disease that probably begins in adolescence, with progression depending upon age, gender, genetic make-up and other risk factors. In some people, atherosclerosis may progress rapidly from their third decade, whilst in others it may not become apparent until later years. Some individuals with atherosclerosis will never experience symptoms or complications from this disease, whilst others may have chronic symptoms. Some may experience sudden acute symptoms with no warning, which may have serious consequences, including death.

Atherogenesis is understood to be influenced by a complex interaction of cardiovascular risk factors (see Chapter 5), inflammation and endothelial dysfunction (Libby and Theroux 2005). Factors such as hypercholesterolaemia, hypertension, smoking and diabetes predispose to both structural and functional damage to the arterial endothelium and initiate the atherosclerotic process.

Endothelial Dysfunction

Endothelium consists of a thin layer of simple, or single-layered, squamous cells that line the interior surface of blood vessels and lymphatic vessels. Endothelium functions as a metabolic and endocrine organ producing a multitude of different molecules, including vasoactive peptide hormones, growth factors, coagulation factors and adhesion molecules (Baumgartner-Parzer and Waldhäusl 2001). Endothelial cells regulate antioxidants, have anti-inflammatory and anticoagulant action, and, thus, control vascular relaxation and contraction, thrombogenesis, fibrinolysis and platelet activation and inhibition. Maintaining the functional integrity of the endothelium is critical to preserving blood flow and preventing thrombosis (Stanek et al. 2018). Endothelial dysfunction is an important early event in the pathogenesis of atherosclerosis that significantly contributes to plaque initiation and progression. It is characterised by impaired vasodilator capacity and disturbances in antithrombotic, profibrinolytic, and anti-inflammatory and antioxidant properties of the normal endothelium (Libby et al. 2016).

Endothelial dysfunction has been observed in relation to ageing, as well as in major lifestyle-related diseases (Stanek et al. 2018). Most forms of cardiovascular disease, including hypertension, CAD, chronic heart failure, and peripheral artery disease, are associated with vascular endothelial dysfunction.

Inflammation

Inflammation has a central role in the pathogenesis and consequences of cardiovascular disease and encompasses a broad range of processes at the site of disease, in the blood, at remote sites and as downstream sequelae of disease. Elevated levels of inflammatory markers such as C-reactive protein (CRP) have been shown to be predictive of future cardiovascular events (Ruparelia et al. 2017).

Myocardial ischaemia results in the activation of the immune response, both locally at the site of injury and in the circulating blood and at remote sites. These processes are important both as mediators of injury and subsequently in repair and recovery. Ischaemia causes initially reversible injury to the cardiac myocytes, impairing both their contraction and relaxation, but if ischaemia is not rapidly resolved, death of cardiomyocytes will occur, and their intracellular contents will be released. This cellular necrotic process will trigger an accentuated inflammatory response with platelet activation, leukocyte infiltration and rapid recruitment of neutrophils to the myocardium. Macrophages serve to scavenge necrotic debris and are then active in promoting reparative processes (Ruparelia et al. 2017). Importantly, it has been shown that chronic suppression of inflammation is effective in reducing the probability of occurrence of acute ischaemic events (Ridker et al. 2017). It is also likely that the effects of statins and some ACE inhibitors in reducing risk of occurrence of acute ischaemia result largely from their anti-inflammatory effects. The activation of the immune system following ACS results in general systemic inflammation, as evidenced by increased plasma levels of inflammatory cytokines, which are positively correlated with adverse outcomes (Valgimigli et al. 2005).

Plaque Rupture and Thrombosis

Most acute coronary events are due to rupture or fissure of an atherosclerotic plaque with associated intra-luminal thrombosis (Libby et al. 2019), while plaque fissure has the more limited exposure of denuding a region of the vascular endothelium from the glycocalyx layer which normally overlies it. Sudden luminal thrombosis may arise from three different plaque morphologies:

- Plaque rupture – responsible for most acute myocardial infarctions (AMI) and sudden cardiac death (SCD)
- Plaque erosion – estimated to cause around a third of ACS cases
- Calcified nodule – an eruptive accumulation of small nodular calcification that accounts for a small percentage of patients with ACS (Lee et al. 2017) and more prevalent in older individuals with tortuous and heavily coronary calcified arteries (Crea et al. 2018).

Plaque Rupture

Plaque rupture is characterised by the presence of a luminal thrombus overlying a thin disrupted fibrous cap. The plaque is often infiltrated by macrophages and T-lymphocytes, and there is an underlying large necrotic core (Otsuka et al. 2016). When endothelium is damaged, macrophages bind to the dysfunctional endothelial wall and can infiltrate the endothelial cell. Activated platelets are likely to aggregate on the damaged surfaces, initiating thrombus formation. Low-density lipoproteins (LDL) also infiltrate the endothelial cell where they are digested by macrophages, becoming foam cells, and thus creating a lipid-filled atherosclerotic plaque. Over time, fats, cholesterol, platelets, cellular debris and calcium are deposited in the damaged artery wall. Smooth muscle proliferation occurs in response to cytokines secreted by the damaged endothelial cells, resulting in the formation of a dense, fibrous extracellular matrix (connective tissue) cap covering the plaque. The integrity of the fibrous cap determines the stability of the atherosclerotic plaque: once the fibrous cap is breached, the thrombogenic lipid core comes into contact with circulating blood (Libby et al. 2019). Even minor damage to the endothelium adjacent to atheromatous plaques, termed plaque fissure, is responsible for the emergence of acute coronary syndromes in a substantial proportion of cases (Libby et al. 2019.)

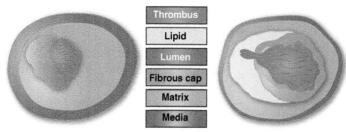

Plaque erosion	Plaque rupture
Lipid poor	Lipid rich
Proteoglyan and glycosaminoglycan rich	Collagen poor, thin fibrous cap
Non-fibrillar collagen breakdown	Interstital collagen breakdown
Few inflammatory cells	Abundant inflammation
Endothelial cell apoptosis	Smooth muscle cell apoptosis
Secondary neutrophil involvement	Macrophage predominance
Female predominance	Male predominance
High triglycerides	High LDL

Figure 13.1 'Contrasts between superficial erosion and fibrous cap rupture as causes of arterial thrombosis. LDL, low-density lipoprotein'. *Source:* Libby and Pasterkamp (2015). Copyright © 2019 European Society of Cardiology.

Foam cells produce large amounts of tissue factor derived from macrophages (Libby et al. 2019). Tissue factor is a transmembrane protein that triggers the primary procoagulant pathway of coagulation. In the absence of injury or inflammatory stimuli, tissue factor is not expressed on cellular surfaces in direct contact with circulating blood, but when inflammation or injury occurs, presentation of tissue factor to the circulation is the event that triggers activation of the clotting cascade (Brummel-Ziedins and Mann 2018). Platelet adhesion, activation and aggregation after plaque rupture or erosion are the major determinants of arterial thrombosis leading to ACS. NSTEMI is frequently characterised by a non-occlusive or transiently occlusive thrombus, whereas a more stable and occlusive thrombus is typical in STEMI.

Plaque Erosion

Plaque erosion is an acute thrombosis without rupture (Libby et al. 2019). The pathogenesis of plaque erosion is not well understood but it is likely mechanistically different from plaque rupture (Libby et al. 2019). Plaque erosion involves an acute thrombus in direct contact with the intima in an area of denuded endothelium (in the absence of a fibrous cap disruption). Unlike plaque rupture, there is no extensive necrotic core, haemorrhage or calcification (Crea et al. 2018). Plaque erosion accounts for over 80% of thrombi occurring in women <50 years of age (Otsuka et al. 2016).

Figure 13.1 shows the differences between the more common causes of ACS: superficial plaque erosion and fibrous cap rupture.

Pathological Characteristics of Myocardial Ischaemia and Infarction

Historically myocardial infarction (MI) has been defined using various clinical, electrocardiographic (ECG), biochemical and

---

Suggested Resource YouTube

Platelet activation and factors for clot formation
Thrombosis Advisor (2014)
https://youtu.be/R8JMfbYW2p4

pathologic characteristics resulting in confusion and controversy (Thygesen et al. 2018). With the introduction of more sensitive cardiac biomarkers, the definition of myocardial infarction became less clear as elevated troponin is often detected in patients who had no evidence of acute coronary thrombosis (see Table 13.1). Criteria to differentiate between myocardial infarction and myocardial injury have been proposed below.

Myocardial injury: 'evidence of elevated cardiac troponin (cTn) values with at least one value above the ninety-ninth percentile upper reference limit (URL). The myocardial injury is considered acute if there is a rise and/or fall of cTn values' (Thygesen et al. 2018, p. 2235).

Universal definitions of myocardial injury and myocardial infarction based on differences in pathophysiology were first introduced in 2000 (Joint European Society of Cardiology/ American College of Cardiology Committee for the Redefinition of Myocardial Infarction 2000) and further refined as shown in Box 13.1. These definitions are useful in refining guidelines for management of MI according to causal mechanism, and in describing or categorising MI in epidemiological studies and clinical trials.

Table 13.1 Reasons for the elevation of cardiac troponin values because of myocardial injury.

Myocardial injury related to acute myocardial ischaemia	
Atherosclerotic plaque disruption with thrombosis	• Takotsubo syndrome
Myocardial injury related to acute myocardial ischaemia because of oxygen supply/demand imbalance	• Coronary revascularisation procedure • Cardiac procedure other than revascularisation • Catheter ablation • Defibrillator shocks • Cardiac contusion
Reduced myocardial perfusion, e.g. • Coronary artery spasm, microvascular dysfunction • Coronary embolism • Coronary artery dissection • Sustained bradyarrhythmia • Hypotension or shock • Respiratory failure • Severe anaemia	*Systemic conditions,* e.g. • Sepsis, infectious disease • Chronic kidney disease • Stroke, subarachnoid haemorrhage • Pulmonary embolism, pulmonary hypertension • Infiltrative diseases, e.g. amyloidosis, sarcoidosis • Chemotherapeutic agents • Critically ill patients • Strenuous exercise
Increased myocardial oxygen demand, e.g. • Sustained tachyarrhythmia • Severe hypertension with or without left ventricular hypertrophy	
Other causes of myocardial injury	
Cardiac conditions, e.g. • Heart failure • Myocarditis • Cardiomyopathy (any type)	

Source: Reprinted from Thygesen et al. (2019). Copyright © 2019 European Society of Cardiology.

Box 13.1   Universal definitions of myocardial injury and myocardial infarction.

Criteria for myocardial injury

The term myocardial injury should be used when there is evidence of elevated cardiac troponin values (cTn) with at least one value above the ninety-ninth percentile upper reference limit (URL). The myocardial injury is considered acute if there is a rise and/or fall of cTn values.

Criteria for acute myocardial infarction (types 1, 2 and 3 MI)

The term acute myocardial infarction should be used when there is acute myocardial injury with clinical evidence of acute myocardial ischaemia and with detection of a rise and/or fall of cTn values with at least one value above the ninety-ninth percentile URL and at least one of the following:

- Symptoms of myocardial ischaemia
- New ischaemic ECG changes
- Development of pathological Q-waves
- Imaging evidence of new loss of viable myocardium or new regional wall motion abnormality in a pattern consistent with an ischaemic aetiology
- Identification of a coronary thrombus by angiography or autopsy (not for type 2 or 3 MIs).

Post-mortem demonstration of acute athero-thrombosis in the artery supplying the infarcted myocardium meets criteria for *type 1 MI*.

Evidence of an imbalance between myocardial oxygen supply and demand unrelated to acute athero-thrombosis meets criteria for *type 2 MI*.

Cardiac death in patients with symptoms suggestive of myocardial ischaemia and presumed new ischaemic ECG changes before cTn values become available or abnormal meets criteria for *type 3 MI*.

Criteria for coronary procedure-related myocardial infarction (types 4 and 5 MI)

Percutaneous coronary intervention (PCI)-related MI is termed type 4a MI.

Coronary artery bypass grafting (CABG)-related MI is termed type 5 MI.

Coronary procedure-related MI $\leq$48 hours after the index procedure is arbitrarily defined by an elevation of cTn values >5 times for type 4a MI and >10 times for type 5 MI of the ninety-ninth percentile URL in patients with normal baseline values. Patients with elevated pre-procedural cTn values, in whom the pre-procedural cTn levels are stable ($\leq$20% variation) or falling, must meet the criteria for a >5 or >10-fold increase and manifest a change from the baseline value of >20%. In addition, with at least one of the following:

- New ischaemic ECG changes (this criterion is related to type 4a MI only)
- Development of new pathological Q-waves
- Imaging evidence of loss of viable myocardium that is presumed to be new and in a pattern consistent with an ischaemic aetiology
- Angiographic findings consistent with a procedural flow-limiting complication such as coronary dissection, occlusion of a major epicardial artery or graft, side-branch occlusion-thrombus, disruption of collateral flow or distal embolisation.

Isolated development of new pathological Q-waves meets the type 4a MI or type 5 MI criteria with either revascularisation procedure if cTn values are elevated and rising but less than the pre-specified thresholds for PCI and CABG.

Other types of 4 MI include type 4b MI stent thrombosis and type 4c MI restenosis that both meet type 1 MI criteria.

Post-mortem demonstration of a procedure-related thrombus meets the type 4a MI criteria or type 4b MI criteria if associated with a stent.

Criteria for prior or silent/unrecognised myocardial infarction

Any one of the following criteria meets the diagnosis for prior or silent/unrecognised MI:

- Abnormal Q waves with or without symptoms in the absence of non-ischaemic causes.

- Imaging evidence of loss of viable myocardium in a pattern consistent with ischaemic aetiology.
- Patho-anatomical findings of a prior MI.

CABG = coronary artery bypass grafting; cTn = cardiac troponin; ECG = electrocardiogram; MI = myocardial infarction; PCI = percutaneous coronary intervention; URL = upper reference limit.
Source: Reprinted from Thygesen et al. (2018). © 2018 The European Society of Cardiology, American College of Cardiology Foundation, American Heart Association, Inc. and the World Heart Federation. All Rights Reserved Published by Elsevier.

Conclusion

Understanding of pathophysiological processes related to atherosclerosis and inflammation and the development of ACS have progressed significantly over the past two decades and continue to evolve. With this further understanding, we can target those individuals at greatest risk for preventative therapies and develop new therapies that may target newly understood pathophysiological processes inherent in the onset of ACS.

Learning Activity 13.1

Consider the process of thrombosis in ACS: what pharmacotherapies do we use in ACS that directly target these processes in clinical practice? Do you know how they work? Visit the suggested resource below for further information.

Suggested resource

Zwart, B., Parker, W. A., & Storey, R. F. (2020). New antithrombotic drugs in acute coronary syndrome. *Journal of Clinical Medicine, 9*(7), 2059. https://www.ncbi.nlm.nih.gov/pmc/articles/PMC7408919/

Learning Activity Answers

Learning Activity 13.1

Answer:
Antiplatelet Therapy
- Aspirin
- P2Y12 inhibitors (usually ticagrelor) is administered with aspirin to provide dual antiplatelet therapy
- GP IIb/IIIa receptor antagonists abciximab, eptifibatide and tirofiban may be used adjunctively at the time of PCI in selected patients with STEMI and NSTE-ACS who are receiving unfractionated heparin, but they are not often used in ACS when patients have dual anti-platelet therapy due to the increased risk of bleeding.

Anticoagulation Therapy:
Unfractionated heparin, low-molecular-weight heparins (e.g. enoxaparin or fondaparinux), Bivalirudin.
    For more comprehensive information about these classes of drugs and how they are used in ACS, see the Suggested Resource below:

Suggested Resource

Janardan, J. and Gibbs, H. (2018). Combining anticoagulation and antiplatelet drugs in coronary artery disease. *Australian Prescriber* 41: 111–115. https://www.nps.org.au/australian-prescriber/articles/combining-anticoagulation-and-antiplatelet-drugs-in-coronary-artery-disease. doi: 10.18773/austprescr.2018.039

References

Baumgartner-Parzer, S.M. and Waldhäusl, W.K. (2001). The endothelium as a metabolic and endocrine organ: its relation with insulin resistance. *Experimental and Clinical Endocrinology and Diabetes* **109** (Suppl. 2): S166–S179.

Crea, F., Kolodgie, F., Finn, A., and Virmani, R. (2018). Mechanisms of acute coronary syndromes related to atherosclerosis. In: (ed. C.P. Cannon, J.C. Kaski, P. Libby, and G. Saperia), *UpToDate*. www.uptodate.com.

Brummel-Ziedins, K. and Mann, K.G. (2018). Chapter 126 – Molecular basis of blood coagulation. In: *Hematology*, 7ee (ed. R. Hoffman, E.J. Benz Jr., L.E. Silberstein, et al.). Elsevier Health Sciences.

Lee, T., Mintz, G.S., Matsumura, M. et al. (2017). Prevalence, predictors, and clinical presentation of a calcified nodule as assessed by optical coherence tomography. *JACC: Cardiovascular Imaging* **10** (8): 883–891. https://doi-org.access.library.unisa.edu.au/10.1016/j.jcmg.2017.05.013.

Libby, P., Bornfeldt, K.E., & Tall, A.R. (2016). Atherosclerosis: successes, surprises, and future challenges. *Circulation Research*, **118**: 531–534. https://doi.org/10.1161/CIRCRESAHA.116.308334.

Libby, P. and Theroux, P. (2005). Pathophysiology of coronary artery disease. *Circulation* **111**: 3481–3488.

Libby, P. and Pasterkamp, G. (2015). Requiem for the 'vulnerable plaque'. *European Heart Journal* **36** (43): 2984–2987.

Libby, P., Pasterkamp, G., Crea, F., & Jang, I.K. (2019). Reassessing the mechanisms of acute coronary syndromes: the 'vulnerable plaque' and superficial erosion. *Circulation Research*, **124** (1), 150–160. https://doi.org/10.1161/CIRCRESAHA.118.311098.

Otsuka, F., Yasuda, S., Noguchi, T., & Ishibashi-Ueda, H. (2016). Pathology of coronary atherosclerosis and thrombosis. *Cardiovascular Diagnosis and Therapy*, **6** (4), 396. doi: https://doi.org/10.21037/cdt.2016.06.01.

Pasupathy, S., Tavella, R., and Beltrame, J.F. (2017). Myocardial Infarction with Nonobstructive Coronary Arteries (MINOCA) the past, present, and future management. *Circulation* **135** (16): 1490–1493.

Ridker, P.M., Everett, B.M., Thuren, T., MacFadyen, J.G., Chang, W.H., Ballantyne, C., . . . & Kastelein, J.J. (2017). Antiinflammatory therapy with canakinumab for atherosclerotic disease. *New England Journal of Medicine*, **377** (12), 1119–1131. DOI: https://doi.org/10.1056/NEJMoa1707914.

Ruparelia, N., Chai, J.T., Fisher, E.A., & Choudhury, R.P. (2017). Inflammatory processes in cardiovascular disease: a route to targeted therapies. *Nature Reviews Cardiology*, **14** (3), 133. doi: https://doi.org/10.1038/nrcardio.2016.185.

Stanek, A., Fazeli, B., Bartuś, S., & Sutkowska, E. (2018). The role of endothelium in physiological and pathological states: new data. *BioMed Research International*, *2018*. https://doi.org/10.1155/2018/1098039.

The Joint European Society of Cardiology/American College of Cardiology Committee (2000). Myocardial infarction redefined – a consensus document of the Joint European Society of Cardiology/American College of Cardiology Committee for the Redefinition of Myocardial Infarction. *European Heart Journal* **21**: 1502–1513.

Thygesen, K., Alpert, J.S., Jaffe, A.S. et al. (2018). Fourth universal definition of myocardial infarction (2018). *Journal of the American College of Cardiology* **72** (18): 2231–2264. https://doi-org.access.library.unisa.edu.au/10.1016/j.jacc.2018.08.1038.

Valgimigli, M., Ceconi, C., Malagutti, P., Merli, E., Soukhomovskaia, O., Francolini, G., . . . & Guardigli, G. (2005). Tumor necrosis factor-α receptor 1 is a major predictor of mortality and new-onset heart failure in patients with acute myocardial infarction: the Cytokine-Activation and Long-Term Prognosis in Myocardial Infarction (C-ALPHA) study. *Circulation*, **111** (7), 863–870. https://doi.org/10.1161/01.CIR.0000155614.35441.69.

Thygesen, K., Alpert, J.S., Jaffe, A.S. et al. (2019). Fourth universal definition of myocardial infarction. *European Heart Journal* **40** (3): 245.

14

Chest Pain Assessment

Angela M. Kucia, John F. Beltrame, and Jan Keenan

Overview

Chest pain is one of the most common present-ing complaints to emergency departments and general practice surgeries. Causes of chest pain can range from benign to life-threatening and potentially serious causes need to be identified and treated. Relatively few patients who pre-sent with a complaint of chest pain will be found to have a cardiac cause, but heart dis-ease is a leading cause of death and disability and so a cardiac cause of chest pain should always be considered and excluded or promptly treated. It is the clinician's expertise in taking a clear history that provides the initial step in achieving an accurate and timely diagnosis for patients with chest pain.

Learning Objectives

After reading this chapter, you should be able to:

- Describe typical features of chest pain associated with myocardial ischaemia and infarction.
- Describe abnormalities on the electro-cardiogram (ECG) associated with myo-cardial ischaemia and infarction and their diagnostic application.

- Describe serum cardiac markers associ-ated with ACSs and their diagnostic application.
- Discuss signs and symptoms of atypical presentations with ACSs and groups of patients in whom these atypical presen-tations are most likely.

Key Concepts

Chest pain assessment; angina; acute coro-nary syndrome

Background

Chest pain is the second most common presen-tation in Emergency Department (ED) and accounts for up to 20% of ED admissions (Parsonage et al. 2013). Ultimately only 10–20% of these patients are diagnosed with acute myocardial infarction (MI) (Wildi et al. 2019). Chest pain is not specific to acute coronary syndrome (ACS) and causes of chest pain range from clinically insignificant to life-threatening. Assessment of patients presenting with chest pain is complex because of the diversity of clinical presentations of ACS and the lack of a single diagnostic test for the entire

---

Cardiac Care: A Practical Guide for Nurses, Second Edition. Edited by Angela M. Kucia and Ian D. Jones.
© 2022 John Wiley & Sons Ltd. Published 2022 by John Wiley & Sons Ltd.

spectrum of the disease (Parsonage et al. 2013). However, a 'missed' diagnosis of ACS in up to 2–5% of patients presenting to ED with chest pain is associated with significant morbidity and mortality and represents a significant proportion of malpractice claims, particularly in the United States (Fernando et al. 2019). Fear of missing an ACS diagnosis and its consequences are key drivers of physician's behaviour in the ED leading to most patients with suspicious symptoms being admitted for prolonged observation (Than et al. 2013). Timely, efficient and accurate evaluation of the patient who presents with chest pain optimises care from an individual, public health and economic perspective (Australian Institute of Health and Welfare 2011; Australian Commission on Safety and Quality in Health Care 2015).

Identification of the 'true positive' ACS patient among the vast number of chest pain presentations to general practitioner (GP) surgeries and EDs is a challenge.

Coronary Heart Disease

Chest pain due to myocardial ischaemia is typically referred to as 'angina pectoris', or simply 'angina'. Angina is the most common manifestation of coronary heart disease (CHD).

Angina Pectoris

Angina may be stable or unstable, both of which result from a perfusion-dependent imbalance between myocardial oxygen supply and demand, though the mechanisms differ. Unstable angina (UA) is classed as an acute coronary syndrome (ACS).

Stable Angina

The classical description of angina pectoris by William Heberden remains as accurate today as the day he penned it in 1772. In his landmark paper entitled 'Some account of a disorder of the breast' he wrote:

> 'They who are afflicted with it, are seized while they are walking, (more especially if it be up hill, and soon after eating) with a painful and most disagreeable sensation in the breast, which seems as if it would extinguish life, if it were to increase or to continue; but the moment they stand still, all this uneasiness vanishes'.

This description captures the essential features of chronic stable angina, namely, its constrictive sensation and relationship to exertion. As this pain is predictable and usually self-limiting once the provocative stimulus has been removed, it is referred to as *stable angina*. Stable angina is not classed as an ACS but is worth mentioning here as it may progress to an unstable phase. The chest pain described by Heberden and summarised in Table 14.1 reflects a

Table 14.1 Characteristics of typical *stable* angina pain.

Type	Definition
Typical angina	(a) Constricting discomfort in the front of the chest, in the neck, shoulders, jaw or arms[a]
	(b) Provoked by exertion[a, b] or emotional stress[a]
	(c) Relieved by rest or sub-lingual nitrates[a, b]
Atypical angina	Pain with two of the above features[a, b, c]
Non-anginal chest pain	Pain with ≤1 of the above features[a, b, c]

- Characteristic quality of the pain is dull, heavy or aching (not sharp or burning).[c]
- Duration should be minutes (not seconds or hours).[c]

[a] National Institute for Clinical Excellence (NICE) characteristics of typical angina.
[b] Gibbons et al. (1999).
[c] Diamond (1983).

predictable pattern of chest pain that occurs in response to a provocative physiological stimulus such as exercise, sexual activity and emotional stress that increases heart rate/blood pressure, and thus myocardial oxygen demand, resulting in ischaemia in the region of myocardium that is supplied by a vessel with an obstructive lesion. Symptoms including pain, shortness of breath, sweating, nausea, vomiting, palpitations and weakness are usually relieved by rest. Table 14.1 summarises characteristics of typical stable angina according to the sources listed beneath the table. It is important to note that these characteristics are commonly seen, but, in some people, myocardial ischaemia may cause different symptoms or different patterns of pain.

The exact aetiology of stable angina is not well defined, but it is thought to be secondary to a mismatch between myocardial supply and demand. While the majority of patients with angina have significant narrowing of one or more epicardial coronary arteries, many patients with stable angina have non-obstructive or even normal coronary arteries. The prognosis for patients with stable angina varies, but there is an annual mortality rate of up to 3.2% (Rousan and Thadani 2019).

Assessment of individuals presenting with suspected stable angina is challenging. Guidelines aim to balance the risk of identifying patients at high risk of future cardiovascular events with efficient diagnostic pathways that minimise unnecessary or inappropriate testing (Adamson et al. 2018).

A change in pattern of stable angina may herald progression to UA. Patients may describe their angina as becoming more frequent, more severe, lasting longer or occurring with less exertion than has previously been the case. It may occur at rest with no obvious precipitating factors and may wake them from sleep. They may describe symptoms limiting their activity which are not responsive to rest or glyceryl trinitrate (GTN).

Acute Coronary Syndrome

ACS refers to ST-segment elevation myocardial infarction (STEMI), non-ST-segment elevation myocardial infarction (NSTEMI) and unstable angina pectoris (UAP), all of which have a shared pathophysiology (see Chapter 13). The most common presenting symptom in ACS is acute chest discomfort. The clinical presentation of ACS is broad and may include cardiac arrest, electrical or haemodynamic instability, cardiogenic shock or mechanical complications such as severe mitral regurgitation. Some patients may have resolution of chest pain by the time of presentation to patients who are already pain free again at the time of presentation (Collet et al. 2021).

Unstable Angina Pectoris

The diagnosis of UA suggests that symptoms are of new onset or depart from the usual pattern of angina. UA is defined as myocardial ischaemia at rest or on minimal exertion in the absence of acute cardiomyocyte injury/necrosis. With the introduction of high sensitivity cardiac troponin (hs-cTn) measurements in ED, there has been an increase in the detection of MI and a reciprocal decrease in the diagnosis of UA (Collet et al. 2021), to the point of UA being a relatively rare diagnosis (Simons and Alpert 2020). Compared with NSTEMI patients those with UA generally have a lower risk of death and do not appear to derive the same benefits from routine intensive antiplatelet therapy or early invasive strategy (Collet et al. 2021).

Key Point

Patients with new onset angina occurring only after heavy physical exertion have a prognosis similar to patients with chronic stable angina. In comparison, new angina occurring after minimal exercise or at rest, particularly if prolonged, carries a worse prognosis in the absence of intervention (Simons and Alpert 2020).

Acute myocardial infarction

Acute myocardial infarction (AMI) may occur with no prior symptoms or may be preceded by a short period of instability characterised by angina. A precipitating factor such as vigorous physical exercise, emotional stress or medical/surgical illness can be present in those who develop AMI, but symptoms often appear at rest. AMI is characterised by ischaemic pain, which is usually prolonged and severe.

Patients with MI are sub-categorised into STEMI and NSTEMI on the basis of their presentation ECG findings (Table 14.2). Studies undertaken more than 25 years ago demonstrated that patients presenting with an AMI who had ST elevation on their presentation ECG frequently had an occluded epicardial coronary artery, whereas those without ST elevation often did not. Strategies to open the occluded vessel in patients with acute ST elevation have developed with substantial success. However, these same strategies, thrombolysis

and immediate angiography appear to be less effective in those patients without ST elevation.

The diagnosis of STEMI and NSTEMI requires knowledge of the presenting symptoms, ECG and troponin (Tn). Urgent management of ACS, particularly STEMI, is of paramount importance for patient prognosis. However, the troponin (Tn) may not be rapidly available; thus, it is not always possible to make an immediate diagnosis of NSTEMI. As a result, two equivalent terms have evolved to define patients on the basis of clinical symptoms and ECG alone. Patients with an ST elevation acute coronary syndrome (STE-ACS) present with rest angina and ST elevation. Most of these patients will evolve into a STEMI and are managed as per STEMI protocols. Patients with a non-ST elevation acute coronary syndrome (NSTE-ACS) will subsequently be classified as NSTEMI if the Tn is positive, or UA if the Tn is negative (Table 14.2). Hence, the diagnoses of NSTE-ACS and STE-ACS are of particular use in the early acute care setting. Furthermore, the term NSTE-ACS is often used

Table 14.2 Clinical classifications of ACS.

Syndrome	Abbreviation	Clinical definition
Unstable angina	UA	• Rest angina >20 min • ECG changes present or absent
Non-ST elevation acute coronary syndrome	NSTE-ACS	• Rest angina >20 min • ST/T changes but no ST elevation • Tn result pending (patients may evolve to UA or NSTEMI)
ST elevation acute coronary syndrome	STE-ACS	• Rest angina >20 min • ST elevation • Tn result pending (most patients will progress to STEMI)
Non-ST elevation myocardial infarction	NSTEMI	• Rest angina >20 min • ST/T changes but no ST elevation • Positive Tn
ST elevation myocardial infarction	STEMI	• Rest angina >20 min • ST-segment elevation • Positive Tn

to categorise UA and NSTEMI together with the exclusion of STEMI.

A universal definition of 'MI' proposed in 2007 is based on differences in pathophysiology, including MI related to percutaneous intervention (PCI) or coronary bypass graft surgery (CABG) (Thygesen et al. 2007). This definition is useful in refining guidelines for the management of MI according to causal mechanism and in describing or categorising MI in epidemiological studies and clinical trials. The universal definition of myocardial infarction (see Chapter 13) is now in its fourth iteration (Thygesen et al. 2018).

Suggested Resource

Reading the following is strongly recommended:
Thygesen, K., Alpert, J. S., Jaffe, A. S. et al. (2018). Fourth universal definition of myocardial infarction (2018). *Journal of the American College of Cardiology* 72 (18): 2231–2264.
https://www.jacc.org/doi/full/10.1016/j.jacc.2018.08.1038

It is important to recognise that there are many conditions other than ACS in which troponin elevation occurs (see Chapter 15).

Myocardial Infarction with Non-Obstructive Coronaries (MINOCA)

In approximately 5–10% of patients fulfilling the universal criteria of an acute MI, coronary angiography reveals no significant obstructive coronary disease. The term MINOCA (Myocardial Infarction with Non-Obstructive Coronaries) has been coined for these patients (Beltrame 2013). A recent systematic literature review reveals that these patients have a significant mortality, equivalent to a patient with single- or double-vessel coronary artery disease (CAD; Pasupathy et al. 2015). Hence, it is important to identify the underlying cause for the clinical presentation in these patients and initiate appropriate therapy (Pasupathy et al. 2015). See Chapter 27 for more information about MINOCA and INOCA.

Presentation with Chest Pain in the Emergency Department

Chest pain is the second most common presenting symptom in the ED, comprising approximately 5% of all ED visits (Johnson and Ghassemzadeh 2020). Symptoms that are suspicious of ACS, most commonly chest pain, are the trigger for individuals to seek emergent care for this potentially life-threatening condition (DeVon et al. 2020). Chest pain can originate from several sources, and it is important to differentiate whether the pain may result from a cardiovascular problem other than myocardial ischaemia. For example, pain that is made worse by lying down, moving or deep breathing and resolving with sitting forward may be caused by pericarditis. Pain that is accompanied by sudden shortness of breath and hypoxia associated with pre-syncope and haemoptysis may be caused by a pulmonary embolism. Abrupt sharp high-intensity chest pain described as stabbing, tearing or ripping in nature at onset is a characteristic of aortic dissection. In evaluating for chest pain, life-threatening causes of chest pain are always considered, including ACS, pulmonary embolism, pneumothorax, pericardial tamponade, aortic dissection and oesophageal perforation. Gastrooesophageal reflux disease and musculoskeletal pain are common non-life-threatening causes of chest pain (Johnson and Ghassemzadeh 2020). See Chapter 15 for more information on differential diagnosis of non-traumatic chest pain and non-MI causes of troponin elevation.

Typical Clinical Presentation of Ischaemic Chest Pain

Chest pain associated with myocardial ischaemia is usually described as tightness, pressure, heaviness, ache or may be mistaken for indigestion. The location of pain can vary, but usually involves the chest and may be central or left sided. It may also involve the epigastrium, left or both arms and/or the throat and may radiate to the jaw, back or shoulder. Chest pain related to myocardial ischaemia is not usually altered by changes in posture or position and is not exacerbated by movement in the region of pain localisation or by deep inspiration. Symptoms that may be associated with the chest pain include dyspnoea, nausea, vomiting, diaphoresis and dizziness. Typical

symptoms of myocardial ischaemia are listed in Table 14.3.

Key Point

It must be remembered that not all people experience 'typical' symptoms. People also may describe pain using alternate words or phrases. For instance, the word 'sharp' may be used to describe a pain that is intense or severe rather than stabbing in nature.

Patients who present with AMI are often anxious and distressed due to severe pain. Associated diaphoresis and peripheral coolness may be present. Although haemodynamic observations may be initially within normal limits, around 25% of patients with anterior wall AMI have associated sympathetic nervous system hyperactivity (tachycardia and/or hypertension), whereas up to half of patients presenting with inferior wall AMI have

Table 14.3 Typical symptoms of myocardial ischaemia.

Stable angina	Unstable angina	Acute myocardial infarction

Typical symptoms:
 • Pain most typically:
   – Central or left-sided chest
   – Left arm
   – Jaw
 	
 May involve or radiate to:
   – Both arms
   – Epigastrium
   – Back
   – Throat
	Typical symptoms:
	 • As for stable angina but may be more severe
		Typical symptoms:
		 • As for stable angina but may be more severe and involve a wider range of the symptoms listed

Typically provoked by: • Exercise • Sexual activity • Emotional stress • Angina is often provoked by the same types of activities and may be predictable	*Typically provoked by:* • May occur during exercise, stress or at rest provoking factors are usually unpredictable	*Typically provoked by:* May occur during exercise, stress or at rest

(Continued)

Table 14.3 (Continued)

Stable angina	Unstable angina	Acute myocardial infarction
Typically occurs: • In the morning • After a heavy meal • In cold weather	*Typically occurs:* • Can occur at any time • May occur with increasing frequency	*Typically occurs:* • Can occur at any time
Typical duration: • 2–10 min	*Typical duration:* • Usually <30 min • Episodes may come and go frequently over a period of time • Patients may describe having had pain for 2 or 3 days, but in fact the pain is not constant – it comes and goes	*Typical duration:* • >30 min
Alleviating factors: • Rest • Sub-lingual nitrate	*Alleviating factors:* • May require • Intravenous nitrates • Anticoagulation • Beta blockers or calcium channel blockers	*Alleviating factors:* • Reperfusion (PCI or thrombolysis)

associated parasympathetic activity (bradycardia and/or hypotension) (Antman and Braunwald 2001).

Atypical Presentations

Approximately 8% of ACS patients do not experience chest pain (Brieger et al. 2004). The major presenting symptoms in these patients include dyspnoea (49%), diaphoresis (26%), nausea/vomiting (24%) and pre-syncope/syncope (19%) (Brieger et al. 2004). Other less-common presentations may result from sudden loss of consciousness, confusion or profound weakness, which may occur as a result of impaired ventricular function or arrhythmia (Antman and Braunwald 2001). Patients with an atypical presentation frequently have poorer outcomes with increased in-hospital mortality (Brieger et al. 2004), and thus an increased vigilance is required for these presentations. Atypical ACS presentations are more likely to occur in women and those with a history of diabetes, heart failure or hypertension. It has been suggested that the older people and those with high alcohol intake may also have an atypical presentation (Canto et al. 2000).

Silent Myocardial Ischaemia

Silent myocardial ischaemia (SMI) is defined as objective evidence of ischaemia without angina (or equivalent symptoms) in the presence of CAD (Indolfi et al. 2020). It is often found during holter monitoring. The mechanism responsible for silent ischaemia is not well understood, but the duration and extent of ischaemia may have a role. Other possible mechanisms may be changes in the perception of painful stimuli with an increased pain threshold, or neuronal dysfunction (Indolfi et al. 2020).

> **Key Point**
>
> Three decades of research suggest that there are moderate gender differences in ACS symptoms, with women more likely to experience 'atypical' symptoms (DeVon et al. 2020).

Chest Pain Assessment

Chest pain can originate from several sources, and it is important to differentiate on the basis of the history, together with the ECG (see Chapter 9), cardiac biomarkers (Chapter 7) and other diagnostic investigations (see Chapter 8), whether the pain may result from a cardiovascular problem or another cause. For example, pain that is made worse by lying down, moving or deep breathing and resolving with sitting forward may be caused by pericarditis. Pain that is retrosternal and accompanied by sudden shortness of breath and hypoxia associated with pre-syncope and haemoptysis may be caused by a pulmonary embolism. Sudden sharp severe chest pain at the onset may be indicative of aortic dissection. Differential diagnosis of chest pain is discussed in more detail in Chapter 15.

Boxes 14.1 and 14.2 outline some of the questions that might be asked to obtain information

---

Box 14.1 PQRST mnemonic applied to chest pain.

P *Precipitating and palliative factors*

Questions that will yield information about what changes the intensity of the pain include:

- What were you doing when the pain started?
- Was there anything that seemed to trigger or cause the pain?
- Was it associated with anything in particular, such as exertion, stress or before, during or after meals?
- Does anything relieve the pain?
- Have you taken anything to relieve the pain?
- Have the ambulance crew given anything that has helped?
- Have you noticed anything that makes the pain worse?
- Have you noticed anything that makes the pain better?
- How did the pain start – gradually or suddenly?

Q *Quality*

- Ask the patient to describe how the pain feels.
- Avoid prompting the patient with descriptors of pain – they will often agree with whatever you are suggesting.
- Watch the patient's body language, hand gestures or affective descriptors.
- Ask the patient whether changing position or taking a deep breath made any difference to the pain.

R *Region and radiation*

- Ask the patient to point to the areas where the pain is located.
- Note the gestures; cardiac pain is for example most likely to be described with hand gestures such as a clenched fist or outstretched hand across the chest area.
- Ask if the pain radiates anywhere, such as the arm, back, neck or jaw.

S *Severity*

- Obtain a baseline assessment of the severity of pain. This baseline can then be used to compare pain intensity at time intervals to see whether it is improving or worsening, and whether therapy is having the desired effect.
- A simple pain-rating scale is often used where 0 is scored as no pain and 10 is the most severe pain ever experienced.

T *Time*

Ask the patient questions that will establish pain onset such as:

- When and how did the pain start?
- Has the pain been continuous since it started or does it come and go?
- Have you had this type of pain before and if so, how often has it occurred?

from a patient presenting with chest pain using either the 'PQRST' or 'OLDCART' mnemonics. Using a mnemonic can help you to remember the questions that need to be asked in assessing a patient with chest pain in order to establish a clear history of the presenting complaint.

Box 14.2 OLDCART mnemonic (Bickley and Szilagyi 2012).

O *Onset*

- When and how did the pain start?
- Was it a sudden or gradual onset?
- Did/does it start with exercise, at rest or at night?

Classically, stable angina discomfort will start predictably with exertion and resolve within 2–5 minutes with rest. Unstable angina pain gradually builds up over the course of a few minutes, is more persistent and not relieved with rest.

L *Location*

- Where is the pain?
- Do you feel it anywhere else?

Cardiac discomfort can radiate to the jaw, neck, shoulders, arms or back. Bear in mind that there is good evidence that women and people from some ethnic minority groups will experience or describe their discomfort quite differently.

D *Duration*

- When and how did the pain start and when did it resolve?
- Did it start suddenly or gradually?
- Has the pain been continuous since it started, or does it come and go?
- When was the worst pain?

C *Character*

- What does the pain feel like?
Typical cardiac chest pain is usually described in terms that indicate heaviness, tightness or pressure. Patients describe the pain in terms that are meaningful to them and may use imagery such as being like 'an elephant sitting my chest'. When asked to show where the pain is, they often use hand gestures that may assist in understanding the nature of the pain, for example using the flat of the hand or a fist rather than a fingertip or pointing.

A *Aggravating or alleviating*

- Does anything make the pain/symptoms better/worse?

If the pain is relieved by sitting forward and made worse by lying flat, with movement and/or inspiration, it may be due to pericarditis or pulmonary embolus. Stable cardiac chest pain will resolve with rest and a decrease in heart rate within 2–5 minutes or more rapidly with sublingual nitrate. Unstable cardiac pain does not completely resolve with rest or sublingual nitrate.

R *Radiation*

- Does the pain go anywhere else/do you have pain anywhere else?

Cardiac pain may radiate to the arm/s, back, neck, jaw or throat.

T *Timing*

- Have you had this pain before and if so, how long ago?
- When did this pain start?
- How long has the pain lasted?
- Is the pain intermittent or continuous?

Setting

- What were you doing when the pain started?

ACS can occur at rest or during exercise. A predictable pattern of exercise-induced pain over recent times may indicate unstable angina

Key Point

Get the patient to sit up – note any grimacing or difficulty in moving and changing position. Ask the patient to take a deep breath in as quickly as they can – if it causes pain in the patient, you often will be able to see by the patient's expression or the patient will be unable to take a deep breath in. A good opportunity to observe this is when you are positioning the patient to auscultate the lungs.

Key Point

A reduction in chest pain after glyceryl trinitrate (GTN) administration is not diagnostically helpful as it may provide relief in other conditions. If symptom relief does occur after GTN, an ECG should be obtained and compared with the ECG obtained during pain to detect any diagnostic changes.

Physical Examination in ACS Patients

The physical examination is an important component in the assessment of patients with an ACS, although it may often be unremarkable. The experienced clinician will rapidly identify the characteristic features of a patient with an AMI from the 'end of the bed'. These patients will appear pale, sweaty and sit/lie motionless often clutching their chest. If associated with dyspnoea, then significant left ventricular dysfunction should be suspected. Examination of the pulse and blood pressure will identify the presence of arrhythmias or shock. This later finding is especially essential, as urgent therapy of shock states is imperative. Examination of the precordium is important to ascertain the presence of ACS haemodynamic consequences (such as acute mitral regurgitation or ventricular septal rupture) or other previous cardiac abnormalities which may impact management

strategies (for instance, severe aortic stenosis). Also, assessment for the presence of cardiac failure is important.

Besides defining the characteristic of the ACS presentation, the clinical examination is useful in considering alternate diagnoses for the presenting chest pain. For example, differential blood pressures between each arm and an aortic regurgitant murmur may indicate aortic dissection. The presence of a pericardial or pleural rub may suggest pericarditis or pleuritis, respectively. Refer to Chapter 6 for more detailed information on physical cardiovascular assessment.

The 12-lead Electrocardiogram in ACS

The ECG is a fundamental clinical tool in the assessment of the ACS patient in many cases and can be instrumental in providing an instantaneous indication as to what the immediate management strategy should be. It should be remembered, however, that electrocardiography does have some limitations: an ECG may suggest that a patient's heart is entirely normal when, in fact, severe and widespread CAD is present. Less than half of patients presenting to hospital with an AMI will have the typical and diagnostic electrocardiographic changes present on their initial ECG, and as many as 20% of patients will have a normal or near-normal ECG (Channer and Morris 2002). Nevertheless, the ECG has stood the test of time to remain one of the most useful clinical tools available in diagnosing abnormal cardiac conditions.

In ACS, acute and evolving ECG changes may provide information that assists the clinician to identify the likely culprit coronary artery; estimate the timing of the ischaemic event in MI and estimate the amount of myocardium at risk according to coronary artery dominance, collateralisation, size and distribution of arterial segments, and location, extent and severity of coronary stenoses (Thygesen et al. 2007). Characteristic abnormalities on the 12-lead ECG indicative of myocardial ischaemia and infarction typically involve the ST segment, T wave and the QRS complex.

ST Segment

The ST segment can become elevated or depressed in myocardial ischaemia/infarction.

ST-segment Depression

ST-segment depression usually indicates sub-endocardial ischaemia. Marked ST-segment depression in the precordial leads, particularly in leads V4 and V5, is often due to extensive ischaemia as a result of stenosis of the left main coronary artery and/or to triple vessel disease, and may produce life-threatening haemodynamic disturbance, both systolic and diastolic (Sclarovsky et al. 1986).

ST-segment Elevation

Taken in context with the patient history and examination to rule out pain from other causes, ST-segment elevation is likely to indicate AMI and requires the urgent application of a reperfusion strategy to minimise myocardial damage.

Learning activity 14.1

Watch the YouTube video below that explains ECG abnormalities associated with acute myocardial infarction. It also explains the correlation of ECG leads to coronary circulation and areas of the heart.

Suggested Resource

Acute coronary syndrome (Part 2) FlippedEM (2013). https://youtu.be/Y_kGJFLljuQ

Key Point

ST-segment elevation can occur for several reasons that are unrelated to fixed coronary artery occlusion such as coronary artery spasm, coronary artery dissection, pericarditis, myocarditis, Takotsubo syndrome, ventricular aneurysm, Brugada syndrome, ventricular paced rhythm, benign early repolarisation, left bundle branch block and left ventricular hypertrophy.

T Waves

T waves may increase in amplitude, become flattened, biphasic or inverted during episodes of myocardial ischaemia. The first ECG sign of sudden narrowing or obstruction of an epicardial artery is often tall, peaked (hyperacute) T waves (Chesebro et al. 1991) that precede the elevation of the ST segment (Thygesen et al. 2007). Biphasic T waves generally are associated with an acute ischaemic episode, and biphasic pattern (terminal T-wave inversion) will usually progress to deep symmetrical T-wave inversion, best seen in the anterior precordial leads (Channer and Morris 2002). 'Pseudonormalisation' or 'normalisation' of the T wave is a phenomenon where the T wave has become inverted following an ischaemic event, and a recurrent ischaemic event results in the inverted T wave first becoming biphasic and then returning to what appears to be a normal configuration. This is usually followed by ST-segment elevation if the ischaemia is not resolved.

The QRS Complex

Pathological Q waves are the most characteristic ECG finding of transmural MI of the left ventricle but are of limited value in the acute setting as the age of the Q wave is often indeterminate.

A pattern of poor R-wave progression in the precordial leads may indicate an anterior MI, but as with Q waves, the age of the infarction may be indeterminate. Observing the pattern of R-wave progression is useful though in patients with a normal ECG but other clinical indicators of AMI, as progressively reduced R-wave amplitude occasionally is seen on serial ECGs in anterior infarction as the only electrocardiographic indicator of recent MI.

The 12-lead ECG assists in the identification of the presence of not only myocardial ischaemia, but also its coronary territory. This is of major importance in the management of the ACS patient as it assists in identifying the culprit coronary artery responsible for the ACS presentation (see Chapter 9).

Troponin

HscTn testing should therefore be considered as just one element of assessing patients with acute cardiac disorders. Results should be evaluated in association with the clinical history, physical examination and ECG findings to reach a definitive diagnosis.

Clinical Assessment and Risk Stratification in ACS

The fundamental purpose of assessing a patient with an ACS is to determine their risk for further events. This is best undertaken by considering the clinical presentation, ECG findings and Tn levels. Several ACS risk stratification models have been established and these are further discussed in Chapter 15.

Another important consideration is the immediate assessment of the ACS patient when they arrive at the ED and are triaged by the triage nurse. This is an important consideration which must be rapidly undertaken without the immediate availability of the standard diagnostic investigations listed earlier. The summarised guidelines for the triage nurse in the rapid assessment of those at risk of ACS are summarised in Table 14.4.

Table 14.4 Guidelines for the identification of ACS patients by ED registration clerks or triage nurses.

Registration/Clerical Staff

Patients with the following chief complaints require immediate assessment by the triage nurse and *should be referred for further evaluation:*

Chief Complaint

Chest pain, pressure, tightness, or heaviness; pain that radiates to neck, jaw, shoulders, back, or one or both arms

Indigestion or 'heartburn'; nausea and/or vomiting associated with chest discomfort

Persistent shortness of breath

Weakness, dizziness, lightheadedness, loss of consciousness

Triage Nurse

Patients with the following symptoms and signs require immediate assessment by the triage nurse *for the initiation of the ACS protocol:*

Chief Complaint

Chest pain or severe epigastric pain, nontraumatic in origin, with components typical of myocardial ischemia or MI:
Central/substernal compression or crushing chest pain
Pressure, tightness, heaviness, cramping, burning, aching sensation
Unexplained indigestion, belching, epigastric pain
Radiating pain in neck, jaw, shoulders, back, or one or both arms

---

(Continued)

Table 14.4 (Continued)

Associated dyspnea

Associated nausea and/or vomiting

Associated diaphoresis

If these symptoms are present, obtain stat ECG.

Medical History

The triage nurse should take a brief, targeted, initial history with an assessment of current or past history of:

CABG, angioplasty, CAD, angina on effort, or AMI

NTG use to relieve chest discomfort

Risk factors, including smoking, hyperlipidemia, hypertension, diabetes mellitus, family history, and cocaine use

This brief history must not delay entry into the ACS protocol.

Special Considerations

Women may present more frequently than men with atypical chest pain and symptoms.

Diabetic patients may have atypical presentations due to autonomic dysfunction.

Elderly patients may have atypical symptoms such as generalized weakness, stroke, syncope, or a change in mental status.

Source: Braunwald et al. (2000). Used with permission.

Conclusion

Acute coronary syndromes represent a wide spectrum of coronary disorders with variable prognosis and management. The clinical presentation is fundamental in the assessment of these patients, and therefore important in their management.

References

Adamson, P.D., Newby, D.E., Hill, C.L. et al. (2018). Comparison of international guidelines for assessment of suspected stable angina: insights from the PROMISE and SCOT-HEART. *JACC: Cardiovascular Imaging* **11** (9): 1301–1310.

Antman, E. and Braunwald, E. (2001). Acute myocardial infarction. In: *Braunwald: Heart Disease: A Textbook of Cardiovascular Medicine*, 6ee, vol. **2** (ed. E. Braunwald), 1114–1231. St. Louis: W.B. Saunders.

Australian Commission on Safety and Quality in Health Care (2015). *Acute Coronary Syndromes – The Case for Improvement.* Sydney: ACSQHC.

Australian Institute of Health and Welfare (AIHW) (2011). *Monitoring Acute Coronary Syndrome Using National Hospital Data: An Information Paper on Trends and Issues.* Cat. no. CVD 57. Canberra: AIHW www.aihw.gov.au/publication-detail/?id=10737420977 (accessed 31 August 2015).

Beltrame, J.F. (2013). Assessing patients with myocardial infarction and nonobstructed coronary arteries (MINOCA). *Journal Internal Medicine* **273** (2): 182–185.

Bickley, L. and Szilagyi, P.G. (2012). *Bates' Guide to Physical Examination and History-Taking.* Lippincott Williams & Wilkins.

Braunwald, E., Antman, E.M., Beasley, J.W. et al. (2000). ACC/AHA guidelines for the management of patients with unstable angina and non-ST-segment elevation myocardial infarction. A report of the American College of Cardiology/American Heart Association Task Force on Practice Guidelines (Committee on the Management of Patients With Unstable Angina). *Journal of the American College of Cardiology* **36**: 970–1062.

Brieger, D., Eagle, K.A., Goodman, S.G. et al. (2004). Acute coronary syndromes without chest pain, an underdiagnosed and undertreated high-risk group: insights from the Global Registry of Acute Coronary Events. *Chest* **126**: 461–469.

Canto, J.G., Shlipak, M.G., Rogers, W.J. et al. (2000). Prevalence, clinical characteristics, and mortality among patients with myocardial infarction presenting without chest pain. *Journal of the American Medical Association* **283**: 3223–3229.

Channer, K. and Morris, F. (2002). ABC of clinical electrocardiography: myocardial ischaemia. *British Medical Journal* **324**: 1023–1026. http://www.bmj.com/cgi/reprint/324/7344/1023.

Chesebro, J.H., Zolhelyi, P., and Fuster, V. (1991). Pathogenesis of thrombosis in unstable angina. *American Journal of Cardiology* **68**: B2–B10.

Collet, J.P., Thiele, H., Barbato, E. et al. (2021). 2020 ESC Guidelines for the management of acute coronary syndromes in patients presenting without persistent ST-segment elevation: the Task Force for the management of acute coronary syndromes in patients presenting without persistent ST-segment elevation of the European Society of Cardiology (ESC). *European Heart Journal* **42** (14): 1289–1367.

DeVon, H.A., Mirzaei, S., and Zègre-Hemsey, J. (2020). Typical and atypical symptoms of acute coronary syndrome: time to retire the terms? *Journal of the American Heart Association* **9** (7): e015539.

Diamond, G.A. (1983). A clinically relevant classification of chest discomfort. *Journal of the American College of Cardiology* **1** (2 Part 1): 574–575.

Fernando, S.M., Tran, A., Cheng, W. et al. (2019). Prognostic accuracy of the HEART score for prediction of major adverse cardiac events in patients presenting with chest pain: a systematic review and meta-analysis. *Academic Emergency Medicine* **26** (2): 140–151.

Gibbons, R.J., Chatterjee, K., Daley, J. et al. (1999). ACC/AHA/ACP-ASIM guidelines for the management of patients with chronic stable angina: a report of the American College of Cardiology/American Heart Association Task Force on Practice Guidelines (Committee on Management of Patients with Chronic Stable Angina). *Journal of the American College of Cardiology* **33**: 2092–2197.

Heberden, W. (1772). Some account of a disorder of the breast. *Medical Transactions* **2**: 59.

Indolfi, C., Polimeni, A., Mongiardo, A. et al. (2020). Old unsolved problems: when and how to treat silent ischaemia. *European Heart Journal Supplements* **22** (Suppl. L): L82–L85.

Johnson, K. and Ghassemzadeh, S. (2020). Chest Pain. In: StatPearls. StatPearls Publishing, Treasure Island (FL). PMID: 29262011. https://europepmc.org/article/nbk/nbk470557.

Parsonage, W.A., Cullen, L., and Younger, J.F. (2013). The approach to patients with possible cardiac chest pain. *Medical Journal of Australia* **199** (1): 30–34.

Pasupathy, S., Air, T., Dreyer, R.P. et al. (2015). Systematic review of patients presenting with suspected myocardial infarction and nonobstructive coronary arteries. *Circulation* **131** (10): 861–870.

Rousan, T.A., & Thadani, U. (2019). Stable angina medical therapy management guidelines: a critical review of guidelines from the European Society of Cardiology and National Institute for Health and Care Excellence. *European Cardiology Review*, **14** (1), 18. doi: https://doi.org/10.15420/ecr.2018.26.1.

Sclarovsky, S., Davidson, E., Strasberg, B. et al. (1986). Unstable angina: the significance of ST segment elevation or depression in patients without evidence of increased myocardial oxygen demand. *American Heart Journal* **112**: 463–467.

Simons, M. and Alpert, J. (2020). Acute coronary syndrome: Terminology and classification. *Uptodate*. (accessed 27 July 2021).

Thygesen, K., Alpert, J.S., White, H.D., and on behalf of the Joint ESC/ACCF/AHA/WHF (2007). Task force for the redefinition of myocardial infarction (2007). *Journal of the American College of Cardiology* **50**: 2173–2195.

Thygesen, K., Alpert, J.S., Jaffe, A.S. et al. (2018). Fourth universal definition of myocardial infarction (2018). *Journal of the American College of Cardiology* **72** (18): 2231–2264.

Wildi, K., Boeddinghaus, J., Nestelberger, T. et al. (2019). Comparison of fourteen rule-out strategies for acute myocardial infarction. *International Journal of Cardiology* **283**: 41–47.

Than, M., Herbert, M., Flaws, D. et al. (2013). What is an acceptable risk of major adverse cardiac event in chest pain patients soon after discharge from the Emergency Department?: a clinical survey. *International Journal of Cardiology* **166** (3): 752–754.

15

Risk Stratification in Acute Coronary Syndromes

Deborah Wright, Cassandra Ryan, and Angela M. Kucia

Overview

Acute coronary syndromes (ACS) are a major health problem resulting in high rates of hospital attendance globally. For patients who present with ischaemic symptoms and evidence of ST-segment elevation acute coronary syndromes (STE-ACS), treatment should progress rapidly following standard reperfusion protocols. In the absence of ST-segment elevation, early risk assessment is required to guide specific treatment to reduce the likelihood of an adverse outcome. There is growing recognition that patients with non-ST-segment elevation acute coronary syndromes (NSTE-ACS), incorporating both non-ST-segment elevation myocardial infarction (NSTEMI) and unstable angina (UA), are at increased risk of death. Moreover, most presentations with acute chest pain result in a non-cardiac diagnosis. Significant resources are consumed in investigating ACS and the challenge for the nurse, as part of the team assessing patients presenting with chest pain or other symptoms suggestive of ACS, is to help identify those patients who need prompt access to specialised and costly cardiac care, as well as those who are sufficiently at low risk to be discharged or cared for in a lower acuity setting.

> **Learning Objectives**
>
> After reading this chapter, you should be able to:
>
> - List the most common differential diagnoses for chest pain presentations
> - Explain why it is important to rapidly differentiate cardiac from non-cardiac pain
> - Explain the concept of risk stratification in patients presenting with undifferentiated chest pain
> - Discuss the merit of currently used tools for risk stratification in patients presenting with undifferentiated chest pain.
> - List potential causes of troponin elevation other than acute coronary syndrome.

> **Key Concepts**
>
> Risk assessment; risk stratification; risk stratification tools; GRACE score; Heart Score

Background

Ischaemic heart disease is the leading cause of death globally and has been so for the last 15 years (World Health Organization 2018). Presentations of ACS are common worldwide.

With the increasing sensitivity of troponin assays, biomarker-negative ACS (UA) is becoming rarer, and this is reflected in current data which reveals that discharge diagnosis of STE-ACS and NSTEMI now exceeds those for UA with a ratio of almost 2:1 (Chew et al. 2013). Early and accurate identification of patients with STE-ACS enables early intervention to restore myocardial perfusion, which has a major impact on outcome (see Chapter 13, Box 13.1 for Universal definitions of myocardial injury and myocardial infarction).

Ischaemic time duration is a major determinant of infarct size in patients with STEMI; thus, prompt recognition and early management of acute STEMI is critical in reducing morbidity and mortality (Scholz et al. 2018). Accurate identification of patients with NSTE-ACS allows for

early initiation of targeted treatment known to improve outcomes in these groups. Accurate exclusion of myocardial infarction in patients with chest pain is essential to minimise the morbidity and mortality associated with missed diagnoses, while avoiding unnecessary overcrowding in the Emergency Department (ED), and the increased costs associated with resource use and over-investigation in those without the disease.

When a patient presents with chest pain or other symptoms suggestive of ACS (see Chapter 14), assessment must progress rapidly. Furthermore, for those without a cardiac cause of chest pain, delay in ruling out AMI defers the diagnosis and management of the actual underlying disease (Wildi et al. 2019), many of which require prompt treatment (see Box 15.1). A large study of patients ≥18 years of age who

---

Box 15.1   A pragmatic differential diagnosis of non-traumatic chest pain[a].

Life-threatening diagnoses that should not be missed:
- Acute coronary syndrome
  - Acute myocardial infarction
  - Unstable angina pectoris
- Acute pulmonary embolism
- Aortic dissection
- Spontaneous pneumothorax

Chronic conditions with an adverse prognosis that require further evaluation:
- Angina pectoris due to stable coronary artery disease
- Aortic stenosis
- Aortic aneurysm
- Lung cancer

Other acute conditions that may benefit from specific treatment:
- Acute pericarditis
- Pneumonia or pleurisy
- Herpes zoster
- Peptic ulcer disease
- Gastrooesophageal reflux
- Acute cholecystitis

Other diagnoses:
- Neuromusculoskeletal causes
- Psychological causes

[a] This differential diagnosis is not intended to be exhaustive.
Source: Reproduced from Parsonage et al. (2013).

presented to an ED with chest pain showed that the most common diagnosis at the completion of ED assessment was non-specific chest pain. When these patients were stratified by age group, the prevalence of serious diagnoses increased with increasing age (Hsia et al. 2016).

The Nature of Risk in Cardiovascular Disease

For almost all risk factors there is no known threshold at which risk begins. Rather, there is an increasing effect as the exposure increases. Individual cardiovascular risk factors alone are poor at predicting the likelihood of developing myocardial ischaemia in an individual patient. Individuals are frequently likely to develop clusters of risk factors and the assessment of disease risk is more accurate when based on the combined effect of multiple risk factors rather than individual risk factors. Risk assessment tools, in the form of algorithms or charts, estimate a person's 10 years ± lifetime risk of developing cardiovascular disease (CVD) and have been developed to identify high-risk people who may benefit from preventative interventions. Risk factors for developing CVD, the concepts of absolute and relative risk and absolute risk calculators are discussed in Chapter 5.

Risk Stratification for Differentiating Between Likely Cardiac-Related Pain and Non-Cardiac Pain

The application of systematic risk stratification models to the patient with chest pain focuses on an overall management strategy in providing estimates of cardiac risk and minimising the potential for cardiovascular complications. Those with objective evidence of ACS or haemodynamic or electric instability are admitted for urgent therapy. Stable patients with no objective evidence of ischaemia (normal or near-normal ECG and negative baseline cardiac injury markers) are deemed

low risk and may be able to be discharged from the ED. Negative results further minimise the probability of ACS, thereby optimising the safety and rationale of discharging these patients, whereas positive results warrant admission and appropriate targeted treatment.

History and Physical Assessment

Patients with suspected ACS undergo a focused history and physical examination. The physical examination is often normal but essential to exclude non-cardiac causes of chest pain (such as pulmonary embolism or musculoskeletal pain) and provide the health care professional with a baseline to work from. The history and physical assessment are used to develop a differential diagnosis (see Box 15.1).

12-lead ECG

The 12-lead ECG is quick, non-invasive and predictive of early risk. Characteristic high-risk ST segment or T-wave abnormalities on the ECG can identify those patients with ACS who require immediate treatment. Characteristic ECG abnormalities associated with NSTE-ACS include ST depression, transient ST elevation and T-wave changes but the ECG is normal in more than one-third of patients in the setting of NSTEACS (Collet et al. 2021).

> **Key Point**
>
> 50% of patients presenting with acute chest pain and LBBB and more than 50% of patients presenting with acute chest pain and RBBB to the ED will ultimately be found to have a diagnosis other than MI. Therefore hs-cTn T/I measurement at presentation should be integrated into decision-making regarding immediate coronary angiography (Collet et al. 2021).

The majority of 'suspected ACS' patients encountered in ED present with undifferentiated chest pain and the diagnosis can be especially difficult if the patient is pain free on presentation, has a normal 12-lead ECG and normal baseline cardiac markers.

> **Key Point**
>
> If the standard 12-lead ECG is inconclusive and the patient has signs or symptoms suggestive of ongoing myocardial ischaemia, additional leads should be recorded:
>
> - Left circumflex artery occlusion may be detected only in V7–V9.
> - Right ventricular MI may only be detected in V3R and V4R (Collet et al. 2021) (see Chapter 9).

Comparison with previous tracings is valuable, particularly in patients with pre-existing ECG abnormalities. Continuous 12-lead ECG monitoring may be warranted in patients whose initial ECG is non-diagnostic and who are at intermediate/high risk of ACS as ECG changes can be dynamic, reflecting the nature of coronary thrombosis and myocardial ischaemia.

> **Key Point**
>
> The resting 12-lead ECG should be obtained within 10 min of the patient's arrival in the emergency room or at first contact with emergency medical services in the prehospital setting and should be immediately interpreted by a qualified physician (Collet et al. 2021).

Biomarkers

Biomarkers reflect inflammation, activation of coagulation, myocyte necrosis, vascular damage and haemodynamic stress. cTn (cTnT or cTnI) is the preferred marker of injury and is the most sensitive and specific biochemical markers of myocardial damage presently available. If the clinical presentation is compatible with myocardial ischaemia, then a dynamic elevation of cardiac troponin (cTn) above the ninety-ninth percentile of healthy individuals indicates MI (Collet et al. 2021). cTn is released into the blood within 3 hours of injury (within 1 hour if using hscTn), peaks at 12–24 hours and remains elevated for up to 14 days (Giannitsis and Katus 2015).

> **Key Point**
>
> Bedside 'point of care' (POC) testing has some advantages, enabling adequately trained staff to obtain information rapidly or when rapid turn-around times are not possible, such as in the rural or remote setting (Aldous et al. 2014). However, the majority of currently used POC assays have lower sensitivity, lower diagnostic accuracy and lower negative predictive value compared with laboratory hscTn assays (Collet et al. 2021).

cTn elevation may be associated with several conditions other than obstructive coronary disease. Other causes include heart failure, hypertensive emergencies, tachyarrhythmias, myocarditis, takotsubo syndrome, valvular heart disease, aortic dissection, cardiac contusion, cardiac procedures (such as cardiac surgery, percutaneous interventions, ablation, pacing, cardioversion), infiltrative disease (amyloidosis, haemochromotosis, sarcoidosis, scleroderma), substances causing myocardial toxicity (some chemotherapy agents, snake venom), pulmonary hypertension, and extreme endurance activities. Illness that is not a primary cardiac condition may also cause cardiac myocyte injury and troponin elevation. These include chronic kidney disease (CKD), critical illness (e.g. shock, burns, sepsis), pulmonary embolus, acute neurological event (e.g. stroke or subarachnoid haemorrhage) hyper-and hypothyroidism, extreme endurance efforts and rhabdomyolysis (Collet et al. 2021).

Chest X-ray

Chest X-ray is recommended in all patients in whom NSTE-ACS is considered unlikely to detect pneumonia, pneumothorax, rib fractures or other thoracic disorders (Collet et al. 2021).

Risk stratification of ACS patients should be based on a combination of clinical presentation and assessment with information derived from ECG, cTn and risk score results. Patients with likely ACS need to be stratified into high, intermediate, or low short-term risk of death or nonfatal MI using validated tools. Determination of the risk of short-term adverse outcomes directs the patient's management strategy in the ED.

Risk Stratification Tools

Several risk-stratifying tools have been developed over the years to differentiate between likely cardiac-related chest pain and non-cardiac chest pain in the ED. Initial ED risk scores were adopted from those created for post-ACS risk stratification such as the Thrombolysis in Myocardial Infarction (TIMI) score (Morrow et al. 2000) and the Global Registry of Acute Coronary Events (GRACE) score (Fox et al. 2006), but as these risk-scoring tools were not specifically designed for chest pain patients in ED, their performance in the

ED has been suboptimal (Liu et al. 2018). In patients with chest pain, the HEART score appears to be superior in discriminating between those with and without MACE and identifies the largest number of patients as low risk without compromising safety (Poldervaart et al. 2017).

Appropriate use of the risk score tools requires an understanding of the variables in the scoring tool. Variables present in GRACE score, HEART score and TIMI score (Six et al. 2008) are shown in Table 15.1

The HEART Score

The History, Electrocardiogram, Age, Risk factors, and initial Troponin (HEART) score (Six et al. 2008) has been well validated for ED prediction of major adverse cardiac events (MACE) and has been widely adopted in the ED environment. It performs well in identifying chest pain patients at high or low risk of developing MACE compared with the previously used risk scores (Liu et al. 2018; Fernando et al. 2019).

The total HEART score is formulated according to the risk of reaching a specific end point including acute MI, percutaneous coronary intervention (PCI), coronary artery bypass graft (CABG) or death within 3 months of ED presentation. In the original study by Six et al. (2008), a scoring system was developed as follows:

- HEART score of 0–3 points holds a risk of 2.5% of reaching an end point and therefore supports a policy of early discharge, and additional diagnostic procedures at the outpatient clinic are unlikely to be useful.
- HEART score of 4–6 points holds a risk of 20.3% for an adverse outcome; therefore, immediate discharge is not an option. These patients should be admitted for clinical observation, treated as an ACS awaiting final diagnosis and subjected to non-invasive investigations, such as repeated troponin, exercise testing and possibly advanced ischaemia detection.

Table 15.1 Variables present in GRACE score, HEART score and TIMI score.

Variables		GRACE score	HEART score	TIMI score
Age		✓	✓	✓
Gender				
History	Suspicious (physicians' opinion)		✓	
	Severe angina (≥ 2 events in last 24 h)			✓
	Use of aspirin last 7 d			✓
	Killip class	✓		
Physical	Heart rate	✓		
Examination	Systolic blood pressure	✓		
ECG	ST deviation	✓	✓	✓
	Repolarisation disorder, LBBB or pacemaker		✓	
	Cardiac arrest at admission	✓		
Laboratory	Creatinine	✓		
results	Positive troponin or creatine kinase	✓	✓	✓
Risk factors	Previous atherosclerotic disease[a]		✓	
	Previous coronary artery disease ≥50%			✓
	Current smoking[b]		✓	✓
	Diabetes mellitus		✓	✓
	Family history of cardiovascular disease		✓	✓
	Hypercholesterolemia		✓	✓
	Hypertension		✓	✓
	Obesity (body mass index >30)		✓	

[a] Previous atherosclerotic disease was defined as myocardial infarction, coronary arterial bypass grafting, percutaneous coronary intervention, stroke or transient ischaemic attack and peripheral artery disease.
[b] Smoking in the HEART – impact trial was defined as smoking currently or stopped <3 months.
Source: Reproduced with permission from Poldervaart et al. (2017). Copyright ©2019 Elsevier Inc. All rights reserved.

- HEART score≥7 points has a risk of 72.7% for an adverse outcome and indicates a need for an early aggressive treatment (including invasive strategies) without preceding non-invasive testing.

An electronic calculator for heart score can be found in the resource link below:

Suggested Resource

Heart score for major cardiac events
MD+ Calc
https://www.mdcalc.com/heart-score-major-cardiac-events

Rule-in/Rule-out Strategies for NSTE-ACS

The assessment process of patients with possible ACS is often challenging and lengthy given the diverse symptoms and signs associated with ACS. The need to avoid unnecessary hospital admissions and to speed up the diagnostic process for patients with chest pain has driven the development of high-sensitivity cardiac troponin (hscTn) assays. With the introduction of hscTn, 'rule-out MI' protocols have grown exponentially, and the time required to rule out MI in the ED with these protocols has reduced considerably (Zhelev et al. 2015). HscTn assays in rapid 'rule-in' and 'rule-out' algorithms for the early detection of MI have been consistently supported in data from large multicentre studies, but multiple approaches are still being tested and the optimal algorithm for ruling out NSTE-ACS is yet to be determined. Three main caveats apply to the use of rule-out algorithms:

- algorithms must be used in conjunction with all available clinical information, including detailed assessment of chest pain characteristics and ECG;
- in patients presenting early (within 1 hour from chest pain onset), the second cTn level should be obtained at 3 hours after pain onset due to the time dependency of troponin release; and
- serial cTn testing should be pursued if the clinical suspicion of ACS remains high or if the patient develops recurrent chest pain as late increases in cTn have been described in 1% of patients (Collet et al. 2021).

In low-risk patients with no recurrence of chest pain, normal ECG findings and normal levels of cTn (preferably Hs), but suspected ACS, a non-invasive stress test (preferably with imaging) for inducible ischaemia is recommended (Roffi et al. 2016). Exercise stress tests (EST) have a well-established role in identifying patients with chest pain who can safely be discharged from the ED (AHA 2010). EST is a relatively safe procedure, with a mortality rate of 1 in 10 000 and a non-fatal MI rate of <4 in 10 000 (CSANZ 2014). Nevertheless, advanced life support-trained staff must be available. A positive EST predicts a sixfold increase in risk of adverse events over the 6 months following attendance. Early EST has a high negative predictive value (Roffi et al. 2016) but does have some limitations.

Other means of evaluating a patient with suspected ACS according to Collet et al. (2021) include:

- Echocardiography to identify abnormalities (segmental hypokinesia or akinesia) suggestive of myocardial ischaemia or necrosis or other conditions including Takotsubo syndrome, acute aortic dissection, pericardial effusion, aortic valve stenosis, hypertrophic cardiomyopathy, or right ventricular dilatation

suggestive of acute pulmonary embolism. Stress imaging can be performed in patients without ischaemic changes on 12-lead ECGs and negative cardiac troponins who are free of chest pain for several hours.

- Single photon emission computed tomography (SPECT) has been shown to be useful for the risk stratification of patients with acute chest pain suggestive of ACS. Fixed perfusion defects suggestive of myocardial necrosis can be detected by myocardial scintigraphy and can be helpful for the initial triage of patients presenting with chest pain without ECG changes or elevated cardiac troponins. Combined stress/rest imaging and/or stress-only imaging may further enhance assessment of ischaemia but is not normally available over 24 hours.
- Cardiac magnetic resonance (CMR) imaging can assess both perfusion and wall motion abnormalities and can facilitate the differential diagnosis between infarction and myocarditis or Takotsubo syndrome.
- Computed tomography coronary angiography (CTCA) allows for visualisation of the coronary arteries. A normal scan excludes coronary artery disease (CAD) but is not helpful in people with known CAD. CT may be useful in excluding other causes of acute chest pain that are associated with high mortality, including pulmonary embolism, aortic dissection, and tension pneumothorax.

Angiography remains the 'gold standard' for assessing coronary anatomy. For further information on cardiac diagnostic procedures, refer to Chapter 8.

Conclusion

Identification of patients presenting with suspected ACS, and particularly those at high risk of adverse events, is a key priority for clinicians in acute cardiac care. The development and use of clinical pathways and new models of care supported by evidence-based guidelines is essential to ensure safe and effective care.

References

Aldous, S., Richards, A.M., George, P.M. et al. (2014). Comparison of new point-of-care troponin assay with high sensitivity troponin in diagnosing myocardial infarction. *International Journal of Cardiology* **177** (1): 182–186.

American Heart Association (AHA) on behalf of American Heart Association Exercise, Cardiac Rehabilitation, and Prevention Committee of the Council on Clinical Cardiology, Council on Cardiovascular Nursing, and Interdisciplinary Council on Quality of Care and Outcomes Research (2010). Testing of low-risk patients presenting to the emergency department with chest pain a scientific statement. *Circulation* **122**: 1756–1776.

Ballocca, F., D'Ascenzo, F., Moretti, C. et al. (2017). High sensitive TROponin levels in patients with chest pain and kidney disease: a multicenter registry – the TROPIC study. *Cardiology Journal* **24** (2): 139–150.

Banerjee, D., Perrett, C., and Banerjee, A. (2019). Troponins, acute coronary syndrome and renal disease: from acute kidney injury through end-stage kidney disease. *European Cardiology Review* **14** (3): 187.

Chesnaye, N.C., Szummer, K., Bárány, P. et al. (2019). Association between renal function and troponin T over time in stable chronic kidney disease patients. *Journal of the American Heart Association* **8** (21): e013091.

Chew, D., French, J., Briffa, T.G. et al. (2013). Acute coronary syndrome care across Australia and New Zealand: the SNAPSHOT ACS study. *The Medical Journal of Australia* **199**: 1–7.

Collet, J.P., Thiele, H., Barbato, E. et al. (2021). 2020 ESC Guidelines for the management of acute coronary syndromes in patients presenting without persistent ST-segment elevation: the Task Force for the management of acute coronary syndromes in patients presenting without persistent ST-segment elevation of the European Society of Cardiology (ESC). *European Heart Journal* **42** (14): 1289–1367.

Fernando, S.M., Tran, A., Cheng, W. et al. (2019). Prognostic accuracy of the HEART score for prediction of major adverse cardiac events in patients presenting with chest pain: a systematic review and meta-analysis. *Academic Emergency Medicine* **26** (2): 140–151.

Fox, K.A., Dabbous, O.H., Goldberg, R.J. et al. (2006). Prediction of risk of death and myocardial infarction in the 6 months after presentation with acute coronary syndrome: prospective multinational observational study (GRACE). *British Medical Journal* **333**: 1091–1094.

Giannitsis, E. and Katus, H.A. (2015). Biomarkers in acute coronary syndromes. In: *The ESC Textbook of Intensive and Acute Cardiovascular Care*, 2e (ed. M. Tubaro, P. Vranckx, S. Price and C. Vrints), 314–320. United Kingdom: Oxford University Press.

Hsia, R.Y., Hale, Z., and Tabas, J.A. (2016). A national study of the prevalence of life-threatening diagnoses in patients with chest pain. *JAMA Internal Medicine* **176** (7): 1029–1032.

Liu, N., Ng, J.C.J., Ting, C.E. et al. (2018). Clinical scores for risk stratification of chest pain patients in the emergency department: an updated systematic review. *Journal of Emergency and Critical Care Medicine* **2** (2): 1–14.

Morrow, D., Antman, E., Charlesworth, A. et al. (2000). TIMI risk score for ST-elevation myocardial infarction: a convenient, bedside, clinical score for risk assessment at presentation. *Circulation* **102**: 2031–2037.

Parsonage, W.A., Cullen, L., and Younger, J.F. (2013). The approach to patients with possible cardiac chest pain. *Medical Journal of Australia* **199** (1): 30–34.

Poldervaart, J.M., Langedijk, M., Backus, B.E., Dekker, I.M.C., Six, A.J., Doevendans, P.A., . . . & Reitsma, J.B. (2017). Comparison of the

GRACE, HEART and TIMI score to predict major adverse cardiac events in chest pain patients at the emergency department. *International Journal of Cardiology*, **227**, 656–661. https://doi.org/10.1016/j. ijcard.2016.10.080.

Roffi, M., Patrono, C., Collet, J.-P. et al. (2016). ESC Scientific Document Group, 2015 ESC Guidelines for the management of acute coronary syndromes in patients presenting without persistent ST-segment elevation: Task Force for the Management of Acute Coronary Syndromes in Patients Presenting without Persistent ST-Segment Elevation of the European Society of Cardiology (ESC). *European Heart Journal* **37** (3): 267–315. https://doi.org/10.1093/eurheartj/ehv320.

Scholz, K.H., Maier, S.K., Maier, L.S. et al. (2018). Impact of treatment delay on mortality in ST-segment elevation myocardial infarction (STEMI) patients presenting with and without haemodynamic instability: results from the German prospective, multicentre FITT-STEMI trial. *European Heart Journal* **39** (13): 1065–1074.

Six, A.J., Backus, B.E., & Kelder, J.C. (2008). Chest pain in the emergency room: value of

the HEART score. *Netherlands Heart Journal*, **16** (6), 191–196. doi: https://doi.org/10.1007/ bf03086144.

The Cardiac Society of Australia and New Zealand (CSANZ) (2014). *Position Statement on Clinical Exercise Stress Testing in Adult*. www. csanz.edu.au/wp-content/uploads/2014/12/ Clinical_Exercise_Stress_Testing_2014- December.pdf (accessed 10 September 2015).

Wildi, K., Boeddinghaus, J., Nestelberger, T. et al. (2019). Comparison of fourteen rule-out strategies for acute myocardial infarction. *International Journal of Cardiology* **283**: 41–47.

World Health Organization (WHO) (2018). Global Health Estimates 2016: Deaths by Cause, Age, Sex and Country and by Region, 2000–2016. https://www.who.int/news- room/fact-sheets/detail/ the-top-10-causes-of-death.

Zhelev, Z., Hyde, C., Youngman, E. et al. (2015). Diagnostic accuracy of single baseline measurement of Elecsys Troponin T high- sensitive assay for diagnosis of acute myocardial infarction in emergency department: systematic review and meta- analysis. *BMJ* **350**: h15.

16

Management of Acute Coronary Syndromes

Christopher J. Zeitz, Ian D. Jones, and Angela M. Kucia

Overview

Acute coronary syndrome (ACS), encompassing ST-elevation myocardial infarction (STEMI), non-ST-elevation myocardial infarction (NSTEMI) and unstable angina (UA), occurs as a result of intracoronary plaque rupture or erosion, and subsequent thrombus formation. The resulting transient or permanent vessel occlusion causes myocardial ischaemia or infarction. The extent and permanency of the occlusion, along with the availability of collateral circulation, will influence the degree of damage that ensues.

The 12-lead electrocardiogram, in conjunction with patient history, guides the initial patient management, which is then supported in the longer term with cardiac biomarkers. Those patients diagnosed with STEMI require immediate access to reperfusion therapy to open the infarct-related artery.

Learning Objectives

After reading this chapter, you should be able to:

- Discuss ECG diagnostic criteria for STEMI and STEMI equivalent patterns.
- Differentiate between the different subgroups of acute coronary syndromes.

- Discuss the management of patients presenting with acute coronary syndromes and implications for nursing care.
- Recognise complications associated with acute coronary syndromes.

Key Concepts

ST-segment elevation myocardial infarction (STEMI); non-ST-segment elevation myocardial infarction (NSTEMI); percutaneous intervention (PCI); fibrinolytic (lytic) therapy

---

Background

The management of patients with suspected ACS, including diagnosis and treatment, starts from the point of first medical contact (FMC). Initial management strategies will be guided by the presence or absence of ST-segment elevation (STE) on the 12-lead electrocardiogram (ECG). Based on the ECG, two groups of ACS patients should be differentiated: those with ST-segment elevation (STE-ACS) and those without ST-elevation (NSTE-ACS).

Cardiac Care: A Practical Guide for Nurses, Second Edition. Edited by Angela M. Kucia and Ian D. Jones.

Considerations in Nursing Care of the Patient with Acute Coronary Syndrome

ACS is a medical emergency and patients with suspected ACS should be managed accordingly. Regular clinical observations including cardiac rhythm, pulse, blood pressure, respirations, oxygen saturation and temperature should be assessed. Refer to Chapter 6 for a review cardiovascular assessment.

Key Point

Continuous ECG monitoring with defibrillator capacity (or a defibrillator immediately available) should be initiated as soon as possible in all patients with suspected STEMI to detect life-threatening arrhythmias and allow prompt defibrillation should they occur (Ibanez et al. 2018).

The nurse should also observe and interpret the cardiac rhythm; detecting arrhythmia early may prevent deterioration. In addition, the pulse should be checked manually. Manual recordings enable the nurse to assess the patient's peripheral perfusion and pulse volume. These are important observations, which are omitted when relying solely on a cardiac monitor.

Continuous 12-lead ECG monitoring should be initiated where possible, to observe for any changes in the ST segments. New ST-segment changes should be reported to the resident medical officer immediately.

Key Point

ECG changes can be dynamic, and it is critical to perform frequent ECGs until such time as the diagnosis and treatment strategy are clear. This is particularly important for patients with ongoing symptoms of ACS and a normal ECG, an ECG with non-specific abnormalities, or subtle STE that does not meet the criteria for a diagnosis of STEMI. If continuous 12-lead ST-segment monitoring is available, this should be used and reviewed regularly.

Changes in blood pressure that are unrelated to pharmacotherapy should be treated with suspicion, and causative factors reviewed and managed. Hypertension increases myocardial workload and oxygen demand, and may be caused by pain, anxiety or omission of medications. Hypotension may indicate the onset of cardiogenic shock and can lead to end-organ failure. In addition to hypotension, cardiogenic shock is associated with resting tachycardia and signs of poor tissue perfusion including oliguria, cyanosis, cool extremities and altered mentation (Ren and Lenneman 2019).

New onset of anxiety and restlessness, difficulty in breathing that worsens with activity or when lying down in the setting of decreasing oxygen saturation, tachycardia and cool, clammy skin may indicate pulmonary oedema.

Key Point

Routine oxygen administration is not recommended as there is some evidence to suggest that hyperoxia may be harmful in patients with uncomplicated myocardial infarction (MI). Oxygen is indicated in hypoxic patients with arterial oxygen saturation (SaO_2) < 90% (Ibanez et al. 2018).

The evolution of the care of patients with ACS has evolved to a point where the duration of inpatient care has become significantly attenuated. Indeed, it is not unusual for such patients to be discharged within 48 hours of presentation, even after presenting with STEMI. As such, it is critical for the nurse to ensure that all necessary interactions and education are delivered early, and that patients are adequately prepared for early discharge. Patients, and family members, are often very anxious at discharge after an ACS and the nurse plays a critical role in allaying any anxieties, with such strategies beginning at the time of admission to prepare the patient for early discharge and subsequent clinic review.

ST Elevation Acute Coronary Syndrome (STE-ACS)

STE-ACS is the most likely diagnosis in patients with acute chest pain and persistent (>20 minutes) STE. STE-ACS generally reflects the presence of a persistent thrombus that totally occludes a coronary artery. The resulting transmural myocardial ischaemia is represented by regional STE on the 12-lead ECG, hence the term STE-ACS. Most patients with STE-ACS will ultimately develop a STEMI as myocyte death occurs.

ST-segment Myocardial Infarction (STEMI)

Where vessel occlusion exists, myocyte death (myocardial infarction) begins within 15 minutes and continues in an exponential fashion such that 50% of the myocardium at risk has died within 4–6 hours (Ibanez et al. 2015), and 80% of the myocardium at risk is permanently damaged by 12 hours (De Luca et al. 2003). The time point at which coronary vessel occlusion has occurred is generally estimated from the time of onset of symptoms (usually chest pain). Time of symptom onset provides a reasonable estimate of the duration of vessel occlusion in this population, but in practice, there is a large degree of variability in symptoms and symptom recognition between individual patients. The size of the myocardial infarction and degree of myocardial salvage are often only determined in retrospect.

Key Point

The terms STE-ACS and STEMI are sometimes used interchangeably, but STE-ACS refers to a patient who presents with ST-segment elevation on the 12-lead ECG and typical symptoms of ACS, but a troponin result is not yet available. The majority of patients with STE-ACS are subsequently found to have an elevated troponin indicating myocardial necrosis and are thus reclassified as STEMI.

An initial working diagnosis of STEMI on patient presentation to an emergency department or health service is based on a combination of patient history and a 12-lead ECG and is subsequently confirmed by elevated troponin levels.

Presenting Symptoms

Presenting symptoms of ACSs are detailed in Chapter 14. Chest pain is the most common presenting symptom in STEMI. Relief of pain is important for comfort reasons but also because pain is associated with sympathetic activation which causes vasoconstriction and increases the workload of the heart. Intravenous opioids are the most commonly used agents in this context, but morphine use is associated with a slower uptake, delayed onset of action and diminished effects of oral antiplatelet agents (clopidogrel, ticagrelor and prasugrel) and may lead to early treatment failure in susceptible individuals.

Patients with STEMI are often anxious and fearful. Reassurance and explanations should be offered to patients and those closely associated with them. A mild sedative should be considered for very anxious patients (Ibanez et al. 2018).

Key Point

Patients with STEMI are dependent on nursing staff to maintain their physical and psychological well-being at a time of great uncertainty. Each patient's needs should be considered on an individual basis rather than routine ritual care.

In the early stages of STEMI many deaths occur out of hospital due to ventricular fibrillation. Urgent angiography should be considered in survivors of cardiac arrest, including unresponsive survivors, when there is a high index of suspicion of ongoing MI. In patients following cardiac arrest and ST-segment elevation on the ECG, primary PCI is the strategy of choice (Ibanez et al. 2018).

ECG Criteria for STEMI and STEMI Equivalents

In the context of a patient history and symptoms suggestive of ACS, the 12-lead ECG diagnostic criteria for STEMI and STEMI equivalents are defined in Table 16.1. STEMI equivalent ECG abnormalities may represent acute coronary occlusion without meeting the traditional ECG STE-ACS/STEMI criteria but may require emergent PCI.

Table 16.1 Diagnostic ECG criteria for STEMI and STEMI equivalents.

Acute ST-segment elevation myocardial infarction (STEMI)

A clinical history of chest pain (>20 min duration) **and** ST-segment elevation (measured at the J-point) in two or more anatomically contiguous (anatomically next to each other) leads as follows:

- *Men aged < 40yr:* ≥ 2.5 mm ST-segment elevation in V2–V3 and/or ≥ 1 mm in the other leads[†]
- *Men aged ≥ 40yr:* 2 mm ST-segment elevation in V2–V3 and/or ≥ 1 mm in the other leads
- *Women (any age)* ≥ 1.5 mm in women in leads V2–V3 and/or ≥ 1 mm in the other leads[†] (Ibanez et al. 2018).

Right ventricular (RV) infarction

Isolated RV infarction is uncommon, but around 30% of patients with inferior STEMI have RV involvement. Right precordial leads (V_3R and V_4R) should be recorded to identify concomitant RV infarction.

- ST-segment elevation in V1 seen with inferior MI may suggest RV MI, but may not be visible if there is concurrent posterior MI.
- ST-segment elevation ≥0.5 mm (≥1 mm in men <30 yr) in V3R or V4R is diagnostic of an RV infarction.
- Absence of elevation in the right-sided leads does not exclude an RV MI (Thygesen et al. 2018).

Posterior myocardial infarction

Marked anterior ST-segment depression in leads V1–V3 may indicate posterior STEMI, especially if the terminal T wave is positive (ST-segment elevation equivalent). Leads V7–V9 should be recorded to identify posterior MI (Ibanez et al. 2018) using the following criteria:

- *Men aged < 40yr:* ≥1 mm ST-segment elevation in leads V7–V9
- *Men aged > 40yr:* ≥0.5 mm ST-segment elevation in leads V7–V9
- *Women:* ≥0.5 mm ST-segment elevation in leads V7–V9

STEMI equivalent ECG abnormalities

Widespread downsloping or horizontal ST depression

Widespread downsloping or horizontal ST-segment depression may indicate left main coronary artery (LMCA) disease, severe triple vessel disease, proximal left anterior descending (LAD) artery occlusion or subendocardial myocardial infarction (MI). ECG findings are:

- Widespread down-sloping or horizontal ST-segment depression most prominent in leads I, II and V4-6
- ST-segment elevation in a VR ≥ 1 mm
- ST-segment elevation in a VR ≥ V1

De Winter T-wave ECG pattern

De Winter T-waves are associated with acute proximal LAD coronary artery occlusion.
ECG findings are:

- Tall, positive, symmetrical T waves in the precordial leads
- Upsloping ST-segment depression >1 mm at the J-point in the precordial leads
- Absence of STE in the precordial leads
- ST-segment elevation (1–2 mm) in a VR (de Winter et al. 2008)

[†] in the absence of left ventricular hypertrophy or left bundle branch block

Wellen's Syndrome

Wellen's syndrome has two patterns: type A has biphasic T-waves, and type B has deep, symmetric T-wave inversions. In addition to the characteristic T-wave morphology, diagnosis requires preserved R-wave progression, no precordial Q-waves and minimal STE (Kreider and Berberian 2019).

In the context of an asymptomatic patient who was recently symptomatic, Wellen's syndrome is indicative of reperfusion in a person with severe proximal LAD coronary artery stenosis. Although the Wellen's pattern does not represent the acute phase of myocardial infarction, it indicates recent myocardial ischaemia and urgent PCI is indicated as the patient is at risk of occluding their proximal LAD coronary artery.

New Bundle Branch Block in the Setting of Acute Symptoms of Myocardial Ischaemia

Left Bundle Branch Block (LBBB)

Acute proximal occlusion of the LAD coronary artery may cause new LBBB, but LBBB is not itself diagnostic of STEMI. Characteristic ST-T wave abnormalities on the ECG changes caused by altered ventricular depolarisation in LBBB make an MI diagnosis difficult. The Sgarbossa criteria (Sgarbossa et al. 1996) (and subsequent criteria modifications to improve sensitivity) may aid diagnosis of MI in LBBB. The modified Sgarbossa criteria (Smith et al. 2012) below have a specificity of 90% and a sensitivity of 91% for detecting myocardial ischaemia in the presence of LBBB.

- ≥1 lead with ≥1 mm of concordant STE (5 points)
- ≥1 lead of V1–V3 with ≥1 mm of concordant ST depression (3 points)
- ≥1 lead anywhere with ≥1 mm STE and proportionally excessive discordant STE, as defined by ≥25% of the depth of the preceding S-wave (2 points).

Right Bundle Branch Block (RBBB)

New STE ≥1 mm or ST-segment or T-wave abnormalities (excluding leads V1–V4) may indicate acute myocardial ischaemia. Recent European Society of Cardiology guidelines state that emergent PCI should be considered when persistent ischaemic symptoms occur in the presence of RBBB (Ibanez et al. 2018) as RBBB is associated with a high risk for mortality in patients with suspected MI, but as with LBBB, RBBB is not itself diagnostic of STEMI.

Key Point

New LBBB due to MI usually results from occlusion of the LAD coronary artery, prior to the first septal perforator and can result in either left or right bundle branch block pattern. Patients with new LBBB due to MI usually have a poor prognosis due to extensive myocardial damage involving a large portion of the distal conduction system and may present in cardiogenic shock (or developing cardiogenic shock).

Ventricular-Paced Rhythm

≥1 lead with ≥1 mm of concordant ST elevation is suggestive of acute MI in right ventricular-paced rhythms (Thygesen et al. 2018). There is some evidence to suggest that Sgarbossa criteria may be useful in detecting myocardial ischaemia. The ECG diagnosis of acute myocardial ischaemia in patients with biventricular pacing is more difficult.

Suggested Resource

The following online resource has more information and examples of ECGs to demonstrate the use of Sgarbossa criteria. Cadogan, M. (2019). Sgarbossa Criteria. *LIFTL*. https://litfl.com/sgarbossa-criteria-ecg-library/

Learning Activity 16.1

Can the computer interpretation of an ECG on the ECG machine be trusted to identify a myocardial infarction? Visit the following website and try out your ECG interpretation skills on some ECGs that were reported as normal by the ECG machine!
McLaren, J. (2019). ECG Cases 1: Missed ischemia – Never trust the ECG computer interpretation. In: *Emergency Medicine Cases* (ed. A. Helman). https://emergencymedicinecases.com/ecg-cases-computer-interpretation-ischemia

Ischaemic ECG Abnormalities not Meeting STEMI Criteria

STEMI ECG criteria were formulated in the era of thrombolytic trials and based upon an area of infarction that was large enough to justify the risk of intracranial haemorrhage with thrombolysis. Such risk-minimising criteria are not relevant to patients undergoing PCI and thus such patients should not be refused timely reperfusion by PCI (if available) even if ECG changes are subtle. A subset of patients presenting with NSTEMI (elevated biomarkers and without classic STE on routine ECG) are found at angiography to have total occlusion of a coronary artery (most often the right coronary artery or left circumflex artery) (Khan et al. 2017). ECG abnormalities (including STE) may be present, but very subtle.

In the absence of STE, a PCI strategy may be indicated in patients with suspected ongoing ischaemic symptoms suggestive of MI and at least one of the following:

- Haemodynamic instability or cardiogenic shock
- Recurrent or ongoing chest pain refractory to medical therapy
- Life-threatening arrhythmias or cardiac arrest
- Mechanical complications of MI
- Acute heart failure
- Recurrent dynamic ST-segment or T-wave changes, especially intermittent STE (Ibanez et al. 2018)

Cardiac Biomarkers in STEMI

Troponin results are often not available prior to reperfusion management as time to reperfusion is of the essence. The utility of cardiac biomarkers in the assessment of chest pain assessment is discussed in Chapter 15.

The mainstay of treatment in patients with STEMI is immediate reperfusion by primary angioplasty or thrombolytic/fibrinolytic (lytic) therapy (Collet et al. 2021).

Principles of Reperfusion Strategies

Reperfusion strategies include pharmacological and mechanical options, and a single strategy will not suit all patients. The reperfusion strategy chosen should seek to address, where possible, the three components of pathophysiology involved: plaque rupture, thrombus formation and vasospasm. While the dominant acute feature is thrombus formation, plaque vulnerability and vasospasm are particularly strong determinants of early adverse events. The key goal of any reperfusion strategy is to restore normal myocardial tissue perfusion as rapidly as possible with the aims of preventing further myocyte loss and restoring normal myocyte function by minimising the time interval from vessel occlusion to reperfusion; thus, the reperfusion strategy needs to be available and effective in a very short time frame. Patients most frequently present within 2 hours of symptom onset, a time when more than 50% of the threatened myocardium can still be salvaged by rapid reperfusion (Ängerud et al. 2019). Hence the concept, time is muscle.

The dilemma facing clinicians when patients present with acute STEMI is the need to balance the time taken to deliver a particular therapy with the likelihood of success of that therapy. Lytic therapy can be delivered easily and rapidly, but it does not confer the same mortality, re-infarction or stroke benefits as PCI. However, the advantages of PCI over lytic therapy are lost if time to PCI is delayed. See Chapter 16 for more information on strategies and benefits of reducing time to treatment for acute myocardial infarction. In making the choice of reperfusion strategy, time of onset of symptoms, availability of skilled PCI operators, risk of bleeding and contraindications to the procedure or pharmacotherapy must also be considered.

When patients give consent to receive either PCI or lytic therapy, they are made aware of the gravity of their situation and the likelihood of treatment success. Whilst this is necessary to secure informed consent, it provides the patients with the stark reality of the situation and is likely to evoke anxiety in the short term, and possible psychological maladaptation in the longer term. Nurses play a key role in providing patients and their families with emotional and psychological support throughout their period of hospitalisation. However, this support is only likely to be meaningful if the messages are provided in a language and a format that patients and their family understand and is based upon their individual needs and concerns rather than a pre-defined agenda.

Mechanical Reperfusion

PCI is superior to lysis in reducing mortality, reinfarction or stroke in high volume, experienced centres where treatment delay is similar. Thus, PCI is the preferred reperfusion strategy in patients with STEMI within 12 hours of symptom onset, provided that it can be performed within 90–120 minutes (depending on the national/international guidelines followed) from STEMI diagnosis by a team of experienced interventional cardiologists and support staff (Ibanez et al. 2018).

Key Point

Routine PCI of an occluded infarct-related artery is not indicated in asymptomatic patients >48 hours after onset of symptoms (Ibanez et al. 2018).

Periprocedural Pharmacotherapy

Management of STEMI patients undergoing PCI involves striking a balance between aggressive inhibition of platelet aggregation and the avoidance of significant bleeding. Patients undergoing PCI should receive dual antiplatelet therapy (DAPT) which is a combination of aspirin and a $P2Y_{12}$ inhibitor, most commonly ticagrelor or prasugrel. Anticoagulant options for PCI include unfractionated heparin, enoxaparin and bivalirudin (Ibanez et al. 2018).

Key Point

Ticagrelor may cause transient dyspnoea at the onset of therapy. Neither prasugrel nor ticagrelor should be used in patients with a previous haemorrhagic stroke, in patients on oral anticoagulants or in patients with moderate-to-severe liver disease (Ibanez et al. 2018).

Periprocedural Considerations During Percutaneous Coronary Intervention

STEMI patients receiving PCI are prone to clinical deterioration as a result of their underlying pathology, the risk of the procedure itself and the additional pharmacotherapy required. It is the nurse's responsibility to closely monitor the patient during and after the procedure for early signs of deterioration. The role of the nurse in preparing the patient for coronary catheterisation is discussed in detail in Chapter 8 and potential complications of PCI can be found in Table 8.3. Nurses in the cardiac catheter laboratory require specialised skills to enable them to provide complex nursing interventions to STEMI patients. The consensus statement below suggests a set of standards for interventional cardiovascular nursing practice.

Suggested resource

White, K., Macfarlane, H., Hoffmann, B. et al. (2018). Consensus statement of standards for interventional cardiovascular nursing practice. *Heart, Lung and Circulation* 27 (5): 535–551. www.csanz.edu.au/wp-content/uploads/2017/07/Standards_Interventional_Cardiovascular_Nursing_Practice_2017.pdf.

Fibrinolytic/Thrombolytic Therapy (Lytics)

A major feature of vessel occlusion in acute STEMI is platelet-rich thrombus. The strategy of using various lytic agents to break down freshly formed thrombus and thus restore flow in the infarct-related artery has resulted in a significant reduction in 30 days mortality for patients presenting with acute STEMI (Second International Study of Infarct Survival [ISIS-2]

Collaborative Group 1988) and was the major therapy for STEMI, with gradual adjustment over time to include agents that were more effective and easier to administer until PCI became available.

There are three major classes of thrombolytic drugs: streptokinase (SK), urokinase (UK) and tissue plasminogen activator (tPA). Fibrin forms a scaffold for platelets and other infiltrating cells to form a clot. Thrombolytic drugs act by converting plasminogen to plasmin, an enzyme that breaks the links between fibrin molecules, thus dissolving the clot. SK, UK and tPA all have the ability to effectively dissolve blood clots, but derivatives of tPA (alteplase, reteplase, tenecteplase) are the most commonly used thrombolytic drugs as they are more selective for clot-bound (rather than circulating) plasminogen than SK and UK; hence, they are referred to as fibrinolytics. Lytic therapy is associated with a risk of bleeding, in particular, intracranial bleeding. Because of the risk of bleeding, lytic therapy is restricted to those patients with clear evidence of significant myocardial infarction as evidenced by the presence of STE on the ECG in accordance with the ECG criteria that have been outlined in Table 16.1. Absolute and relative contraindications to lytic therapy are listed in Table 16.2.

Key Points

Repeat treatment with streptokinase administered more than 5 days and less than 12 months after initial treatment may not be effective because of the increased likelihood of resistance due to antistreptokinase antibodies. Similarly, the therapeutic effect may be reduced in patients with recent streptococcal infections such as streptococcal pharyngitis, acute rheumatic fever and acute glomerulonephritis.

Streptokinase is antigenic and can cause immunologic sensitisation and allergic reactions, particularly with repeat administration, though this is rare.

Table 16.2 Absolute and relative contraindications to thrombolytic/fibrinolytic therapy.

Absolute contraindications	Relative contraindications
• Previous intracranial haemorrhage or stroke of unknown origin • Known structural cerebral vascular lesion • Ischaemic stroke in the preceding 3 mo • Central nervous system damage, neoplasms or arteriovenous malformation • Recent (within 3 mo) major trauma, head or facial injury • Active bleeding or bleeding diathesis (excluding menses) • Suspected aortic dissection • Recent gastrointestinal bleeding	• Severe uncontrolled hypertension at presentation • History of chronic, severe, poorly controlled hypertension (SBP >180 mm Hg or DBP >110 mm Hg) • Transient ischaemic attack in the preceding 6 mo • History of ischaemic stroke more than 3 mo prior • Prolonged (> 10 min) or traumatic CPR • Oral anticoagulant therapy with elevated international normalised ratio (INR) >1.7 or prothrombin time (PT) >15 s • Pregnancy or within 1 wk postpartum • Recent (within 2–4 wk) internal bleeding • Pericarditis or pericardial fluid • Advanced liver disease • Infective endocarditis • Active peptic ulcer • Recent invasive procedures • Uncompressible vascular punctures • Age > 75 yr • Diabetic retinopathy

Role of the Nurse when Caring for a Patient Receiving Thrombolysis

The nurse should be familiar with the specific care that is required when caring for a patient receiving lytic therapy. Nurses are usually responsible for mixing and delivering lytic therapy, monitoring patients during and after lytic delivery and detecting and managing complications.

Prior to lytic therapy:

• Ensure that the patient has no contraindications to lytic therapy (Table 17.2).
• Explain the proposed benefit of the therapy versus known risks (bleeding, stroke) to the patient. It may be necessary to contextualise this for some patients to balance the risks of not having the therapy (heart failure, death) with the risks of therapy.
• Obtain blood for cardiac biomarkers, full blood count (FBC), group and save (in case of need for transfusion), blood glucose, electrolytes, urea, creatinine and lipid screen.

• Provide continuous arrhythmia monitoring (and continuous 12-lead ST-segment monitoring if available).
• Frequent blood pressure checks and report hypo- or hypertension promptly to the responsible medical officer prior to commencing lytic therapy.
• Ensure dual intravenous access.
• Administer prescribed adjunct pharmacotherapies as ordered.

During lytic therapy:

• Observe for allergic reaction to therapy.
• Observe for signs of hypotension (altered conscious state, frequent yawning).
• Monitor blood pressure frequently but be aware that frequent hyperinflation of blood pressure cuff can lead to pain and bruising at the site.
• Continuous cardiac monitoring to identify signs of life-threatening reperfusion arrhythmia and immediate access to the defibrillator.
• Observe and report signs of bleeding at puncture sites.

- Observe and report changes in neurological state that may indicate stroke.
- Observe and report signs or symptoms of gastrointestinal bleed.

Following lytic therapy:

- Provide ongoing psychological support to ensure the patient and family members are conversant with the need for ongoing care.
- Continue to observe for signs and symptoms of internal or external bleeding.
- Serial ECGs to assess reperfusion status (continuous ST-segment monitoring or frequent 12-lead ECG).

Non-reperfusion within 90 minutes of lytic therapy (<50% ST-segment resolution) or continued haemodynamic instability necessitates immediate rescue PCI (Ibanez et al. 2018). Where reperfusion has been achieved (>50% ST-segment resolution), follow-up PCI should be undertaken within 2–24 hours (Ibanez et al. 2018).

Complications of STEMI

Re-occlusion of the Infarct-Related Artery

Re-occlusion of the infarct-related artery remains a significant risk for at least 24 hours regardless of the reperfusion strategy adopted. Acute STEMI involves active thrombus formation in a setting where there is ongoing significant stimulus for thrombus formation, even after intervention. Drug-eluting stents have reduced the incidence of early stent thrombosis following PCI (Sabaté et al. 2016); there is still a possibility that this may occur.

Patient's symptoms, although useful, are not always a reliable guide to vessel patency with some re-occlusion being relatively clinically silent. Detection of re-occlusion relies upon ongoing monitoring of the ECG. Ideally, this should involve continuous monitoring of the ST segments, particularly in the lead where STE was maximal. Patients who re-occlude

following initial successful thrombolysis or PCI should receive emergency PCI. Repeat thrombolysis is no longer recommended.

Heart Failure

The most frequent complication of STEMI is heart failure. Most commonly this is due to left ventricular dysfunction. Other possible causes are rhythm disturbances, mechanical complications and valve dysfunction (see Chapter 23).

Acute Pulmonary Oedema

Acute pulmonary oedema (APO) in the setting of ACS is a consequence of elevated cardiac filling pressure leading to rapid accumulation of fluid within the lung's interstitial and/or alveolar spaces. Clinical symptoms include extreme dyspnoea worse on any activity or lying down, cough, anxiety and restlessness and a feeling of drowning. Cough is a frequent complaint and in severe cases, pink, frothy sputum may be present. Clinical signs reflect evidence of hypoxia and increased sympathetic tone (tachycardia and vasoconstriction causing cool and clammy peripheries).

The goals of therapy are to improve oxygenation, maintain an adequate blood pressure for perfusion of vital organs and reduce excess extracellular fluid. Drugs used in the management of APO include nitrates, diuretics and inotropes. Some patients will require ventilatory support, usually non-invasive positive pressure ventilation in the first instance (Purvey and Allen 2017). See Chapter 23.

Suggested Resource

Noninvasive positive-pressure ventilation
The New England Journal of Medicine (2018)
https://youtu.be/TK9xtbOU2xs

Right Ventricular Infarction

Right ventricular (RV) infarction seldom occurs in isolation but is a concomitant finding in around one-third of patients with inferior wall myocardial infarction (Ali et al. 2020) and is associated with haemodynamic and electrophysiological complications and higher mortality (Namana et al. 2018). RV ischaemia impairs RV stroke volume and leads to reduced left ventricular (LV) filling and cardiac output, despite normal LV contractility. Dilatation of the RV eventually reduces LV compliance and contractile function. Right atrial (RA) ischaemia is present in around 20% of cases of RV infarction, resulting in further decreases in RV preload and cardiac output. RA ischaemia is also associated with rate and rhythm disturbances.

Patients with RV infarction often present with hypotension and an elevated jugular venous pressure (JVP) in the absence of pulmonary congestion. Symptoms typically include chest pain, diaphoresis, nausea and vomiting. Signs and symptoms that may indicate impending haemodynamic instability include Kussmaul's sign (paradoxical rise in JVP on inspiration, or lack of appropriate fall of the JVP with inspiration indicating limited RV filling); pulsus paradoxus (an exaggerated decrease of systolic blood pressure during inspiration) and a murmur indicating tricuspid regurgitation (Namana et al. 2018). A right-sided precordial lead ECG is useful in diagnosing RV infarction in the setting of inferior wall myocardial infarction (see Table 16.1). To perform a right-sided precordial ECG, precordial leads V4-6 are placed in the same anatomical position but on the right side of the chest wall. ST-elevation in V4R is sensitive and specific for RV infarction and is a strong predictor of major complications including cardiogenic shock, ventricular fibrillation and complete heart block (Ali et al. 2020).

Treatment of myocardial ischaemia is the first consideration. As patients with RV infarction are preload dependent, therapies that reduce pre-load, such as nitrates and diuretics, should be avoided. An initial volume challenge with isotonic saline is appropriate if the patient has clear lungs, hypotension and a low JVP, but excessive volume loading may further dilate the RV, causing a further decrease in LV compliance. Inotropic agents such as dobutamine may also be required to support systolic function (Namana et al. 2018). AV dyssynchrony (atrial fibrillation) should be corrected. Atrioventricular heart block may require AV sequential pacing.

Cardiogenic Shock

Cardiogenic shock (CS), defined as decreased cardiac output and evidence of tissue hypoxia in the presence of adequate intravascular volume, is the leading cause of death in acute MI (Ren and Lenneman 2019). CS includes severe myocardial ischaemia that leads a reduction in cardiac output, systemic hypotension and systemic tissue hypoperfusion that can affect all organs (Zeymer et al. 2020). CS is usually due to extensive LV infarction, in which case signs of pulmonary congestion are also present. CS can also occur with right ventricular (RV) infarction and is associated with the typical triad of hypotension, clear lung fields and increased jugular venous pressure (Ibanez et al. 2018). Mechanical circulatory support devices are increasingly used in CS to support unstable patients, but exactly when, whether, and how to incorporate them in shock care remains controversial. Devices that have been used include: (1) Intra aortic balloon pump (IABP) counterpulsation; (2) Impella; (3) Tandemheart and (4) Veno-arterial extra corporeal oxygenation (ECMO). 57% patients receiving ECMO survive (DeChambrun 2020). A classification system has been developed for the stages of CS: (A) at risk; (B) beginning shock; (c) classic CS; (D) deteriorating; and (E) extremis (Baran et al. 2019). The system aims to facilitate clear communication regarding patient status which has potential to streamline management and allows for clinical trials to appropriately differentiate the heterogeneous CS patient subsets when trialling therapies.

Suggested Resource

Baran, D. A., Grines, C. L., Bailey, S., Burkhoff, D., Hall, S. A., Henry, T. D., ... & Naidu, S. S. (2019). SCAI clinical expert consensus statement on the classification of cardiogenic shock: this document was endorsed by the American College of Cardiology (ACC), the American Heart Association (AHA), the Society of Critical Care Medicine (SCCM), and the Society of Thoracic Surgeons (STS) in April 2019. *Catheterization and Cardiovascular Interventions*, 94(1), 29–37.
https://doi.org/10.1002/ccd.28329

Arrhythmias and Conduction Disturbances

Arrhythmias and conduction disturbances are common and potentially life-threatening in the context of STEMI. Refer to Chapter 12 for information on the management of arrhythmias.

Key Point

Around 5% of patients with acute MI will have ventricular tachycardia (VT) or ventricular fibrillation (VF), most commonly within 48 hours of presentation. Sustained ventricular arrhythmias in the setting of ACS is more often polymorphic VT or VF than monomorphic VT (Al-Khatib et al. 2018, p. e101). Accelerated idioventricular rhythm is commonly seen in patients with acute MI, including patients with STEMI who are treated with mechanical (Al-Khatib et al. 2018) or pharmacological reperfusion therapy.

Mechanical Complications

Sudden hypotension, recurrence of chest pain, new cardiac murmurs, pulmonary congestion or jugular vein distension following STEMI may indicate a life-threatening mechanical complication that requires prompt assessment and treatment (Ibanez et al. 2018).

Free Wall Rupture

Rupture of the LV free wall is relatively rare with the highest incidence in those of older age, with late lysis or failed reperfusion and generally occurs in the first week following transmural MI. Clinical signs and symptoms include sudden pain and/or cardiovascular collapse with or without electromechanical dissociation. The development of haemopericardium and tamponade leads to profound shock and is usually rapidly fatal unless partial sealing of the ruptured site by thrombus formation occurs and permits time for pericardiocentesis and haemodynamic stabilisation followed by immediate surgery (Ibanez et al. 2018).

Ventricular Septal Rupture

Ventricular septal rupture may occur within 24 hours to several days after MI with mortality rates between 20 and 75%. It is usually associated with sudden clinical deterioration and acute heart failure or cardiogenic shock. A loud systolic murmur can be heard during the subacute phase. Echocardiography is required to confirm the diagnosis and assess the size of the rupture and the degree of left to right shunt, which may result in signs and symptoms of right heart failure. Heart failure therapy and an intraaortic balloon pump (IABP) may be used to stabilise the patient and reduce cardiac workload until surgery can be performed (Ibanez et al. 2018).

Papillary Muscle Rupture

Rupture of the papillary muscle or chordae tendineae usually presents as sudden haemodynamic deterioration with acute dyspnoea, pulmonary oedema and/or cardiogenic shock two to 7 days following acute MI. Supportive treatment is similar to that of ventricular septal rupture with emergency surgery being the treatment of choice and mortality rates of 20–25% (Ibanez et al. 2018).

Pericarditis

Post MI pericardial complications include early pericarditis, Dressler syndrome (late

Suggested Resource:

Acute coronary syndromes
NICE guideline [NG185]Published: 18 November 2020.
https://www.nice.org.uk/guidance/ng185

pericarditis one to 2 weeks after STEMI) and pericardial effusion. Symptoms are pleuritic chest pain and signs may include pericardial friction rub, typical ECG changes (see Chapter 9) and pericardial effusion. Anti-inflammatory therapy is recommended with aspirin being the first choice post STEMI and colchicine as an adjunct to aspirin if required. Pericardiocentesis for pericardial effusion is rarely required unless there is haemodynamic compromise with signs of tamponade (Ibanez et al. 2018).

Non-ST-segment Elevation Acute Coronary Syndrome (NSTE-ACS)

The diagnosis of NSTE-ACS is based primarily on the patient history and presenting ECG. The two subtypes of NSTE-ACS (UA and NSTEMI) can only be differentiated once the results of cardiac biomarkers are available. UA is confirmed when signs of cardiac ischaemia are present but cardiac myocyte necrosis is absent (evidenced by normal troponin levels). NSTEMI is confirmed in the presence of both cardiac ischaemia and cardiac myocyte necrosis (evidenced by elevated troponin levels) (see Chapter 15). The clinical presentation is similar to that of STE-ACS, but unlike STE-ACS, there is an absence of STE on the ECG. The characteristics of the ECG in NSTE-ACS include ST-segment depression and T-wave abnormalities, though

Suggested Resource:

Ibanez, B., James, S., Agewall, S. et al. (2018). 2017 ESC Guidelines for the management of acute myocardial infarction in patients presenting with ST-segment elevation. *European Heart Journal* 39: 119–177. https://doi.org/10.1093/eurheartj/ehx393

Table 16.3 Risk criteria guiding invasive strategy in NSTE-ACS.

Very high-risk criteria (Collet et al. 2021).
- Recurrent or ongoing chest pain refractory to medical treatment
- Haemodynamic instability/cardiogenic shock
- Mechanical complications of MI
- Acute heart failure clearly related to NSTE-ACS
- Life-threatening arrhythmias or cardiac arrest
- ST-segment depression >1mm in 6 leads plus ST segment elevation in leads aVr and/ or V1

High-risk criteria
- Established NSTEMI diagnosis
- Dynamic new or presumably new contiguous ST-segment or T-wave changes (symptomatic or silent)
- Resuscitated cardiac arrest without ST-segment elevation or cardiogenic shock
- GRACE score > 140 (Collet et al. 2021).

Low-risk criteria
- Characteristics not mentioned above

the ECG may be normal. Patients with ST-segment depression have a poorer prognosis than those with a normal ECG (Ibanez et al. 2018).

The timing of PCI in patients with NTE-ACS is based on patient risk (see Table 16.3). For those deemed to be very high risk, an immediate invasive strategy (<2 hours) is advised. For those deemed to be high risk, an early invasive strategy is advised (<24 hours) (Collet et al. 2021). Lytic therapy is not used in NSTE-ACS, but pharmacological management is otherwise similar to that in STE-ACS. Patients with suspected NSTE-ACS require rapid evaluation to identify high-risk individuals. Once the initial pharmacotherapy regime is administered, further management of the patient is based on responsiveness to anti-anginal treatment and risk assessment. For those at lowest risk with no further pain or changes in haemodynamic status, a non-invasive strategy using imaging techniques such as stress echocardiography or cardiac MR can be considered (Collet et al. 2021).

Convalescence and Secondary Prevention

Discharge planning, convalescence and secondary prevention following ACS are discussed in Chapters 17 and 18.

Suggested Resource:

The GRACE Risk Score is a well-validated tool for estimating short- and long-term risk in acute coronary syndromes (ACS). The GRACE 2.0 ACS Risk Calculator is a tool to help clinicians assess the future risk of death or myocardial infarction (MI), as a guide to treatment options, in a patient with ACS. GRACE Risk Scores 1 and 2 can be found at https://www.outcomes-umass-med.org/grace/acs_risk.aspx

Suggested Resource:

Collet, J.P., Thiele, H., Barbato, E., Barthélémy, O., Bauersachs, J., Bhatt, D.L., Dendale, P., Dorobantu, M., Edvardsen, T., Folliguet, T. and Gale, C.P. (2021). 2020 ESC Guidelines for the management of acute coronary syndromes in patients presenting without persistent ST-segment elevation: the Task Force for the management of acute coronary syndromes in patients presenting without persistent ST-segment elevation of the European Society of Cardiology (ESC). *European Heart Journal* 42 (14): 1289–1367. https://doi.org/10.1093/eurheartj/ehaa575

Conclusion

ACS remains a significant cause of premature death. The restoration of early, complete and sustained myocardial reperfusion continues to be the primary goal in acute STEMI care and with the advent of PCI and antiplatelet agents, this goal is being achieved in more cases. However, the benefits of PCI are only realised if administered within a limited timeframe and therefore, thrombolysis continues to play a major part in STEMI care in some areas of the world. Furthermore, the improved sensitivity of cardiac biomarkers has identified an increasing number of people diagnosed with non-STEMI. These patients require antiplatelet therapy with follow-up coronary revascularisation as per risk profile. This increasing evidence base for coronary intervention in ACS has transformed patient care in many ways over recent decades but the importance of high-quality nursing care remains a constant.

Learning Activity 16.2

MCQs

1) STEMI is diagnosed in which one of the following circumstances:
   a) The patient has chest pain, the ECG has ST-segment depression and the troponin levels are abnormally elevated.
   b) The patient has no chest pain, the ECG is normal and the troponin levels are abnormally elevated.
   c) The patient has chest pain, the ECG has STE and the troponin levels are abnormally elevated.
   d) The patient has chest pain, the ECG has STE and the troponin level is not elevated.

2) Thrombolysis is justified in which one of the following circumstances:
   a) The patient has chest pain, the ECG has STE and the nearest PCI centre is 180 minutes away.
   b) The patient has chest pain, the ECG has STE and the nearest PCI centre is 60 minutes away.
   c) The patient has chest pain, the ECG has ST-segment depression and the nearest PCI centre is 60 minutes away.
   d) The patient has chest pain, the ECG has ST-segment depression and the nearest PCI centre is 180 minutes away.

3) Immediate PCI is justified in which one of the following circumstances:
   a) The patient has a normal troponin, no further pain and is haemodynamically stable.
   b) The patient has an abnormally elevated troponin, but no further pain.
   c) The patient has an abnormally elevated troponin, no further pain and has type 2 diabetes.
   d) The patient has an abnormally elevated troponin, is complaining of

pain and has signs of acute heart failure.

4) What percentage of ST-segment resolution on the ECG is considered to be a sign of reperfusion?
   a) 20%
   b) 40%
   c) 50%
   d) 60%

5) Which of the following medications is not commonly used in acute coronary syndromes?
   a) Unfractionated heparin
   b) Warfarin
   c) Low molecular weight heparin
   d) Ticagrelor

Learning Activity Answers

Learning Activity 16.2 Multiple Choice Questions

Answers: 1 (c); 2 (a); 3 (d); 4 (c); 5 (b)

References

Ali, H., Sarfraz, S., Fawad, M., & Shafique, Z. (2020). Frequency of right ventricular infarction in inferior wall myocardial infarction. *Cureus*, **12** (5): e8238. doi: https://doi.org/10.7759/cureus.8238.

Al-Khatib, S.M., Stevenson, W.G., Ackerman, M.J. et al. (2018). 2017 AHA/ACC/HRS guideline for management of patients with ventricular arrhythmias and the prevention of sudden cardiac death: a report of the American College of Cardiology/American Heart Association Task Force on Clinical Practice Guidelines and the Heart Rhythm Society. *Journal of the American College of Cardiology* **72** (14): e91–e220.

Ängerud, K.H., Sederholm Lawesson, S., Isaksson, R.M. et al. (2019). Differences in symptoms, first medical contact and pre-hospital delay times between patients with ST-and non-ST-elevation myocardial infarction. *European Heart Journal: Acute Cardiovascular Care* **8** (3): 201–207.

Baran, D.A., Grines, C.L., Bailey, S., Burkhoff, D., Hall, S.A., Henry, T.D., ... & Naidu, S.S. (2019). SCAI clinical expert consensus statement on the classification of cardiogenic shock: this document was endorsed by the American College of Cardiology (ACC), the American Heart Association (AHA), the Society of Critical Care Medicine (SCCM), and the Society of Thoracic Surgeons (STS) in April 2019. *Catheterization and Cardiovascular Interventions*, **94** (1), 29–37.

Collet, J.P., Thiele, H., Barbato, E. et al. (2021). 2020 ESC Guidelines for the management of acute coronary syndromes in patients presenting without persistent ST-segment elevation: the Task Force for the management of acute coronary syndromes in patients presenting without persistent ST-segment elevation of the European Society of Cardiology (ESC). *European Heart Journal* **42** (14): 1289–1367.

de Chambrun, M.P., Brechot, N., & Combes, A. (2020). The place of extracorporeal life support in cardiogenic shock. *Current Opinion in Critical Care*, **26** (4), 424–431.

De Luca, G., Suryapranata, H., Zijlstra, F., van't Hof, A.W., Hoorntje, J.C., Gosselink, A.M., ... & Zwolle Myocardial Infarction Study Group. (2003). Symptom-onset-to-balloon time and mortality in patients with acute myocardial infarction treated by primary angioplasty. *Journal of the American*

College of Cardiology, **42** (6), 991–997. https://doi.org/10.1016/S0735-1097(03)00919-7.

Ibanez, B., Heusch, G., Ovize, M., and Van de Werf, F. (2015). Evolving therapies for myocardial ischemia/reperfusion injury. *Journal of the American College of Cardiology* **65**: 1454–1471.

Ibanez, B., James, S., Agewall, S., Antunes, M.J., Bucciarelli-Ducci, C., Bueno, H., . . . & Hindricks, G. (2018). 2017 ESC Guidelines for the management of acute myocardial infarction in patients presenting with ST-segment elevation: the task force for the management of acute myocardial infarction in patients presenting with ST-segment elevation of the European Society of Cardiology (ESC). *European Heart Journal*, **39** (2), 119–177. https://doi.org/10.1093/eurheartj/ehx393.

ISIS-2 (Second International Study of Infarct Survival) Collaborative Group (1988). Randomized trial of intravenous streptokinase, oral aspirin, both, or neither among 17 187 cases of suspected acute myocardial infarction: ISIS-2. *Lancet* **2** (8607): 349–360.

Khan, A.R., Golwala, H., Tripathi, A. et al. (2017). Impact of total occlusion of culprit artery in acute non-ST elevation myocardial infarction: a systematic review and meta-analysis. *European Heart Journal* **38** (41): 3082–3089.

Kreider, D. & Berberian J. (2019). STEMI equivalents: Cannot miss patterns. *EM Resident*. https://www.emra.org/emresident/article/stemi-equivalents.

Namana, V., Gupta, S.S., Abbasi, A.A. et al. (2018). Right ventricular infarction. *Cardiovascular Revascularization Medicine* **19** (1): 43–50.

Purvey, M. and Allen, G. (2017). Managing acute pulmonary oedema. *Australian Prescriber* **40** (2): 59.

Ren, X. & Lenneman A. (2019). Cardiogenic shock. In: *Medscape* (ed. H.H. Ooi). https://emedicine.medscape.com/article/152191-overview.

Sgarbossa, E.B., Pinski, S.L., Barbagelata, A. et al. (1996). Electrocardiographic diagnosis of evolving acute myocardial infarction in the presence of left bundle-branch block. *New England Journal of Medicine* **334** (8): 481–487.

Smith, S.W., Dodd, K.W., Henry, T.D. et al. (2012). Diagnosis of ST-elevation myocardial infarction in the presence of left bundle branch block with the ST-elevation to S-wave ratio in a modified Sgarbossa rule. *Annals of Emergency Medicine* **60** (6): 766–776.

Tehrani, B.N., Truesdell, A.G., Psotka, M.A., Rosner, C., Singh, R., Sinha, S.S., ... & Batchelor, W.B. (2020). A standardized and comprehensive approach to the management of cardiogenic shock. *Heart Failure*, **8** (11), 879–891. https://doi.org/10.1016/j.jchf.2020.09.005

Thygesen, K., Alpert, J.S., Jaffe, A.S. et al. (2018). Fourth universal definition of myocardial infarction (2018). *Journal of the American College of Cardiology* **72** (18): 2231–2264.

de Winter, R.J., Verouden, N.J., Wellens, H.J., and Wilde, A.A. (2008). A new ECG sign of proximal LAD occlusion. *New England Journal of Medicine* **359** (19): 2071–2073.

Zeymer, U., Bueno, H., Granger, C.B., Hochman, J., Huber, K., Lettino, M., ... & Thiele, H. (2020). Acute Cardiovascular Care Association position statement for the diagnosis and treatment of patients with acute myocardial infarction complicated by cardiogenic shock: A document of the Acute Cardiovascular Care Association of the European Society of Cardiology. *European Heart Journal: Acute Cardiovascular Care*, **9** (2), 183–197.

17

Discharge Planning and Convalescence

David R. Thompson, Patricia M. Davidson, and Rosemary A. Webster

Overview

This chapter outlines the common reactions to and needs of patients and their partners after an acute cardiac event, the process and elements of discharge planning and strategies to facilitate convalescence. Although this chapter focuses on the role of the nurse, it does so on the basis that the nurse serves as a key member of the multidisciplinary healthcare team, acknowledging that it is the nurse who usually has more frequent and closer contact with the patient and family.

Learning Objectives

After reading this chapter, you should be able to:

- Describe the common reactions to and needs of patients and their partners after an acute cardiac event.
- Describe the process and elements of discharge planning.
- Discuss the importance of the multidisciplinary team in discharge planning.
- Identify strategies to facilitate convalescence.
- Discuss the need to identify patients at higher risk for adverse outcomes following discharge.

Key Concepts

Patient and partner reactions and needs; discharge planning; convalescence, health behaviour

---

Hospitalisation

Hospitalisation for an acute cardiac event can evoke a range of emotions and responses for patients and their families, particularly partners. Undeniably, hospitalisation for an acute cardiac event is stressful for patients and their loved ones and is often a time for revisiting and appraising life goals and plans. Nurses play an important role in not only assisting patients in coping and adjusting to their diagnosis, but also planning their discharge from hospital and assisting them in their subsequent convalescence (Hayman et al. 2015). This can be especially challenging nowadays with the short hospital stay that many patients with an acute cardiac event increasingly face. In addition, many of these patients experience frequent changes in their condition and multiple transitions between care settings and providers (Thompson et al. 2019). In many instances, patients are expected to make significant changes in their lifestyles and considerable adjustments to their circumstances that

Cardiac Care: A Practical Guide for Nurses, Second Edition. Edited by Angela M. Kucia and Ian D. Jones.
© 2022 John Wiley & Sons Ltd. Published 2022 by John Wiley & Sons Ltd.

can impact not only themselves, but also their family members and friends. An important issue for cardiac nurses to consider is that this situation of crisis can often cause new, and evoke latent, conflicts and stressors among family members, particularly partners (Saltmarsh et al. 2016). Associated disability and time off work mean that many families face economic loss and uncertainty. Although the illness course can seem straightforward and commonplace to the cardiac nurse, these events can be very distressing to patients, and unless they and their families adjust appropriately, a range of physical, social and psychological disabilities can ensue.

Patient and Partner Reactions and Needs after an Acute Cardiac Event

An acute cardiac event is usually a sudden, unexpected, frightening and stressful occurrence for most patients and for their partners and family members. Their reactions will be influenced by their individual unique knowledge, attitudes, values and experiences, factors that are in turn influenced by their cultural and socio-economic standpoint as well as physiological and psychological characteristics. Patients and their partners will typically initially often experience not only fear (of what is happening to them or of another event or potential death) but also anxiety (particularly in the first few hours) and depression (particularly over the following few days or weeks), but then, over the next few days, begin a reappraisal of their life circumstances, search for a sense of control and certainty in changing circumstance, look for continuity and coordination of care and seek reassurance. Many people experience psychological difficulties after a cardiac event including anxiety, depressed mood, adjustment difficulties and feelings of grief and loss. The immediate post-discharge phase is certainly a period of vulnerability (Tran et al. 2019). Feelings of perceived control are important for psychosocial recovery after a cardiac event. For

example, self-blame attributions do not aid adjustment or enhance control (Bennett et al. 2013). Therefore, these factors should be key concerns for the nurse when facilitating the patient's discharge from hospital and designing strategies to promote successful convalescence. Simple measures such as providing brief advice or more detailed psychological support to allay anxiety and depression in patients and partners can be effective (Reid et al. 2013; Richards et al. 2018). Health behaviour change techniques, such as motivational interviewing, can also be useful here (Thompson et al. 2011; Chair et al. 2012).

> **Key Point**
>
> Patients and their partners often experience significant distress, particularly fear, anxiety and depressed mood following an acute cardiac event.

Discharge Planning

Discharge planning provides support, follow-up and other interventions that span the transition from hospital to home or community settings. If discharge planning is accomplished properly, it can reduce initial hospital length of stay and subsequent hospital readmission (Gonçalves-Bradley et al. 2016). Effective communication is central to the discharge planning process and communication interventions at discharge are significantly associated with fewer hospital admissions, higher treatment adherence and higher patient satisfaction (Becker et al. 2021). Discharge planning should begin from the time of admission and be a coordinated effort by the multidisciplinary team, including nurses, physicians, dieticians, pharmacists, physiotherapists, occupational therapists and social workers. The broad goals during the hospital discharge phase are to prepare the patient for as normal activities as possible and use the acute cardiac event as an opportunity to re-evaluate the plan of care, particularly regarding psychosocial issues, lifestyle adjustments and risk factor modification (Amsterdam et al. 2014). For example, the medical regimen should be individualised to each patient based on in-hospital findings, coronary risk factors, drug tolerability and recent interventions. The mnemonic 'ABCDE' (Assessment of risk, Antiplatelet therapy, Blood pressure management, Cholesterol management, Cigarette/ tobacco cessation, Diet and weight management, Diabetes prevention and treatment, and Education and Exercise) is a useful guide (Hsu et al. 2013). Before hospital discharge, patients and partners should be provided with easily understood and culturally sensitive verbal and written instructions about medication type, purpose, dose, frequency, side effects and duration of use. Health literacy is an important component of care but often overlooked, even though many patients (particularly older, male and non-white ethnic) and family members may have low health literacy, which is associated with hospital readmissions, low health-related quality of life, higher anxiety levels and lower social support (de Melo Ghisi et al. 2018). If the pattern or severity of symptoms such as pain changes, patients should contact their doctor without delay to assess the need for additional treatment or testing. Patients and partners should be educated about modification of cardiovascular risk factors and referred routinely to a comprehensive cardiac rehabilitation programme, ideally before hospital discharge or during the first outpatient visit. These programmes, which typically provide patient education, enhance regular exercise, monitor risk factors and address lifestyle modification, are highly effective (Anderson et al. 2016). Daily walking can be encouraged soon after discharge for most patients. Regular physical activity reduces symptoms, enhances functional capacity, improves other risk factors such as insulin resistance and glucose control and is important in weight control. Equal attention should be paid to assessing and addressing psychosocial issues – particularly anxiety,

depression and social support – that many of these patients and family members commonly present with but which are often overlooked (Pogosova et al. 2015; Thompson et al. 2018).

Patient and partner education should consider appropriate cholesterol management, blood pressure, smoking cessation and lifestyle management. Patients who have undergone percutaneous coronary intervention or coronary artery bypass grafting benefit from risk factor modification and should be counselled that revascularisation does not obviate the need for lifestyle changes. Test results should be discussed with the patient and partner in an understandable manner.

It should be acknowledged that many patients with an acute cardiac event may present with other morbidities, and these must be considered when planning discharge or designing service delivery. Also, the nurse needs to consider contextual factors such as community resources and policies; healthcare system features and delivery system elements such as congruence between the nurse and the patient around health goals that promote effective, efficient, evidence-based and culturally appropriate care and self-management by patients. Self-management is essential but often compromised because of inadequate social support, personal characteristics such as age, social deprivation, race/ethnicity and lack of health insurance (Pilkerton et al. 2017).

The decision about when to discharge a patient will depend on the patient's diagnosis, their clinical and psychosocial state, the risk of complications and/or other cardiac events as well as their prognosis. The discharge planning process will also be influenced by the individual's physical, social and family circumstances. It is important that patients are discharged from hospital with a clear plan of treatment that is appropriate for their condition as well as for their social and psychological circumstances. For those patients recovering from an acute cardiac event, episodes of an acute coronary syndrome are most likely to occur in the first 3 months after their discharge. Therefore, it is important to initiate interventions in hospital which are designed to reduce this immediate risk as well as to develop a strategy to reduce the longer-term adverse events and prepare the patient with realistic expectations and goals for recovery. For example, special attention needs to be paid to patients who have an implantable cardioverter defibrillator (ICD) and to their partners, who may find adjustment to life challenging and benefit from efforts to bolster social support (Rottmann et al. 2018), perceived control and, in turn, their health-related quality of life (Hammash et al. 2019). For patients with atrial fibrillation, a brief mindfulness-based cognitive behavioural therapy programme may improve their health-related quality of life and sense of coherence (Malm et al. 2018).

Learning Activity 17.1

Identify the members of the MDT that might be included in the discharge of a cardiac patient. What is the contribution of each of the MDT members?

High-Risk Groups

As the cardiac nurse works with the patient and their family in planning for discharge, it is important to consider both individuals and groups at higher risk of adverse outcomes and particularly re-hospitalisation. The ageing of the population, increasing numbers of co-morbid conditions, shortened lengths of stay and the increased complexity of treatment highlight the importance of identifying those at higher risk. Figure 24.1 summarises the key signs to indicate potential poor adjustment and higher risk for adverse health outcomes (Preyde and Brassard 2011; Borenstein et al. 2013; Glozier et al. 2013; Gonçalves-Bradley et al. 2016; Morath et al. 2017). In addition, cardiac patients taking oral anticoagulation, who are elder people, or who have renal dysfunction

---

Box 17.1   High-risk factors for adverse health outcomes.

Prolonged and complicated hospital stay
Recent hospitalisation
Poor social support
Cognitive impairment
Socio-economic disadvantage
Depression, anxiety and stress
Polypharmacy
Low health literacy
Financial challenges
Physical disability
Poor prognosis

---

or diabetes or are non-reperfused, will require special consideration (Ibanez et al. 2018). High-risk factors for adverse health outcomes are listed in Box 17.1.

The optimal length of stay in the CCU and hospital should be determined on an individual basis, according to the patient's cardiac risk, comorbidities, functional status and social support (Ibanez et al. 2018) Early discharge (within 48–72 hours) should be considered appropriate in selected low-risk patients if early rehabilitation and adequate follow-up are arranged (Ibanez et al. 2018). A short hospital stay is challenging for nurses to provide proper patient education and up-titration of secondary prevention measures; thus, these patients should have early post-discharge consultations and be rapidly enrolled in a formal rehabilitation programme (Ibanez et al. 2018).

Key Point

Hospital stays for acute coronary syndrome patients are becoming shorter and therefore there is a need to ensure strategic initiatives to prepare the patient for discharge and arrange CR enrolment. Nurses are in a key position to manage the patient journey including discharge (Smith et al. 2018).

Prior to discharge the patient and their family need to receive face-to-face information that is backed up with written advice sheets which they can refer to once they are at home. This face-to-face communication is critical in ensuring that the patient and their family understand the discharge plan. Nurse-led telephone-based follow-up, particularly in the early days after discharge, can reinforce the information that has been given in hospital and also serve as a method for answering questions, addressing concerns, monitoring progress and engaging the patient as well as increasing adherence to secondary prevention measures (Huber et al. 2017). Both the patient and their family will need to know what to expect during recovery and what to do if cardiac symptoms reoccur. They will also need information about the importance of hospital follow-up, lifestyle modification, exercise, drug therapy and practical advice on return to work and resuming normal activity. For example, they need to be informed about sexual matters and prepared for decreased sexual function that commonly occurs after an acute cardiac event (Arenhall et al. 2018). This period often marks the beginning of a patient's secondary prevention input and as such needs to set the tone for future intervention from healthcare professionals.

As lengths of hospital stay following an acute cardiac event continue to decrease, traditional models of in-hospital cardiac rehabilitation become difficult to achieve. Despite this challenge, the following important information should be provided to patients and their families. Where time is limited, the emphasis should be on providing initial contact and introduction, basic information and reassurance, supportive counselling, guidelines for increasing physical activity and information on pharmacotherapy. A useful patient guide to discharge planning (Goodman et al. 2013) provides the following prompts to them:

- Know *where you will go* after you are discharged.
- You may need *special care*.

- Some new *medications* may have been started in the hospital.
- Know what *activities* you can do.
- Know which *healthcare professionals* you will see after you are discharged.

Appropriate discharge planning should include arranging follow-up by the general practitioner/primary care provider and referral to a secondary prevention programme.

Careful, systematic and well-implemented discharge planning for patients with acute coronary syndrome can result in improvements in health outcomes, including adherence to lifestyle changes and medication guidance as cardiovascular and psychological assessment and satisfaction (Lu et al. 2013).

Convalescence

Convalescence refers to the process of recuperation and recovery following an acute illness. Consequently, this requires the cardiac nurse to look beyond the confines of the coronary care unit and consider key factors impacting the individual's life experience. The period of convalescence is a time of recuperation and adjustment and often marks a life-transition phase. Sustaining an acute cardiac event such as a myocardial infarction or acute heart failure often marks a period of transition from a perception of invincibility to adjusting to living with a chronic condition. Successful transition from hospital to home requires a structured approach, preferably nurse led (Bumpus et al. 2017). The key goals following an acute cardiac event are listed as follows:

- Promote physical, social, psychological and existential well-being.
- Prevent or manage deterioration.
- Assist the individual to achieve optimal physical, social and psychological functioning.
- Support the individual and their families to make the necessary adjustments to cope with a potentially life-limiting chronic illness.

- Facilitate the adoption of effective secondary prevention initiatives.
- Ensure communication and continuity of care across care provider settings.

Approaches should be tailored to best suit the local context and needs of the patient but ideally integrated into a chronic care model that recognises the importance of patient-centred care and self-management as part of a multidimensional approach to improving chronic care and recognising that nurses play a critical role in delivering effective chronic care. Various chronic care models have been developed and implemented. While the most common elements are self-management and delivery system design there is considerable variation regarding which elements are included and how they are delivered (Davy et al. 2015). The key elements of a chronic care model are listed as follows:

- Facilitated community support to meet the needs of patients.
- Facilitated unpaid/informal family support to meet the needs of patients.
- Self-management support to meet the needs of patients.
- Health system improvement to meet the needs of healthcare providers.
- Delivery system design to meet the needs of healthcare providers.
- Enhanced healthcare professional case management support to meet the needs of patients.
- Decision support to meet the needs of healthcare providers.
- Clinical information systems to meet the needs of healthcare providers.

Key Point

It is essential that patient preferences and cultural values are considered when designing an individual's chronic care plan.

Many patients leave hospital with a misconception that they are 'cured'. Cardiac nurses are only too aware that heart disease is a chronic condition, and our challenge is to engage our patients and their families as partners in chronic disease management strategies. Self-care and self-management (see later) strategies aim to empower individuals with the confidence, resources and strategies to be active participants in managing their condition. Through active participation, self-management may increase the patient's independence of their activities of daily living, improve adherence with treatment recommendations and promote optimal health outcomes, all being important strategies in promoting a successful convalescence. However, self-management interventions can be complex and tend to be led by professionals rather than patients, and the effectiveness of self-management interventions among people with ACS remains inconclusive (Guo and Harris 2016).

As part of the discharge process and planning for convalescence, it is vital that nurses reinforce the importance of adopting healthy behaviours (e.g. where appropriate, quitting smoking, beginning ambulatory exercise, eating healthily), intensive risk factor modification (e.g. controlling hypertension, managing diabetes mellitus) and adherence to proven cardioprotective medications (e.g. anti-platelet drugs, beta-blockers, statin, angiotensin co-enzyme inhibitors/angiotensin receptor blockers). Often people's medication behaviours are associated with past experiences, such as taking antibiotics for an infection, and they do not understand the significance of long-term pharmacotherapy. In addition, models of nursing care are commonly configured to the needs of people with acute illnesses; therefore, a range of strategies have been undertaken to introduce models related to chronic care. The individual's response to a cardiac event is dependent on prior experiences, individual psychological characteristics, level of social support and disease prognosis. The responses of patients and their families in this situation range from a flat affect relating to processing the impact of an acute cardiac event, to a debilitating depression.

Adverse psychological reactions to cardiac conditions have significant implications for treatment and health-related outcomes. Clinical depression can delay the recovery process, exacerbate functional impairment and have adverse outcomes on health-related quality of life (Thompson et al. 2018). In addition to depression (or depressive symptoms), anxiety is also associated with worse prognosis, lower compliance and poorer quality of life. Beyond the psychological and social distress associated with anxiety and depression, these factors are associated with increased risk for recurrent cardiac events and mortality. An increasing body of research demonstrates the importance of psychosocial adjustment in the recovery process and underscores the importance of nurses' interventions in planning the convalescent phase (Reid et al. 2013; Ski et al. 2016). An important goal of both planning for discharge and convalescence is supporting patients and their families to incorporate self-management strategies. If the individual appears to have an inability to self-care, either due to cognitive impairment, physical, psychological or social issues, a long-term case-management plan is recommended. This involves liaising with community-based services, general practitioners and other health providers.

Key Point

Advice given should be clearly documented in the discharge communication to the patient, carers (including family members) and all relevant health professionals.

Promoting Self-Care and Self-Management in the Convalescent Phase

An important strategy of preparing people for the convalescent phase is planning for self-care, the naturalistic decision-making process addressing prevention and management of cardiac disease (Riegel et al. 2017), with the core elements of self-care maintenance (adhering to behaviours needed to maintain physical and emotional stability), self-care monitoring (observing oneself for changes in signs and symptoms) and self-care management (responding to signs and symptoms when they occur). Thus, knowledge, skills, confidence and motivation are needed to perform self-care effectively. Though self-care is often thought of as solely an individual-level behaviour, it occurs at the individual (e.g. diet, exercise), family (e.g. facilitating medication adherence, symptom monitoring) and community (e.g. access to services, healthy food) levels.

Individual-level, family-level and community-level factors similarly influence self-care (Riegel et al. 2017). For example, at the individual level this includes anxiety, depression, poor self-efficacy, cognitive decline and multimorbidity; at the family level this includes social network or capital (informal support connections, help and information) and at the community level this includes community centers, transport, health fairs and gyms.

Although for many decades health professionals, particularly nurses, have sought to involve the patient in their own health, this has moved beyond purely providing information to engaging in active partnerships and empowering the individual to participate in their care plans. Patient, carer and family engagement involves the nurturing of collaborative relationships and fostering mutual respect and partnerships. This occurs at both an individual level, for example, between patients, their families and health professionals, and a systems-based level with managers and policy makers.

The terms 'self-care' and 'self-management' are often used interchangeably or together though these constructs are discrete entities; self-care refers to the everyday decisions people make regarding their health, whereas self-management is a deliberate, active decision-making process whereby a person with an illness engages in either maintenance or management of their condition and is part of the broader construct of self-care. Self-management involves working with health professionals to assist in making informed choices and developing problem-solving skills.

Suggested Resource: Website

Supported self-management
NHS England
https://www.england.nhs.uk/personalised-care/supported-self-management

Suggested Resource: Reading

Riegel, B., Moser, D. K., Buck, H. G. et al. (2017). Self-care for the prevention and management of cardiovascular disease and stroke: a scientific statement for healthcare professionals from the American Heart Association. *Journal of the American Heart Association* 6 (9): e006997. https://www.ahajournals.org/doi/10.1161/JAHA.117.006997

Learning Activity 17.2

After engaging with the resources above, consider which of these strategies you have used in your practice to support self-management for patients. Consider which of these strategies you may be able to adopt or adapt for patients in the future.

The principles of self-management rely on a partnership between the health professional, patients, partners, families and carers. Carers are generally family members, volunteers and friends who actively engage in supporting patients and health professionals in providing care. The role of the cardiac nurse is to facilitate the development of knowledge and skills, so that the patient may engage in self-management practices. The use of a traditional education-delivery approach, which involves didactic teaching methods with little follow-up to assess how well the patient has understood the information, is often ineffective as they fail

to engage the patient in a meaningful relationship and employ principles of adult learning. Failing to provide individuals with an opportunity to make informed decisions and relate these to their lifestyle circumstances minimises information acquisition and, more importantly, decreases engagement in recommended healthcare behaviours. To improve knowledge and promote engagement in health-seeking behaviours, nurses need to adopt the role of facilitator, rather than instructor, promoting the individual's self-efficacy to manage their condition. Self-efficacy, the level of confidence an individual has in their ability to perform a task, is an important consideration in self-management strategies.

Self-management may be particularly challenging when patients have, for example, substantial cognitive impairment. Therefore, partners and other caregivers play an important role, which needs to be recognised and supported. This support involves home- and community-based services to provide interventions such as home-based physical activity and support to reduce the severity of depressive symptoms. It is important to recognise that nurses are dealing with a growing ageing population who are presenting with multi-morbidities and long-term conditions, which present multiple challenges to the patient and family as well as to the healthcare system. Many patients and families have low or no confidence in how to manage their condition and they need tailored guidance, coaching and support from the nurse. This may require a range of approaches such as education, motivation, pacing and goal setting, either from a nurse in person or from using an eHealth approach or a case manager. For example, nurse-led case management is particularly promising in people with multi-morbidity (García-Fernández et al. 2014) with benefits such as better patient self-rated health, satisfaction and self-efficacy, lower readmission rates and reduced consumption of primary care resources.

In summary, the process of self-management, including self-care, is dynamic and includes a range of values, attitudes, behaviours and skills directed towards managing the impact of a condition(s) on daily living. Important considerations for the nurse planning convalescence following an acute cardiac event are:

- Providing the patient and their family with knowledge of their heart condition, the management plan and likely outcomes.
- Participating in decision-making with health professionals, family members and/or carers.
- Negotiating a self-management care plan in partnership with health professionals, family members and/or carers.
- Providing the patient with strategies for monitoring and managing signs and symptoms of their heart condition.
- Minimising the impact of the condition on physical, emotional, occupational and social functioning.
- Adopting lifestyles that promote favourable health behaviours and minimise risk of complications, adverse events and unplanned admissions to hospital and the emergency department.
- Facilitating access to support services in the community.
- Empowering the patient with the confidence to participate in their care planning.

Common Concerns of Partners and Family Members

Many partners of patients who have had an acute cardiac event experience psychological distress and report stressors relating to living with a partner with heart disease. A range of factors can contribute to marital and family discord in the convalescent phase. This can range from over-vigilance and over-protectiveness to emotional distancing. Often, care-giving family members are concerned about what to do in case another event happens or if another medical emergency occurs once they have brought their family member home. For instance, wound sites or implantation of implantable cardioverter defibrillators may cause caregivers to be fearful of hurting the patient or themselves. In addition, many couples experience concern regarding their capacity to engage in sexual activity.

In some instances, a health crisis can bring a family or couple closer together and in others it can evoke long-simmering conflicts and exacerbate existing difficulties. An acute cardiac event can alter the dynamics within families and also promote distress. Both the patient and their family must adjust to either temporary or longer-term changes in roles of household members. The inability to resume previous roles may cause the patient psychological distress, which may in turn affect the family members. If caregivers take on too many roles, they may suffer physical and psychological exhaustion. A loss of income is an important concern, particularly given the associated costs related to medication and healthcare. Marital and family concerns need to be addressed as soon as possible through referral to appropriate counselling services.

Facilitating Convalescence

Cardiac rehabilitation is an effective treatment shown to improve health outcomes for people with cardiovascular disease (Anderson et al. 2016). Nevertheless, despite robust evidence obtained from well-designed, controlled trials to support its benefits and the endorsement of peak cardiovascular bodies, such as the American Heart Association and National Heart Foundation of Australia, low participation rates continue to be a challenge internationally. The barriers to cardiac rehabilitation have been replicated in many studies. Factors associated with low participation rates include system-related factors such as lack of availability of programmes, provider factors such as physician's endorsement and individual patient-related factors such as limited access to transport, low self-efficacy for exercise and the need to return to work. Participation is particularly low among women, older people, ethnic minority groups and people living in rural communities (Resurrección et al. 2019). To address the barriers to standardised models of cardiac rehabilitation, a range of innovative solutions to address promoting effective convalescence and the facilitation of chronic disease management have been implemented. A number of models that support the needs of people who cannot or do not want to attend a hospital-based service include home-based and tele-health technology-based ones (Blair et al. 2011; Dalal and Taylor 2016). Cardiac rehabilitation is discussed in more detail in Chapter 18.

An interdisciplinary team is required to produce the best outcomes in the convalescence phase. Team members include the patient's physicians, both specialist and general practitioners, ideally working with a team of nurses, physiotherapists or exercise physiologists, dieticians, social workers, psychologists, occupational therapists and others depending on an individual's needs. Unfortunately, the choice of service provision is often dictated by availability rather than appropriateness to the patient's clinical condition. Therefore, to facilitate convalescence, the cardiac nurse has to be aware of services available to patients and their families in their local community. Simple strategies such as calling the patient in the early post-discharge phase can be reassuring and can also identify potential problems early.

Home-Based Services

Home-based cardiac rehabilitation is just as effective as traditional hospital-based rehabilitation (Taylor et al. 2019; Thomas et al. 2019, Krishnamurthi et al. 2019), including for heart failure (Dalal et al. 2019). Improvements in exercise participation and exercise capacity as well as in lipid and blood pressure profiles have been reported as participants can incorporate physical activity in their daily routine. In addition, home-based programmes show reductions in hospital readmission and improvements in psychological well-being, knowledge, satisfaction, return to work, resumption of driving and improved quality of life. Home-based cardiac rehabilitation also promotes physical activity and facilitates convalescence at similar or lower costs than hospital-based programmes (Anderson et al. 2017).

Nurse-Led Clinics

Increasingly, nurse-led/coordinated/directed/managed clinics are used to manage people with heart disease in a community-based setting. These clinics demonstrate significant improvements in a variety of health outcomes and are particularly effective in managing patients with heart failure in primary and secondary care settings (Thompson et al. 2019). They reduce the need for in-hospital care and provide high quality patient-centred care (Liljeroos and Strömberg 2019).

Community Health Workers

Liaising with community health workers within the target community can be useful in gaining access to vulnerable populations. Culture and ethnicity influence an individual's views of both illness and health, help-seeking behaviour and the capacity to adhere to healthcare recommendations (Ski et al. 2018). A range of cultural values and beliefs dictate an individual's view of convalescence. For example, in many cultures, bed rest is advocated which is in stark contrast to evidence-based recommendations. Bilingual healthcare workers are valuable resources who understand the cultural elements associated with particular conditions and can assist in formulating culturally competent care plans. Engaging health workers is particularly important in indigenous communities. Collaborating with these health workers is particularly useful because of not only their knowledge, resources and skill base, but also their standing within their communities (LeGrande et al. 2017).

Information Technology

Advances in information technology (e.g. e-health and m-health) have expanded the capacity of nurses and other health professionals to engage with people with heart disease at home, in the community and remotely. Mobile technologies are developing rapidly, and their effectiveness, acceptability and usefulness can vary, though they are particularly useful for cardiac patients. For example, in relation to self-management, cardiac patients using mobile applications (apps) benefit from improvements in knowledge, quality of life, psychosocial well-being, blood pressure, body mass index, waist circumference, cholesterol and exercise capacity as well as physical activity, medication adherence and smoking cessation (Coorey et al. 2018). This is a rapidly evolving area of practice with the potential to complement and enhance interventions and communication strategies. There is the potential for people with mobile devices to use apps with sensors and machine-learning algorithms to self-diagnose and treat but also for them to bypass the healthcare system.

Nursing Strategies to Promote Convalescence

As discussed above, a range of models of interventions are available to assist patients and their families in the convalescence phase. To achieve a seamless transition and ensure that coordination of care is optimal, communication across healthcare settings is critical. Therefore, strategies such as clinical pathways, discharge planning meetings and other integrated patterns of follow-up can facilitate optimal patient outcomes. To prepare the patient and the family for the convalescence phase, it is important that people know:

- What to expect – including a realistic view of their prognosis.
- Important issues to follow-up and their timing.
- Where to get information and assistance.

Palliative Care

Although improvements in cardiovascular care over recent decades have been remarkable, in many instances the prognosis for many individuals remains poor. This is particularly the case for those with heart failure. Unfortunately, a growing literature describes the limitations of health systems in delivering palliative and supportive care in heart failure (Schallmo et al. 2019). These limitations range from failing to meet the physical, social, emotional and existential needs of patients and their families to ethical dilemmas. Professional bodies are increasingly recognising the role of palliative and supportive care in cardiovascular care, and this is reflected in recent clinical practice guidelines. As part of preparing for discharge and convalescence, the notion of living with a potentially life-limiting illness needs to be considered. Effective and honest communication is an important strategy in ensuring that patients and their families are well prepared for the future. For example, skilled, ethical communication is paramount in addressing decisions regarding the use of an implantable cardioverter-defibrillator (Clark et al. 2011). Failing to address the patient's prognosis and discuss available treatment choices and the options to develop advance care plans can often lead to an unnecessary burden on patients and their family's healthcare systems.

Conclusion

As discussed earlier and illustrated in the case studies, preparing the patient for convalescence requires the nurse to undertake a comprehensive patient assessment and knowledge of community-based resources. As the population ages and lengths of hospital stays shorten, the significance of this planning increases in importance to optimise health outcomes and minimise burden on healthcare systems because of unnecessary hospitalisation.

Learning Activity 17.3

Reflective Case Study 1

Felicity is a 64-year-old widow, living alone, who recently experienced a cardiac arrest while having dinner at a local restaurant with friends. Fortunately, she was resuscitated by bystanders and taken to her local hospital where she under-went primary percutaneous coronary intervention. Following the procedure, Felicity had a further cardiac arrest. Echocardiography revealed impaired systolic dysfunction and she had an automated ICD implanted. Other post-procedural complications included a urinary tract infection and pneumonia. Felicity has two children living abroad who are concerned for her well-being. Understandably, Felicity is anxious regarding her future and this anxiety is likely exacerbated by dealing with stopping smoking. Felicity also tells you that she has experienced some 'weird' feelings about the cardiac arrests she has suffered. It is Day 4 and you are being told by the discharge services that Felicity should be discharged by Day 7.

Reflect on the information provided within this chapter and the text and consider:

- What are the important strategies to consider in planning Felicity's discharge and convalescent period?
- What information would you consider providing to Felicity and her family to assist them in planning for the future?
- How would you approach discussing the emotions and existential issues surrounding the cardiac arrest?
- What services could you mobilise to support Felicity in her convalescence?
- What sort of follow-up and support do you think will be appropriate to support Felicity?

References

Amsterdam, E.A., Wenger, N.K., Brindis, R.G. et al. (2014). 2014 AHA/ACC guideline for the management of patients with non–ST-elevation acute coronary syndromes: a report of the American College of Cardiology/American Heart Association Task Force on Practice Guidelines. *Journal of the American College of Cardiology* **64** (24): e139–e228.

Anderson, L., Thompson, D.R., Oldridge, N. et al. (2016). Exercise-based cardiac rehabilitation for coronary heart disease. *Cochrane Database of Systematic Reviews* (1). https://doi.org/10.1002/14651858.CD001800.pub3.

Anderson, L., Sharp, G.A., Norton, R.J. et al. (2017). Home-based versus centre-based cardiac rehabilitation. *Cochrane Database of Systematic Reviews* **6**: https://doi.org/10.1002/14651858.CD007130.pub4.

Arenhall, E., Eriksson, M., Nilsson, U. et al. (2018). Decreased sexual function in partners after patients' first-time myocardial infarction. *European Journal of Cardiovascular Nursing* **17** (6): 521–526.

Becker, C., Zumbrunn, S., Beck, K., Vincent, A., Loretz, N., Müller, J., Amacher, S.A., Schaefert, R., & Hussler, S. (2021). Interventions to improve communication at hospital discharge and rates of readmission: a systematic review and meta-analysis. *JAMA Network Open* **4** (8), e2119346.

Bennett, K.K., Howarter, A.D., and Clark, J.M. (2013). Self-blame attributions, control appraisals and distress among cardiac rehabilitation patients. *Psychology and Health* **28** (6): 637–652.

Blair, J., Corrigall, H., Angus, N.J. et al. (2011). Home versus hospital-based cardiac rehabilitation: a systematic review. *Rural and Remote Health* **11** (2): 190–206.

Borenstein, J., Aronow, H.U., Bolton, L.B. et al. (2013). Early recognition of risk factors for adverse outcomes during hospitalization among medicare patients: a prospective cohort study. *BMC Geriatrics* **13** (1): 1–9.

Bumpus, S.M., Krallman, R., Kline-Rogers, E., et al. (2017). Transitional care to reduce cardiac readmissions: 5-year results from the BRIDGE Clinic. *Journal of Family Medicine and Disease Prevention*, **3** (3). DOI: https://doi.org/10.23937/2469-5793/1510062.

Chair, S.Y., Chan, S.W.C., Thompson, D.R. et al. (2012). Short-term effect of motivational interviewing on clinical and psychological outcomes and health-related quality of life in cardiac rehabilitation patients with poor motivation in Hong Kong: a randomized controlled trial. *European Journal of Preventive Cardiology* **19** (6): 1383–1392.

Clark, A.M., Jaarsma, T., Strachan, P. et al. (2011). Effective communication and ethical consent in decisions related to ICDs. *Nature Reviews Cardiology* **8** (12): 694–705.

Coorey, G.M., Neubeck, L., Mulley, J., and Redfern, J. (2018). Effectiveness, acceptability and usefulness of mobile applications for cardiovascular disease self-management: Systematic review with meta-synthesis of quantitative and qualitative data. *European Journal of Preventive Cardiology* **25** (5): 505–521.

Dalal, H.M. and Taylor, R.S. (2016). Telehealth technologies could improve suboptimal rates of participation in cardiac rehabilitation. *Heart* **102** (15): 1155–1156.

Dalal, H.M., Taylor, R.S., Jolly, K. et al. (2019). The effects and costs of home-based rehabilitation for heart failure with reduced ejection fraction: The REACH-HF multicentre randomized controlled trial. *European Journal of Preventive Cardiology* **26** (3): 262–272.

Davy, C., Bleasel, J., Liu, H. et al. (2015). Effectiveness of chronic care models: opportunities for improving healthcare practice and health outcomes: a systematic review. *BMC Health Services Research* **15** (1): 1–11.

García-Fernández, F.P., Arrabal-Orpez, M.J., Rodríguez-Torres, M.D.C. et al. (2014). Effect of hospital case-manager nurses on the level of dependence, satisfaction and caregiver burden in patients with complex chronic disease. *Journal of Clinical Nursing* **23** (19–20): 2814–2821.

Glozier, N., Tofler, G.H., Colquhoun, D.M. et al. (2013). Psychosocial risk factors for coronary heart disease. *Medical Journal of Australia* **199** (3): 179–180.

Gonçalves-Bradley, D.C., Lannin, N.A., Clemson, L.M. et al. (2016). Discharge planning from hospital. *Cochrane Database of Systematic Reviews* (1): CD000313.

Goodman, D.M., Burke, A.E., and Livingston, E.H. (2013). Discharge planning. *JAMA* **309** (4): 406–406.

Guo, P. and Harris, R. (2016). The effectiveness and experience of self-management following acute coronary syndrome: a review of the literature. *International Journal of Nursing Studies* **61**: 29–51.

Hammash, M., McEvedy, S.M., Wright, J. et al. (2019). Perceived control and quality of life among recipients of implantable cardioverter defibrillator. *Australian Critical Care* **32** (5): 383–390.

Hayman, L.L., Berra, K., Fletcher, B.J., and Houston Miller, N. (2015). The role of nurses in promoting cardiovascular health worldwide: the global cardiovascular nursing leadership forum. *JACC* **66** (7): 864–866.

Hsu, S., Ton, V.K., Dominique Ashen, M. et al. (2013). A clinician's guide to the ABCs of cardiovascular disease prevention: the Johns Hopkins Ciccarone Center for the Prevention of Heart Disease and American College of Cardiology Cardiosource Approach to the Million Hearts Initiative. *Clinical Cardiology* **36** (7): 383–393.

Huber, D., Henriksson, R., Jakobsson, S., and Mooe, T. (2017). Nurse-led telephone-based follow-up of secondary prevention after acute coronary syndrome: 1-year results from the randomized controlled NAILED-ACS trial. *PLoS One* **12** (9): e0183963.

Ibanez, B., James, S., Agewall, S. et al. (2018). 2017 ESC Guidelines for the management of acute myocardial infarction in patients presenting with ST-segment elevation: the task force for the management of acute myocardial infarction in patients presenting with ST-segment elevation of the European Society of Cardiology (ESC). *European Heart Journal* **39** (2): 119–177.

Krishnamurthi, N., Schopfer, D.W., Ahi, T. et al. (2019). Predictors of patient participation and completion of home-based cardiac rehabilitation in the Veterans Health Administration for patients with coronary heart disease. *American Journal of Cardiology* **123** (1): 19–24.

LeGrande, M., Ski, C.F., Thompson, D.R. et al. (2017). Social and emotional wellbeing assessment instruments for use with Indigenous Australians: a critical review. *Social Science and Medicine* **187**: 164–173.

Liljeroos, M. and Strömberg, A. (2019). Introducing nurse-led heart failure clinics in Swedish primary care setting. *European Journal of Heart Failure* **21** (1): 103–109.

Lu, M., Tang, J., Wu, J. et al. (2013). Discharge planning for acute coronary syndrome patients in a tertiary hospital: a best practice implementation project. *JBI Database of Systematic Reviews and Implementation Reports* **13** (7): 318–334.

Malm, D., Fridlund, B., Ekblad, H. et al. (2018). Effects of brief mindfulness-based cognitive behavioral therapy on health-related quality of life and sense of coherence in atrial fibrillation patients. *European Journal of Cardiovascular Nursing* **17** (7): 589–597.

de Melo Ghisi, G.L., da Silva Chaves, G.S., Britto, R.R., and Oh, P. (2018). Health literacy and coronary artery disease: a systematic review. *Patient Education and Counseling* **101** (2): 177–184.

Morath, B., Mayer, T., Send, A.F.J. et al. (2017). Risk factors of adverse health outcomes after hospital discharge modifiable by clinical pharmacist interventions: a review with a systematic approach. *British Journal of Clinical Pharmacology* **83** (10): 2163–2178.

Pilkerton, C.S., Singh, S.S., Bias, K.T.K. et al. (2017). Healthcare resource availability and cardiovascular health in the USA. *BMJ Open* **7** (12): e016758.

Pogosova, N., Saner, H., Pederesen, S.S. et al. (2015). Psychosocial aspects in cardiac rehabilitation: from theory to practice. A position paper from the Cardiac Rehabilitation Section of the European Association of Cardiovascular Prevention and Rehabilitation of the European Society of Cardiology. *European Journal of Preventive Cardiology* **22** (10): 1290–1306.

Preyde, M. and Brassard, K. (2011). Evidence-based risk factors for adverse health outcomes in older patients after discharge home and assessment tools: a systematic review. *Journal of Evidence-Based Social Work* **8** (5): 445–468.

Reid, J., Ski, C.F., and Thompson, D.R. (2013). Psychological interventions for patients with coronary heart disease and their partners: a systematic review. *PLoS One* **8** (9): e73459.

Resurrección, D.M., Moreno-Peral, P., Gomez-Herranz, M. et al. (2019). Factors associated with non-participation in and dropout from cardiac rehabilitation programmes: a systematic review of prospective cohort studies. *European Journal of Cardiovascular Nursing* **18** (1): 38–47.

Richards, S.H., Anderson, L., Jenkinson, C.E. et al. (2018). Psychological interventions for coronary heart disease: Cochrane systematic review and meta-analysis. *European Journal of Preventive Cardiology* **25** (3): 247–259.

Riegel, B., Moser, D.K., Buck, H.G. et al. (2017). Self-care for the prevention and management of cardiovascular disease and stroke. A scientific statement for healthcare professionals from the American Heart Association. *Journal of the American Heart Association* **6** (9): e006997.

Rottmann, N., Skov, O., Andersen, C.M., et al. (2018). Psychological distress in patients with an implantable cardioverter defibrillator and their partners. *Journal of Psychosomatic Research*, **113**, 16–21.

Saltmarsh, N., Murphy, B., Bennett, P. et al. (2016). Distress in partners of cardiac patients: relationship quality and social support. *British Journal of Cardiac Nursing* **11** (8): 397–405.

Schallmo, M.K., Dudley-Brown, S., and Davidson, P.M. (2019). Healthcare providers' perceived communication barriers to offering palliative care to patients with heart failure: an integrative review. *Journal of Cardiovascular Nursing* **34** (2): E9–E18.

Ski, C.F., Jelinek, M., Jackson, A.C. et al. (2016). Psychosocial interventions for patients with coronary heart disease and depression: a systematic review and meta-analysis. *European Journal of Cardiovascular Nursing* **15** (5): 305–316.

Ski, C.F., Thompson, D.R., Fitzsimons, D., and King-Shier, K. (2018). Why is ethnicity important in cardiovascular care? *European Journal of Cardiovascular Nursing* **17** (4): 294–296.

Smith, A.E., Parkinson, S., Johnston, I. et al. (2018). An acute coronary syndrome nurse service. *British Journal of Cardiac Nursing* **13** (4): 173–180.

Taylor, R.S., Sadler, S., Dalal, H.M. et al. (2019). The cost effectiveness of REACH-HF and home-based cardiac rehabilitation compared with the usual medical care for heart failure with reduced ejection fraction: a decision model-based analysis. *European Journal of Preventive Cardiology* **26** (12): 1252–1261.

Thomas, R.J., Beatty, A. L, Beckie, T.M., et al. (2019). Home-based cardiac rehabilitation: A Scientific Statement from the American Association of Cardiovascular and Pulmonary Rehabilitation, the American Heart Association, and the American College of Cardiology. *Circulation*, **140** (1), e69–e80.

Thompson, D.R., Chair, S.Y., Chan, S.W. et al. (2011). Motivational interviewing: a useful approach to improving cardiovascular health? *Journal of Clinical Nursing* **20** (9–10): 1236–1244.

Thompson, D.R., Ski, C.F., and Saner, H. (2018). Psychosocial assessment and intervention – are we doing enough? *Heart and Lung* **47** (4): 278–279.

Thompson, D.R., Ski, C.F., and Clark, A.M. (2019). Transitional care interventions for heart failure: what are the mechanisms? *The American Journal of Medicine* **132** (3): 278–280.

Tran, H., Byatt, N., Erskine, N. et al. (2019). Impact of anxiety on the post-discharge outcomes of patients discharged from the hospital after an acute coronary syndrome. *International Journal of Cardiology* **278**: 28–33.

18

Prevention Strategies in Cardiovascular Disease

Rosemary A. Webster, Patricia M. Davidson, Praba Rabasse, and Angela M. Kucia

Overview

Atherosclerotic cardiovascular disease (CVD) is the leading cause of morbidity and mortality globally and has a significant economic cost in terms of healthcare delivery, medications and lost productivity. Although there has been some improvement in outcomes for patients with CVD, implementation of prevention strategies and control of risk factors for CVD is suboptimal (Arnett et al. 2019). Prevention strategies are targeted both at the population level to encourage healthy behaviours and at the level of individuals who may have subclinical or established disease using a patient-centred approach that addresses all aspects of an individual's lifestyle habits and estimated risk of a future CVD event. Healthcare teams that deliver prevention services can be hospital or community based and may include chronic disease management teams as well as cardiac rehabilitation (CR). Cardiac nurses have an important role in integrating hospital and community CVD prevention services and in moving the delivery of these prevention services forward.

Learning Objectives

After reading this chapter, the reader will be able to:

- Recognise the significance of the evidence-based guidelines that inform CVD prevention plans.

- Identify key strategies to promote effective CVD prevention for people following an acute cardiac event.
- Describe the aims and principles of CR.
- Describe various models of CR and evidence of efficacy.
- Identify population groups who have poor CR attendance patterns and reasons why this may be so.

Key Concepts

Primary prevention; secondary prevention; tertiary prevention; CR

Prevention Strategies

Preventative strategies are often described in terms of primary, secondary and tertiary prevention. Over the years the distinctions between the three stages of prevention have become blurred and cause confusion, particularly in CVD prevention. Where primary prevention once referred to strategies such as counseling healthy individuals about the risk of developing CVD, primary prevention now includes interventions such as prescribing antihypertensive medication and statins to prevent CVD.

- Primary prevention targets healthy populations and consists of measures to prevent

---

Cardiac Care: A Practical Guide for Nurses, Second Edition. Edited by Angela M. Kucia and Ian D. Jones.

disease in a susceptible population by removing the cause. A typical example of this is immunisation.

- Secondary prevention refers to early detection of disease and targets individuals who appear to be healthy but may have subclinical disease pathology in the absence of overt symptoms. Secondary disease aims to prevent the onset of illness. A typical example of this is blood pressure or cholesterol screening.

- Tertiary prevention is implemented in symptomatic patients to reduce the severity of disease and prevent further adverse events. Tertiary prevention aims to reduce the effects of an established disease in an individual. A typical example of tertiary prevention is CR (Kisling and Das 2019).

Key Point

In some disciplines, such as cardiology, the term 'secondary prevention' is used when discussing tertiary prevention (Fletcher and Fletcher 2020). In this chapter, we will refer to primary and secondary prevention in the context that it is currently used in Cardiology guidelines.

Primary Prevention in Cardiovascular Disease

Primary prevention in cardiovascular health is focused on preventing atherosclerotic vascular disease, heart failure and atrial fibrillation by promoting a healthy lifestyle for all the population throughout life. Prevention strategies have a strong focus on lifestyle optimisation to minimise the risk of atherosclerotic CVD events and include improvements in diet, physical activity and avoidance of tobacco use and exposure to secondhand smoke. Primary prevention in an individual requires a comprehensive patient-centred approach that addresses all aspects of a patient's lifestyle habits. Assessing the risk of

future events is the first step in deciding whether pharmacotherapy, such as antihypertensive therapy, a statin or aspirin, is indicated (Arnett et al. 2019). The concepts of absolute and relative risk and CVD risk assessment calculators are discussed in Chapter 5.

Suggested Resource

Arnett, D. K., Blumenthal, R. S., Albert, M. A. et al. (2019). 2019 ACC/AHA guideline on the primary prevention of cardiovascular disease: a report of the American College of Cardiology/American Heart Association Task Force on Clinical Practice Guidelines. *Journal of the American College of Cardiology* 74 (10): e177–e232. https://doi.org/10.1016/j.jacc.2019.03.010

Secondary Prevention in Cardiovascular Disease

Comprehensive secondary prevention aims to decrease the need for interventional procedures such as angioplasty and bypass grafting, reduce the incidence of subsequent cardiac events, improve quality of life and extend overall survival (Ibanez et al. 2018). The rationale for secondary prevention in CVD assumes that the progression of vascular lesions, arterial thrombosis and the occurrence of arrhythmias, in those with existing CVD, can be influenced by a variety of metabolic and cardiovascular factors. A comprehensive management approach to secondary prevention is often necessary and may employ different strategies depending on the cardiovascular risk assessment and the presence of concomitant diseases (Piepoli et al. 2016a). Interventions to reduce risk in CVD comprise many components, and it is often difficult to establish if a single intervention produces a positive outcome or if the effect is greater than the sum of its parts. The interplay of risk factors for CVD and CVD risk scores is discussed in Chapter 5. The question of whether risk stratification is appropriate for people with previous CVD has not yet been answered. Risk among such persons is heterogeneous and some risk assessment models that have been developed to date suggest that predictors of risk may be quite different from those used in primary prevention (Piepoli et al. 2020).

Target Population for Secondary Prevention

Effective targeting of secondary prevention is a significant challenge, particularly as the number of individuals identified as being eligible for such an intervention increases. This is in part due to the improved survival rates from acute cardiac events and a demographic shift towards a higher proportion of older people. As populations age they take on the increased risk of CVD with older individuals being more likely to experience a cardiac event, arrhythmia or heart failure. Older people often have multiple pathology and complex social circumstances and therefore there is the potential to put increased demand on secondary prevention services. Patients with documented CVD are at very high risk of recurrent cardiovascular events. High-risk individuals are more likely to benefit from preventative treatments (Piepoli et al. 2016a). Intensive risk factor modification is recommended for all patients with established CVD; though for varying reasons, a large proportion of CVD patients do not achieve their lifestyle, risk factor or therapeutic targets (Kotseva et al. 2016). Identifying and modifying risk factors is the main driver in reducing cardiac events in this population. Preventative care with a simple structured approach can enable clinicians to provide appropriate lifestyle and pharmacological interventions (Jones et al. 2018). The core components of secondary prevention include a structured base line assessment, including assessment for risk of adverse cardiovascular

events and monitoring related outcome measures (improvement in functional capacity, blood pressure control, intervention for tobacco use and response to therapy and program effectiveness) (Thomas et al. 2019).

Learning Activity 18.1

Populations at highest risk of future cardiovascular events derive the greatest benefit from aggressive secondary prevention. Consider the population of patients in your workplace. Are there any specific risk factors that are common in your patient population? Refer to Chapter 5 for information about risk factors and identifying people who at higher risk.

Cardiac Rehabilitation

CR is a multi-factorial and comprehensive secondary prevention intervention, designed to limit the physiological and psychological effects of CVD, manage symptoms and reduce the risk of future cardiovascular events (Piepoli et al. 2016b). The World Health Organization (WHO) defines CR as 'the coordinated sum of activities required to influence favourably the underlying cause of CVD, as well as to provide the best possible physical, mental and social conditions, so that the patients may, by their own efforts, preserve or resume optimal functioning in their community and through improved health behaviour, slow or reverse progression of disease' (WHO 1993). CR has been shown to reduce mortality, hospital readmissions, healthcare costs, improve exercise capacity, quality of life and psychological well-being (Anderson et al. 2016). Evidence suggests that CR is cost-effective, particularly with an added exercise component (Shields et al. 2018). Consequently, CR is recommended in international guidelines for patients following ST-elevation acute myocardial infarction (STEMI), non-ST-elevation myocardial infarction (NSTEMI) and those with stable coronary artery disease. It has been proposed that other groups of patients with other cardiac conditions may benefit from CR, such as those who have had revascularisation procedures (coronary artery bypass grafts or percutaneous transluminal coronary angioplasty [PTCA]), heart transplant, ventricular assist devices, implantable cardioverter-defibrillator (ICD) therapy, cardiac resynchronisation therapy (CRT), heart valve replacement and those with stable angina, heart failure, cardiomyopathies or arrhythmia (Dalal et al. 2015). Exercise training is a core component of most CR programs.

Key Point

CR following a cardiac event decreases morbidity and mortality and improves quality of life for patients with CVD. CR is now indicated for patients with a range of cardiac disorders, leading to a diverse array of CR services tailored to an individual's needs and capabilities (Woodruffe et al. 2015).

CR programs usually have both an inpatient and an outpatient phase.

Inpatient Cardiac Rehabilitation

As the average length of stay following a cardiac event continues to decrease, there are limited opportunities for in-hospital CR. CR should therefore start as soon as is practical following admission. Where time is limited, the emphasis should be on providing:

- initial contact and introduction
- basic information and reassurance
- supportive counselling
- guidelines for mobilisation
- information on pharmacotherapy and use of sub-lingual nitrates
- appropriate discharge planning, including follow-up by the general practitioner/primary care provider and referral to outpatient CR

(National Heart Foundation [NHF] 2004).

Outpatient Cardiac Rehabilitation

A structured outpatient CR program aims to empower the patient to adopt self-management strategies. The length and content of the program will depend upon the needs of the patient and the resources available; but typically commences at discharge and lasts from four to 12 weeks, and can be provided in a range of settings, such as hospitals, community health centres and general medical practices, or a combination thereof. Outpatient CR can also be provided on an individual basis in the patient's home, using a combination of home visits, telephone support, telemedicine or specifically developed self-education materials. The main elements of outpatient CR are:

- assessment, review and follow-up
- low or moderate intensity physical activity
- education, discussion and counselling (NHF 2004).

The core components of CR align with those of secondary prevention and include equity and access to services; assessment and short-term monitoring; lifestyle/behavioural modification and medication adherence; recovery and longer-term maintenance and evaluation and quality improvement (Woodruffe et al. 2015).

Equity and Access

Despite the evidence of benefit of CR participation, CR uptake is suboptimal and ranges from 10 to 60% globally (Hinde et al. 2019). Reasons for underuse relate to both personal and organisational barriers. At the inpatient stage of the pathway, the most common reasons for not participating among both men and women were related to the service (63.9 and 60.7% respectively). At the outpatient stage, the reasons for not participating were more likely to be personal to the individual patient for both men and women (57.3 and 59.5%, respectively) (British Heart Foundation 2018). It has been suggested that participation rates may improve if CR commences before discharge from the hospital and if CR sessions commence within 10 days of hospital discharge (National Institute for Health and Care Excellence [NICE] Guidelines 2020). Commencing CR when the patient is in a hospital lays a strong foundation for education and support and targets the patient when they are potentially most likely to appreciate the need for long-term treatment and lifestyle change. However, the hospital may not always be the most appropriate environment or provide the best time for detailed teaching and discussion, which is often more effective when continued after discharge and in the community setting.

CR can be tailored and offered in various settings to improve equity and access to programs. Programs may be offered face-to-face, over the telephone, on the internet, in a group or one-to-one. CR may be delivered in the hospital, community settings, clinics or in the home.

Key Point

Demand for CR is often greater than resource availability and with rapid discharge of cardiac patients, many do not receive early counseling about secondary prevention. Cardiac nurses should commence CR as soon as practical for cardiac patients on the wards. It is not just the responsibility of designated CR nurses.

Home-based CR

Home-based CR (HB-CR) programs have been increasingly introduced to improve access and participation. HB-CR can include supervised and unsupervised elements and utilise strategies such as e-learning, telemonitoring, structured telephone support, telerehabilitation and teleconsultation (Frederix et al. 2019). HB-CR seems to be as effective as centre-based programs in terms of mortality, morbidity, short-term exercise capacity, blood pressure, smoking cessation and health-related quality of life (Anderson et al. 2017). Consumer mobile health applications (apps) have the potential to enhance patient care and education through low-cost, around-the-clock access to health information to end users on a global scale; however, health information in most apps has not been scrutinised by regulatory bodies and may not offer accurate information or information that applies to all patient circumstances (Kao and Liebovitz 2017).

Assessment and Short-Term Monitoring

Patient assessment involves a comprehensive review incorporating a full medical history to identify cardiovascular problems, interventions, co-morbidities (physical and psychological) and symptoms. Physical examination incorporates a full cardiovascular assessment (see Chapter 6). A cardiovascular risk profile will help quantify the patient's risk and help prioritise secondary prevention strategies (see Chapter 5).

Lifestyle/Behavioural Modification

Age, gender and a family history of CVD are risk factors for CVD that cannot be modified. It should be emphasised to the patient that these are risks for CVD and thus reducing risk by modifying additional risk factors that are amenable to change is particularly important.

Modifiable Biomedical Risk Factors

Hypertension
Hypertension (HT) is discussed in Chapter 5. Lifestyle interventions such as weight control

and regular physical activity may be sufficient to control high normal and grade-1 HT in some patients. To maintain a healthy blood pressure, in addition to medication, people should initiate and maintain a lifestyle that incorporates weight control, appropriate physical activity, alcohol in moderation, sodium reduction and an emphasis on increased consumption of fresh fruits, vegetables and low-fat dairy products. Patients with HT should be advised to avoid added salt and high-salt food. As the BP-lowering effect of increased potassium has been well documented in the DASH diet (rich in fruits, vegetables and low-fat dairy products with a reduced content of dietary cholesterol as well as saturated and total fat), patients with HT should generally be advised to eat more fruits and vegetables and to reduce their intake of saturated fat and cholesterol (Piepoli et al. 2016a).

> **Key Point**
>
> Achieving target BP control is multifactorial. Lifestyle changes are recommended in all patients with suboptimal BP control, including for those on antihypertensive medications. The decision to start antihypertensive treatment depends on the BP level and total CV risk (NHFA 2016).

When pharmacological management is required, the lowest recommended dose of the selected first-line drug should be used initially. Angiotensin-converting enzyme (ACE) inhibitors (or angiotensin II receptor antagonists), calcium channel blockers and low-dose thiazide diuretics are effective for first-line use in initial and maintenance therapy for HT. If monotherapy does not achieve the target BP, it is preferable to add a low-dose second agent from a different pharmacological class rather than increasing the dose of the first agent to minimise the chance of side effects (NHFA 2016).

> **Key Point**
>
> Several medications and complementary therapies influence blood pressure and can interfere with antihypertensive medications. Health professionals should be aware of medications that may influence BP before prescribing them. Patients need to be aware that some over-the-counter medications may influence BP (NHFA 2016, p. 22).

> **Suggested Resources**
>
> Hypertension clinical information and guidelines.
> Heart Foundation of Australia.
> https://www.heartfoundation.org.au/conditions/hypertension
>
> National Institute for Health and Care Excellence (NICE) (2019). Hypertension in adults: diagnosis and management
> NICE guideline [NG136]Published: 28 August 2019 Last updated: 18 March 2022.
> https://www.nice.org.uk/guidance/ng136
>
> Williams, B., Mancia, G., Spiering, W. et al. (2018). 2018 ESC/ESH Guidelines for the management of arterial hypertension: the task force for the management of arterial hypertension of the European Society of Cardiology (ESC) and the European Society of Hypertension (ESH). *European Heart Journal* 39, 3021–3104.
> https://doi.org/10.1093/eurheartj/ehy339

Dyslipidaemia

Dyslipidaemia is a metabolic derangement resulting from elevation of plasma cholesterol and/or triglycerides (TGS), or a low high-density lipid (HDL) level that contributes to the development of atherosclerosis (see Chapter 5). Atherosclerotic lesions that occur because of endothelial cell dysfunction are more likely to develop in the presence of increased levels of low-density lipoprotein cholesterol (LDL-C) (Ference et al. 2017). The evidence that reducing plasma LDL-C reduces CVD risk is unequivocal. Statins, ezetimibe and PCSK9 inhibitors have been shown to reduce the risk of adverse cardiovascular events.

> **Key Point**
>
> People with CVD and a history of ACS are at very high risk and need to receive long-term, intensive lipid-lowering therapy irrespective of baseline LDL-C level. Guidelines may vary slightly. The European Society of Cardiology guidelines recommend a therapeutic regimen that achieves ⩾50% LDL-C reduction from baseline and an LDL-C goal of <1.4 mmol/l (<55 mg/dl) (Mach et al. 2020).

Statins are the first choice in virtually all patients with elevated LDL-C. The results of epidemiological studies and clinical trials with and without statins using angiographic or clinical endpoints confirm that reducing LDL-C is essential in the CVD prevention. All patients with known CVD are treated with proven lifestyle interventions and high-intensity statin therapy, irrespective of baseline LDL cholesterol (Ibanez et al. 2018). In patients who do not tolerate one statin because of myopathy, another statin may be better tolerated or alternative dosing regimens, such as giving the drug every other day, often using low doses may be tried. In most patients, target levels are achievable through statin monotherapy (Rosenson et al. 2020). Ezetimibe is co-administered with a statin when LDL-C is not appropriately controlled. This may be administered after either appropriate dose titration or when the titration is limited by intolerance to the initial statin therapy (Hammersley and Signy 2017). Nicotinic acid (niacin) raises HDL-C and inhibits the production of LDL-C. It is used in combination therapy with statins and for treating hyperlipidaemia in those with normal or low HDL-C levels (Keenan 2018).

> **Key Point**
>
> Lipid profiles need to be repeated 4–6 weeks after an acute event to determine whether the target levels have been reached (Ibanez et al. 2018). For patients in whom the target LDL is not achieved after prescribed high-intensity statin therapy, possible non-adherence should be considered before adding a second drug, given that non-adherence to statin therapy is frequent (Rosenson et al. 2020).

> **Suggested Resources**
>
> Lipid disorders
> NICE
> www.nice.org.uk/guidance/conditions-and-diseases/cardiovascular-conditions/lipid-disorders
> Mach, F., Baigent, C., Catapano, A. L. et al. (2020). 2019 ESC/EAS Guidelines for the management of dyslipidaemias: lipid modification to reduce cardiovascular risk: the task force for the management of dyslipidaemias of the European Society of Cardiology (ESC) and European Atherosclerosis Society (EAS). *European Heart Journal* 41 (1): 111–188. https://doi.org/10.1093/eurheartj/ehz455

Overweight/Obesity

Being overweight is associated with raised plasma lipids, glucose intolerance and HT. Multicomponent interventions are required to tackle obesity. Weight management programs should incorporate behaviour change strategies to promote physical activity levels, decrease inactivity, improve eating behaviour and nutrition and reduce energy intake.

Strategies for effective weight loss include:

- Calculating the BMI and/or waist circumference on each visit and encouraging weight maintenance/reduction through an appropriate balance of physical activity, caloric intake and formal behavioural programs as appropriate to maintain/achieve a BMI between 18.5 and 24.9 kg/m^2.
- Setting weight-loss targets that are realistic and achievable. The initial goal should be to reduce body weight by approximately 10% from baseline. Weight loss of around 0.5 kg/wk is a realistic target and is best achieved through regular and slow eating of meals and regular physical activity.
- Initiating appropriate treatment of metabolic syndrome if a patient has a waist circumference over the target size.

Suggested Resources

NICE (2021). Obesity: identification, assessment and management.
www.nice.org.uk/guidance/CG189

Diabetes/Insulin Resistance

Type 2 diabetes mellitus (T2DM) and pre-diabetes mellitus (DM) are common in patients with ACS and chronic cardiac disease and are associated with an impaired prognosis (Cosentino et al. 2020). DM is associated with other risk factors associated with CVD including dyslipidaemia, HT and overweight/obesity. Intensive secondary prevention is indicated in patients with DM and CVD and must include vigorous modification of risk factors including physical activity and optimal management of weight, BP control and lipid levels.

As poor glycaemic control contributes to worse cardiovascular outcomes, current treatment recommendations for patients with DM place a heavy emphasis on closely monitoring and controlling glycaemic levels to improve cardiac outcomes. The exact glycaemic level that should be targeted for diabetics varies somewhat depending on the organisational guidelines, but setting a goal of haemoglobin A1c (HbA1c) less than or equal to 6.5–7% is common. Glycaemic goals may be adjusted based on factors such as age, years with the disease and cardiovascular risk (Leon and Maddox 2015). For further information on diabetes in cardiovascular disease refer to Chapter 5.

Suggested Resource

NICE Guideline [NG28]. (2015, updated 2022). Type 2 diabetes management in adults: management.
https://www.nice.org.uk/guidance/ng28

Modifiable Behavioural Risk Factors

The long-term changes in behaviour and lifestyle that are recommended for reducing CVD risk are not always easy for patients to accommodate. Unless they acknowledge the need for change and fully understand the change that is required, change is unlikely to be embraced. A regime that fosters ownership, encouragement and positive feedback and allows the patient to progress at a realistic pace is most likely to be successful. The family should be involved at all stages and advised on how best to support the patient by encouraging changes in risk behaviour. Family members may be identified as having risk factors themselves, and so a family approach to lifestyle change is a positive way forward. Identifying patient characteristics such as communication difficulties, education barriers and mobility problems can also help in developing individualised delivery of secondary prevention. Identifying family networks, social support structures, work and social roles is also important in individualising care. It is important to assess the patient's understanding of health problems, health beliefs, expectations, goals, misconceptions, and to have an appreciation of the patient's motivation and ability to engage in the process of secondary prevention. Behavioural risk factors for CVD include tobacco use, physical inactivity, poor nutrition and excessive alcohol consumption (see Chapter 5).

Behaviour change is a complex phenomenon. Health behaviours can be defined as 'overt behavioural patterns, actions and habits that relate to health maintenance, to health restoration and to health improvement' (Gochman 1997, p. 3). Health behaviours include smoking, alcohol use, diet, physical activity, physician visits and medication adherence (Conner and Norman 2017). Changing people's health-related behaviour can have a major impact on cardiovascular mortality and morbidity, but attempts to modify harmful behaviours are often unsuccessful. One reason why this may be so is that theories and principles of successful planning, delivery and evaluation of behavioural change theories have not been considered when introducing an intervention.

Key Point

Effective communication between health practitioner and patient and an understanding that each patient is unique with personal needs and experiences and ability to change behaviours facilitates the process of behaviour change.

Suggested resources

Behaviour change: general approaches NICE 2007.
www.nice.org.uk/guidance/PH6/chapter/introduction

Smoking

Smoking cessation is more effective in reducing cardiovascular risk than any pharmaceutical treatment of major risk factors (van den Berg et al. 2019) and therefore is a major focus for secondary prevention in patients with CVD and should be a key objective for patients with vascular disease.

Key Point

A recent study found that patients who quit smoking after their first cardiovascular event were found to live on average 5 years longer than patients who continued to smoke and lived on average 10 more years without recurrent cardiovascular events (van den Berg et al. 2019).

Brief interventions with advice to stop smoking (Piepoli et al. 2016a) and individual counselling have been shown to be an effective way of helping patients to stop smoking (Lancaster and Stead, 2017). Patients may also require pharmacological support. Nicotine-replacement therapy (NRT) is an established and safe method of facilitating the weaning-off process and is more effective if a patch is combined with a short acting form. Varenicline or bupropion may also be considered except in pregnant women or people at higher risk of seizures. People on these medications should be monitored for adverse psychological reactions. When prescribing smoking cessation drugs, the importance of commitment to total abstinence from the quit day onwards must be emphasised. Adding behavioural support increases the chances of success (Hartmann-Boyce and Aveyard 2016).

Many initiatives designed to help smokers stop smoking are being led by nurses and include smoking-cessation clinics in both secondary and primary care. Nurse-led stage-matched cessation counselling resulted in successful abstinence and smoking reduction (Lu et al. 2019).

An effective smoking cessation intervention should incorporate:

- Asking the patient about their tobacco use at every visit.
- Advising the patient and family members to give up alongside the patient in order to provide encouragement and support.
- Assessing the patient's willingness to quit and identify psychological factors that may inhibit success.

- Stressing the benefits of stopping smoking including feeling healthier, improved sense of taste/smell, avoidance of nicotine-stained fingers, fresher home environment, improved lung function, easier breathing, increased self-esteem, better example to children, financial advantages, preventing harm to others through passive smoking.
- Assistance through counselling, motivational strategies and developing a stepwise plan for quitting.
- Arranging follow-up and ongoing contact, referral to special programs and/or pharmacotherapy.
- Suggesting supplementary strategies if desired – for example, acupuncture, hypnosis.
- Advising against exposure to environmental tobacco smoke at work and home.

Most countries will have a service devoted to quitting smoking and contact details available online for those who require information and support. For more information on the cardiovascular effects of cigarette smoking see Chapter 5.

Suggested Resources

Quit Smoking
National Health Service
https://www.nhs.uk/live-well/quit-smoking/

Smoking and Tobacco Resources
Australian Government Department of Health
https://www.health.gov.au/health-topics/smoking-and-tobacco/smoking-and-tobacco-resources

---

Physical Inactivity

Physical inactivity is a major risk factor for the development of CVD and contributes to the development of other CVD risk factors including obesity, HT, dyslipidaemia and diabetes. It is recommended that physical activity should occur at a frequency of at least 3–5 sessions/wk, but preferably every day. Individuals should accumulate at least 30 min/d, 5 d/wk of moderate intensity of physical activity (150 min/wk) or 15 min/d, 5 d/wk of vigorous intensity

physical activity (75 min/wk) or a combination of both, performed in sessions with a duration of at least 10 minutes. Shorter exercise sessions that are less than 10 minutes may also be appropriate, especially in very deconditioned individuals (Piepoli et al. 2016a; Piercy et al. 2018). Aerobic physical activity includes cycling, walking, heavy household work, includes everyday activity, including active travel (cycling or walking), heavy household work, gardening, occupational activity and leisure time activity or exercise such as brisk walking, Nordic walking, hiking, jogging, or running, cycling, cross-country skiing, aerobic dancing, skating, rowing or swimming (Piepoli et al. 2016a).

Suggested Resource

Physical activity
NICE
www.nice.org.uk/guidance/lifestyle-and-wellbeing/physical-activity

WHO Guidelines for Physical Activity
Bloom Allied Health (2020)
https://youtu.be/87uIyAFcYMY

Sedentary Behaviour

Sedentary behaviour (SB) is defined as 'any waking behaviour characterised by an energy expenditure ≤ 1.5 metabolic equivalents of task (METs), while in a seated, reclined or lying posture' (Tremblay et al. 2017). SB (such as excessive watching of television, reading, computer work and driving) is an independent risk factor for CVD and is therefore considered separately to physical activity, body weight and diet (Lavie et al. 2019). Patients may be physically active for the recommended 150–300 min/wk, yet they may sit for several hours a day in a sedentary occupation or during their leisure time (Lavie et al. 2019). Sitting is associated with all-cause and CVD mortality risk among the least physically active adults. Moderate-to-vigorous physical activity within current recommendations reduces or eliminates this association (Stamatakis et al. 2019). Patients can reduce the time they spend being sedentary by undertaking activities such as frequent standing and stretching, taking walks during lunch breaks, using a standing desk in the workplace, regularly undertaking chores around the house, taking stairs instead of an elevator or spending time gardening. There are apps for smartphones or watches that prompt people to change position regularly. Some work computers have programs to prompt people to stand and stretch frequently.

Nutrition

Nutritional counselling includes the following advice to patients:

- Reduce intake of saturated fat to <7% of calories and *trans*-fatty acids and cholesterol to <200 mg dietary cholesterol per day as reducing dietary saturated fatty acid lowers cardiovascular events by 17% (Hooper et al. 2015).
- Add plant stanol/sterols (2 g/d) and viscous fibre (more than 10 g/d) to further lower LDL-C.
- Promote daily PA and weight management.
- Consume a Mediterranean-style diet with more fruit, bread, vegetables and fish (Jones et al. 2018).

Key Point

Eating and drinking are often embedded in social, family-centred and culturally defined behaviours that over time become established as normal routine. Changing such established behaviour is a challenge and can be difficult for patients and their families.

Suggested Resources

Food and nutrition
Heart Foundation (Australia)
https://www.heartfoundation.org.au/heart-health-education/healthy-eating
Nutrition Basics
American Heart Association
https://www.heart.org/en/healthy-living/healthy-eating

Ever-changing information via the media and from family and friends can be confusing to patients and makes them uncertain of the best way forward. Health professionals need to provide dietary advice that is easy to understand and sets realistic targets for long-term healthy eating. Patients need to understand the basic principles of dietary content, such as calories, fat, cholesterol and nutrients. All patients with CVD should adopt a diet that contains protein, complex carbohydrates, fruits, vegetables, nuts and whole grains, and is restricted in saturated fat and cholesterol (NICE 2013).

Alcohol Consumption

Alcohol consumption is a major risk factor for many diseases. The relationship between alcohol consumption and cardiovascular risk (or potential benefit with low-to-moderate alcohol consumption) is uncertain as data are derived from epidemiologic studies. Therefore, healthcare professionals should not recommend alcohol consumption as a primary or secondary lifestyle intervention. There is evidence of harm from long-term heavy alcohol use and binge drinking. Heavy alcohol use may lead to alcoholic cardiomyopathy. Binge drinking is associated with a heightened risk of HT, stroke, atrial fibrillation, myocardial infarction (MI) and sudden death (Piano 2017). For people with alcohol dependence, abstinence should be advised.

Suggested Resources

National Health and Medical Research Council, Australian Research Council and Universities Australia (2020) Australian Guidelines to Reduce Health Risks from Drinking Alcohol. Commonwealth of Australia, Canberra.
https://www.nhmrc.gov.au/file/15923/download?token=t0Hrxdvq

National Institute for Health and Care Excellence (NICE) (2011). *Alcohol-use Disorders: Diagnosis, Assessment and Management of Harmful Drinking and Alcohol Dependence.* London: NICE.
https://www.nice.org.uk/guidance/cg115

Psychosocial Risk Factors

Psychological coping responses to a cardiac event, in particular anxiety and depression, can hamper recovery irrespective of the patient's physical condition. Other psychological problems include anger or hostility, social isolation, marital and family distress, sexual dysfunction and alcohol and other substance abuse. Major depression has been found to be an independent risk factor for cardiac events after ACS (Lichtman et al. 2014). Anxiety is an acceptable adaptive response to a perceived threat such as a cardiac event, but it can become maladaptive and be a precursor to depression in certain circumstances. Patients often feel that stress has contributed to their condition, although its precise role as a risk factor is unclear. Relaxation has been shown to enhance recovery from ischaemic cardiac events and has a role to play in secondary prevention.

Strategies designed to reduce stress and anxiety and improve overall psychological well-being include:

- Planned periods of rest and relaxation
- Frequent exercise
- Avoidance of polyphasic activities (not doing more than one thing at once)
- Instruction in anticipating/recognising emotions and how to manage them – encouraging self-help
- Group sessions to offer social and peer support
- Individual sessions on counselling and education on adjustment to heart disease, stress management and lifestyle change
- Including family members in the support
- Referring patients experiencing clinically significant psychosocial distress to appropriate specialists for further evaluation, support and antidepressant medication if required.

Medication Adherence

As well as medication prescribed to reach lipid, blood pressure and glucose targets and control ischaemic symptoms, other drugs are used in secondary prevention to reduce morbidity and mortality. A patient's drug regimen will need to be individualised and depend on cardiac events, the results of diagnostic tests, procedural interventions and coronary artery disease risk factors. Current international guidelines for the management of patients following MI are derived from a large body of evidence, showing the beneficial effects of several single-drug therapies such as dual antiplatelet therapy (DAPT) with aspirin and a $P2Y_{12}$ inhibitor (prasugrel, ticagrelor or clopidogrel), lipid-lowering drugs (LLDs), ACE inhibitors or angiotensin receptor blockers (ARBs) and beta-blockers (BBs). Despite better outcomes for patients who take prescribed medications for secondary prevention following MI, non-adherence to medication regimes is a common and costly problem in a significant proportion of patients (Huber et al. 2019). Non-adherence to medications may take the form of:

- non-fulfillment in which prescriptions are never filled (primary non-adherence)
- non-persistence where patients stop their medication without being advised by a health professional to do so
- non-conforming, encompassing ways that medications are not taken as described (such as skipping doses, taking incorrect doses or doses at incorrect times or taking more than prescribed (Gellad et al. 2009)).

Suggested Resource

Ma, T.T., Wong, I.C.K., Man, K.K.C. et al. (2019). Effect of evidence-based therapy for secondary prevention of cardiovascular disease: systematic review and meta-analysis. *PLoS One* 14 (1): e0210988. https://journals.plos. org/plosone/article?id=10.1371/journal. pone.0210988

Adherence to evidence-based secondary prevention pharmacotherapy in patients after an acute coronary syndrome is suboptimal (Chen et al. 2015). Non-adherence to medications can be influenced by several factors as shown in Table 18.1. Given the complexities associated

Table 18.1 Factors influencing medication adherence.

Patient factors

Illness representation
- Heath beliefs (including beliefs about medications), knowledge about the illness.

Cognitive function
- Memory and ability to understand information.

Health Literacy
- Ability to read, comprehend and critically analyse health information.

Demographics
- Age, gender, ethnicity, culture, physical limitations, socio-economic situation.

Co-existing illness
- Medical and mental health conditions, smoking, alcohol and illicit drug use.

Difficulty with medication administration
- Visual or hearing impairment, inability to open medication containers.

Impact of medical regimes
- Complexity of the regime, side effects.

Organisational and provider factors

Access to care
- Rural and remote access.
- Availability of general practitioner (GP) appointments.

Fragmentation of care
- Communication between healthcare providers (for example, between hospital, specialist and GP).
- Poor communication between healthcare providers and the patient.
- System failures (no follow-up appointments).

Patient–provider trust and satisfaction
- Consideration of a patient's individual situation, time spent with the patient, respect shown to the patient, education about medical therapies.
- Patient's past experiences of healthcare provision.

---

with medication non-adherence, it is likely that many of these factors contribute and overlap with one another (Crawshaw et al. 2016).

Efforts to improve adherence is an important component of effective patient management and it is essential that medication adherence is followed up regularly in scheduled follow-up appointments with health providers, including the CR nurse, GP and cardiologist. The first follow-up appointment in ACS patients within several weeks after hospital discharge represents an important opportunity to identify patient's medication non-adherence, and opportunities to jointly develop patient-specific solutions to non-adherence by healthcare providers and their patients (Gellad et al. 2009).

Recovery and Longer-Term Maintenance

Patients need to be informed about specific targets for risk factor modification and other appropriate lifestyle changes. Goals should be agreed with the patient for the short term (wk/mo) after which follow-up plans are developed. These plans should be discussed with the patient and appropriate family members in collaboration with the primary health-care team. Services must be flexible enough to accommodate an individual's clinical condition and psychological state and consider their lifestyle, health beliefs, goals and expectations. Thought needs to be given to presenting information in a way that renders them both relevant and accessible for the patient.

Suggested Resource

Motivational interviewing is a communication style that aims to lead patients to make change commitments and take action to adopt healthy lifestyles. The link below takes you to a series of videos about the principles, mechanisms and skills associated with motivational interviewing that you can incorporate into your practice.
Motivational interviewing
Heart Foundation (2012)
https://youtu.be/lufiDGl1ckM

Conclusion

A comprehensive program of behaviour change is required for patients with established CVD. Prevention strategies should incorporate education, risk factors reduction and drug therapy and lifestyle changes that are tailored to individual patients. It is important that the cardiac nurse be aware of available resources and current evidence-based guidelines to assist in developing tailored CR programs in practice.

References

Anderson, L., Thompson, D.R., Oldridge, N. et al. (2016). Exercise-based cardiac rehabilitation for coronary heart disease. *The Cochrane Database of Systematic Reviews* 1: CD001800. doi: https://www.cochranelibrary.com/cdsr/doi/10.1002/14651858.CD001800.pub3/full.

Anderson, L., Sharp, G.A., Norton, R.J. et al. (2017). Home-based versus centre-based cardiac rehabilitation. *Cochrane Database of Systematic Reviews* 6: CD007130. https://www.cochranelibrary.com/cdsr/doi/10.1002/14651858.CD007130.pub4/full.

Arnett, D.K., Blumenthal, R.S., Albert, M.A., Buroker, A.B., Goldberger, Z.D., Hahn, E.J., . . . & Michos, E.D. (2019). 2019 ACC/AHA guideline on the primary prevention of cardiovascular disease: a report of the American College of Cardiology/American Heart Association Task Force on Clinical Practice Guidelines. *Journal of the American College of Cardiology*, **74** (10), e177–e232. DOI: https://doi.org/10.1016/j.jacc.2019.03.010.

van den Berg, M.J., van der Graaf, Y., Deckers, J.W. et al. (2019). Smoking cessation and risk of recurrent cardiovascular events and mortality after a first manifestation of arterial disease. *American Heart Journal* 213: 112–122.

British Heart Foundation (2018). The National Audit of Cardiac Rehabilitation (NACR). Quality and Outcomes Report. www.bhf.org.uk/informationsupport/publications/statistics/national-audit-of-cardiac-rehabilitation-quality-and-outcomes-report-2018 (accessed 04 January 2020).

Chen, H.Y., Saczynski, J.S., Lapane, K.L. et al. (2015). Adherence to evidence-based secondary prevention pharmacotherapy in patients after an acute coronary syndrome: a systematic review. *Heart and Lung* **44** (4): 299–308.

Conner, M. and Norman, P. (2017). Health behaviour: Current issues and challenges. *Psychology & Health* **32** (8): 895–906.

Cosentino, F., Grant, P.J., Aboyans, V. et al. (2020). 2019 ESC guidelines on diabetes, pre-diabetes, and cardiovascular diseases developed in collaboration with the EASD: the task force for diabetes, pre-diabetes, and cardiovascular diseases of the European Society of Cardiology (ESC) and the European association for the study of diabetes (EASD). *European Heart Journal* **41** (2): 255–323.

Crawshaw, J., Auyeung, V., Norton, S., and Weinman, J. (2016). Identifying psychosocial predictors of medication non-adherence following acute coronary syndrome: a systematic review and meta-analysis. *Journal of Psychosomatic Research* **90**: 10–32.

Dalal, H.M., Doherty, P., and Taylor, S.R. (2015). Cardiac rehabilitation – clinical review. *BMJ* 351: h5000. https://www.bmj.com/content/bmj/351/bmj.h5000.full.pdf (accessed 04 January 2020).

Ference, A.B., Ginberg, N.H., Graham, I. et al. (2017). Low–density lipoproteins cause atherosclerotic cardiovascular disease. Evidence from genetic, epidemiologic, and clinical studies. A consensus statement from the European Atherosclerosis society Consensus panel. *European Heart Journal* **38**: 2459–2472.

Fletcher, S.W. and Fletcher, R.H. (2020). Evidence-based approach to prevention. [Updated 2020 March 5]. In: *UpToDate* [Internet]. https://www.uptodate.com/contents/evidence-based-approach-to-prevention.

Frederix, I., Caiani, E.G., Dendale, P. et al. (2019). ESC e-Cardiology Working Group Position Paper: overcoming challenges in digital health implementation in cardiovascular medicine. *European Journal of Preventive Cardiology* **26** (11): 1166–1177.

Gellad, W.F., Grenard, J., and McGlynn, A. (2009). *Review of Barriers to Medication Adherence: A Framework for Driving Policy Options*. Santa Monica, CA: RAND Corporation [Internet] https://www.rand.org/pubs/technical_reports/TR765.html.

Gochman, D.S. (ed.) (1997). *Handbook of Health Behavior Research (vols 1–4)*. New York, NY: Plenum.

Hammersley, D., & Signy, M. (2017). Ezetimibe: an update on its clinical usefulness in specific patient groups. *Therapeutic Advances in Chronic Disease*, **8** (1), 4–11. https://doi.org/10.1177/2040622316672544.

Hartmann-Boyce, J. and Aveyard, P. (2016). Drugs for smoking cessation. *BMJ* **352**: i571.

Hinde, S., Bojke, L., Harrison, A., and Doherty, P. (2019). Improving cardiac rehabilitation uptake: potential health gains by socioeconomic status. *European Journal of Preventive Cardiology* **26** (17): 1816–1823.

Hooper, L., Martin, N., Abdelhamis, A., and Davey Smith, G. (2015). Reduction in saturated fat intake for cardiovascular disease. *Cochrane database Systematic Review* June **10** (6): Cd 011737. https://doi.org/10.1002/14651858.CD011737 (accessed 8 January 2019).

Huber, A.C., Meyer, M., Blozik, E. et al. (2019). Post-myocardial infarction (MI) care: medication adherence for secondary prevention after MI in a Large real-world population. *Clinical Therapeutics* **41** (1): 107–117.

Ibanez, B., James, S., Agewall, S. et al. (2018). 2017 ESC guidelines for the management of acute myocardial infarction in patients presenting with ST–segment elevation: the task Force for the management of acute myocardial infarction in patients presenting with ST–elevation of the European Society of Cardiology(ESC). *European Heart Journal* **39** (2): 119–177.

Jones, R., Arps, K., Davis, M.D., and Blumenthal, R.S. (2018). *Clinician Guide to the ABC of Primary and Secondary Prevention of Atherosclerotic Cardiovascular Disease*. American College of Cardiology https://www.acc.org/latest-in-cardiology/articles/2018/03/30/18/34/clinician-guide-to-the-abcs (accessed 04 January 2020).

Kao, C.K. and Liebovitz, D.M. (2017). Consumer mobile health apps: current state, barriers, and future directions. *PM&R* **9** (5): S106–S115.

Keenan, M.J. (2018). The role of Niacin in the management dyslipidemia. *IntechOpen*, DOI: https://doi.org/10.5772/intechopen.81725.

Kisling, L.A. and Das, J.M. (2019). Prevention strategies. [Updated 2019 January 31]. In:

StatPearls [Internet]. Treasure Island (FL): StatPearls Publishing; 2020 January-. https://www.ncbi.nlm.nih.gov/books/NBK537222.

Kotseva, K., De Bacquer, D., De Backer, G. et al. (2016). Lifestyle and risk factor management in people at high risk of cardiovascular disease. A report from the European Society of Cardiology European Action on Secondary and Primary Prevention by Intervention to Reduce Events (EUROASPIRE) IV cross-sectional survey in 14 European regions. *European Journal of Preventive Cardiology* **23**: 2007–2018.

Lancaster, T. & Stead, L.F. (2017). Individual behavioral counseling for smoking cessation. *Cochrane Database Systematic Review*, 3:CD001292.DOI: https://doi.org/10.1002/14651858.CD001292.pub3.

Lavie, C.J., Ozemek, C., Carbone, S. et al. (2019). Sedentary behavior, exercise, and cardiovascular health. *Circulation Research* **124** (5): 799–815.

Leon, B.M. and Maddox, T.M. (2015). Diabetes and cardiovascular disease: epidemiology, biological mechanisms, treatment recommendations and future research. *World Journal of Diabetes* **6** (13): 1246.

Lichtman, J.H., Froelicher, E.S., Blumenthal, J.A. et al. (2014). Depression as a risk factor for poor prognosis among patients with acute coronary syndrome: systematic review and recommendations: a scientific statement from the American Heart Association. *Circulation* **129** (12): 1350–1369.

Lu, C.C., Hsiao, Y.C., Huang, H.W. et al. (2019). Effects of a nurse-led, stage-matched, tailored program for smoking cessation in health education centers: a prospective, randomized, controlled trial. *Clinical Nursing Research* **28** (7): 812–829.

Mach, F., Baigent, C., Catapano, A.L. et al. (2020). 2019 ESC/EAS Guidelines for the management of dyslipidaemias: lipid modification to reduce cardiovascular risk: the task force for the management of dyslipidaemias of the European Society of Cardiology (ESC) and European Atherosclerosis Society (EAS). *European Heart Journal* **41** (1): 111–188.

National Heart Foundation of Australia, Australian Cardiac Rehabilitation Association (2004). *Recommended Framework for Cardiac Rehabilitation '04*. Canberra: National Heart Foundation of Australia, Australian Cardiac Rehabilitation Association.

National Heart Foundation of Australia (2016). *Guideline for Diagnosis and Management of Hypertension on Adults – 2016*. Melbourne: National Heart Foundation of Australia [NHFA] www.heartfoundation.org.au/images/uploads/publications/PRO-167_Hypertension-guideline-2016_WEB.pdf.

National Institute for Health and Care Excellence. (2014). *Obesity: Identification, assessment and management* (NICE guideline NG189) https://www.nice.org.uk/guidance/cg189/chapter/1-Recommendations

National Institute for Health and Care Excellence. (2020). *Acute coronary syndromes* (NICE guideline NG185). https://www.nice.org.uk/guidance/ng185/chapter/Recommendations#drug-therapy-for-secondary-prevention

Piano, M.R. (2017). Alcohol's effects on the cardiovascular system. *Alcohol Research: Current Reviews* **38** (2): 219.

Piepoli, F.M., Hoes, W.A., Agewell, S. et al. (2016a). European Guidelines on cardiovascular disease prevention in clinical practice: the Sixth Joint Taskforce of the European Society of Cardiology and other societies on cardiovascular disease prevention in clinical practice. Developed with the special contribution of The European Association for Cardiovascular Prevention and Rehabilitation (EACPR). *European Heart Journal* **37** (29): 2315–2381.

Piepoli, M.F., Corrà, U., Dendale, P. et al. (2016b). Challenges in secondary prevention after acute myocardial infarction: a call for action. *European Journal of Preventive Cardiology* **23**: 1994–2006.

Piepoli, M.F., Abreu, A., Albus, C. et al. (2020). Update on cardiovascular prevention in clinical practice: a position paper of the European Association of Preventive Cardiology of the European Society of Cardiology. *European Journal of Preventive Cardiology* **27** (2): 181–205. https://journals.sagepub.com/doi/pdf/10.1177/2047487319893035.

Piercy, K.L., Troiano, R.P., Ballard, R. et al. (2018). The physical activity guidelines for americans. *Journal of the American Medical Association* **320** (19): 2020–2028.

Rosenson, R.S., Hayward, R.A., and Lopez-Sendon, J. (2020). Management of low-density lipoprotein cholesterol (LDL-C) in the secondary prevention of cardiovascular disease. In: (ed. Freeman, E.W., Cannon. C.P., Kaski, J.C., and Saperia, G.M.). *UpToDate* [website]. www.uptodate.com.

Shields, E.J., Wells, A., Doherty, P. et al. (2018). Cost-effectiveness of cardiac rehabilitation: a systematic review. *Heart* **104**: 1403–1410.

Stamatakis, E., Gale, J., Bauman, A. et al. (2019). Sitting time, physical activity, and risk of mortality in adults. *Journal of the American College of Cardiology* **73** (16): 2062–2072.

Thomas, J.R., Beatty, L.A., Beckie, M.T. et al. (2019). Home-based cardiac rehabilitation: a scientific statement from the American Association of Cardiovascular and Pulmonary Rehabilitation, the American Heart Association, and the American College of Cardiology. *Journal American College of Cardiology* **74** (1): 133–153.

Tremblay, M.S., Aubert, S., Barnes, J.D. et al. (2017). Sedentary behavior research network (SBRN)–terminology consensus project process and outcome. *International Journal of Behavioral Nutrition and Physical Activity* **14** (1): 75.

Woodruffe, S., Neubeck, L., Clark, R.A. et al. (2015). Australian Cardiovascular Health and Rehabilitation Association (ACRA) core components of cardiovascular disease secondary prevention and cardiac rehabilitation 2014. *Heart, Lung and Circulation* **24** (5): 430–441.

World Health Organization (1993). *Needs and Action Priorities in Cardiac Rehabilitation and Secondary Prevention in Patients with Coronary Heart Disease*. Geneva: WHO Regional Office for Europe 1993.

Part V

Cardiac Arrest

19

Sudden Cardiac Death

Pete Gregory and Angela M. Kucia

Overview

Sudden cardiac death (SCD) can be defined as 'death resulting from abrupt cessation of cardiac function due to sudden cardiac arrest'. The principal risk factor for SCD is coronary heart disease (CHD), particularly in the presence of left ventricular (LV) dysfunction with reduced ejection fraction (EF). There has been a dramatic decrease in age-adjusted death rates due to coronary artery disease (CAD) in the past 30 years due to progress in prevention and treatment, but SCD remains a major public health challenge, accounting for close to one-fifth of all mortality in developed countries (Junttila et al. 2016; Wong et al. 2019). There are several non-CHD conditions including genetic factors and structural heart defects, which increase the risk of SCD. Moreover, SCD can occur in the absence of any identified cardiac abnormality. The ability to predict the likelihood of SCD remains elusive as SCD seems to result from the interaction of a vulnerable substrate (genetic or acquired changes in the electrical or mechanical properties of the heart) with multiple transient factors that serve to trigger the event (Priori et al. 2015). Risk-reduction strategies include revascularisation for ongoing ischaemia, beta-blockade and use of implantable cardioverter defibrillators (ICDs), although it is not an exhaustive list. A major aspect of care, irrespective of the identified risk factor, is the support for those identified as 'at risk' and their families; for bereaved relatives who have lost a close family member to SCD, further assessment of risk is required together with appropriate therapies and ongoing psychological support.

> **Learning Objectives**
>
> After reading this chapter, you should be able to:
>
> - Describe conditions commonly associated with SCD.
> - Identify the inherited primary arrhythmia syndromes.
> - List the key aspects of patient assessment and risk stratification and strategies to reduce the risk of SCD.
> - Discuss the support needs of 'at risk' patients and their families.

> **Key Concepts**
>
> Sudden cardiac death; sudden cardiac arrest; arrhythmia; channelopathies; structural heart disease

Background

Sudden cardiac arrest (SCA) can be defined as 'sudden cessation of cardiac activity so that the victim becomes unresponsive, with no normal breathing and no signs of circulation' (Al-Khatib et al. 2018, p. e97). If corrective measures are not taken to rapidly reverse cardiac arrest it will result in SCD. SCD can be defined as 'the unexpected death of an individual not attributable to an extracardiac cause, usually within 1 hour of symptom onset (or within 24 hours of last being seen in good health if the death is unwitnessed)' (Isbister and Semsarian 2019, p. 826). A death can also be classified as sudden if a patient was resuscitated after a cardiac arrest, survived on life support for a limited period and then died due to irreversible brain damage (Basso et al. 2017).

> **Key Point**
>
> Cardiac arrest is the term used to signify an event that can be reversed, usually by cardiopulmonary resuscitation (CPR), administration of medications and/or defibrillation or cardioversion (Al-Khatib et al. 2018).

The most common electrical event associated with SCD is ventricular fibrillation (VF), often preceded by ventricular tachycardia (VT), though there are substantial numbers of SCA where bradyarrhythmias or asystole are the underlying rhythm. The majority of SCD fatal events occur in the community and most of these in patients' homes. Since most SCD occurs in the non-monitored patient, the mechanism can only be inferred from limited retrospective series. In a classic report of 157 patients who had SCD while undergoing ambulatory ECG monitoring it was found that 8% had primary VF, 62% VT/VF, 13% polymorphic VT or torsade de pointes and 16% bradycardia. Increased premature ventricular beats preceding the terminal arrhythmia were observed in 70% of these patients, and ST-segment abnormalities suggestive of myocardial ischaemia were seen in 13% (Bayés de Luna et al. 1989). Recognition and management of cardiac arrhythmias that are found in SCA are reviewed in Chapters 11 and 12.

> **Key Point**
>
> In out-of-hospital cardiac arrest, asystole may often be the first rhythm observed, but this is probably a marker of the duration of the arrest and delay in getting an ambulance to the patient, rather than an indication of the primary arrhythmia.

Burden of Disease

Estimates of the incidence of SCD in a general population vary according to the epidemiological methods used, but SCD accounts for over half of all cardiac deaths and 20% of natural deaths in Western societies (Tan et al. 2018). SCD is the first symptomatic cardiac event in approximately 25% of those patients with SCD. Survival statistics following out of hospital (OOH) cardiac arrest continue to be poor, with approximately 10% of people with OOH cardiac arrest surviving to hospital discharge (Al-Khatib et al. 2018; Beck et al. 2018). 70% of OOH cardiac arrests occur in the home and survival rates for this subgroup are even poorer at 6%. Factors associated with better survival rates are highly developed and publicly visible emergency rescue response in a public location, bystander cardiopulmonary resuscitation (CPR), quick arrival of first responders, availability of an automated external defibrillator (AED), shockable rhythm at initial contact and possibly telecommunication-directed CPR. Survival to discharge following in-hospital cardiac arrest is approximately 24%. Again, survival rates are higher for those in a shockable rhythm compared with those with pulseless electrical activity (PEA) or asystole (Al-Khatib et al. 2018).

Risk Factors for Sudden Cardiac Death

Table 19.1 shows conditions that are commonly associated with SCD. It is difficult to predict an individual's risk for SCA and SCD as currently there are no adequately tested and validated methods in the general population. SCD is more common in males than in females. Increasing age is a strong predictor of risk for SCD, but the relationship between advancing age and incidence of SCD is not linear. SCD has an initial peak between 0 and 5 years of age before a much larger second peak between 75 and 85 years of age (Isbister and Semsarian 2019). Underlying causes of SCD differ between younger and older aged individuals; in younger people there is a predominance of channelopathies, cardiomyopathies, myocarditis and substance abuse; in older individuals, chronic degenerative conditions including CHD, valvular disease and heart failure (HF) are more common (Priori et al. 2015).

CHD is the most common underlying cause of SCD, though the incidence of CHD-related SCD seems to be decreasing, while various forms of cardiomyopathy leading to SCD seem to be increasing (Al-Khatib et al. 2018). The proportion of SCDs associated with hypertensive heart disease and left ventricular hypertrophy (LVH) in the absence of CHD is increasing, as is SCD related to myocardial fibrosis in the

Table 19.1 Conditions associated with sudden cardiac death.

Coronary heart disease	*Valve disease*
• Myocardial infarction	Aortic stenosis
• Anomalous coronary artery origin	Bicuspid aortic valve
• Coronary artery spasm	Mitral valve prolapse
• Spontaneous coronary artery dissection (SCAD)	
	Congenital diseases
	Tetralogy of Fallot
Heart failure	
• LV dysfunction with EF less than 35%	*Other*
	Aortic dissection
Cardiomyopathies	Vasculitis
Alcoholic	Electrolyte imbalance (potassium and magnesium)
Arrhythmogenic right ventricular cardiomyopathy (ARVC)	Recreational drug use
Fibrotic	Pro-arrhythmic drugs
Hypertrophic	Wolff-Parkinson-White syndrome
Dilated	Marfan's syndrome
Idiopathic	Takotsubo syndrome
Obesity-related	Pulmonary embolism
Myocarditis	Intracranial haemorrhage
Infiltrative (amyloidosis, sarcoidosis, Fabry disease)	Commotio cordis
	Blunt trauma to the head/neck
Inherited channelopathies	Drowning
Brugada syndrome	Electrocution
Catecholaminergic polymorphic ventricular tachycardia (CPVT)	Status asthmaticus
Early repolarisation syndrome	Heat stroke
Long QT syndrome (LQTS)	
Short QT syndrome (SQTS)	

absence of myocarditis or other known pathologies (Junttila et al. 2016). SCD accounts for over half of all cardiac deaths and may be the first manifestation of underlying CHD. Recent trends suggest that patients surviving out of hospital (OOH) cardiac arrest are more likely to have a high-risk profile for CHD than manifest disease (Al-Khatib et al. 2018). As the population ages and more patients survive acute myocardial infarction (MI), the burden of chronic heart failure (HF) increases and with it the risk of SCD associated with reduced EF.

Patients with genetic abnormalities, such as those resulting in long QT syndrome (LQTS), account for a small fraction of the overall population at risk of SCD, but the presence of such abnormalities places the affected individual at very high risk of SCD. Several studies have demonstrated a genetic predisposition to SCD (Friedlander et al. 1998; Jouven et al. 1999; Dekker et al. 2006), but there is no single method for risk stratification for SCD in the various inheritable channelopathies and cardiomyopathies. Genetic information is only useful in a few inheritable diseases (Priori et al. 2015).

Social and economic stress has been shown to increase the risk of a coronary event, and this is said to be particularly striking in relation to SCD. Behavioural and emotional factors are probable triggers of events in vulnerable individuals, although precise mechanisms and strategies to reduce risk are not yet fully understood (Strike and Steptoe 2005). Patients with CHD and depressive symptoms are associated with increased risk of SCD independent of other clinical risk factors and LV function (Lahtinen et al. 2017).

Screening in the General Population for Risk of Sudden Cardiac Death

Electrocardiographic (ECG) and echocardiographic signs of inheritable arrhymogenic diseases may contribute to the early identification of people at risk of SCD, but there does not seem to be any evidence that routine screening in the general population will change incident rates for SCD (Priori et al. 2015). Abnormal findings in an ECG and/or echocardiogram during scheduled examinations may alert the clinician to an individual at increased risk of SCD. ECG findings associated with an increased risk of SCD are discussed in Chapter 11.

Mechanisms of Sudden Cardiac Death

Ventricular Arrhythmias

The most common electrical event associated with SCD is VF, often preceded by VT. Mechanisms of ventricular arrhythmias (VAs) include enhanced automaticity, triggered activity induced by early or late afterdepolarisations, and reentry. These mechanisms are discussed in Chapter 11.

Assessment of patients with suspected arrhythmia is discussed in Chapter 12. Table 19.2 lists important considerations in the evaluation of patients with known or suspected VAs.

Management of VAs is discussed in Chapter 12. Comprehensive guidelines for the management of patients with VAs and prevention of SCD can be found below:

Suggested Resource

Al-Khatib et al. (2018). 2017 AHA/ACC/HRS guideline for management of patients with ventricular arrhythmias and the prevention of sudden cardiac death: a report of the American College of Cardiology/American Heart Association Task Force on Clinical Practice Guidelines and the Heart Rhythm Society. *JACC* 72 (14): e91–e220. https://doi.org/10.1016/j.jacc.2017.10.054

Table 19.2 Important considerations in the evaluation of patients with known or ventricular arrhythmias.

Component	Assessment and findings relevant for VA and/or SCD risk

History	1) Symptoms/events related to arrhythmia: palpitations, lightheadedness, syncope, dyspnoea, chest pain, cardiac arrest
	2) Symptoms related to underlying heart disease: dyspnoea at rest or on exertion, orthopnoea, paroxysmal nocturnal dyspnoea, chest pain, oedema
	3) Precipitating factors: exercise, emotional stress
	4) Known heart disease: coronary, valvular (e.g. mitral valve prolapse), congenital heart disease, others
	5) Risk factors for heart disease: hypertension, diabetes mellitus, hyperlipidaemia, and smoking
	6) Medications:
	  • Antiarrhythmic medications
	  • Other medications with potential for QT prolongation and torsades de pointes
	  • Medications with potential to provoke or aggravate VA
	    – Stimulants including cocaine and amphetamines
	    – Supplements including anabolic steroids
	  • Medication–medication interaction that could cause QT prolongation and torsades de pointes
	7) Past medical history:
	  • Thyroid disease
	  • Acute kidney injury, chronic kidney disease or electrolyte abnormalities
	  • Stroke or embolic events
	  • Lung disease
	  • Epilepsy (arrhythmic syncope can be misdiagnosed as epilepsy)
	  • Alcohol or illicit drug use
	  • Use of over-the-counter medications that could cause QT prolongation and torsades de pointes
	  • Unexplained motor vehicle crashes

Family history	1) SCD, SCA or unexplained drowning in a first-degree relative
	2) SIDS or repetitive spontaneous pregnancy losses given their potential association with cardiac channelopathies
	3) Heart disease
	  • Ischaemic heart disease
	  • Cardiomyopathy: Hypertrophic, dilated, ARVC
	  • Congenital heart disease
	  • Cardiac channelopathies: Long QT, Brugada, Short QT, CPVT
	  • Arrhythmias
	  • Conduction disorders, pacemakers/ICDs
	4) Neuromuscular disease associated with cardiomyopathies
	  • Muscular dystrophy
	5) Epilepsy

Examination	1) Heart rate and regularity, blood pressure 2) Jugular venous pressure 3) Murmurs 4) Pulses and bruits 5) Oedema 6) Sternotomy scars

ARVC indicates arrhythmogenic right ventricular cardiomyopathy; CPVT, catecholaminergic polymorphic ventricular tachycardia; IHD, ischaemic heart disease; SCA, sudden cardiac arrest; SCD, sudden cardiac death; SIDS, sudden infant death syndrome and VA, ventricular arrhythmia.

Source: Reprinted with permission. Al-Khatib et al. (2018). Copyright © 2020 Elsevier B.V. or its licensors or contributors.

Sudden Cardiac Death in Structural Heart Disease

Studies of survivors of SCA show apparently normal hearts in 5–10%, but the overwhelming majority have cardiac pathology including CHD. For those with SCD, most have hypertrophy or scarring, serving as substrate for lethal arrhythmias at autopsy. Farb et al. (1995) reported active coronary lesions at autopsy in around half of SCD cases where myocardial scarring was found in the absence of acute infarction.

Key Point

The term 'structural heart disease' encompasses cardiac conditions other than coronary artery disease. It includes valvular heart disease and defects in the muscular structure of the heart that may be congenital or acquired.

Coronary Heart Disease

In up to 50% of patients with SCA there is no known history of CHD, but most have concealed heart disease. VF is a complication of ST-segment-elevation myocardial infarction (STEMI) in approximately 10% of patients (Jabbari et al. 2015) and may be the first underlying symptom of CHD (Jacobsen et al. 2020). Thus, managing risk factors associated with CHD (see Chapter 5) in the general population may reduce risk of SCD in the general population. For patients with CHD who survive SCA, PCI or coronary artery bypass surgery (CABG) is the appropriate treatment where indicated. The only reliable indicator for risk of SCD in the setting of myocardial infarction is persistent LV dysfunction and reduced EF, for which ICD implantation is recommended if criteria are met (Priori et al. 2015).

Key Point

Potassium disturbances (hypokalaemia and hyperkalaemia) among STEMI patients may increase the risk of VF before primary percutaneous coronary intervention and subsequent death during acute ischaemia (Jacobsen et al. 2020).

Valvular Heart Disease

Valvular heart disease poses a risk of VAs prior to and following valvular surgery.

Inflammatory Heart Disease

Myocarditis

Myocarditis results from myocardial infection and/or an autoimmune response that causes active destruction of myocytes. Acute fulminant myocarditis with refractory malignant VAs in the context of severe heart failure has a poor prognosis. Longer-term inflammatory cardiomyopathy with LV dysfunction carries a high risk of SCD. Antiarrhythmic therapy should be considered for VAs during the acute course of the disease and ICD implantation may be considered after resolution of the acute episode if the patient is expected to survive >1 year with good functional status (Priori et al. 2015).

Pericarditis

SCD can occur in pericarditis but usually has a haemodynamic rather than an arrhythmic cause.

Endocarditis

Endocarditis may be associated with first- or second-degree heart block which raises the suspicion of abscess formation in the valve annulus. Acute haemodynamic compromise in endocarditis may cause VT and is an indication for early surgery (Priori et al. 2015).

Cardiomyopathies and Sudden Cardiac Death

Dilated Cardiomyopathy

Dilated cardiomyopathy (DCM) is defined as 'LV dilatation and systolic dysfunction in the absence of abnormal loading conditions or CAD sufficient to cause global systolic impairment' and presents in people of all ages and ethnicities (Priori et al. 2015, p. 1635). In adults it is more common in men than in women. SCD is a major cause of death in people with DCM with VAs being common mechanisms for SCD. Optimal medical therapy including angiotensin-converting enzyme (ACE) inhibitors, beta-blockers and aldosterone receptor antagonists (MRAs) is recommended in patients with DCM to reduce the risk of sudden death and progressive heart failure (HF). An ICD or catheter ablation may be recommended for selected patients with DCM.

Hypertrophic Cardiomyopathy

Hypertrophic cardiomyopathy (HCM) refers to left wall thickness without an obvious cause and is usually hereditary. Patients with HCM are advised not to participate in competitive sports and intense physical activity. While medical treatment alone does not prevent disease progression (and is not indicated therefore in asymptomatic patients), and no randomised trials of ICD use have demonstrated efficacy in reducing SCD, patients with multiple risk factors are considered at sufficient risk to 'merit consideration' of ICD. Aborted cardiac arrest or sustained VT are associated with a high risk of subsequent lethal cardiac arrhythmias, though SCD is often the first manifestation of HCM (Priori et al. 2015). Genetic testing may contribute to risk stratification and counselling of relatives.

Arrhythmogenic Right Ventricular Cardiomyopathy

Arrhythmogenic right ventricular cardiomyopathy (ARVC), sometimes known as arrhythmogenic right ventricular dysplasia, is a genetic progressive heart muscle disorder where cardiomyocytes are replaced by adipose and fibrous tissue. While AVRC is defined by this abnormality in the right ventricle, LV involvement occurs in approximately 50% of patients (Priori et al. 2015). SCD is often the first manifestation and an important cause of death in athletes and young people. As with DCM, competitive sports should be avoided. Beta blockers are recommended as the first line of therapy for patients with frequent premature ventricular contractions (PVCs) and non-sustained VT. ICD implantation is considered in selected patients.

Other Cardiomyopathies

Less common cardiomyopathies associated with SCD include cardiac amyloidosis, restrictive cardiomyopathies and Chaga's disease.

Takotsubo Syndrome

The incidence of life-threatening arrhythmias in Takotsubo syndrome (TTS) is significant (El-Battrawy et al. 2018). SCD due to arrhythmia is the initial presentation for TTS in some people.

Anomalous Coronary Arteries

The coronary arteries arise from the aortic sinuses. Normally, there are three main coronary arteries, the right coronary artery (RCA), left circumflex artery (LCX) and left anterior descending (LAD), with the LCX and LAD arteries arising from a common stem, the left main coronary artery (LMCA) (see Chapter 4).

Coronary artery anomalies (CAAs) are congenital disorders with various clinical manifestations. Although rare, they are the second most common cause of SCD among young athletes. It is uncertain whether incidental findings of CAAs in middle age or elderly individuals are associated with risk (Villa et al. 2016).

The clinical symptoms of a patient with a coronary anomaly will vary according to which group the anomaly belongs. In some cases, they can cause severe myocardial ischaemia, arrhythmias and SCD (Villa et al. 2016).

Inherited Primary Arrhythmia Syndromes

Brugada Syndrome

The Brugada syndrome (BS) was first described in 1953, but the genetic basis of BS was identified in a cohort of patients with the characteristically abnormal ECG and high risk for SCD with a structurally normal heart (Brugada and Brugada 1992). The syndrome is rare, having a prevalence of less than 5 in 10 000. Although men and women and are equally likely to inherit the genetic mutation, 90% of those affected with a diagnostic ECG are men.

> **Key Point**
>
> Brugada syndrome is most prevalent in young men of Southeast Asian origin and is the main cause of death among young healthy men in Southeast Asia (Nademanee et al. 1997).

Syncope or SCA associated with BS occurs predominantly in men in their 30s or 40s, often with fever as a predisposing factor. The ECG in BS typically shows incomplete right bundle branch block (RBBB) with ST-segment elevation in leads V1–V3, although there have been reports of ST-segment elevation in inferior leads. The ECG pattern can be present intermittently, possibly reflecting sporadic periods of vulnerability to SCD. ST-segment elevation can occur spontaneously or be revealed by the administration of drugs such as flecainide, procainamide or ajmaline; those with spontaneously occurring ST-segment elevation are regarded as having a worse prognosis. Patients with BS who have experienced syncope and have spontaneous ECG changes have a sixfold higher risk of SCA. Identification of those at risk is highly dependent on symptoms, including syncope, spontaneous ST-segment elevation or sustained VAs and family history of SCD. However, it is important to note that those without a family history are not at reduced risk, nor are family members of a victim of SCD necessarily at increased risk. Despite the identification of 18 associated genes, an identifiable genetic cause is not found in 65–70% of clinically diagnosed cases of BS (Sarquella-Brugada et al. 2016).

> **Suggested Resource**
>
>
>
> ECG of the week: Brugada syndrome
> RCSI Cardiovascular Society (2020)
> https://youtu.be/7A-JLgDYmA8

Long QT Syndrome

Long QT syndrome is an inherited disease characterised by prolonged ventricular repolarisation and ventricular tachyarrhythmias that are mainly triggered by adrenergic activation (Priori et al. 2015). Mutations in 13 genes have been found to be associated with LQTS. The three subtypes of LQTS are shown in Table 19.3.

Of the two identified patterns of inheritance for LQTS, the autosomal-dominant syndromes (Romano–Ward and Timothy syndromes) are more common than the often more severe autosomal-recessive syndrome (Jervell Lange-Nielsen syndrome). The genetic variants of the disease are used alongside factors such as gender and QT interval to inform risk stratification.

Table 19.3 LQTS subtypes.

LQTS type/gene mutation	ECG characteristics	Associated features
Romano-Ward syndrome LQT1–6 and LQT9–13	• Prolonged QT interval	
Anderson-Tawil syndrome LQT7	• Prolonged QT interval • Prominent U wave • Polymorphic or bidirectional VT	• Facial dysmorphisms • Hyper–/hypokalaemic periodic paralysis
Timothy syndrome LQT8	• Prolonged QT interval	• Webbed fingers or toes • Cardiac malformations • Autism spectrum disorder • Dysmorphisms
Jervell and Lange-Neilson syndrome KCNE1 and KCNQ1	• Extremely prolonged QT interval	• Congenital deafness

Presentations of LQTS range from near-syncope to syncope and SCD, with the average age of first manifestation being 14 years (Priori et al. 2015). Arrhythmias may be provoked by stress, physical exertion and emotion, but it can also occur during sleep. LQTS survivors of SCA have a poor outlook with relative risk of further SCA. Syncope is mostly (but not exclusively) due to malignant ventricular tachyarrhythmias. Torsade de pointes has been identified when ECG monitoring has been available at the time of an attack. Individuals with LQTS are advised to avoid competitive sports and, for those with the LQT1 form, swimming should only be undertaken with close supervision, if not avoided altogether. Those with LQT2 should be advised to avoid sudden noises such as telephones and alarm clocks. Medications known to prolong QT interval or potassium/magnesium depletion should also be avoided. Beta blockers may be useful on empiric grounds as prophylaxis against life-threatening arrhythmias (Priori et al. 2015).

An acquired form of LQTS is well recognised. Drug-induced torsade de pointes is a rare, but potentially lethal, side effect of some commonly prescribed drugs, including many non-cardiac agents such as antihistamines, antipsychotics and some antibiotics (Fitzgerald and Ackerman 2005). There is also evidence that genetic differences in drug metabolism may be a risk factor for acquired LQTS, especially if multiple drugs are involved (Aerssens and Paulussen 2005). Causes for acquired LQTS are shown in Table 19.4.

Table 19.4 Causes of acquired LQTS.

Medications

Common classes of drugs:

Antiarrhythmic drugs, some antimicrobials psychotropic medications and gastric motility agents.

A more comprehensive list of medications that are known to cause QT prolongation can be found at www.crediblemeds.org. Free registration is required.

Electrolyte imbalance

Hypokalaemia, hypomagnesaemia and hypocalcaemia

Structural heart disease

Myocardial ischaemia/infarction, heart failure, diastolic dysfunction, LVH

Bradyarrhythmias

The likelihood of developing QT prolongation and TdP is increased by bradycardia, but it is less clear whether bradycardia alone causes TdP (Berul 2020).

Suggested Resource

Advanced EKGs - The QT interval and long QT syndrome
Strong Medicine (2016)
https://youtu.be/UTek1i23yuQ

Suggested Resource

Advanced EKGs: Sudden Cardiac Death (Hypertrophic cardiomyopathy, ARVD, Brugada syndrome, and CPVT)
Strong Medicine (2016)
https://youtu.be/Lm1HAmCnr9A

Sudden Cardiac Death Related to Special Populations

Young People

SCD is rare in infants, children, adolescents and young adults, but it still amounts to many thousands of deaths each year in those under 20 years of age. While CHD is the common cause of SCD in older populations, genetic (inherited) cardiac disorders comprise a substantial proportion of SCD cases aged 40 years and less (Semsarian et al. 2015). Figure 19.1 shows causes of sudden cardiac death in the young.

SADS, sudden arrhythmic death syndrome; LQTS, long-QT syndrome; CPVT1, catecholaminergic polymorphic ventricular tachycardia type 1; HCM, hypertrophic cardiomyopathy; ARVC, arrhythmogenic right ventricular cardiomyopathy. Others includes SIDS cases. Approximate proportion of cases shown as (%) within each category.

Key Point

No cause of death is identified in approximately 30% of young SCD victims and this causes additional distress in an already tragic situation. Postmortem genetic testing of the deceased's blood sample involving deoxyribonucleic acid (DNA) extraction, followed by DNA analysis of selected genes responsible for the main primary arrhythmogenic diseases, may identify an underlying cause of SCD and may have implications for surviving at-risk family members (Semsarian et al. 2015).

Athletes

SCD in athletes, though rare, is often highly publicised. The precise incidence is unknown but is estimated between one in 40 000 and one in 80 000 per year (Harmon et al. 2014). Older studies have suggested that SCD in athletes have predominantly been due to inherited cardiomyopathies (HCM and ARVC in particular), but a more recent study from Canada found that SCA due to structural heart disease occurred infrequently during competitive sports (Landry et al. 2017). Other potential mechanisms of SCD in athletes are anomalous coronary arteries and acquired causes such as commotion cordis, myocarditis, substance misuse and trauma (Maron et al. 2009).

Pregnancy

The risk of SCA and SCD is significantly higher during the 9 months after delivery, particularly among women with LQT2. Beta blockers during pregnancy are associated with decreased risk of SCD (Al-Khatib et al. 2018).

Impact of Sudden Cardiac Death on Families and Loved Ones

Sudden unexpected death (SUD) is defined as a 'death, non-violent and not otherwise explained, occurring less than 24 hours from

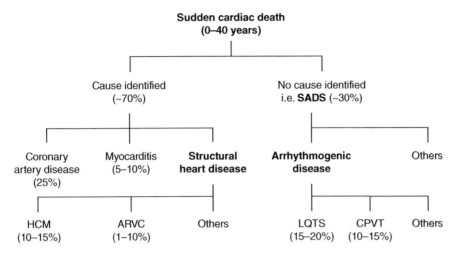

Figure 19.1 Causes of sudden cardiac death in the young (0–40 years). Based on postmortem findings. *Source:* Reprinted with permission. Semsarian et al. (2015). Copyright © 2020 Oxford University Press.

the onset of symptoms' (World Health Organization [WHO] 2016). Common causes of SUD are cardiac conditions (acute myocardial infarction or arrhythmia), neurological emergencies (such as stroke or epilepsy), pulmonary embolus or aortic dissection, but there are many other causes. SUD has a devastating impact on the families of the person who has died. They may exhibit a range of emotional responses including shock, disbelief, helplessness, confusion, anger, guilt, regret, depression, rage, apathy and loneliness (Rosenfeld and Gilbert 2013). In cases where the cause of death is not clear, identifying a definitive cause of death may help in understanding and acceptance of their loss. An autopsy presents the only opportunity to establish and register an accurate cause of SUD, but the proportion of autopsies that take place following SUD varies among countries (Fellmann et al. 2019). Expert cardiac autopsy improves diagnostic accuracy and retention of appropriate material for post-mortem genetic testing (molecular autopsy) may provide a genetic diagnosis in up to a third of cases of SADS (Isbister and Semsarian 2019). An algorithm for the assessment of SCD has been proposed by Isbister and Semsarian (2019) in Figure 19.2.

Family Screening

Family screening of first-degree relatives of victims of SUD is important to identify individuals at risk, advise on available treatment and adequately prevent SUD. Various protocols have been proposed for screening family members of sudden death victims, most of which follow a stepwise approach, starting with lower-cost and higher-yield investigations and moving on to further examinations based on both the initial findings and the family history (Priori et al. 2015).

SCD broadly falls into three categories: coronary artery disease, cardiomyopathies and no causative pathology (Fellmann et al. 2019). Sudden unexplained death in the context of a normal heart at post-mortem and negative toxicological analysis is deemed to be sudden arrhythmic death syndrome (SADS), and is often due to cardiac genetic disease, particularly channelopathies (Mellor and Behr 2014; Fellmann et al. 2019). The risk that many of these deaths confer upon surviving relatives compounds the grief that they are experiencing due to death of a loved one (Isbister and Semsarian 2019). Assessment of family members of SADS victims will usually reveal at least one affected individual in up to half of families. Screening surviving relatives and instituting

Algorithm for assessment of SCD

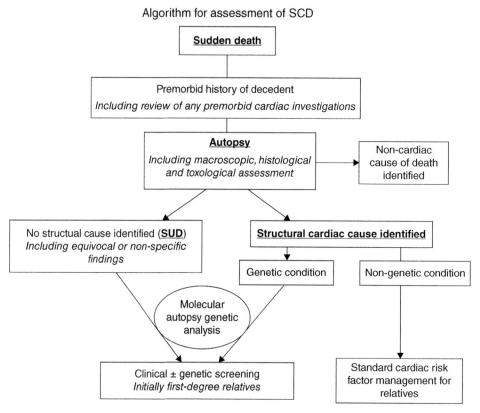

Figure 19.2 Clinical pathway for assessment of sudden cardiac death. *Source:* Reprinted with permission. Isbister and Semsarian (2019). Copyright © 1999–2020 John Wiley & Sons, Inc. All rights reserved.

therapy to reduce SCD risk is needed (Isbister and Semsarian 2019). Clinical assessment of families of SADS victims initially comprises a 12-lead ECG with high right ventricular leads, echocardiogram and exercise testing. Additional investigations may be required and include sodium channel blocker and epinephrine provocation tests. Family members with a diagnosis should be managed as per guidelines, while with negative investigations can generally be discharged unless they are young and/or symptomatic (Isbister and Semsarian 2019).

Suggested Resource

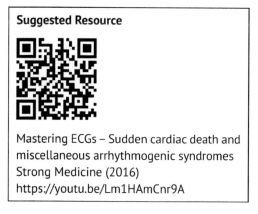

Mastering ECGs – Sudden cardiac death and miscellaneous arrhythmogenic syndromes
Strong Medicine (2016)
https://youtu.be/Lm1HAmCnr9A

Learning Activity 19.1

Identify local, national and international support mechanisms for relatives of patients who have suffered SCD. Review identified resources and websites and discuss the relative merits of these (with colleagues or fellow students) and how best to make use of such resources in your practice. Some examples are:

Cardiac Arrest in the Young https://www.c-r-y.org.uk/

Arrhythmia Alliance: https://www.heart rhythmalliance.org/aa/uk

Sudden Arrhythmia Deaths Syndrome (SADS) Foundation: https://www.sads.org

---

Suggested Resource: Reading

Tan, H. L., Dagres, N., Böttiger, B. W. et al. (2018). European Sudden Cardiac Arrest network: toward Prevention, Education and New Effective Treatments (ESCAPE-NET) A major European Horizon 2020 project focused on cardiac arrest. *European Heart Journal* 39 (2): 86–88. https://doi.org/10.1093/eurheartj/ehx758

Conclusion

SCD is a major public health problem and associated with tragedy affecting hundreds of thousands of individuals and families. While most SCDs are associated with CHD, there are many rarer, but important, associated conditions placing individuals at risk. The evidence base for risk stratification (often based on genetics) and treatment (increasingly involving implantable devices) has grown in recent years, but more work is needed to improve access to early diagnosis and treatment, and to appropriate support for individuals and their families.

References

Aerssens, J. and Paulussen, A.D. (2005). Pharmacogenomics and acquired long QT syndrome. *Pharmacogenomics* **6**: 259–270.

Al-Khatib, S.M., Stevenson, W.G., Ackerman, M.J. et al. (2018). 2017 AHA/ACC/HRS guideline for management of patients with ventricular arrhythmias and the prevention of sudden cardiac death: a report of the American College of Cardiology/American Heart Association Task Force on Clinical Practice Guidelines and the Heart Rhythm Society. *Journal of the American College of Cardiology* **72** (14): e91–e220.

Basso, C., Aguilera, B., Banner, J. et al. (2017). Association for European Cardiovascular Pathology. Guidelines for autopsy investigation of sudden cardiac death: 2017 update from the Association for European Cardiovascular Pathology. *Virchows Archiv* **471** (6): 691–705.

Bayés de Luna, A., Coumel, P., and Leclercq, J.F. (1989). Ambulatory sudden cardiac death: mechanisms of production of fatal arrhythmia on the basis of data from 157 cases. *American Heart Journal* **117** (1): 151–159.

Beck, B., Bray, J., Cameron, P. et al. (2018). Aus-ROC Steering Committee Regional variation in the characteristics, incidence and outcomes of out-of hospital cardiac arrest in Australia and New Zealand: results from the Aus-ROC Epistry. *Resuscitation* **126**: 49–57.

Berul, C. (2020). Acquired long QT syndrome: definitions, causes, and pathophysiology. In: (ed. S. Asirvatham, P.J. Zimetbaum, and B.C. Downey). *UpToDate*. www.uptodate.com.

Brugada, P. and Brugada, J. (1992). Right bundle branch block, persistent ST segment elevation and sudden cardiac death: a distinct clinical and electrocardiographic syndrome.

A multicenter report. *Journal of the American College of Cardiology* **20**: 1391–1396.

Dekker, L.R., Bezzina, C.R., Henriques, J.P. et al. (2006). Familial sudden death is an important risk factor for primary ventricular fibrillation. *Circulation* **114** (11): 1140–1145.

El-Battrawy, I., Lang, S., Ansari, U. et al. (2018). Prevalence of malignant arrhythmia and sudden cardiac death in takotsubo syndrome and its management. *EP Europace* **20** (5): 843–850.

Farb, A., Tang, A.L., Burke, A.P. et al. (1995). Sudden coronary death. Frequency of active coronary lesions, inactive coronary lesions, and myocardial infarction. *Circulation* **92**: 1701–1709.

Fellmann, F., Van El, C.G., Charron, P. et al. (2019). European recommendations integrating genetic testing into multidisciplinary management of sudden cardiac death. *European Journal of Human Genetics* **27** (12): 1763–1773.

Fitzgerald, P.T. and Ackerman, M.J. (2005). Drug-induced torsades de pointes: the evolving role of pharmacogenetics. *Heart Rhythm* **2** (Suppl): S30–S37.

Friedlander, Y., Siscovick, D.S., Weinmann, S. et al. (1998). Family history as a risk factor for primary cardiac arrest. *Circulation* **97** (2): 155–160.

Harmon, K.G., Drezner, J.A., Wilson, M.G., and Sharma, S. (2014). Incidence of sudden cardiac death in athletes: a state-of-the-art review. *Heart* **100** (16): 1227–1234.

Isbister, J. and Semsarian, C. (2019). Sudden cardiac death: an update. *Internal Medicine Journal* **49** (7): 826–833.

Jabbari, R., Engstrøm, T., Glinge, C. et al. (2015). Incidence and risk factors of ventricular fibrillation before primary angioplasty in patients with first ST-elevation myocardial infarction: a nationwide study in Denmark. *Journal of the American Heart Association* **4** (1): e001399.

Jacobsen, E.M., Hansen, B.L., Kjerrumgaard, A. et al. (2020). Diagnostic yield and long-term outcome of nonischemic sudden cardiac arrest survivors and their relatives: results from a tertiary referral center. *Heart Rhythm* **17** (10): 1679–1686.

Jouven, X., Desnos, M., Guerot, C., and Ducimetière, P. (1999). Predicting Sudden Death in the Population: The Paris Prospective Study I. *Circulation* **99** (15): 1978–1983.

Junttila, M.J., Hookana, E., Kaikkonen, K.S., Kortelainen, M.L., Myerburg, R.J., & Huikuri, H.V. (2016). Temporal trends in the clinical and pathological characteristics of victims of sudden cardiac death in the absence of previously identified heart disease. *Circulation: Arrhythmia and Electrophysiology*, **9** (6), e003723. https://doi.org/10.1161/CIRCEP.115.003723.

Lahtinen, M., Kiviniemi, A.M., Junttila, M.J. et al. (2017). Depressive symptoms and risk for sudden cardiac death in stable coronary artery disease. *European Heart Journal* **38** (suppl. 1): 317.

Landry, C.H., Allan, K.S., Connelly, K.A. et al. (2017). Sudden cardiac arrest during participation in competitive sports. *New England Journal of Medicine* **377** (20): 1943–1953.

Maron, B.J., Doerer, J.J., Haas, T.S. et al. (2009). Sudden deaths in young competitive athletes: analysis of 1866 deaths in the United States, 1980–2006. *Circulation* **119** (8): 1085–1092.

Mellor, G. and Behr, E.R. (2014). Sudden unexplained death–treating the family. *Arrhythmia and Electrophysiology Review* **3** (3): 156.

Nademanee, K., Veerakul, G., Nimmannit, S. et al. (1997). Arrhythmogenic marker for the sudden unexplained death syndrome in Thai men. *Circulation* **96** (8): 2595–2600.

Priori, S.G., Blomström-Lundqvist, C., Mazzanti, A. et al. (2015). 2015 ESC Guidelines for the management of patients with ventricular arrhythmias and the prevention of sudden cardiac death: The Task Force for the Management of Patients with Ventricular Arrhythmias and the Prevention of Sudden

Cardiac Death of the European Society of Cardiology (ESC) Endorsed by: Association for European Pediatric and Congenital Cardiology (AEPC). *EP Europace* **17** (11): 1601–1687.

Rosenfeld, A.G. and Gilbert, K. (2013). Lives forever changed: family bereavement experiences after sudden cardiac death. *Applied Nursing Research* **26** (4): 168–173.

Sarquella-Brugada, G., Campuzano, O., Arbelo, E. et al. (2016). Brugada syndrome: clinical and genetic findings. *Genetics in Medicine* **18** (1): 3–12.

Semsarian, C., Ingles, J., and Wilde, A.A. (2015). Sudden cardiac death in the young: the molecular autopsy and a practical approach to surviving relatives. *European Heart Journal* **36** (21): 1290–1296.

Strike, P.C. and Steptoe, A. (2005). Behavioral and emotional triggers of acute coronary syndromes: a systematic review and critique. *Psychosomatic Medicine* **67** (2): 179–186.

Tan, H.L., Dagres, N., Böttiger, B.W. et al. (2018). European Sudden Cardiac Arrest network: towards Prevention, Education and New Effective Treatments (ESCAPE-NET) A major European Horizon 2020 project focused on cardiac arrest. *European Heart Journal* **39** (2): 86–88.

Villa, A.D., Sammut, E., Nair, A., Rajani, R., Bonamini, R., & Chiribiri, A. (2016). Coronary artery anomalies overview: the normal and the abnormal. *World Journal of Radiology*, **8** (6), 537. doi: https://doi.org/10.4329/wjr.v8.i6.537.

Wong, C.X., Brown, A., Lau, D.H. et al. (2019). Epidemiology of sudden cardiac death: global and regional perspectives. *Heart, Lung and Circulation* **28** (1): 6–14.

World Health Organization (2016). International statistical classification of diseases and related health problems (10th Revision), 6th edition. https://icd.who.int/browse10/2016/en#/R96.1.

20

Pre-hospital Management of Cardiac Emergencies

Pete Gregory and Angela M. Kucia

Overview

Out-of-hospital cardiac arrest (OHCA) is a major public health problem that incurs significant mortality. Successful resuscitation of victims of OHCA depends upon many factors, and much has been done to establish the predictors of survival to maximise the number of successful outcomes. There is a general agreement that the likelihood of a successful resuscitation is improved where the presenting cardiac arrest rhythm is ventricular fibrillation (VF), the cardiac arrest is witnessed and bystander cardiopulmonary resuscitation (CPR) is implemented, and where there is early access to defibrillation. Additionally, there is a positive relationship between the return of spontaneous circulation in the out-of-hospital environment and survival to hospital discharge.

Strategies to improve survival from OHCA include education to raise community awareness and response to OHCA. The 'chain of survival' approach has been adopted by many communities; this seeks to promote early recognition and notification of emergency services, early initiation of CPR, early defibrillation, and early advanced care. The proliferation of automated external defibrillators (AED) in public areas is improving survival from OHCA.

This chapter will cover the major recommendations of international guidelines as they relate to basic life support (BLS, including AED use) in OHCA. The reader is encouraged to access full guidelines for more detailed information, as national guidelines may have subtle differences.

Learning Objectives

After reading this chapter, you should be able to:

- Explain the aetiology and burden of OHCA.
- Identify hazards to the victim and the rescuer and discuss circumstances that make management of OHCA different to in-hospital resuscitation.
- Recognise cardiac arrest and examine the procedures for performing BLS.
- Establish the value of early defibrillation in the management of VF and pulseless ventricular tachycardia (VT).
- Discuss the principles and factors affecting defibrillation.

Cardiac Care: A Practical Guide for Nurses, Second Edition. Edited by Angela M. Kucia and Ian D. Jones.
© 2022 John Wiley & Sons Ltd. Published 2022 by John Wiley & Sons Ltd.

Key Concepts

Pre-hospital care; basic life support; cardiopulmonary resuscitation; airway management; automated external defibrillation

Introduction

Cardiac arrest (CA) refers to the cessation of cardiac mechanical activity, as confirmed by the absence of signs of circulation (Benjamin et al. 2019). OHCA can be categorised into events with external causes (drowning, trauma, asphyxia, electrocution and drug overdose) or medical causes (Perkins et al. 2015c). OHCA is a major public health problem across the more economically developed areas of the world. Estimates of the numbers of OHCA per year are 65 000, 275 000, 356 000 and 61 000 in the United Kingdom, Europe, the United States and Australia respectively (Gräsner et al. 2020). Resuscitation is commenced in fewer than half of these cases (approximately 28 000) (Perkins et al. 2015b). It is a similar figure in Australia where resuscitation is attempted in around 43% of the 25 000 OHCA cases each year (Nehme et al. 2014). The main reasons that Emergency Medical Services (EMS) personnel do not initiate CPR in all cases are that the person has been dead for a prolonged period or has not received bystander CPR so has effectively died by the time the EMS arrive.

Survival rates from OOH CA vary significantly between countries and even between regions within countries. It is not always easy to make direct comparisons, but the extent of the variation can be seen in some recent studies. In England, successful resuscitation to discharge from hospital was recorded as 7–8% between 2011 and 2014 (NHS England 2015), and in the United States around 10.6% (Kolte et al. 2015).

Analysis of these variations may be helpful in generating strategies to improve outcomes for victims of CA.

The chances of survival vary according to the availability and quality of interventions carried out immediately following the CA.

Key Point

Any type of CPR is associated with doubled survival rates in comparison with cases not receiving CPR before emergency medical services arrival, but there is significantly higher chance of survival after CPR with compression and ventilation in comparison with compression-only CPR (Riva et al. 2019).

OHCA may present as either a shockable rhythm (VF or pulseless VT) or a non-shockable rhythm (asystole or pulseless electrical activity [PEA]) (Soar et al. 2021). Unless a reversible cause can be found and treated effectively, the prognosis for both asystole and PEA is poor despite advanced life support (ALS); however, with both VF and pulseless VT there is an opportunity to terminate the arrhythmia with defibrillation and increase the chances of survival. It has been known for over two decades that the time to the first defibrillation shock is a key predictor of outcome, with chances of survival to discharge falling by 10–15% for every minute of delay to defibrillation (Weaver et al. 1988; Valenzuela et al. 1997). Unsurprisingly, delays in the initiation of both BLS and ALS have been shown to affect the outcome from OHCA negatively. A study from Sweden showed that a 30-day survival rate of 10.5% was achieved when CPR was performed before arrival of EMS, versus a rate of just 4.0% when CPR was not performed prior to EMS arrival (Hasselqvist-Ax et al. 2015). They also showed a clear correlation between the number of people trained in performing CPR and the number of cases where CPR was performed before the arrival of EMS.

Key Point

Studies have shown that telephone-assisted CPR (usually EMS despatcher assisted) is independently associated with improved survival and improved functional outcomes following CA (Ro et al. 2017).

Hazards to the Victim and Rescuer

Out-of-hospital CA differs significantly from in-hospital CA in terms of risks to the rescuer and the resources available. These differences need to be considered when managing a CA, as failure to do so can lead to suboptimal patient management and unnecessary risk-taking by the practitioner. The practitioner should ensure their own safety, the safety of the patient and the safety of bystanders.

Scene Safety

Ensuring that the scene is as free from hazards and dangers as possible is always the first step in the management of OHCA and should be a conscious element of the approach to any casualty. A rescuer who becomes injured is less able to help the patient and is likely to increase the work of the Emergency Medical Services (EMS). It may not be possible to eliminate all dangers, so the risks should be assessed and reduced to a level that is acceptable to the individual rescuer. Risk assessment is a very personal assessment, and the degree of acceptable risk will vary according to factors such as health care experience (particularly out-of-hospital experience), gender and age. If the risks cannot be eliminated or brought within the rescuer's own personal scope of safety, then the patient should not be approached, and further assistance should be sought. Risk is a fluid situation and circumstances may change; it is essential that the rescuer ensures that there is safe egress from the scene if the risk level increases.

Risks to the Rescuer

EMS workers are at risk of occupational injuries from overexertion, transportation-related incidents, assaults, falls, harmful exposures and contact with objects and equipment (Reichard et al. 2017). Risks may be inherent in the environment, related to the patient or bystanders on scene, or to the treatments that need to be administered. Examples of these risks are shown in Box 20.1.

Resuscitation During the COVID-19 Pandemic

Recently published data in regions with high prevalence of COVID-19 show significant increases in OHCA incidence and changes to Utstein factors associated with survival. More CAs are occurring at home, fewer CAs are witnessed, emergency medical services (EMS) response times are longer and there is a decrease in bystander CPR rates (Bray et al. 2020). The willingness of the community to commence chest compressions and defibrillation is critical for even a narrow chance of survival (Couper et al. 2020), but there is a reluctance to commence CPR in the community for fear of contracting COVID.

Suggested Resource

Resuscitation Council UK Statement on COVID-19 in relation to CPR and resuscitation in first aid and community settings (2020) https://www.resus.org.uk/covid-19-resources

---

Key Point

In developing practice recommendations, guideline writers must balance an unknown potential infection risk to rescuers against the known risk to the patient from treatment delays.

Box 20.1 Hazards to rescue workers.

Physical injury
Rare occurrences of muscle strain, back symptoms, shortness of breath, hyperventilation, pneumothorax, chest pain, myocardial infarction and nerve injury have been reported in training and performing CPR (Peberdy et al. 2006; Cheung et al. 2009)

Infection
The hazard of greatest concern to the rescuer is the perceived risk of infection from performing CPR. It is likely that the Severe Acute Respiratory Syndrome Coronavirus two (SARS-CoV-2), referred to as COVID-19, will have an impact on the way CPR is delivered in the community. There is a risk of contagion during aerosol-generating procedures. At the time of writing, there has been some discordance between the World Health Organization (WHO) and other guidelines as to whether chest compressions or defibrillation causes aerosol generation or potential transmission of the (COVID-19) to rescuers. The WHO has categorised CPR as an aerosol-generating procedure (AGP), requiring the wearing of respirator masks and other personal protective equipment (PPE) (WHO 2020a, 2020b). Delaying the delivery of chest compressions and defibrillation for up to several minutes for a patient infected

with COVID-19 while healthcare workers on PPE will reduce the likelihood of patient survival; however, chest compressions may generate aerosols and simultaneous exposure to airway manoeuvres during resuscitation attempts that may place rescuers at risk. The safety of the rescuer is tantamount (Couper et al. 2020).

Environmental hazards
Potential hazards include traffic, gas leaks, electricity, poisons, trip hazards, confined spaces, pets and weather.

Patient/bystander hazards
Occasionally there may be the risk of violence from persons at the scene. This may be related to the stress of the situation, drug or alcohol intoxication, mental illness or another less obvious cause.

Hazards associated with treatment
Defibrillation is a potentially hazardous intervention that may result in injury to any person on scene; it is essential that all appropriate safety procedures are applied when carrying out defibrillation. In addition, it may be necessary to move the patient in order to place them on a firm, flat surface, which produces a risk of injury to both the rescuer and the patient.

Learning Activity 20.1

Review the information in the webpage below and watch the video on OHCA guidance during the COVID-19 pandemic. https://www.resus.org.uk/covid-19-resources/covid-19-resources-general-public/resuscitation-council-uk-statement-covid-19

Risks to the Victim

CPR is associated with a broad spectrum of iatrogenic injuries to the victim that range from skin abrasions and bruising, to rib and sternal fractures, and serious intrathoracic injuries (ITI). Skeletal chest fractures are the most common injury with rib fractures being reported in 60–85% of patients and sternal fractures in 15–58% (Rudinská et al. 2016). CPR-associated skeletal chest fractures may contribute to death by causing pneumothorax, haemothorax or cardiac lacerations (Rudinská et al. 2016) but more often are limited to post-resuscitation pain and discomfort in survivors. Serious ITI include lung contusion or laceration, cardiac contusion or rupture, pneumothorax and aortic rupture (Rudinská et al. 2016; Milling et al. 2019). Intra-abdominal injuries include liver or spleen contusion (Milling et al. 2019). Mechanical CPR as an adjunct to manual CPR is associated with both a higher number of injuries per patient and a significantly higher number of visceral injuries (Milling et al. 2019). The requirement for CPR and ensuring that compressions are deep enough to generate the pressure changes required to move blood around the body overrides the potential for injuries, but it may accentuate the need for CPR training.

Learning Activity 20.2

What considerations would you need to give to ensuring scene safety? Consider strategies for reducing the risk of injury to yourself as a rescuer, the patient and bystanders in an OHCA.
The resource below may be of assistance:

Suggested Resource

Resuscitation Council (UK) 2021. Guidance for safer handling during cardiopulmonary resuscitation in healthcare settings.
https://www.resus.org.uk/library/publications/publication-guidance-safer-handling

---

Circumstances that make OHCA Different from Hospital Resuscitation

Delay

In a hospital, recognition of CA and arrival of personnel skilled in resuscitation presents challenges, but these are less complex than for OHCA, where emergency personnel may have to travel several miles to the patient, inevitably delaying definitive treatment. The availability of AEDs is increasing in the more economically developed areas so the time delay to defibrillation can be reduced if trained people are available. The guidelines state that CPR should be continued up until the point where an AED has been connected to the patient, but the imperative to undertake a period of 3 minutes CPR prior to defibrillation has been removed due to a lack of robust evidence (Soar et al. 2015).

Resource Issues

In OHCA, a nurse may be the only person available with a health care or first-aid background and, in such circumstances, will be expected to take the lead in patient management. The problems associated with the management of OHCA are often compounded by a lack of the equipment normally available in hospital. It may be that little more than a pocket mask is available or, in many cases, no equipment at all prior to the arrival of emergency services. To manage the situation effectively, an action plan is required to overcome these problems.

Learning Activity 20.3

Create an action plan of how you will manage an OHCA using only the equipment you would normally have with you. Consider the following points:

- Who you would call and when you would call them – how would you manage if you were in an area with poor mobile phone reception?
- How would you manage the airway; what if the patient had vomited?
- What are the risks of infection associated with mouth-to-mouth ventilation? Do you have a pocket mask?

- How would you adapt your actions during the COVID-19 pandemic?
- How would you minimise the interruptions to chest compressions?

Suggested Resource

Teen's cardiac arrest and life-saving rescue caught on video
Jeff Hill (2016)
https://youtu.be/1z1_z2l0u6c

Recognition of Cardiac Arrest and BLS

The sequence used for recognition of CA will be dependent upon the rescuer's level of training and their experience of assessing respiration and circulation in sick patients. Checking the carotid pulse has been shown to be inaccurate as a method of assessing circulation in both lay persons and healthcare professionals (Bahr et al. 1997; Nyman and Sihvonen 2000), and it has also been demonstrated that both groups have difficulty in determining the presence or absence of adequate breathing. It should be noted that agonal breathing (described as occasional gasps, slow, laboured or noisy breathing) (Clark et al. 1992) occurs in up to 40% of CA cases and, if responded to as a sign of CA, is associated with higher survival rates (Bobrow et al. 2008).

Key Point

Current guidelines suggest that resuscitation should be commenced in an unconscious patient who is not breathing normally (Olasveengen et al. 2021).

Basic life support is a key skill in which every healthcare professional should be adept. The immediate commencement of CPR has been shown to double or even quadruple the probability of survival from CA (Wissenberg et al. 2013; Hasselqvist-Ax et al. 2015). CPR provides a small but essential flow of blood to the heart and the brain and increases the likelihood that the heart will resume an effective rhythm and contraction. Chest compressions are especially important if a shock cannot be delivered within the first few minutes after collapse. For every minute of delay to defibrillation, the probability of survival to discharge reduces by 10–12% but when CPR is provided, the decline is more gradual and averages only 3–4% per minute of delay to defibrillation (Deakin and Nolan 2005).

Learning Activity 20.4

The link to Australian Resuscitation Council is shown below. Ensure that you understand and can apply these guidelines in your practice.

The ARC Guidelines
Australian and New Zealand Committee on Resuscitation (2021)
https://resus.org.au/guidelines/

2021 Resuscitation Guidelines
Resuscitation Council UK (2021)
https://www.resus.org.uk/library/2021-resuscitation-guidelines

---

This section is not intended to teach BLS procedures; rather it is designed to provide a rationale for the actions to be taken. The reader is advised to access the published guidelines.

Pauses in Chest Compressions

Minimising pauses in chest compressions is associated with improved outcomes for patients in CA (Christenson et al. 2009; Sell et al. 2010; Vaillancourt et al. 2011; Cheskes et al. 2014). It is essential to minimise any gaps between chest compressions as a result of ventilation of the patient or pre- and post-shock.

Continuous compressions can be applied when advanced airway management techniques are available, but these are often not accessible in OHCA. Where advanced airway management is not available, efforts should be made to resume compressions as quickly as possible; this can be facilitated by:

- Giving rescue breaths over 1 second to reduce delay between compressions.
- Placing hands in the centre of the chest rather than measuring for correct position.
- Using a ratio of 30:2 compressions: ventilations.
- Commencing chest compressions immediately after CA is established (in the adult patient) (Pierce et al. 2015).

Key Point

It has been suggested that compression-only CPR may be effective in eliminating pauses and may be useful for those not wishing to use a mouth-to-mouth technique; however, it is believed that this may only be viable for a short period in non-asphyxial CA and should not be used routinely by healthcare professionals (Olasveengen et al. 2021), except where there are concerns about infection such as in COVID-19.

Automated External Defibrillation

The incidence of VF as the initial rhythm in OHCA has been falling and an increasing number of patients are now presenting in non-shockable rhythms (Keller and Halperin 2015); however, survival rates from shockable rhythms are significantly better than any other CA arrhythmia. Examples include (Nadkarni et al. 2006; Meaney et al. 2010; Chan et al. 2014).

The only effective therapy for CA caused by VF is the early application of defibrillation which, if applied within 3–5 minutes of collapse, can produce survival rates as high as 50–70% (Perkins et al. 2015a). The survival benefit to be gained by those treated with CPR plus AED compared with those treated with CPR alone is significant, and this has led to the development of numerous public access defibrillator schemes. Given that AEDs can be used safely and effectively by lay people with minimal training, it seems incumbent upon the healthcare professional to consider the use of an AED as being integral to BLS.

Defibrillation is commonly available in EMS systems across the economically developed world. As CPR and defibrillation need to be administered as early as possible to maximise chances of survival, it is incumbent upon bystanders and health professionals to initiate the opening links of the 'chain of survival'. AEDs use voice and visual prompts to guide the practitioner in the delivery of defibrillatory shocks to patients in CA as a result of VF or pulseless VT. They have become more sophisticated and safer over recent years and are suitable for use by lay people as well as healthcare professionals.

Practical Factors Affecting Defibrillation

Transthoracic Impedance

Transthoracic impedance is the resistance to the passage of electricity created by the chest; it is a key factor in determining the amount of energy that passes through the myocardium during defibrillation. The greater the impedance, the less energy is delivered to the myocardium, which reduces the chances of successful defibrillation. Transthoracic impedance is influenced by factors such as the contact between skin and pad, the size of the pad and the phase of ventilation.

Contact Between Pad and Skin

Chest hair will interfere with electrical contact, but hair should be shaved only if excessive, to reduce delay in shock delivery. Often a razor is kept with the AED, but if no razor is immediately available, defibrillation should not be delayed finding one.

Pad Position

Successful defibrillation is achieved by the passage of an electrical current between two external electrodes (pads), resulting. In a current of sufficient magnitude to defibrillate a critical mass of myocardium. Pad position has been the subject of much discussion, but no new high-quality evidence was established between the 2105 and 2021 resuscitation guidelines. As such, the recommendations remain the same. The sternal pad is normally placed to the right of the sternum just below the border of the clavicle; the apical pad should be placed in the mid-axillary line approximately level with the V6 ECG electrode position (Perkins et al. 2015a). It is important that the position used is clear of breast tissue; in large-breasted patients it is acceptable to place the apical pad lateral to or underneath the left breast (Olasvgeengen et al. 2021). An anterior–posterior configuration is the other commonly used placement and side-to-side placement. A further recommendation is that the apical pad be placed in a longitudinal rather than transverse position (Deakin et al. 2003). Most AED defibrillation pads carry a diagram indicating recommended placement. It is not important if the pads are placed in reverse positions.

All new defibrillators deliver shocks using a biphasic waveform, which means that the current flows initially in a positive direction and then, after a predetermined time reverses to a negative direction. Defibrillation energy is predetermined when using an AED, so should not cause any concerns for the rescuer.

Even when all of the above factors are optimal, the survival chances of the victim will be heavily influenced by the delay between defibrillation and recommencement of chest compressions. The use of AEDs will inevitably involve a period of delay whilst rhythms are being analysed, but human factors are also associated with postshock delay and should be eliminated from the process. As soon as defibrillation has been delivered, chest compressions should be restarted immediately, irrespective of changes observed in the cardiac rhythm.

Chest Compressions Following Defibrillation

Following defibrillation, chest compressions remain important. If the heart is in a viable condition following defibrillation, then there should be a resumption of pacemaker activity followed by organised contraction. However, the force of contraction is likely to be weak and the heart rhythm may be slow. Chest compressions must be continued until adequate cardiac function returns (Perkins et al. 2015a).

Conclusion

Out-of-hospital CA is a major public health problem that affects hundreds of thousands of people each year. Programmes that incorporate early BLS and the use of an AED show significant benefit in terms of survival to discharge from hospital. Health professionals should be competent in performing BLS, should have a strategy for managing OHCA and should be proficient in the use of an AED.

References

Bahr, J., Klingler, H., Panzer, W. et al. (1997). Skills of lay people in checking the carotid pulse. *Resuscitation* **35** (1): 23–26.

Benjamin, E.J., Muntner, P., Alsonso, A. et al. (2019). Heart disease and stroke statistics – 2019 update: a report from the American Heart Association. *Circulation* **139** (10): e56–e528. https://www.ahajournals.org/doi/full/10.1161/CIR.0000000000000659.

Bobrow, B.J., Zuercher, M., Ewy, G.A. et al. (2008). Gasping during cardiac arrest in humans is frequent and associated with improved survival. *Circulation* **118** (24): 2550–2554.

Bray, J., Cartledge, S., and Scapigliati, A. (2020). Bystander CPR in the COVID-19 pandemic. *Resuscitation Plus* **4**: 100041.

Chan, P.S., McNally, B., Tang, F. et al. (2014). Recent trends in survival from out-of-hospital cardiac arrest in the United States. *Circulation* **130** (21): 1876–1882.

Cheung, W., Gullick, J., Thanakrishnan, G. et al. (2009). Injuries occurring in hospital staff attending medical emergency team (MET) calls – a prospective, observational study. *Resuscitation* **80** (12): 1351–1356.

Cheskes, S., Schmicker, R.H., Verbeek, P.R. et al. (2014). The impact of peri-shock pause on survival from out-of-hospital shockable cardiac arrest during the Resuscitation Outcomes Consortium PRIMED trial. *Resuscitation* **85** (3): 336–342.

Christenson, J., Andrusiek, D., Everson-Stewart, S. et al. (2009). Chest compression fraction determines survival in patients with out-of-hospital ventricular fibrillation. *Circulation* **120** (13): 1241–1247.

Clark, J.J., Larsen, M.P., Culley, L.L. et al. (1992). Incidence of agonal respirations in sudden cardiac arrest. *Annals of Emergency Medicine* **21** (12): 1464–1467.

Couper, K., Taylor-Phillips, S., Grove, A. et al. (2020). COVID-19 in cardiac arrest and infection risk to rescuers: a systematic review. *Resuscitation* **151**: 59–66.

Deakin, C.D. and Nolan, J.P. (2005). European Resuscitation Council Guidelines for Resuscitation 2005: Section 3. Electrical therapies: automated external defibrillators, defibrillation, cardioversion and pacing. *Resuscitation* **67**: S25–S37.

Deakin, C.D., Sado, D.M., Petley, G.W., and Clewlow, F. (2003). Is the orientation of the apical defibrillation paddle of importance during manual external defibrillation? *Resuscitation* **56** (1): 15–18.

Gräsner, J.T., Wnent, J., Herlitz, J. et al. (2020). Survival after out-of-hospital cardiac arrest in Europe-Results of the EuReCa TWO study. *Resuscitation* **148**: 218–226.

Hasselqvist-Ax, I., Riva, G., Herlitz, J. et al. (2015). Early cardiopulmonary resuscitation in out-of-hospital cardiac arrest. *New England Journal of Medicine* **372** (24): 2307–2315.

Keller, S.P. and Halperin, H.R. (2015). Cardiac arrest: the changing incidence of ventricular fibirrllation. *Current Treatment Options in Cardiovascular Medicine* **17** (7): 392.

Kolte, D., Khera, S., Aronow, W.S. et al. (2015). Regional variation in the incidence and outcomes of in-hospital cardiac arrest in the United States. *Circulation* **131** (16): 1415–1425.

Meaney, P.A., Nadkarni, V.M., Kern, K.B. et al. (2010). Rhythms and outcomes of adult in-hospital cardiac arrest. *Critical Care Medicine* **38**: 101–108.

Milling, L., Astrup, B.S., and Mikkelsen, S. (2019). Prehospital cardiopulmonary resuscitation with manual or mechanical chest compression: a study of compression-induced injuries. *Acta Anaesthesiologica Scandinavica* **63** (6): 789–795.

Nadkarni, V.M., Larkin, G.L., Peberdy, M.A. et al. (2006). First documented rhythm and clinical outcome from in-hospital cardiac arrest among children and adults. *JAMA* **295**: 50–57.

Nehme, Z., Andrew, E., Cameron, P.A. et al. (2014). Population density predicts outcome from out-of-hospital cardiac arrest in Victoria,

Australia. *Medical Journal of Australia* **200** (8): 471–475.

NHS England (2015) Ambulance Quality Indicators. Secondary Ambulance Quality Indicators, 2015. http://www.england.nhs.uk/statistics/statistical-work-areas/ambulance-quality-indicators (accessed 4 November 2015).

Nyman, J. and Sihvonen, M. (2000). Cardiopulmonary resuscitation skills in nurses and nursing students. *Resuscitation* **47** (2): 179–184.

Olasveengen, T.M., Semeraro, F., Ristagno, G., Castren, M., Handley, A., Kuzovlev, A., ... & Perkins, G.D. (2021). European Resuscitation Council Guidelines 2021: Basic life support. *Resuscitation*, **161**, 98–114.

Peberdy, M.A., Van Ottingham, L., Groh, W.J. et al. (2006). Adverse events associated with lay emergency response programs: the public access defibrillation trial experience. *Resuscitation* **70** (1): 59–65.

Perkins, G.D., Handley, A.J., Koster, R.W. et al. (2015a). European Resuscitation Council Guidelines for Resuscitation 2015: Section 2. Adult basic life support and automated external defibrillation. *Resuscitation* **95**: 81–99.

Perkins, G.D., Lockey, A.S., de Belder, M.A., Moore, F., Weissberg, P., Gray, H. (2015b) National initiatives to improve outcomes from out of hospital cardiac arrest in England. *Emergency Medicine Journal* doi: https://doi.org/10.1136/emermed-2015-204847.

Perkins, G.D., Jacobs, I.G., Nadkarni, V.M. et al. (2015c). Cardiac arrest and cardiopulmonary resuscitation outcome reports: update of the Utstein resuscitation registry templates for out-of-hospital cardiac arrest: a statement for healthcare professionals from a task force of the International Liaison Committee on Resuscitation (American Heart Association, European Resuscitation Council, Australian and New Zealand Council on Resuscitation, Heart and Stroke Foundation of Canada, InterAmerican Heart Foundation, Resuscitation Council of Southern Africa . . .). *Circulation* **132** (13): 1286–1300.

Pierce, A.E., Roppolo, L.P., Owens, P.C. et al. (2015). The need to resume chest compressions immediately after defibrillation attempts: an analysis of post-shock rhythms and duration of pulselessness following out-of-hospital cardiac arrest. *Resuscitation* **89**: 162–168.

Reichard, A.A., Marsh, S.M., Tonozzi, T.R. et al. (2017). Occupational injuries and exposures among emergency medical services workers. *Prehospital Emergency Care* **21** (4): 420–431.

Riva, G., Ringh, M., Jonsson, M. et al. (2019). Survival in out-of-hospital cardiac arrest after standard cardiopulmonary resuscitation or chest compressions only before arrival of emergency medical services: nationwide study during three guideline periods. *Circulation* **139** (23): 2600–2609.

Ro, Y.S., Do Shin, S., Lee, Y.J. et al. (2017). Effect of dispatcher-assisted cardiopulmonary resuscitation program and location of out-of-hospital cardiac arrest on survival and neurologic outcome. *Annals of Emergency Medicine* **69** (1): 52–61.

Rudinská, L.I., Hejna, P., Ihnát, P. et al. (2016). Intra-thoracic injuries associated with cardiopulmonary resuscitation–Frequent and serious. *Resuscitation* **103**: 66–70.

Sell, R.E., Sarno, R., Lawrence, B. et al. (2010). Minimizing pre-and post-defibrillation pauses increases the likelihood of return of spontaneous circulation (ROSC). *Resuscitation* **81** (7): 822–825.

Soar, J., Böttiger, B.W., Carli, P., Couper, K., Deakin, C.D., Djärv, T., Lott, C., Olasveengen, T., Paal, P., Pellis, T., Perkins, G.D., Sandroni, C., & Nolan, J.P. (2021). European Resuscitation Council Guidelines 2021: Adult advanced life support. *Resuscitation*, **161**, 115–151. https://doi.org/10.1016/j.resuscitation.2021.02.010.

Soar, J., Nolan, J.P., Böttiger, B.W. et al. (2015). European resuscitation council guidelines for resuscitation 2015: section 3. Adult advanced life support. *Resuscitation* **95**: 100–147.

Vaillancourt, C., Everson-Stewart, S., Christenson, J. et al. (2011). The impact of increased chest compression fraction on return of spontaneous circulation for out-of-hospital cardiac arrest patients not in ventricular fibrillation. *Resuscitation* **82** (12): 1501–1507.

Valenzuela, T.D., Roe, D.J., Cretin, S. et al. (1997). Estimating effectiveness of cardiac arrest interventions: a logistic regression survival model. *Circulation* **96** (10): 3308–3313.

Weaver, W.D., Hill, D., Fahrenbruch, C.E. et al. (1988). Use of the automatic external defibrillator in the management of out-of-hospital cardiac arrest. *New England Journal of Medicine* **319** (11): 661–666.

Wissenberg, M., Lippert, F.K., Folke, F. et al. (2013). Association of national initiatives to improve cardiac arrest management with rates of bystander intervention and patient survival after out-of-hospital cardiac arrest. *JAMA* **310** (13): 1377–1384.

World Health Organization (2020a). *Modes of Transmission of Virus Causing COVID-19: Implications for IPC Precaution Recommendations: Scientific Brief, 27 March 2020* (No. WHO/2019-nCoV/Sci_Brief/Transmission_modes/2020.1). World Health Organization.

World Health Organization (2020b). *Infection Prevention and Control During Health Care when COVID-19 is Suspected: Interim Guidance, 19 March 2020* (No. WHO/2019-nCoV/IPC/2020.3). World Health Organization.

21

In-Hospital Resuscitation

Angela M. Kucia and Melanie Rushton

Overview

Despite advances in systems of care and therapeutic interventions, survival rates for in-hospital cardiac arrest (CA) remain relatively low, especially outside critical care environments. As most in-hospital cardiac arrests are predictable, early recognition and effective treatment may prevent CA and help identify those individuals for whom resuscitation is not appropriate or against their wishes. To aid in early detection of critical illness, many hospitals now utilise early warning scores, and in most areas a Medical Emergency Team (MET) enables patients to be treated as soon as a deterioration in their condition is detected, rather than waiting for CA to occur. Of patients resuscitated, over half die before leaving hospital, signifying the vital role that post-resuscitation care plays in the process. Nurses must be proficient in both assessment and resuscitation to maximise the patient's chances of a successful outcome.

Learning Objectives

After reading this chapter, you should be able to:

- Discuss factors contributing to outcomes of in-hospital cardiac arrest.
- Understand the importance of identifying patients at risk of cardiac arrest.

- Describe the in-hospital resuscitation process and understand how it might differ from a pre-hospital situation.
- Recognise the importance of post-resuscitation care.
- Discuss the need to adopt uniform reporting of outcome after cardiac arrest.

Key Concepts

In-hospital cardiac arrest; outreach service/medical emergency teams; advanced life support; resuscitation education; data collection and quality improvement

---

Introduction

CA refers to the cessation of cardiac mechanical activity, as confirmed by the absence of signs of circulation. From an operational perspective, sudden cardiac arrest (SCA) refers to unexpected CA that results in attempts to restore circulation. If resuscitation attempts are unsuccessful, sudden cardiac death (SCD) results (Benjamin et al. 2019). The global incidence of in-hospital cardiac arrest (IHCA) in adults has not been well described. The majority of data are derived from the American Heart Association's Get with the Guidelines-Resuscitation (GWTG-R) registry, the National Cardiac Arrest Audit from the Resuscitation Council (UK) and the Intensive Care National Audit and Research Centre (Andersen et al. 2019).

Table 21.1 Definitions for the aetiology of cardiac arrest.

An arrest is presumed to be of the following aetiology if its cause can be primary related to:

Cardiac
Heart diseases such as coronary heart disease, arrhythmic mechanism or other types of structural heart disease (e.g. congenital coronary artery anomalies, myocarditis, hypertrophic cardiomyopathy, arrhythmogenic right ventricular cardiomyopathy), hypertension.

Pulmonary
Chronic obstructive pulmonary disease (COPD) characterised by airflow limitation that is not fully reversible, a chronic inflammatory disorder of the airways, pulmonary embolism, central airway obstruction.

Aortic dissection/rupture
Tear in the aortic intima with or without blood passing into the aortic media.

Intoxication and adverse drug reactions
Accidental and intentional poisonings or iatrogenic or accidental drug overdose, adverse reactions to medications.

Exsanguination
Bleeding (gastrointestinal, iatrogenic or spontaneously vascular, excl. Spontaneous aortic rupture, etc.)

Metabolic
Electrolyte disorders (hypo-/hyperkalaemia), hypoglycaemia, hyperglycaemia, lactic acidosis, hepatic disorders, uraemia, etc.

Cerebral
Intracranial/subarachnoid haemorrhage, cerebral vascular occlusion/thrombosis, contusion, tumour, meningitis/encephalitis, seizures/status epilepticus, heat stroke, etc.

Sepsis
The clinical syndrome that results from a dysregulated inflammatory response to an infection with signs of hypoperfusion or organ dysfunction.

Accidental hypothermia
Defined as a core temperature below 35 °C (95 °F) caused by evaporation, radiation, conduction and/or convection leading to heat loss with altered cell membrane function, efflux of intracellular fluid, enzymatic dysfunction and electrolyte imbalances.

Other or unknown causes
Cause of arrest is known and documented such as reactions to foods and/or insect stings capable of producing a sudden, systemic degranulation of mast cells or basophils into an acute, potentially lethal, multisystem syndrome (anaphylaxis) and is not one of the available options above and such as trauma

Source: Reprinted with permission. Wallmuller et al. (2012). Copyright © 2020 Elsevier B.V. or its licensors or contributors.

Reported estimates of cardiac arrest range from 1.6 to 8.27 per thousand hospital admissions (Benjamin et al. 2019). According to the GWTG-R of unpublished data, the mean age of cases is 66 years, there are slightly more males than females and the presenting rhythm for adult IHCA in over 80% of cases is non-shockable (asystole or pulseless electrical activity) 2017; cited in Andersen et al. (2019). Approximately half of IHCA occur in critical care areas with the other half in general wards (Andersen et al. 2019).

IHCA results from many disease processes (see Table 21.1) with around 50-60% of cases being cardiac and 15–40% being of pulmonary origin (Andersen et al. 2019).

Despite the resources and opportunity to intervene early when a CA occurs in the hospital, survival to hospital discharge following

IHCA is estimated, to be less than 25% (Andersen et al. 2019; Benjamin et al. 2019).

Factors associated with survival can be divided into two groups: (i) those relating to the patient and (ii) those related to the event. Factors associated with a decreased chance of survival following IHCA include increased age (above 70 years), presence of pre-existing medical and surgical conditions such as malignancy, sepsis, poor functional status prior to the cardiac arrest, pneumonia, hypotension, renal dysfunction and hepatic dysfunction (Andersen et al. 2019). Causes of IHCA associated with poor outcomes include aortic dissection or rupture, sepsis, exsanguination (predominantly gastrointestinal bleeding) and cerebral pathologies (intracerebral or subarachnoid haemorrhage or status epilepticus) (Wallmuller et al. 2012). System factors associated with poorer outcomes include IHCA at night or weekends (Ofoma et al. 2018) and lower nurse-to-patient ratios (McHugh et al. 2016).

Patients with a shockable rhythm (ventricular tachycardia or fibrillation) have two to three times higher survival to hospital discharge compared with patients with a non-shockable rhythm and this may reflect the potential for more effective treatment (defibrillation) of these patients (Andersen et al., 2019). Only around 15–20% of IHCA patients have a recorded shockable rhythm at the onset of CA (Benjamin et al. 2019; Andersen et al. 2019). System factors associated with an improved chance of survival following IHCA include witnessed events, CA in monitored areas, short time between collapse and arrival of the resuscitation team, and short duration of cardiopulmonary resuscitation (CPR) (Andersen et al. 2019) and decreased patient-to-nurse ratios on medical and surgical units (McHugh et al. 2016).

> **Key Point**
>
> Reasonable nurse workloads and good hospital work environments are associated with higher odds of patient survival after an IHCA (McHugh et al. 2016). Registered Nurse (RN), but not Nurse Assistant (NA) staffing levels, influence the rates of failure to respond for patients with the most abnormal vital signs (Smith et al. 2020).

Prevention: Systems for Identifying Patients at Risk of Cardiac Arrest

Vulnerable Patients

Hospitals have experienced an increase in acuity over recent years, resulting from a larger volume of patients presenting with more complex disease states and healthcare needs. Patients are often elderly with multiple comorbidities and require a higher level of care to reduce the risk of adverse events. Acutely ill patients (and those identified as at-risk of physiological decline) should be admitted to hospital areas where high acuity care can be managed (Smith 2005).

> **Key Point**
>
> Patients at high risk of CA should be cared for in a well-staffed monitored area, with facilities for immediate resuscitation.

Use of Treatment Limitation Plans

For many patients who are admitted to hospital, CA may be a terminal event. Early assessment of high-risk patients should be undertaken to identify those in whom resuscitation measures may not be appropriate (such as those with terminal illness or trauma where death is imminent), as resuscitation attempts may not prolong life but cause unnecessary pain and trauma. The default position is to undertake resuscitation measures if there has been no directive from the patient not to do so. Discussions with at-risk patients about the benefits and risks of CPR are a form of informed consent and should be addressed well in advance of the potential need for the CPR. Issues related to quality of life and chance of survival, and specifically, likelihood of survival to discharge with intact cognitive function, need to be discussed to enable them to participate in shared decision-making (Rubins et al. 2019). This discussion should take place early in the admission to allow time for the patient and family members to process the information rather than having to make quick decisions in the case of acute deterioration and critical illness. In some cases, resuscitation efforts may ultimately be a medical decision based on multiple factors, including whether or not resuscitation efforts are likely to be futile, but the patients views and involvement in the discussion are important. The nurse has the role of providing information and support to the patient and their family and implementation of palliative care if required. See Chapter 22 for more information.

> **Key Point**
>
> Ensure that Advanced Directives (AD) and Do Not Resuscitate (DNR)/Do Not Attempt Resuscitation (DNAR) orders are in place where appropriate. A patient's wishes may change over time so AD and DNR/DNAR orders should be reviewed with the patient at each opportunity.

Recommended Strategies for the Prevention of Avoidable Cardiac Arrest

As survival rates following IHCA are poor, strategies for CA prevention assume great importance. Several strategies to facilitate the early detection of critically ill patients and reduce the risk of CA have been proposed.

Acute clinical deterioration can occur at any phase of a patient's hospitalisation. Early recognition of deterioration is essential and should be accompanied by an appropriate response. Early indicators of critical illness are often missed by healthcare professionals. Failure to recognise and appropriately manage deteriorating patients is a contributing factor to adverse patient outcomes.

Rapid Response Systems (RRS)

Rapid response systems (RRS) have been implemented internationally as the standard structure for recognising and managing deteriorating patients, though supporting evidence for RRS is weak because there are few rigorous randomised clinical trials and heterogeneity between hospital systems (Andersen et al. 2019). Rapid Response Teams (RRTs) (also known as Critical Care Outreach Teams) respond to hospitalised patients with acute clinical deterioration with the goal of preventing IHCA and mortality (Lyons et al. 2019). Common elements include early recognition and detection of patients with potential or established critical illness, timely attendance by appropriately skilled staff and admission to intensive care services where needed (Gao et al. 2007).

RRS may also be referred to as track and trigger systems with tracking denoting periodic observation of physiology and trigger being a predetermined response by criteria (Kramer et al. 2019). RRS have four components: the afferent limb (event detection and response trigger); the efferent limb (response resources including personnel and equipment); the quality improvement limb and the administrative limb. The afferent limb is one of the most important components as many failures of RRS are attributed to an inability to recognise patient deterioration and seek assistance. In the event of patient deterioration, a chain of events occurs, leading to a call for assistance from a response team (Figure 21.1).

Each step in the chain of event recognition and response triggering can be easily broken, leading to failure to respond to a patient in crisis and an adverse outcome (Rao and Devita 2017). In the sense that the afferent limb is responsible for identifying a crisis and triggering a response, it may be the most important component because without it there can be no response.

Components of RRS include early warning score (EWS) systems, medical emergency teams (MET), 'patient at-risk' teams (PART), intensive care liaison nurses and integrated outreach programs.

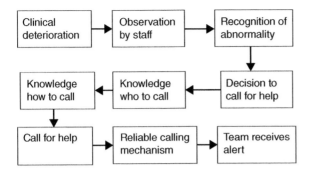

Figure 21.1 The afferent limb of rapid response systems. *Source:* Reproduced with permission. Rao and DeVita (2017). © 2019 Springer Nature Switzerland AG.

Early Warning Scoring (EWS) Systems RRTs

Clinical deterioration is common prior to in-hospital CA and many in-hospital cardiac arrests are considered preventable or avoidable on retrospective review (Andersen et al. 2019). The impetus behind the development of RRTs was to intervene and halt clinical deterioration before CA occurs. To this end, usable criteria (EWS) for general ward staff to use in the early recognition of impending deterioration was developed and ward staff empowered to call for help from a team of critical care physicians and/or nurses, to improve outcomes for deteriorating patients and avoid admission to the Intensive Care Unit (ICU), where possible (Winters and DeVita 2017).

Changes in vital signs (temperature, respiratory rate, heart rate, blood pressure and SaO_2) are the first and most easily detectable parameters of clinical decline. Such changes can be used singularly or in combination with other measures, such as mental status to help detect deterioration of the patient's condition (Kramer et al. 2019). These are mostly used in clinical areas other than critical care units to detect early changes in patient's vital signs prior to physiological decline (Kramer et al. 2019). EWS are usually part of track and trigger systems and are used extensively in clinical practice, though some question the methodology behind them (Gerry et al. 2017).

> **Key Point**
>
> In recent years, observation charts that incorporate specific features such as EWS have been introduced to assist in the identification of patients who are deteriorating (Green et al. 2018).

Modified Early Warning Score (MEWS), National Early Warning Score (NEWS) and NEWS2

The Modified Early Warning Score (MEWS) was introduced in the UK in 1996 (Morgan et al. 1997) and its clinical utility reported in numerous studies. MEWS is based on allocating a certain number of points to six clinical measurements based on how far each deviates from normality. The score includes systolic blood pressure, heart rate, respiratory rate, body temperature and urine output. MEWS also incorporates a measure of consciousness known as the AVPU score (Alert, responds to Voice, responds to Pain, Unresponsive). Each parameter is based on the degree of abnormality and the sum of these values yields a MEWS score upon which the need for further clinical action is based (Kramer et al. 2019). MEWS was superseded by the UK National Early Warning Score (NEWS) (Williams et al. 2012) and NEWS 2 (Royal College of Physicians 2017), each of which modified the inclusion or exclusion of the physiological parameters used to form the aggregate score upon which clinical action was based.

Various EWS systems have been proposed, but the efficacy of EWS depends upon organisational dynamics, resources, professional skills and heterogeneity of the patient cohort (Le Lagadec and Dwyer 2017). Human factors largely influence whether MER/RRS are activated appropriately. The main reasons for lack of appropriate action include staff thinking that they have the situation under control, fear of reproach, inadequate patient monitoring and poor communication (Shearer et al. 2012). EWS efficacy is also dependent on establishing the correct threshold scores for at-risk patients and an appropriate response to prevent patient deterioration (Le Lagadec and Dwyer 2017).

Key point

RRS rely on an objective set of calling criteria, though there is regional and interhospital variability in the types of criteria and the actual limits used: in some systems an EWS is calculated from a number of physiological variables whereas others may have single-parameter triggers (Rao and DeVita 2017).

Medical Emergency Teams

Studies of the impact of METs have reported mixed results (Rao and Devita 2017) though meta-analyses have concluded that there is a benefit in both mortality and CA rate in hospitalised patients outside the ICU (Chan et al. 2010).

The 'Chain of Survival' concept (Cummins et al. 1991) has influenced the development of in-hospital resuscitation strategies. Resuscitation should be regarded as a continual process with interventions that may vary depending on the underlying cause of CA. Traditionally, resuscitation teams comprise individuals within the hospital or health setting who are competent in

resuscitation. In the hospital setting, resuscitation involves both basic life support (BLS) and advanced life support (ALS), with some overlap between the two. BLS aims to maintain coronary and cerebral perfusion through support of the airway, breathing and circulation until more definitive treatment can be initiated (see Chapter 20). ALS combines BLS with the added use of drugs, specialist techniques and equipment to maintain circulation and respiration.

Critical Care Outreach and Intensive Care Liaison Nurses

Critically ill patients are increasingly managed outside of ICUs. As a result, Critical Care Outreach Teams (CCOTs) and intensive care liaison nurse (ICLN) roles have emerged, and these comprise clinicians trained in critical care with support from experienced medical staff. The focus is on early detection and intervention for the acutely ill ward patient, in addition to taking an active role in supporting discharge from the ICU and facilitation of timely admission. Team composition, working patterns and activity vary, and a number of different service models have emerged to suit local needs.

Key Point

It is important for health professionals to understand their role in resuscitation. Clinicians who are not trained in advanced life support (ALS) play an important role even after the arrival of the resuscitation team, such as ensuring accurate handover of details of the patient's diagnosis and events leading up to the acute event, assistance with chest compressions, attaching monitoring equipment and defibrillation under direction from the resuscitation team leader, documenting the event, moving and collecting required equipment and liaising with family members and other staff involved in the patient's care (American Association of Respiratory Care 2004).

Rescuer Safety

Risks to the rescuer have some similarities to those discussed in Chapter 20, though the environment is different. See Table 21.2 that outlines risks to in-hospital resuscitation teams and potential preventive strategies to mitigate risk.

In-hospital Resuscitation in COVID19

Resuscitation for patients with COVID 19 has resulted in confusion and concern for many healthcare workers (HCWs) about the safety of normal life-saving procedures. It is generally agreed that early defibrillation saves lives and is not considered an aerosol-generating procedure. All other resuscitative procedures are considered aerosol generating and require the use of airborne personal protective equipment (PPE) (Craig et al. 2020).

It is critical to ensure that HCWs receive basic life support training incorporating PPE use and that resuscitation equipment is readily available together with appropriate PPE. The level of resuscitation procedures will be guided by available PPE. Chest compressions only

Table 21.2 Risks to in-hospital resuscitation teams and potential preventive strategies to mitigate risk.

Risk category	Specific risks and potential exposures	Potential preventive actions and solutions
Infectious	• Percutaneous/needlestick injuries • Respiratory/airborne exposures • Contact exposures • Emerging/re-emerging infections	• Convenient sharps disposal • Use of needles with safety features • Blood-borne pathogens training for all employees • Reporting of needlestick injuries with post-exposure medical evaluations and prophylaxis • Breathing filter during mask ventilation • Clearly defined roles for staff regarding who is responsible for blood draw, central line placement, etc.
Electrical	• Shock during defibrillation • ICD misfiring • Fire generation near oxygen-rich atmospheres	• Standard maintenance of defibrillators • Training of resuscitation team members on the use of defibrillators • Placing a donut magnet over ICDs; consider including on code cart • Clear announcement of impending defibrillation • Preferential use of gel-adhesive pads instead of hand-held paddles. If paddles are used, avoidance of excess amounts of conduction gel • Consider removal of supplemental oxygen from bed prior to defibrillation
Musculoskeletal	• Neck/back injuries during/ following chest compressions • Falls while running to code situations	• Training to providers on proper posture and chest compression technique • Adjust height of bed during chest compressions and/or use of step stools • Adequate number of chest compressors to allow recovery and reduce resuscitator fatigue
Chemical	• Risks of chemical warfare	• Programs for decontamination of victims of chemical warfare

(Continued)

Table 21.2 (Continued)

Risk category	Specific risks and potential exposures	Potential preventive actions and solutions
Irradiative	• Exposure during cross-table cervical spine radiographs with manual cervical spine stabilisation, generally in trauma patients • Brachytherapy patients	• Maximise distance between provider and radiation beam • Use of lead-lined gloves, lead aprons, thyroid shields and glasses
Psychological	• Traumatic stress with short- and long-term mental and physical impact	• Stress management programs • De-briefing following resuscitation efforts, ideally within less than 72 h and in a non-threatening manner • Counseling and related programs for depression, PTSD and overall mental health well-being • Implementation of 'death rounds'

Source: Vindigni et al. (2017). This article is distributed under the terms of the Creative Commons Attribution 4.0 International License (http://creativecommons.org/licenses/by/4.0)

CPR may be used until HCWs are appropriately protected with PPE to manage the airway (Cochrane Australia 2021).

Suggested Resource

Adult resuscitation of a COVID patient Learn with NUH (2020)
https://youtu.be/1SSiflULeRY

Resuscitation Council UK Statement on COVID-19 in relation to CPR and resuscitation in acute hospital settings Resuscitation Council UK (2020, Reviewed August 2021)
https://www.resus.org.uk/covid-19-resources/statements-covid-19-hospital-settings/resuscitation-council-uk-statement-covid

Suggested Resource

Cardiopulmonary resuscitation of adults with covid-19 in healthcare settings National COVID-19 Clinical Evidence Taskforce (2021)
https://covid19evidence.net.au/wp-content/uploads/FLOWCHART-6-CPR-IN-HOSPITAL.pdf

Suggested Resource

Jevon, P. (2020). How to ensure safe and effective resuscitation for patients with Covid-19. *Nursing Times* 116 (27): 26–30.
https://www.nursingtimes.net/clinical-archive/infection-control/how-to-ensure-safe-and-effective-resuscitation-for-patients-with-covid-19-22-06-2020/

Experience from previous coronavirus outbreaks, notably severe acute respiratory syndrome (SARS) in 2003, has shown that HCWs are at risk of acquiring infection, particularly when involved in aerosol-generating critical care procedures. Fatalities of HCWs in other countries resulting from the COVID-19 suggest an even greater risk of infection (Craig et al. 2020).

The traditional approach of rushing to provide life-saving resuscitation must now be balanced with the risk of acquiring a potentially fatal illness, highlighting an ethical tension between the duty to treat and a HCW's right to protection (Craig et al. 2020). HCWs are also at risk for moral injury, that is psychological distress derived from actions (or the impossibility of implementing actions) that violate their personal ethical and moral code (Benfante et al. 2020). As stated by Benfante et al. (2020, p.2)

> 'Healthcare workers (HCWs) have been faced with unprecedented demands, both professionally and personally, in efforts to manage a disease with unclear etiology and pathology, no cure, no vaccine, and a high mortality rate. They are obliged to make difficult ethical decisions and function professionally under conditions of fear for themselves and their loved ones'.

A recent systematic review and meta-analysis by Li et al. (2021) identified a high prevalence of moderate depression, anxiety and post-traumatic stress disorder (PTSD) among HCWs during the COVID-19 pandemic. Another systematic review of post-traumatic stress symptoms in HCWs during the COVID pandemic showed young age, low work experience, female gender, heavy workload, working in unsafe settings and lack of training and social support as predictors of PTSS (d'Ettorre et al. 2021). Both authors flagged the need for urgent interventions aimed at protecting HCWs from the psychological impact of traumatic events related to the pandemic and leading to PTSS and its sequelae, PTSD.

Equipment

All clinical areas must have immediate access to functioning resuscitation equipment, including defibrillators, airway adjuncts and pharmacologic agents in order to facilitate timely response and intervention in the event of cardiac arrest. Equipment used should be consistent across the institution where possible. Regardless of scope of practice, skill level and training, all clinicians should have a thorough understanding of the location and nature of equipment available in their clinical setting to implement prompt resuscitation. Ward and resuscitation team members have a responsibility to check that equipment is in working order, with a standard checking procedure completed on a regular basis (Resuscitation Council [UK] 2020).

Basic Life Support

For clinicians working in the acute care setting, the ability to implement BLS is essential, and BLS accreditation is mandatory in most institutions, with annual mandatory updates for all clinical staff. When a CA occurs in the hospital environment, it is expected that the staff involved in the care of the patient are able to carry out a series of standard actions. These form the basis of the first three links in the chain of survival and include:

- Immediate recognition of cardiac arrest.
- Alert other staff and call for help (MET) using a predetermined emergency number.
- Commence CPR (using simple airway devices).
- Defibrillate within 3–5 minutes using an automated external defibrillator (AED).

CPR includes delivery of chest compressions over the lower half of the sternum at a depth of at least 5 cm, and at a rate of approximately 100–120 per minute, and at a ratio of 30 chest compressions to two breaths, while minimising interruptions to compressions. Interruptions to CPR decrease the chance of survival from cardiac arrest. The person delivering compressions should change every 2 minutes or sooner if the compressor becomes fatigued.

Key Point

As the quality of chest compressions and CPR in general have been associated with better outcomes in patients with cardiac arrest, optimisation of CPR quality is a priority. CPR training for all hospital personnel has, therefore, been mandatory in many hospital systems for decades (Andersen et al. 2019).

An automated external defibrillator (AED) should be applied as soon as available and follow the prompts. If a rhythm compatible with spontaneous circulation is observed, the defibrillator should be disarmed and the pulse checked (Australian Resuscitation Council/New Zealand Resuscitation Council [ANZCOR] 2018).

Key Point

Although only approximately 20% of patients with IHCA have an initial shockable rhythm, rapid defibrillation is associated with improved outcomes for these patients (Andersen et al. 2019).

Advanced Life Support

ALS refers to a set of skills, techniques and use of drugs and equipment that extend BLS to further support the airway, ventilation and circulation. During ALS, cardiac compressions continue as for BLS. The cardiac compression/ventilation ratio continues until advanced airway management is instituted, and then one breath is given every 6 seconds (Panchal et al. 2018). ALS consists of cycles of CPR,

rhythm checks and defibrillation for shockable rhythms, and drug therapy including epinephrine for asystole and pulseless electrical activity.

Key Point

It is not clear whether AEDs have any advantage over manual defibrillators for IHCA (Andersen et al. 2019) but in observing their use in practice in a team setting where interpretation of cardiac rhythms may cause delay in decision-making as to whether a shock is required, AED use may save time.

Data supporting the efficacy of medications during in-hospital CA are sparse (Andersen et al. 2019), though current evidence suggests that administration of epinephrine in IHCA patients with a non-shockable rhythm is associated with better outcomes, whereas early epinephrine for patients with a shockable rhythms is associated with worse outcomes (Andersen et al. 2019). Antiarrhythmic drugs (amiodarone or lignocaine) are used in the case of recurrent arrhythmia but are unlikely to convert pulseless ventricular tachycardia or ventricular fibrillation to a perfusing rhythm. Rather, they are used to facilitate successful defibrillation and reduce the risk of recurrent arrhythmia.

During prolonged resuscitation, attempts should be made to identify and treat potential reversible underlying causes of CA and this should include consideration of the five Hs and five Ts:

- Hypovolaemia
- Hypoxia
- Hydrogen ion (acidosis)
- Hypo-/hyperkalaemia
- Hypothermia
- Tension pneumothorax
- Tamponade (cardiac)
- Toxins
- Thrombosis (pulmonary)
- Thrombosis (coronary)

The optimal sequence of ALS interventions, including administration of antiarrhythmic drugs during resuscitation, and the preferred manner and timing of drug administration in relation to shock delivery are still not known.

Over the past 30 years, many large randomised clinical trials for specific CA treatments have found no demonstrated benefit (Graham et al. 2015) and current CA guidelines have limited high-quality scientific evidence to support recommendations (Panchal et al. 2018). Guidelines are frequently reviewed and updated and sometimes differ slightly between countries. Hence, the guidelines from your national organisation that guides resuscitation practice should be followed, and institutional practices updated accordingly.

Resuscitation should continue until return of spontaneous circulation (ROSC) is achieved and signs of life restored, in which case post-resuscitation care commences. If ROSC is not achieved, resuscitation attempts should continue until the appropriate senior medical officer determines that continuing interventions are futile. Once resuscitation efforts have ceased, events should be carefully documented, and the process and performance of those involved reviewed and assessed (AARC 2004). There is limited guidance in contemporary guidelines for when to stop CPR during CA and it is a difficult decision. Although longer duration of resuscitation is associated with worse outcomes, survival with good neurological outcome is possible with prolonged CPR (Andersen et al. 2019).

Suggested Resources: Guidelines

Guidelines for BLS and ALS are reviewed and updated periodically following detailed evaluation of published evidence and are available from international and national resuscitation organisations.
International Liaison Committee on Resuscitation (ILCOR)
https://www.ilcor.org
Australian Resuscitation Council/New Zealand Resuscitation Council (ANZCOR)
https://resus.org.au
European Resuscitation Council
https://www.erc.edu
Resuscitation Council UK
www.resus.org.uk

Key Point

Clinicians involved in resuscitation in the hospital setting have different levels of competence and should only work within their scope of practice, utilising the skills in which they are proficient. Clinicians and institutions must accept accountability for annual training, evaluation and performance monitoring of resuscitation procedures and skills. This should occur at frequent intervals to ensure safe and effective care.

Post-Resuscitation Care

Post-resuscitation care generally focuses on the precipitating cause of CA, haemodynamic and respiratory support, neuroprotective care (Andersen et al. 2019) and assessment and mitigation of ischaemia–reperfusion injury to multiple organ systems (Callaway et al. 2015). Multiorgan dysfunction following CA is the primary driver of mortality in those with IHCA, but neurological death occurs in around a quarter of patients with IHCA (Benjamin et al. 2019). The high mortality rate of patients who initially achieve ROSC after CA can be attributed to a pathophysiological process involving multiple organs which is often referred to as 'post-cardiac arrest syndrome' (PCAS) (Neumar et al. 2008). The key components of PCAS are post-CA brain injury, post-CA myocardial dysfunction, systemic ischaemia/reperfusion response and persistent issues from the pathology that precipitated the CA and other underlying co-morbities (Milonas et al. 2017). The severity of these disorders after ROSC will vary in individuals based on the severity of the ischaemic insult, the cause of CA and the patient's prearrest state of health. If ROSC is achieved rapidly after onset of cardiac arrest, the post-CA syndrome will not occur. Management strategies for patients following resuscitation include targeted temperature management (TTM) (previously known as therapeutic hypothermia), glycaemic control, controlled ventilation, oxygenation, controlled haemodynamic support, prognostication consideration and timeliness of interventions (Milonas et al. 2017).

> **Key point**
>
> Neurological prognosis based on physical examination findings should be deferred until at least 72 h after ROSC or rewarming (if targeted temperature management is used), and longer if effects of sedation or neuromuscular blockade may still be present.

Survivors of CA experience multiple medical problems related to critical illness (Benjamin et al. 2019). As many as 40% of adult survivors of IHCA have moderate to severe functional impairment at hospital discharge that results in reduced quality of life and shortened lifespan (Benjamin et al. 2019).

Audit and Data Collection

Survival rates from CA vary considerably between healthcare systems, but most reported outcome figures are poor. To improve outcomes, all potential risk factors and interventions must be carefully assessed, but this process has been hindered by lack of accurate data on structure, process and outcome of care, which Jacobs et al. (2004) suggest is due, in part, to the lack of uniformity in defining and reporting results. Inconsistent reporting makes reliable comparison of results from different studies and healthcare systems impossible.

The International Liaison Committee on Resuscitation (ILCOR) produced guidelines for the uniform reporting of data for out-of-hospital and in-hospital cardiac arrest: the Utstein Guidelines (Cummins et al. 1991) with the aim of providing clear and precise definitions of interventions, intervals and outcomes,

and the production of templates for reporting of resuscitation attempts. The Utstein template was used extensively and contributed significantly to a better understanding of resuscitation practices and has had several updates to the original guideline, including the update to the template to include data for IHCA (Nolan et al. 2019).

The Utstein guidelines have become an important tool for quality assurance and improvement in both pre-hospital and in-hospital settings. The in-hospital version recommends a set of uniform data and 'gold standard' process indicators (such as time to defibrillation), and several outcome indicators to be assessed at regular intervals. Hospitals can incorporate these indicators into a program for quality monitoring and improvement, which provides feedback, education and training to staff involved in resuscitation.

It is now widely acknowledged that the quality of post-resuscitation care is an important determinant of outcome following cardiac arrest, and many critical care units are involved in the collection and analysis of data on survivors of cardiac arrest. An Utstein template has recently been devised to define the way in which this data is collected, which will allow meaningful comparison. The science of resuscitation continues to develop and the gathering of data throughout the process is essential to improve the outcome of CA.

Conclusion

In-hospital cardiac arrests may result from a variety of causes. However, there is evidence to suggest that these events do not occur in isolation, and they may be predictable and preceded by a period of acute deterioration. Despite technological advancements and improvements in therapeutic interventions, survival rate from CA to discharge remains low. The notion that early recognition and prevention of deterioration is of paramount importance has influenced the development and implementation of a range of strategies for detecting and managing impending physiological collapse, though the efficacy of such strategies in the clinical setting remains to be fully demonstrated.

There is a need for clinicians to become proactive and proficient in their approach to patient assessment, and the implementation of resuscitation and post-resuscitation care. This may assist in the reduction of associated deaths from in-hospital CA and provide the potential for successful patient outcomes.

References

American Association of Respiratory Care (2004). *AARC Clinical Practice Guideline Resuscitation and Defibrillation in the Health Care Setting—2004 Revision & Update.* https://www.aarc.org/wp-content/uploads/2014/08/08.04.1085.pdf (accessed 4 February 2022).

Andersen, L.W., Holmberg, M.J., Berg, K.M. et al. (2019). In-hospital cardiac arrest: a review. *JAMA* **321** (12): 1200–1210.

Australian Resuscitation Council/New Zealand Resuscitation Council (ANZCOR) (2018). ANZCOR Guideline 11.2 Protocols for Adult Advanced Life Support. file:///C:/Users/hp./Downloads/anzcor-guideline-11-2-protocols-august-2018.pdf.

Benfante, A., Di Tella, M., Romeo, A., and Castelli, L. (2020). Traumatic stress in healthcare workers during COVID-19 pandemic: a review of the immediate impact. *Frontiers in Psychology* **11**: 2816.

Benjamin, E.J., Muntner, P., Alsonso, A. et al. (2019). Heart disease and stroke statistics – 2019 update: a report from the American Heart Association. *Circulation* **139** (10): e56–e528. https://www.ahajournals.org/doi/full/10.1161/CIR.0000000000000659.

Callaway, C.W., Donnino, M.W., Fink, E.L. et al. (2015). Part 8: post–cardiac arrest care: 2015 American Heart Association guidelines update for cardiopulmonary resuscitation and emergency cardiovascular care. *Circulation* **132** (18_suppl_2): S465–S482.

Chan, P.S., Jain, R., Nallmothu, B.K. et al. (2010). Rapid response teams: a systematic review and meta-analysis. *Archives of Internal Medicine* **170** (1): 18–26.

Cochrane Australia 2021. Saving lives safely during COVID-19: new CPR flowcharts issued by COVID Taskforce. https://australia.cochrane.org/news/saving-lives-safely-during-covid-19-new-cpr-flowcharts-issued-covid-taskforce (accessed 1 August 2021).

Craig, S., Cubitt, M., Jaison, A. et al. (2020). Management of adult cardiac arrest in the COVID-19 era: consensus statement from the Australasian College for Emergency Medicine. *Medical Journal of Australia* **213** (3): 126–133.

Cummins, R., Ornato, J., Thies, W., and Pepe, P. (1991). Improving survival from sudden cardiac arrest: the 'chain of survival' concept. A statement for health professionals from the Advanced Life Support Subcommittee and the Emergency Cardiac Care Committee, American Heart Association. *Circulation* **83**: 1832–1847.

d'Ettorre, G., Ceccarelli, G., Santinelli, L. et al. (2021). Post-traumatic stress symptoms in healthcare workers dealing with the COVID-19 pandemic: a systematic review. *International Journal of Environmental Research and Public Health* **18** (2): 601.

Gao, H., McDonnell, A., Harrison, D.A. et al. (2007). Systematic review and evaluation of physiological track and trigger warning systems for identifying at-risk patients on the ward. *Intensive Care Medicine* **33** (4): 667–679.

Gerry, S., Birks, J., Bonnici, T. et al. (2017). Early warning scores for detecting deterioration in adult hospital patients: a systematic review protocol. *BMJ Open* **7** (12): 1–5.

Graham, R., McCoy, M.A., and Schultz, A.M. (ed.) (2015). *Strategies to Improve Cardiac Arrest Survival: A Time to Act.* Washington, DC: National Academies Press.

Green, M., Lander, H., Snyder, A. et al. (2018). Comparison of the between the flags calling criteria to the MEWS, NEWS and the electronic Cardiac Arrest Risk Triage (eCART) score for the identification of deteriorating ward patients. *Resuscitation* **123**: 86–91.

Jacobs, I., Nadkani, V., Bahr, J. et al. (2004). Cardiac arrest and cardiopulmonary resuscitation outcome reports: update and simplification of the Utstein templates for resuscitation registries. A statement for healthcare professionals from a taskforce of the International Liaison Committee on Resuscitation. *Resuscitation* **63**: 233–249.

Kramer, A.A., Sebat, F., and Lissauer, M. (2019). A review of early warning systems for prompt detection of patients at risk for clinical decline. *Journal of Trauma and Acute Care Surgery* **87** (1S): S67–S73.

Le Lagadec, M.D. and Dwyer, T. (2017). Scoping review: the use of early warning systems for the identification of in-hospital patients at risk of deterioration. *Australian Critical Care* **30** (4): 211–218.

Li, Y., Scherer, N., Felix, L., and Kuper, H. (2021). Prevalence of depression, anxiety and post-traumatic stress disorder in health care workers during the COVID-19 pandemic: A systematic review and meta-analysis. *PLoS One* **16** (3): e0246454.

Lyons, P.G., Edelson, D.P., Carey, K.A., and American Heart Associatin's Get With the Guidelines–Resuscitation Investigators (2019). Characteristics of rapid response calls in the United States: an analysis of the first 402 023 adult cases from the get with the Guidelines Resuscitation-Medical Emergency Team

Registry. *Critical Care Medicine* **47** (10): 1283–1289.

McHugh, M.D., Rochman, M.F., Sloane, D.M. et al. (2016). Better nurse staffing and nurse work environments associated with increased survival of in-hospital cardiac arrest patients. *Medical Care* **54** (1): 74.

Milonas, A., Hutchinson, A., Charlesworth, D. et al. (2017). Post resuscitation management of cardiac arrest patients in the critical care environment: a retrospective audit of compliance with evidence based guidelines. *Australian Critical Care* **30** (6): 299–305.

Morgan, R.J.M.W.F., Lloyd-Williams, F., Wright, M.M., & Morgan-Warren, R.J. (1997). An early warning scoring system for detecting developing critical illness. https://www.scienceopen.com/document?vid=28251d22-8476-40a6-916d-1a34796816e4.

Neumar, R.W., Nolan, J.P., Adrie, C. et al. (2008). Post–cardiac arrest syndrome: epidemiology, pathophysiology, treatment, and Prognostication a consensus statement from the international liaison committee on resuscitation (American Heart Association, Australian and New Zealand Council on Resuscitation, European Resuscitation Council, Heart and Stroke Foundation of Canada, International American Heart Foundation, Resuscitation Council of Asia, and the Resuscitation Council of Southern Africa); the American Heart Association Emergency Cardiovascular Care. *Circulation* **118** (23): 2452–2483.

Nolan, J.P., Berg, R.A., Andersen, L.W. et al. (2019). Cardiac arrest and cardiopulmonary resuscitation outcome reports: update of the Utstein resuscitation registry template for in-hospital cardiac arrest: a consensus report from a task force of the international Liaison committee on resuscitation (American heart association, European resuscitation Council, Australian and New Zealand Council on resuscitation, heart and stroke foundation of Canada, InterAmerican Heart Foundation, Resuscitation Council of Southern Africa,

Resuscitation Council of Asia). *Circulation* **140** (18): e746–e757.

Ofoma, U.R., Basnet, S., Berger, A. et al. (2018). Trends in survival after in-hospital cardiac arrest during nights and weekends. *Journal of the American College of Cardiology* **71** (4): 402–411.

Panchal, A.R., Cash, R.E., Crowe, R.P. et al. (2018). Delphi analysis of science gaps in the 2015 American Heart Association cardiac arrest guidelines. *Journal of the American Heart Association* **7** (13): e008571.

Rao, A.D. and DeVita, M.A. (2017). RRS's general principles. In: *Textbook of Rapid Response Systems* (ed. M.A. DeVita, K. Hillman, R. Bellomo, et al.), 25–30. Cham: Springer.

Resuscitation Council UK (2020). Quality standards: Acute Care. Published November 2013; last updated May 2020. https://www.resus.org.uk/library/quality-standards-cpr/quality-standards-acute-care (accessed 4 February 2022)

Royal College of Physicians (2017). National Early Warning Score (NEWS) 2: Standardising the assessment of acute-illness severity in the NHS. In: *Updated Report of a Working Party.* London: RCP https://www.rcplondon.ac.uk/file/8636/download.

Rubins, J.B., Kinzie, S.D., and Rubins, D.M. (2019). Predicting outcomes of in-hospital cardiac arrest: retrospective US validation of the good outcome following attempted resuscitation score. *Journal of General Internal Medicine* **34** (11): 2530–2535.

Shearer, B., Marshall, S., Buist, M.D. et al. (2012). What stops hospital clinical staff from following protocols? An analysis of the incidence and factors behind the failure of bedside clinical staff to activate the rapid response system in a multi-campus Australian metropolitan healthcare service. *BMJ Quality and Safety* **21** (7): 569–575.

Smith, G. (2005). Prevention of in-hospital cardiac arrest and decisions about cardiopulmonary resuscitation. In: *Resuscitation Council (UK), Resuscitation Guidelines 2005*. Resuscitation Council UK www.resus.org.uk/pages/poihca.pdf.

Smith, G.B., Redfern, O., Maruotti, A. et al. (2020). The association between nurse staffing levels and a failure to respond to patients with deranged physiology: a retrospective observational study in the UK. *Resuscitation* **149**: 202–208.

Vindigni, S.M., Lessing, J.N., and Carlbom, D.J. (2017). Hospital resuscitation teams: a review of the risks to the healthcare worker. *Journal of Intensive Care* **5** (1): 1–8. URL: https://rdcu.be/cqZVX.

Wallmuller, C., Meron, G., Kurkciyan, I. et al. (2012). Causes of in-hospital cardiac arrest and influence on outcome. *Resuscitation* **83** (10): 1206–1211.

Williams, B., Alberti, G., Ball, C. et al. (2012). *Royal College of Physicians, National Early Warning Score (NEWS), Standardizing the Assessment of Acute-Illness Severity in the NHS*. London: RCP https://www.rcplondon.ac.uk/file/8636/download (accessed 4 February 2022).

Winters, B.D. and DeVita, M.A. (2017). Rapid response systems: history and terminology. In: *Textbook of Rapid Response Systems* (ed. M.A. DeVita, K. Hillman, R. Bellomo, et al.), 17–24. Cham: Springer.

22

Ethical Issues in Resuscitation and end of Life Care

Angela M. Kucia and Annabella S. Gloster

Overview

The last few decades have produced a diverse range of pharmacological and technological advancements in healthcare. The general public is better educated about healthcare, and with this increased understanding comes higher expectations of healthcare workers and the healthcare system. Unfortunately, in the setting of finite resources, there are limitations as to what can be provided in healthcare, and perhaps, questions about what should reasonably be expected and provided. Ethical tensions exist across the healthcare spectrum, with resuscitation and end-of-life issues producing some of the most difficult problems faced by health professionals. This chapter discusses some contemporary ethical issues that arise when dealing with end-of-life issues and resuscitation.

- Discuss how patient-centred care can be promoted in resuscitation decisions.
- Detail the nature of advanced directives (AD) and when they should be used.
- Explore the emotional responses of health professionals in resuscitation situations.

Key Concepts

Resuscitation; ethical issues; end-of-life care; autonomy; futility

Guiding Ethical Principles in Resuscitation

Cardiopulmonary resuscitation (CPR) is appropriate when it is associated with a reasonable chance of a good outcome, but in many cases, outcomes are poor and not in accordance with the values and treatment goals of the patient and family (Marco 2005). A person's wishes about end-of-life care should be upheld wherever possible if their wishes are known, but in the event that a patient is not in a position to express their wishes, it is often the healthcare team that must make decisions on the course of action that they believe is in the patient's best interest. Patients and their families often rely upon the expertise of health professionals to recommend appropriate therapy, particularly in

Learning Objectives

After reading this chapter, you should be able to:

- Discuss the factors in ethical decision-making related to commencing or withholding resuscitation.
- Contrast patients' understanding of resuscitation issues with that of the health professional.

emergencies requiring rapid assessment and initiation of treatment (Marco et al. 2000).

Key Point

Personal values of healthcare workers have the potential to influence decision-making about resuscitation. When presenting information to patients and families to aid in decision-making about end-of-life care, the information provided should include potential and likely outcomes based upon scientific evidence.

Decisions about resuscitation are often emotive and difficult, particularly as the outcome cannot always be predicted, and health professionals often experience dilemmas about the best course of action. Employing an ethical decision-making process using the ethical principles of beneficence (do only good), non-maleficence (do no harm), justice (fairness and equity) and autonomy (self-determination) may appear to be straightforward, but when we incorporate factors such as patient and family preferences, physician and institutional characteristics and attitudes, availability and cost of treatments, religion, culture and law, decision-making becomes very complex.

Suggested Resource

The Ethics of Resuscitation and End-of-Life Decisions
ercEuroResusCouncil (2015)
https://youtu.be/P-ndeE3ZlqY

Mentzelopoulos, S.D., Couper, K., Van de Voorde, P. et al. (2021). European Resuscitation Council Guidelines 2021: ethics of resuscitation and end of life decisions. *Resuscitation* 161: 408–432.
https://doi.org/10.1016/j.resuscitation.2021.02.017

Medical Futility

The World Medical Association defines futile medical treatment as a treatment that 'offers no reasonable hope of recovery or improvement' or from which 'the patient is permanently unable to experience any benefit' (Williams 2015). Futile resuscitation attempts only delay death for a short time, causing added suffering for the patient. Resuscitation is considered futile when the chances of good quality survival are minimal (Kidd et al. 2014) and it is generally accepted that medical futility involves both quantitative and qualitative considerations, but there is no consistent consensus among physicians about the definition of futility. The best outcome for a person is 'to be cognitively unimpaired and with an acceptable quality of life, or to report no significant deterioration when compared to the pre-morbid state' (Bossaert et al. 2015). A number of studies have attempted to define pre-arrest criteria for predicting functional status following resuscitation, but there is no assured method of predicting outcome. Pre-arrest variables that have been consistently associated with less than 3% survival in multiple studies include malignancy, age ≥80 years and dependent status at admission (Ebell et al. 2013).

Key Point

If a treating clinician considers that CPR would be futile, the patient cannot require him/her to provide it. However, the patient is entitled to know that the clinical decision has been taken and given the opportunity to seek a second opinion (Etheridge and Gatland 2015).

It is difficult to define an optimal duration for resuscitation attempts. A study by Iqbal et al. (2015) found that the proportion of patients with good functional status fell exponentially with every minute of resuscitation; conversely, resuscitation ≤3 minutes in duration predicted a more favourable functional status. Although there is evidence to show that 88% of patients who achieved sustained return of spontaneous circulation did so within 30 minutes (Goldberger et al. 2012) there are always exceptions to this rule. Whilst predictive models to assist clinicians in making resuscitation decisions may be a useful guide, decisions should not be made on a single factor such as age or duration of resuscitation. There will always be variability in condition and circumstances for individual patients requiring good clinical judgment in resuscitation decisions.

Learning Activity 22.1

A single resuscitation attempt can cost thousands of dollars and monopolise the time and efforts of several healthcare professionals (Marco 2005). Escalating healthcare costs have led to debate over whether the patient (and their family) should have total autonomy in decision-making about resuscitation, particularly if a positive outcome is unlikely. Should the greater emphasis be placed on individual patient autonomy or should the benefits to society at large outweigh the autonomy of the individual when choosing resuscitation options? Explore your thoughts on this and consider the factors that contribute to your view.

Resuscitation Orders

Various terms and abbreviations are used in the documentation of resuscitation orders, and this may cause some confusion to health professionals and the public. Table 22.1 shows commonly used terminology.

The aims of resuscitation orders are to avoid distressing interventions and promote dignity and comfort at the end of life. Orders to withhold resuscitation strategies are appropriate in the following circumstances:

- When a patient makes an informed decision to decline resuscitation measures
- In situations where resuscitation measures are known to be ineffective

Table 22.1 Terminology used for resuscitation orders.

Abbreviation	Full term
AND	Allow natural death
DNACPR	Do not attempt cardiopulmonary resuscitation
DNAR	Do not attempt resuscitation
DNR	Do not resuscitate
NFCPR	Not for cardiopulmonary resuscitation
NFR	Not for resuscitation

- When the doctor and the patient (or relative if they are unconscious) together feel the burden of resuscitation measures would outweigh the potential benefit (Mockford et al. 2015).

Provisions to protect human rights, including the right to life, protection from inhuman or degrading treatment, respect for privacy and family life, freedom of expression (including the right to hold opinions and to receive information) and freedom from discriminatory practice, must always be observed when health professionals are involved in making decisions about resuscitation (Council of Europe 2010). The Liverpool Care Pathway, a set of guidelines developed in the United Kingdom with the aim of assisting hospital staff to provide quality palliative care to terminally ill patients, were phased out after an independent review in 2013, following complaints from patients and their families that they were not consulted before being put on the pathway (Hill et al. 2015). If patients are able to communicate and make decisions, they must be involved in decision-making about resuscitation unless there is a clear indication that the discussion would cause the patient physical or psychological harm. Resuscitation decisions must be made in accordance with a clear and accessible policy so that patients and their families are aware of the criteria used in reaching a decision and can challenge the decision if they choose to.

Many people have an unrealistic view of the success rate of CPR and a poor understanding of potential adverse outcomes such as hypoxic brain injury, increased physical disability and undignified death (Mockford et al. 2015). They tend to focus on life-sustaining therapies rather than long-term goals (Anderson et al. 2011) and may choose CPR because of uncertainty and fear that a 'do not resuscitate' order may result in withdrawal of all treatment and care. Information about the care that they can expect to receive, and the likely outcome of resuscitation attempts applied to their personal health situation is essential for patients to make an informed decision.

Learning Activity 22.2

Some healthcare professionals are uncomfortable about initiating discussion about resuscitation with patients, particularly when it comes to describing what resuscitation actually involves. Why do you think this may be so? Consider patients with advanced heart disease – how might you overcome some of the barriers in initiating this type of discussion with these patients?

Suggested Resource

Denvir, M.A., Murray, S.A., and Boyd, K.J. (2015). Future care planning: a first step to palliative care for all patients with advanced heart disease. *Heart* 101 (13): 1002–1007.

The decision to start or discontinue resuscitation is particularly challenging when it occurs suddenly and a patient's wishes and baseline health status are not known (Bossaert et al. 2015), but the default position should be that the patient is for attempted CPR (Fritz et al. 2014).

Suggested Resource

Fritz, Z., Cork, N., Dodd, A., and Malyon, A. (2014). DNACPR decisions: challenging and changing practice in the wake of the Tracey judgment. *Clinical Medicine* 14 (6): 571. https://doi.org/10.7861/clinmedicine. 14-6-571

Advanced Care Planning and Advanced Directives

Advanced care planning (ACP) is a process whereby a mentally competent and informed adult expresses their preferences for future health and end-of-life care. Some of the terminology and documents used in ACP are listed in Table 22.2.

AD are the voluntarily documented instructions for future health and end-of-life care. AD may also name a surrogate decision maker to provide direction in decision-making about personal healthcare if a person is unable to

Table 22.2 Terminology and documents used in advanced care planning.

Abbreviation	Full term
ACP	Advanced care planning
AD	Advanced directives
	Living Will
MOLST	Medical orders for life-sustaining treatment
POLST	Physician orders for life-sustaining treatment
PPC	Preferred priorities for care

make decisions for themselves. AD are protected by legislation in several countries (Bosseart et al. 2015), but AD do have some limitations. Healthcare providers may not be aware of their existence and nominated surrogate decision-makers may not feel confident in representing the patient's wishes (Tanner 2015). In an unexpected event, health professionals may hesitate to honour AD as a person's perception of quality of life and desired duration of life may change, particularly as they decline or recover from an illness, or when faced with imminent death.

> **Key Point**
>
> AD should be reviewed periodically and with each hospital admission or change in the patient's condition in an effort to ensure that the patients' wishes about resuscitation are implemented with consideration given to their current health status.

Newer models of ACP including programs such as 'Respecting Patient Choices' have been implemented with varying degrees of success in many countries. The program involves training of ACP facilitators, education of healthcare providers and patients and integration of ACP into ongoing clinical care (Tanner 2015).

Suggested Resources

Treatment escalation plans and resuscitation
Health Education England (2020)
https://youtu.be/vXrRp7AW5E4

Advanced Care Planning Australia
www.advancecareplanning.org.au

End of Life Care
National Health Service (NHS) (2018)
https://www.nhs.uk/conditions/end-of-life-care/

> **Key Point**
>
> ACP for patients with end-stage heart failure is now a fundamental aspect of care. There are also other groups of patients with advanced heart disease who are at increased risk of death due to their primary cardiac disorder or associated co-morbidities who need to consider ACP.

Withdrawal of Treatment

Withdrawal of life-sustaining treatment, once initiated, can be a vexed issue. Despite consensus that there is no ethical or legal distinction between withholding and withdrawing treatment (Reynolds et al. 2007), some find it difficult to make the distinction between withdrawing a burdensome treatment and euthanasia. The cause of death is considered to be the medical condition that necessitates the treatment that is withheld or withdrawn (Sprung et al. 2014) rather than the withdrawal of treatment itself.

It is becoming increasingly common to limit life-sustaining treatments, though internationally there is a lot of variability as practices are influenced in some cases by law, religion and culture. It has also been found that there are wide variations within a country (Sprung et al. 2014).

The ability to withdraw life-sustaining treatment that is not assisting recovery is important as clinicians may be reluctant to implement a therapy knowing that it will be difficult to withdraw if not beneficial. It is essential that patients are not deprived of life-sustaining treatment when there is a chance that it may be effective. A therapy can be tried for a predefined period of time with an assessment of whether it has been of benefit and should be continued or ceased (Wilkinson and Savulescu 2014). In this way, healthcare workers, patients and their families know that every effort has been made to preserve life.

When it is certain that death is inevitable and imminent, the healthcare team need to advise and discuss the rationale for treatment withdrawal with the patient and their family. This gives the patient and family an opportunity to participate in the treatment plan, but relieves the family of the burden of responsibility and feelings of guilt that may be involved in making a decision themselves to withdraw treatment.

Witnessed Resuscitation

Family members being present during the resuscitation process has become an accepted practice in many countries. Family members have reported that having the opportunity to share the last minutes of their loved one's life has helped with the grieving process, acceptance of death (Walker 2013) and feeling that everything reasonable had been done (Baskett et al. 2005). Initial concerns that family members would be traumatised by witnessing CPR seem to be unfounded (Clark et al. 2013). There is no evidence to suggest that family members interfere with medical care procedures, get in the way during the resuscitation process (Bosseart et al. 2015) or change the focus of care from what is in the best interests of the patient to what is the best way of avoiding litigation (Chapman et al. 2013).

Key Point

Relatives should be offered the choice to be present during a resuscitation attempt where possible, but cultural and social variations in acceptance of this practice must be managed with sensitivity. An experienced member of staff should provide explanations and support the relatives during the resuscitation attempt whenever possible (Mentzelopoulos et al. 2021).

Organ Donation

Transplantation is the only therapeutic option for terminal organ failure. Despite campaigns to raise public awareness, the annual number of organ transplants performed represents less than 10% of the global need (Citerio et al. 2016). Organ donation may occur after brain death is confirmed by neurological criteria; following the planned withdrawal of life-sustaining treatments and with subsequent confirmation of death using cardio-respiratory criteria; or following an unexpected cardiac arrest and death is confirmed using cardio-respiratory criteria after resuscitation efforts have been unsuccessful (Citerio et al. 2016). Minimum clinical standards for brain death determination include:

- unresponsive coma with an established aetiology
- absence of reversible conditions
- absence of cortical or brainstem-mediated motor responses
- absent brainstem reflexes
- loss of the capacity to breathe (Shemie and Baker 2015).

Consent to organ donation varies around the world. Current models of consent include explicit opt-in organ donation where an individual expresses consent to become a potential donor; or explicit opt-out systems that presume consent unless an individual expresses their refusal to become a potential donor. Some countries encourage opt-in organ donation by giving consenting potential donors priority for transplant receipt (Zúñiga-Fajuri 2015).

Organ donation is fraught with ethical issues involving difficult decisions and uncertainties, which may contribute to the low number of organ transplants performed. One example is the 'dead donor rule' stating that vital organs can only be retrieved after an individual has died and that retrieval of donated organs shall not cause the donor's death (Citerio et al. 2016). In practice, it is not always possible to draw a line between physical death and organ procurement. The living body of a person in whom brain death has been determined is supported until the required organs have been removed. Where circulatory determination of death is used, the dying process is driven by the procurement of the organs, often involving surgical procedures and non-therapeutic medications (Truog 2016).

Key Point

The COVID-19 pandemic has negatively impacted organ donation and transplantation in countries that have experienced high rates of infection, including the United States, France and the United Kingdom, all reporting >50% reductions in transplant activity (Chadban et al. 2020).

Training and Research with the Newly Dead

Allowing healthcare professionals to perform posthumous procedures on the newly deceased will ultimately decrease patients' morbidity and mortality as they gain and perfect their procedural skills (Rajagopal and Champney 2020). The use of the newly dead for the benefit of training and research raises ethical questions in terms of autonomy, consent, the need for disclosure and justification of practice (Abraham 2015). In some countries, the newly dead are used for teaching techniques such as endotracheal intubation, CPR and evaluation of pharmacologic treatments and mechanical devices (Abramson et al. 2001). It has been argued that the practice of using the newly dead for training in endotracheal intubation is justifiable because it is non-mutilating, brief and an effective teaching technique that ultimately is beneficial to others. In most cases, endotracheal intubation training takes place without consent from the patient prior to death, or the

family following death. It has been claimed by some that obtaining consent for this practice from the family is unnecessary because corpses are 'non-persons' and thus have no autonomy (Abramson et al. 2001). Others argue a case for 'presumed consent' which implies that a reasonable person would give consent to being involved in this practice under the same circumstances.

Research to test commonly used interventions with uncertain efficacy or new and potentially beneficial treatments in resuscitation is essential, but obtaining consent to participation in research from a patient who is undergoing a resuscitation attempt is not possible prior to study inclusion. Deferred consent or exception to informed consent with prior community consultation are considered ethically acceptable alternatives for respecting autonomy (Bosseart et al. 2015).

Suggested Resource

Mentzelopoulos, S.D., Bossaert, L., Raffay, V. et al. (2016). A survey of key opinion leaders on ethical resuscitation practices in 31 European Countries. *Resuscitation* 100: 11–16.
https://www.resuscitationjournal.com/article/S0300-9572(16)00012-5/fulltext

---

Conclusion

Actions taken by health professionals need to take into consideration the situational context and patient and family wishes when dealing with issues relating to end of life care. End of life care wishes are personal and differ according to the beliefs and situational understanding of a patient (or their decision maker if they do not have decision-making capacity). Introducing conversations about end of life care may be confronting for the patient and family who may not have previously considered the need to make these plans.

There are times when death may be unexpected and health professionals may have to lead decisions about resuscitation based upon the likelihood of benefit or futility, particularly in the setting of cardiac arrest or where there are no further valid options for treatment.

Good communication between health practitioners, the patient and their family is paramount in order to reach agreement on resuscitation or end of life care and should be based on an understanding of what is possible and in the patient's best interests.

References

Abraham, J. (2015). Practicing on newly dead. *SAGE Open* **5** (3): 2158244015595270. https://journals.sagepub.com/doi/full/10.1177/2158244015595270 (accessed 15 September 2015).

Abramson, N., de Vos, R., Fallat, M.E. et al. (2001). Ethics in emergency cardiac care. *Annals of Emergency Medicine* **37** (4): S196–S200.

Anderson, W.G., Chase, R., Pantilat, S.Z. et al. (2011). Code status discussions between attending hospitalist physicians and medical patients at hospital admission. *Journal of General Internal Medicine* **26** (4): 359–366.

Baskett, P.J.F., Steen, P.A., and Bossaert, L. (2005). European Resuscitation Council Guidelines for Resuscitation 2005: Section 8. The ethics of resuscitation and end-of-life decisions. *Resuscitation* **67** (Suppl. 1): S171–S180.

Bossaert, L.L., Perkins, G.D., Askitopoulou, H. et al. (2015). European Resuscitation Council Guidelines for Resuscitation 2015: Section 11. The ethics of resuscitation and end-of-life decisions. *Resuscitation* **95**: 302–311.

Chadban, S.J., McDonald, M., Wyburn, K. et al. (2020). Significant impact of COVID-19 on organ donation and transplantation in a low-prevalence country: Australia. *Kidney International* **98** (6): 1616.

Chapman, R., Watkins, R., Bushby, A., and Combs, S. (2013). Assessing health professionals' perceptions of family presence during resuscitation: a replication study. *International Emergency Nursing* **21**: 17–25.

Citerio, G., Cypel, M., Dobb, G.J. et al. (2016). Organ donation in adults: a critical care perspective. *Intensive Care Medicine* **42** (3): 305–315.

Clark, A.P., Guzzetta, C.E., and O'Connell, K.J. (2013). Family presence during resuscitation attempts is associated with positive psychological effects for the observers. *Evidence Based Mental Health* **16**: 78.

Council of Europe (2010). *Biomedicine Human Rights – The Oviedo Convention its Additional Protocols*. Strasbourg: Council of Europe.

Ebell, M.H., Afonso, A.M., Geocadin, R.G., and American Heart Association (2013). Prediction of survival to discharge following cardiopulmonary resuscitation using classification and regression trees*. *Critical Care Medicine* **41** (12): 2688–2697.

Etheridge, Z. and Gatland, E. (2015). When and how to discuss "do not resuscitate" decisions with patients. *BMJ* **350**: h2640. doi: https://doi.org/10.1136/bmj.h2640.

Fritz, Z., Cork, N., Dodd, A., and Malyon, A. (2014). DNACPR decisions: challenging and changing practice in the wake of the Tracey judgment. *Clinical Medicine* **14** (6): 571–576.

Goldberger, Z.D., Chan, P.S., Berg, R.A. et al. (2012). American Heart Association get with the Guidelines – Resuscitation (formerly National Registry of Cardiopulmonary Resuscitation) Investigators. Duration of resuscitation efforts and survival after in-hospital cardiac arrest: an observational study. *Lancet* **380** (9852): 1473–1481.

Hill, L., McIlfatrick, S., Taylor, B. et al. (2015). Patients' perception of implantable cardioverter defibrillator deactivation at the end of life. *Palliative Medicine* **29** (4): 310–323.

Iqbal, M.B., Al-Hussaini, A., Rosser, G. et al. (2015). Predictors of survival and favorable functional outcomes after an out-of-hospital cardiac arrest in patients systematically brought to a dedicated heart attack center (from the Harefield Cardiac Arrest Study). *The American Journal of Cardiology* **115** (6): 730–737.

Kidd, A.C., Honney, K., Myint, P.K. et al. (2014). Does medical futility matter in 'do not attempt CPR'decision-making? *International Journal of Clinical Practice* **68** (10): 1190–1192.

Marco, C.A. (2005). Ethical issues of resuscitation: an American perspective. *Postgraduate Medical Journal* **81**: 608–612.

Marco, C.A., Larkin, G.L., Moskop, J.C., and Derse, A.R. (2000). Determination of 'futility' in emergency medicine. *Annals of Emergency Medicine* **35** (6): 604–612.

Mentzelopoulos, S.D., Couper, K., Van de Voorde, P. et al. (2021). European Resuscitation Council Guidelines 2021: ethics of resuscitation and end of life decisions. *Resuscitation* **161**: 408–432. https://www. sciencedirect.com/science/article/pii/ S0300957221000708.

Mockford, C., Fritz, Z., George, R. et al. (2015). Do not attempt cardiopulmonary resuscitation (DNACPR) orders: a systematic review of the barriers and facilitators of decision-making and implementation. *Resuscitation* **88**: 99–113.

Rajagopal, A.S., & Champney, T.H. (2020). Teaching without harm: the ethics of performing posthumous procedures on the newly deceased. *Cureus*, **12** (12):e11855. doi: https://doi.org/10.7759/cureus.11855.

Reynolds, S., Cooper, A.B., and McKneally, M. (2007). Withdrawing life-sustaining treatment: ethical considerations. *Surgical Clinics of North America* **87** (4): 919–936.

Shemie, S.D. and Baker, A. (2015). Uniformity in brain death criteria. *Seminars in Neurology* **35** (2): 162–168.

Sprung, C.L., Paruk, F., Kissoon, N. et al. (2014). The Durban world congress ethics round table conference report: I. differences between withholding and withdrawing life-sustaining treatments. *Journal of Critical Care* **29** (6): 890–895.

Tanner, C. (2015). Decision making about end of life care: advance directives, durable power of attorney for healthcare, and talking with patients with heart disease about dying. In: *End-of-Life Care in Cardiovascular Disease* (ed. S.J. Goodlin and M.W. Rich), 21–32. London: Springer.

Truog, R. (2016). The price of our illusions and myths about the dead donor rule. *Journal of Medical Ethics* medethics-2015.

Walker, W. (2013). Emergency care staff experiences of lay presence during adult cardiopulmonary resuscitation: a phenomenological study. *Emergency Medicine Journal* **31**: 453–458.

Wilkinson, D. and Savulescu, J. (2014). A costly separation between withdrawing and withholding treatment in intensive care. *Bioethics* **28** (3): 127–137.

Williams, J.R. (2015). *WMA Medical Ethics Manual*, 3ee. The World Medical Association, Inc https://www.wma.net/what-we-do/ education/medical-ethics-manual/ (accessed 8 January 2016).

Zúñiga-Fajuri, A. (2015). Increasing organ donation by presumed consent and allocation priority: Chile. *Bulletin of the World Health Organization* 2015 (93): 199–202.

Part VI

Chronic Cardiac Conditions

23

Heart Failure

Salimah Hassan, Christopher Nicholson, Robyn Lotto, and Angela M. Kucia

Overview

The main function of the heart is to pump blood through the circulatory system to meet systemic needs. Heart failure (HF) is a clinical syndrome that is characterised by typical signs and symptoms that are caused by a structural and/or functional cardiac abnormality resulting in a reduced cardiac output (CO) and/or elevated intracardiac pressures at rest or during stress (Ponikowski et al. 2016). To compensate for this inefficiency, several physiological processes are initiated. These compensatory mechanisms, whilst maintaining function in the short term, can cause longer-term problems. HF may present as an acute problem or as a chronic condition and may be reversible or irreversible, depending on the underlying cause. A multidisciplinary framework that includes discharge planning, patient education and frequent outpatient assessment is required to optimise the care of patients with HF (Hajouli and Ludhwani 2020). It is important that patients have access to expert treatment as HF outcomes can significantly improve when managed by HF specialists (British Society for Heart Failure 2017).

Key Point

The latest and most comprehensive guideline is the '2021 ESC Guidelines for the diagnosis and treatment of acute and chronic heart failure'. These guidelines are very detailed and advise on HF management across a range of contexts. It is strongly advised that you review the most current guidelines for HF as they incorporate the most recent available evidence. HF management guidelines are similar for most countries but may have some subtle differences and are updated regularly as new evidence emerges.

Suggested Resource

McDonagh, T.A., Metra, M., Adamo, M., Gardner, R.S., Baumbach, A., Böhm, M., Burri, H., Butler, J., Čelutkienė, J., Chioncel, O., and Cleland, J.G (2021). 2021 ESC Guidelines for the diagnosis and treatment of acute and chronic heart failure: Developed by the Task Force for the diagnosis and treatment of acute and chronic heart failure of the European Society of Cardiology (ESC) With the special contribution of the Heart Failure Association (HFA) of the ESC. *European Heart Journal* 42 (36): 3599–3726. https://doi.org/10.1093/eurheartj/ehab368

Learning Objectives

After reading this chapter and completing the learning activities, the reader will be able to:

- Discuss the epidemiology and pathophysiology of HF.
- Explain the process of assessment of patients with suspected HF and the role of diagnostic tests used to investigate patients with suspected HF.
- Describe current pharmacological and non-pharmacological management strategies for acute and chronic HF.
- Discuss the roles of multidisciplinary team members in HF management.
- Discuss the impact of conditions associated with HF on patient care.
- Locate evidence-based resources to assist with care planning for people with HF.

Key Concepts

Heart failure; heart failure with reduced ejection fraction; heart failure with preserved ejection fraction; self-management; decompensated heart failure

Definition of Heart Failure

HF is defined as "a complex clinical syndrome with typical symptoms and signs that generally occur on exertion but can also occur at rest (particularly when recumbent). It is secondary to an abnormality of cardiac structure or function that impairs the ability of the heart to fill with blood at normal pressure or eject blood sufficient to fulfil the needs of the metabolising organs" (Atherton et al. 2018, p. 1136). The cardiac cycle can be affected during contraction (systolic dysfunction), during relaxation (diastolic dysfunction) or both phases. There can be anatomical changes within the heart including chamber dilation, muscle hypertrophy or cardiac valve disorders. The disorder may predominantly affect the left side of the heart, the right side or both (Ponikowski et al. 2016).

Heart Failure Terminology

New onset or de novo *HF* refer to the first presentation and diagnosis of HF in a patient who has not previously received HF treatment. The history of symptoms may be short (hours to days) or long (weeks to months) (Atherton et al. 2018).

Chronic HF (CHF) is used to describe HF in patients who have had the condition for some time (arbitrarily a period of 3 months) and have usually received HF treatment (Atherton et al. 2018). Chronic HF is a clinical syndrome of events leading to abnormal LV dysfunction and neurohormonal regulation resulting in episodes of shortness of breath and fatigue. Treated patients with clinical signs and symptoms that have remained generally unchanged for at least 1 month are said to be *'stable'* (Ponikowski et al., 2016).

Acute HF refers to the acute onset or significant worsening of symptoms of HF which requires treatment intervention. Specific subgroups of acute HF include the following:

- *Acute decompensated HF (ADHF)* refers to clinical deterioration in a stable HF patient. Decompensation may happen quickly or take time to develop. Decompensation often leads to hospital admission and is of prognostic importance (Ponikowski et al. 2016). The precipitants of decompensation often require attention concurrently with the management of the HF (Atherton et al. 2018).

- *Acute (cardiogenic) pulmonary oede*ma (APO) is a medical emergency with pulmonary oedema as the dominant clinical feature of left HF with redistribution of fluid into the pulmonary interstitium and alveolar flooding. Without intervention APO results in the rapid development of life-threatening respiratory failure (Atherton et al. 2018).
- *Cardiogenic shoc*k is a medical emergency with poor prognosis that is characterised by the acute development of reduced CO and hypotension (systolic blood pressure (BP) < 90 mm Hg) in the setting of HF that compromises end-organ perfusion. Without intervention, multiorgan failure and death ensues. Cardiogenic shock most commonly results from a large acute myocardial functional insult (such as myocardial infarction (MI)) or a catastrophic cardiac structural insult (such as torrential valvular regurgitation). Cardiogenic shock may also be the manifestation of end-stage CHF (Atherton et al. 2018).

Right Heart Failure

Right HF (RHF) refers to solitary or predominant failure of the right heart. RHF is associated with a diverse array of conditions and may be acute or chronic. Although HF is predominantly discussed in the context of left-sided HF, RHF is a serious condition that is generally associated with a poor prognosis (Atherton et al. 2018).

Conditions associated with RHF include:

- Pulmonary hypertension (PH)
- RV myocardial ischaemia or infarction (see Chapter 17)
- Myocarditis
- Arrhythmogenic right ventricular cardiomyopathy (ARVC) (see Chapter 12)
- Tricuspid or pulmonary valve regurgitation
- Congenital heart disease (see Chapter 24)
- Acute LV failure
- Pulmonary embolism
- Acute lung injury/hypoxia
- RV outflow tract obstruction

RVH management depends upon treatment of the underlying causative condition.

Biventricular Failure

Biventricular HF indicates that both sides of the heart are affected. Symptoms may include those that are typical of both left-sided and right-sided HF and are often encountered in end-stage HF.

Heart Failure with Preserved Ejection Fraction (HFpEF)

HFpEF (previously referred to as 'systolic HF') is a clinical syndrome in which patients have signs and symptoms of HF with a normal or near normal LVEF (≥50%) (Borlaug and Colucci 2019). A common pattern of structural change that leads to HF is LV hypertrophy. This is often (though not exclusively) due to chronic hypertension. In hypertrophic hearts, the left ventricle may be smaller in volume due to thickening of the chamber wall and as a result, the LVEDV is reduced. If the SV remains the same (or only slightly less) despite the reduction in the LVEDV, the LVEF is likely to be preserved. In this case, the patients are classified as having HFpEF. In patients with HFpEF it is likely that the underlying diseases and natural progression will mean that eventually HF with reduced EF will develop.

Heart Failure with Reduced Ejection Fraction (HFrEF)

When the LVEF is reduced and the heart does not contract efficiently, patients are classified as having *HF with reduced ejection fraction* (HFrEF). The European Society of Cardiology (ESC) define HFrEF as a LVEF of 40% or less (McDonagh et al. 2021), whereas the National Heart Foundation of Australia (NHFA)/ Cardiac Society of Australia and New Zealand (CSANZ) diagnostic criteria are symptoms (with or without signs of HF) and an

LVEF <50% (Atherton et al. 2018). HFrEF begins with an insult to the heart, such as MI. Subsequently, areas of myocardium may become akinetic (not contract), hypokinetic (contract poorly) or dyskinetic (contract in an uncoordinated fashion). When contractility is impaired, areas of the heart muscle may change shape over time (remodeling), often leading to dilation. An enlarged heart (cardiomegaly) is less efficient than a normal-sized heart. Cardiac physiology and regulation of cardiovascular function are discussed in Chapters 1 and 2.

Heart Failure with Mildly Reduced Ejection Fraction

A new category termed *heart failure with mildly reduced ejection fraction* (HFmrEF) has been proposed where the LVEF is between 40 and 49% (McDonagh et al. 2021). This new category has not been endorsed by the Cardiac Society of Australia and New Zealand (Atherton et al. 2018).

Key Points

Approximately half of all patients with signs and symptoms of HF have an LVEF that is not markedly abnormal (Pfeffer et al. 2019). Functional HF can occur with or without the structure of the heart being impaired.

Epidemiology

The prevalence of HF continues to rise over time. In part, the increasing prevalence is a result of people with HF surviving longer due to better treatments, as opposed to an increasing number of cases of new onset HF. Figures for the incidence and prevalence of HF vary and are subject to problems of diagnostic and coding accuracy (Quach et al. 2010), but it is estimated that HF currently affects at least thirty-eight million people worldwide (Atherton et al. 2018). Prevalence of HF in Australia, Europe and North America ranges between 1.3 and 2.2% (Sahle et al. 2016). As HF is caused by a wide range of underlying diseases (see Box 23.1), the prevalence of those underlying conditions influences the incidence of HF. In high-income countries, ischaemic heart disease (IHD) is the most common cause of HF in adults and is more common in older age, whereas in low- and middle-income countries, HF is mainly due to hypertensive heart disease and cardiomyopathies. Paediatric HF in low- and middle-income countries is predominantly due to acquired and preventable causes of HF, including rheumatic heart diseases (RHD), endomyocardial fibrosis, nutritional deficiencies and other tropical diseases. RHD is the first cause of cardiovascular mortality in children and young adults (Sibetcheu et al. 2018).

HF is a highly prevalent condition, and the incidence rises in older people. With improved treatment, there are signs that HF mortality is falling (Roger 2013; Taylor et al. 2019a).

Box 23.1 Left ventricular ejection fraction (LVEF) measurement.

HF assessment and diagnosis are aided by the measurement of the LV ejection fraction (LVEF). LVEF is a measurement of how much blood is pumped out of the left ventricle during systole. LVEF is calculated by dividing the stroke volume (SV) by the LV end diastolic volume (LVEDV) (i.e. the ratio of blood that leaves the left ventricle during a contraction divided by the total amount of blood that was present in the left ventricle prior to contraction). The lower limit of normal LVEF is between 50 and 55% (52% in men and 54% in women) (Butler et al. 2019). LVEF is usually measured in patients with HF using echocardiography. LVEF is an imperfect measure of ventricular function because measurement is influenced by various factors including sex, age, volume status, BP, method used for imaging, quality of images and intraobserver and interobserver variability in the estimation of LVEF, but it is the best non-invasive measure available (Butler et al. 2019).

In high-income countries, lower acute mortality rates mean that more patients survive for longer with chronic HF; however, in low-income countries this is not the case as patients are often unable to access services and treatment due to severely limited financial, human and infrastructural resources.

Significance

HF is associated with high mortality and significant morbidity, as well as consumption of substantial resources to manage the condition. Treating HF has been calculated to cost $32 billion in the United States (Monza et al. 2015) and $108 billion worldwide annually (Cook et al. 2014). HF is associated with one of the longest average lengths of hospital stay of any condition, which means admissions are expensive and have a significant effect on bed-flow management. Avoiding unnecessary admissions is therefore both clinically appropriate and cost effective (British Society for Heart Failure 2017). HF also takes a huge personal toll on the person with the condition. In addition to learning to cope with debilitating chronic physical symptoms, a diagnosis of HF can destabilise the life balance and mental health of an individual, and place enormous stress on their carers and loved ones. Quality of life (QoL) is impacted by limitations in daily activities, dietary restrictions, drug side effects, changes in sexual life, inability to work and earn an income, changes in interpersonal relationships and dependence, and frequent hospitalisations. Anxiety and depression triggered by stress are commonly compounded by the complexity of the disease, with high mortality rates and disease burden (Korkmaz et al. 2019).

Prognosis

HF mortality data in contemporary studies show that about 10% of patients hospitalised with HF do not survive to discharge (Parenica et al. 2013). Survival rates for chronic HF range from 81 to 91% at 1 year and from 52 to 63% at 5 years (Atherton et al. 2018). It is difficult to estimate the actual number of deaths attributed to HF alone as HF is commonly categorised as an intermediate stage of an underlying condition such as coronary artery disease (CAD) rather than the actual cause of death (Ziaeian and Fonarow 2016).

HF patients usually die from pump failure or from sudden cardiac death (SCD). The mode of death depends upon the severity of the HF: the risk of dying suddenly is greater in patients with mild HF, whereas with more severe HF, the risk of dying from pump failure is greater. SCD is generally assumed to be due to arrhythmia, but autopsies have shown that ischaemic events may be present. Autopsies are seldom performed in patients with HF, and thus the incidence of acute MI as a cause of death may be underestimated (Dahlström 2019).

> **Key Point**
>
> There are several prognostic markers of death and/or HF-related hospitalisation for patients with HF. Multivariable risk scores (some of which are available online) may help predict death in patients with HF, but remain less useful for the prediction of subsequent HF hospitalisations (Ponikowski et al. 2016).

Aetiology

Determining the cause of a patient's HF is important because different causes require distinct treatments. For example, a patient with IHD may require coronary revascularisation; a patient with valvular heart disease may require some form of surgical intervention and a patient with alcoholic dilated cardiomyopathy will require interventions to support alcohol abstinence. In patients with known HF, it is important to consider triggers that might provoke an acute episode. For example, a patient with chronic HF may not cope with the increased metabolic demands of acute illness such as pneumonia, which may precipitate acute HF. A common cause of deterioration in patients with chronic HF is non-adherence with treatment (Corotto et al. 2013; Ruppar et al. 2016), particularly with diuretics and beta-blockers (Viana et al. 2014). Aetiologies of HF are shown in Table 23.1. Takotsubo syndrome (TTS) (not included in this table) is another potential cause of acute HF which generally resolves following the acute phase of TTS.

Diagnosis

Diagnosing HF can be challenging due to the broad spectrum of associated signs and symptoms and the overlap of these symptoms with other diseases, especially in obese individuals, the older patients and patients with chronic lung disease. Younger patients with HF often have a different aetiology, clinical presentation and outcome compared with older patients (Ponikowsi et al. 2016). History and physical assessment are the cornerstone of HF diagnosis as there is no universal single highly sensitive sign for the positive diagnosis of HF. In isolation, signs lack specificity but when several signs are present diagnostic accuracy improves. Signs of HF have patterns of low CO, compensatory processes to maintain CO, fluid retention and structural heart changes (Clerkin et al. 2019).

Table 23.1 Aetiologies of heart failure.

Diseased myocardium		
Ischaemic heart disease	Myocardial scar	
	Myocardial stunning	
	Epicardial coronary artery disease	
	Abnormal coronary microcirculation	
	Endothelial dysfunction	
Toxic damage	Recreational substance abuse	Alcohol, cocaine, methamphetamine anabolic steroids
	Heavy metals	Copper, iron, lead, cobalt
	Medications	Cytostatic drugs (e.g. anthracyclines), immunomodulating drugs (e.g. interferons, monoclonal antibodies such as trastuzumab and cetuximab), antidepressant drugs, antiarrhythmics, non-steroidal anti-inflammatory drugs, anaesthetics
	Radiation	
Immune-mediated and inflammatory damage	Related to infection	Bacteria, spirochaetes, fungi, protozoa, parasites (Chaga's disease), rickettsiae, viruses (HIV/AIDS)
	Not related to infection	Lymphocytic/giant cell myocarditis, autoimmune disease (Grave's disease, rheumatoid arthritis, connective tissue disorders, mainly systemic erythematosus), hypersensitivity, eosinophilic myocarditis (Churg-Strauss).
Infiltration	Related to malignancy	Direct infiltrations and malignancies
	Not related to malignancy	Amyloidosis, sarcoidosis, haemochromatosis (iron), glycogen storage diseases (e.g. Pompe disease), lysosomal storage diseases (e.g. Fabry's disease).

Table 23.1 (Continued)

Diseased myocardium		
Metabolic disorders	Hormonal	Thyroid disease, parathyroid diseases, acromegaly, GH deficiency, hypercortisolaemia, Conn's disease, diabetes, Addison's disease, metabolic syndrome, pheochromocytoma, pathologies related to pregnancy and peripartum.
	Nutritional	Deficiencies in thiamine, L-carnitine, selenium, iron, phosphates, calcium, complex malnutrition (malignancy, AIDS, anorexia nervosa), obesity.
Genetic abnormalities	Diverse forms	HCM, DCM, LV non-compaction, ARVC, restrictive cardiomyopathy (for details see respective expert documents), muscular dystrophies and laminopathies.

Abnormal loading conditions		
Hypertension		
Valve and myocardium structural defects	Acquired	Mitral, aortic, tricuspid and pulmonary valve diseases.
	Congenital	Atrial and ventricular septum defects and others (for details see respective expert documents).
Pericardial and endomyocardial pathologies	Pericardial	Constrictive pericarditis Pericardial effusion.
	Endomyocardial	HES, EMF, endocardial fibroelastosis.
High-output states		Severe anaemia, sepsis, thyrotoxicosis, Paget's disease, arteriovenous fistula, pregnancy.
Volume overload		Renal failure, iatrogenic fluid overload.

Arrhythmias	
Tachyarrhythmias	Atrial, ventricular arrhythmias.
Bradyarrhythmias	Sinus node dysfunctions, conduction disorders.

Source: Reproduced with permission. Ponikowski et al. (2016).

Heart Failure Assessment

Aspects of general cardiac assessment are covered in Chapter 6. Examining a patient with HF has additional complexities and requires advanced assessment skills. Symptoms and signs of HF are listed in Box 23.2.

Key Point

HF is a heterogeneous syndrome with various phenotypic presentations, comorbidities, precipitating factors and management strategies which makes prognostication challenging for clinicians (Cameli et al. 2019).

Typical Symptoms

Dyspnoea (breathlessness) is one of the most common presenting symptoms for patients with HF. Dyspnoea is defined as the subjective sensation of abnormal breathing. Patients commonly describe a sensation of 'inadequate breathing' or 'air hunger'. Dyspnoea in patients with HF can be both acute and chronic. Patients may be short of breath at rest or on exertion and may take an increased time to recover from exercise. *Orthopnoea* (shortness of breath when recumbent) often develops secondary to increased venous return from lower extremities and increased pulmonary venous pressures leaving patients unable to lie flat due

---

Box 23.2   Causes of dyspnoea.

Cardiac
- Increased left-sided intracavity filling pressure
  - HF due to myocardial dysfunction (HFrEF, HFpEF)
  - Left-sided valvular dysfunction (aortic or mitral stenosis or regurgitation)
- Myocardial ischaemia
- Arrhythmia
  - Low CO (left-sided):
  - pulmonary hypertension
  - hypovolaemia
  - cardiac shunt
  - cardiac compression (pericardial constriction, cardiac tamponade, tension pneumothorax)

Respiratory
- Hypoxia
  - pulmonary parenchymal abnormality: infection (pneumonia), fibrosis, destruction (emphysema), oedema, alveolar haemorrhage and compression (pleural effusion and pneumothorax)
  - airway obstruction (asthma, bronchitis, upper airway) – ventilation–perfusion mismatch (pulmonary embolus and pulmonary shunt)
- Central respiratory drive abnormality (pharmacological, metabolic)
- Musculoskeletal respiration abnormality
  - skeletal myopathy
  - respiratory muscle fatigue
  - chest wall abnormality (kyphoscoliosis, thoracic skeletal pain and obesity)

Peripheral muscle oxygen extraction abnormality or insufficiency
- Poor physical fitness
- Myopathy

Anxiety

Anaemia, iron deficiency

Hyperventilation
- Acidosis (renal failure, ketoacidosis, shock)
- Pharmacological cause
- Thyrotoxicosis

Source: Reproduced with permission. Atherton et al. (2018).

---

to breathlessness or to wake up suddenly acutely breathless from sleep (*paroxysmal nocturnal dyspnoea*). It is common for patients to have to use extra pillows or need to sleep in a chair. They may have sleep-disordered breathing or a cough productive of copious frothy sputum (Alpert et al. 2017). The subjective nature of dyspnoea can be difficult for the clinician to interpret. Moreover, there are many different pathological and physiological states besides HF that may cause dyspnoea (see Box 23.2) (Atherton et al. 2018).

Less common respiratory symptoms of HF include nocturnal cough, wheezing, and bendopnoea (McDonagh et al. 2021)

Fatigue

Reduced exercise tolerance, increased time to recover from exercise, fatigue and tiredness are also common in HF. Decreased CO and skeletal muscle dysfunction are frequently found in patients with HF. Patients with chronic HF often experience sleep disturbances compounded by increased frequency of urination at night. Reversible causes of fatigue may include hypothyroidism, anaemia and depression (Clerkin et al. 2019).

Other Symptoms

Less common symptoms include feeling bloated and poor appetite, palpitations, dizziness and syncope, depression and confusion (especially in the older people) (McDonagh et al. 2021).

Physical Examination

Cardiac examination is discussed in more detail in Chapter 6. Common abnormalities found in HF are discussed below.

Basic Vital Signs

Tachycardia is common in HF (especially if acute). If CO falls, there is a compensatory increase in heart rate (via the sympathetic nervous system) resulting in sinus tachycardia. Faster heart rates increase CO, but if the SV remains constant or increases, tachycardia reduces the diastolic filling time, in turn increasing the risk of a reduction in LVEDV with a subsequent reduction in SV. Arrhythmia may also be present, particularly atrial fibrillation (AF).

Key Point

The combination of loss of the atrial kick and irregular fast heart rhythm in AF can reduce CO by up to 30% (Atherton et al. 2018). In a patient with reduced LVEF, this is poorly tolerated and can lead to acute pulmonary oedema.

Low CO may cause persistent hypotension. Patients with HF frequently have cool peripheries. This is partly an effect of reduced CO but may also be made worse by HF medications. In patients with HF hypotension may have systemic effects: for example, in the renal system there may be reduced urine output (*oliguria*) or even no urine at all produced (*anuria*) at the end of life. Liver function may decline. There may be cardiac ischaemia if the CO is not sufficient to perfuse the myocardium adequately. Confusion, dizziness and cognitive impairment may occur if cerebral perfusion is inadequate. Chronic hypotension is an important negative prognostic sign.

Malignant hypertension suggests aetiology of hypertensive cardiomyopathy (Clerkin et al. 2019).

Inspection and Palpation of the Precordium

Cardiac examination begins with palpation of the precordium. The point of maximal impulse (PMI) that should be felt on the chest wall over the apex of the heart will be displaced to a more left lateral position if left ventricular enlargement is present. Patients with chronic HF may have a diffuse PMI or a non-palpable PMI due to decrease in contractility. An LV heave may be present suggesting LVH.

Jugular Venous Pressure

Jugular venous pressure (JVP) is assessed. An elevated JVP (defined as venous pulsation height greater than 4 cm) has been shown to correlate with a pulmonary capillary wedge pressure (PCWP) above 18 mmHg (Clerkin et al. 2019). Hepatojugular reflux (distension of the neck veins precipitated by placing firm pressure over the liver) may be present.

Cardiac Auscultation

Cardiac auscultation may reveal various abnormalities. A patient with dyspnoea due to HF may include a gallop (S3 or S4) and/or a new or worsened murmur (e.g. acute mitral regurgitation, severe aortic stenosis). HFrEF is classically associated with an S3 gallop indicating an abnormal relation between the rate of rapid filling and the ventricle's ability to accommodate its increasing diastolic volume (Clerkin et al. 2019).

Pulmonary Examination

Typical findings are those of rales or pulmonary crackles, resulting from the opening of fluid compressed alveoli; however, these findings are not always present in chronic HF due to lymphatic compensation. Wheezing or 'cardiac asthma' may be present in up to a third of older patients with acute HF resulting from bronchospasm secondary to elevated pulmonary venous pressure in acute HF (Clerkin et al. 2019).

Pulmonary vascular congestion may lead to pleural effusions that tend to be greater on the right side (Clerkin et al. 2019). Tachypnoea, inability to lie flat, and varying degrees of respiratory distress may be present. Cheyne-Stokes respiration (CSR), a form of central sleep-disordered breathing in which there are cyclical fluctuations in breathing that lead to periods of central apnoea/hypopnoea alternating with periods of hyperpnoea, is associated with increased mortality and morbidity in subjects with variable degrees of HF. The crescendo-decrescendo pattern of respiration in CSR is a compensation for the changing levels of blood oxygen and carbon dioxide (AlDabal and BaHammam 2010).

Peripheries

Lower extremities are examined for oedema. Congestion or symptoms of systemic volume overload are common in HF, the most frequent of which is *peripheral oedema* (Clerkin et al. 2019). Peripheral oedema in HF is bilateral, pitting and begins to build in the most dependent areas. While peripheral oedema is a common consequence of HF, it may occur in other disease states and is common in older people. When fluid retention is due to HF other signs of higher preload may also be present, such as a raised JVP, tricuspid regurgitation, ascites and liver enlargement (*hepatomegely*).

Key Point

The JVP is usually elevated if peripheral oedema is due to HF (Colluci 2020).

Peripheral oedema in HF tends to build over several weeks and is influenced by gravity so that in mobile patients, it accumulates first in the feet, ankles and lower legs. It is hard to see oedema in the knees and thighs but more visible if it occurs in the genitalia, as may happen as volume overload increases. The abdomen is assessed for hepatomegaly or free fluid in the abdomen (*ascites*). In severe volume overload, fluid can build in the abdomen leading to symptoms of bloating, loss of appetite and pain and may lead to poor absorption from the gastrointestinal tract and reduced bioavailability of oral medications (Bowman et al. 2016). In immobile patients, fluid may settle around the sacrum. Inactivity impairs the ability of the venous system to mechanically return the fluid to the heart.

Key Point

Oedema results from an imbalance between hydrostatic pressure, oncotic pressure and vascular permeability. Traditionally this has

---

been explained as resulting from increases in venous hydrostatic pressure leading to fluid accumulation in the lungs, abdomen and periphery. More recently it has been recognised that oedema in HF is caused by systemic processes that lead to a catabolic state with decreased serum albumin (oncotic pressure) and increased pro-inflammatory cytokines (vessel permeability) that add to extravascular fluid accumulation (Clerkin et al. 2019).

Assessment of the skin may demonstrate mottling and coolness, both suggestive of low CO (Clerkin et al. 2019). Patients with chronic severe HF can have muscle-wasting (*cachexia*) through several pathophysiological processes (Lavie et al. 2014).

Heart Failure Classification

The severity of symptoms can be quantified using classification systems. The most commonly used is the New York Heart Association Classification (NYHA) scheme (Levin et al. 1994) (see Table 23.2). Although symptom severity correlates poorly with many measures of LV function there is a clear relationship between severity of symptoms and survival (Ponikowski et al. 2016).

Patients can move backward and forward between stages in the NYHA classification scheme.

The American College of Cardiology (ACC)/American Heart Association (AHA) HF Classification (Yancy et al. 2013) has four stages and differs from the NYHA classification in that it is based on HF progression and there is no moving backwards to prior stages of classification (see Table 23.3).

Whilst some patients present in severe acute HF requiring hospitalisation (see later section), an initial diagnosis of chronic HF is more common. Patients with chronic HF often present with varying patterns of symptoms and signs (see Box 23.1) suggestive of HF, prompting investigations

Table 23.2 New York Heart Association Classification (NYHA) scheme.

NYHA Class	Symptoms
I	No limitation of physical activity. Ordinary physical activity does not cause undue fatigue, palpitation, dyspnoea.
II	Slight limitation of physical activity. Comfortable at rest. Ordinary physical activity results in fatigue, palpitation, dyspnoea.
III	Marked limitation of physical activity. Comfortable at rest. Less than ordinary activity causes fatigue, palpitation or dyspnoea.
IV	Unable to carry on any physical activity without discomfort. Symptoms of HF at rest. If any physical activity is undertaken, discomfort increases.

Table 23.3 ACC/AHA heart failure classification.

Stage	Criteria
A	Patients at risk for HF who have not yet developed structural heart changes (i.e. those with diabetes, those with coronary disease without prior infarct)
B	Patients with structural heart disease (i.e. reduced EF, LVH, chamber enlargement) who have not yet developed symptoms of HF
C	Patients who have developed clinical HF
D	Patients with refractory HF requiring advanced intervention (i.e. biventricular pacemakers, LV assist device, transplantation)

leading to a definitive diagnosis. It is important though to remember that some patients, if well compensated or on treatment, may have a dysfunctional or structurally damaged heart without overt clinical presentation for HF. Absence of clinical signs and symptoms does not exclude a HF diagnosis. Conversely, the presence of certain signs and symptoms, such as breathlessness or leg oedema, does not confirm HF, as other conditions can also produce those symptoms. Severity of patient symptoms does not always correlate with the degree of objective cardiac dysfunction. For a diagnosis of HF, it is therefore necessary to confirm clinical symptoms and signs with objective investigations (NICE 2018).

Key Point

Patients with new onset HF may delay seeking help for symptoms as they may attribute them to another cause such as smoking. Increased public awareness of HF symptoms may help patients to recognise the disease and seek medical help earlier (Taylor et al. 2017)

Investigations

Transthoracic echocardiography (TTE) is the method of choice for assessment of myocardial systolic and diastolic function of both left and right ventricles (Ponikowsi et al. 2016) and is very important in the assessment and diagnosis of HF (see Chapter 8). It shows the shape and function of the heart through the cardiac cycle; the sizes of the chambers; the muscle function and shape; valve structure and flow; volumes, haemodynamics, pericardial effusions and thrombus. Further testing is sometimes necessary if echocardiogram images are sub-optimal or more detail is needed. Cardiac magnetic resonance (CMR) imaging (see Chapter 8) is acknowledged as the gold standard for the measurements of volumes, mass and EF of both the left and right ventricles, and is the best alternative cardiac imaging modality for patients with non-diagnostic echocardiographic studies (Ponikowski et al. 2016).

In patients who are suspected to have HF without a history of MI, a screening test is recommended prior to echocardiogram. This is a practical, staged approach, to contextualise results and avoid unnecessary investigations. A normal electrocardiogram (ECG) or *brain natriuretic peptide* (BNP) blood test can be used to rule out HF because both tests have a negative predictive value of around 95–98% (Ponikowski et al. 2016). If these tests are positive it does not confirm the patient has HF, but it does indicate heart disease is likely, so an echocardiogram is warranted. If the tests are negative, then alternative diagnosis should be explored. If another diagnosis is not found, then HF can be reconsidered, and testing arranged.

A 12-lead ECG is recommended in patients with either a suspected diagnosis or a new diagnosis of HF to assess cardiac rhythm, QRS duration and the presence of underlying conditions such as myocardial ischaemia or LVH (Atherton et al. 2018). Whilst no single ECG abnormality universally indicates HF, HF is unlikely in patients presenting with a completely normal ECG (sensitivity 89%); thus, the routine use of an ECG is recommended to rule out HF (McDonagh et al. 2021).

Brain natriuretic peptides (BNP) are hormones secreted by cardiomyocytes when the ventricle is strained. There are several types of BNP blood tests available, but the most common in clinical practice are BNP and NTproBNP (Saenger et al. 2016). Brain natriuretic peptides tests possess a high negative predictive value of 0.94–0.98, so a normal test almost rules out HF (McDonagh et al. 2021). A high BNP suggests that the heart is under strain but does not explain why: thus, an echocardiogram is needed. Caution needs to be exercised as BNPs also reduce with treatment and in obesity. Additionally, baseline BNP can rise above the normal range with other chronic conditions, such as renal and respiratory diseases. A very high BNP is an indicator of poor prognosis (Roberts et al. 2015).

Other investigations for patients with suspected HF are included in Box 23.3.

Key Point

Patients may present with asymptomatic structural or functional cardiac abnormalities that are precursors of HF. These precursors are related to poor outcomes and starting treatment at the precursor stage may reduce mortality in patients with asymptomatic systolic LV dysfunction (Ponikowski et al. 2016).

Suggested Resource:

The following website explains radiological evidence of HF on the CXR with examples:
Heart failure
Radiology assistant
https://radiologyassistant.nl/chest/chest-x-ray/heart-failure

---

Chronic Heart Failure Management

The treatment of chronic HF requires a multi-disciplinary approach and includes medications, management of contributing factors and associated conditions, cardiac rehabilitation and lifestyle modification, devices and cardiac surgery if indicated and palliative care at the end of life.

Medication Management

The evidence supporting medication management for patients with HFrEF has been in place for many years, but there is less evidence available for HFmrEF and HFpEF. For patients with HFpEF, diuretics are used to manage congestion and comorbidities including hypertension, IHD, diabetes and AF are actively managed (Atherton et al. 2018). Most drugs that have been shown to improve survival and reduce hospital admissions for patients with HFrEF are those that work to counteract the over-active compensatory neurohormonal pathways discussed earlier in this chapter.

Box 23.3   Investigations for patients presenting with dyspnoea.

Basic investigations	Rationale
Basic observations and cardiovascular examination (see Chapters 5 and 6)	• Assess for hypertension • Baseline values to aid in diagnosis, monitor treatment and progress of disease • Establish risk profile for heart disease (cardiovascular, rheumatic, congenital, inflammatory)
12-lead ECG (see Chapter 9)	• Detect evidence of chamber enlargement, prior infarction, arrhythmia, increased muscle mass (HCM), low voltage (infiltration e.g. amyloidosis) or conduction system abnormality (Clerkin et al. 2019). *Patients with HF almost always have an abnormal ECG, though these changes are often non-specific.*
CXR (see Chapter 8)	• Detect signs of cardiomegaly (cardiac silhouette occupies >50% of the thoracic diameter); upper lobe pulmonary venous diversion (cephalisation); interstitial opacities (peribronchovascular cuffing; Kerley B lines); airspace opacification (filling of alveoli with fluid – may have a 'perihilar' or 'batwing distribution); pleural effusion. • Identify alternative cardiac or non-cardiac cause of dyspnoea *A normal CXR does not rule out HF*
Laboratory tests • Biochemistry (E; U, Cr, LFTs) • CBE (FBE) (see Chapter 7)	• Provide baseline values to guide treatment and monitor progress of disease • Detect and assess comorbid conditions • Detect potential alternative causes for fluid overload

Further investigations	Rationale
Natriuretic peptides (BNP and NTproBNP) (see Chapter 7)	• Rule out HF in patients with undifferentiated dyspnoea in emergency and primary care settings. *Patients with normal BNP or NT proBNP are unlikely to have HF.*
Cardiac troponin (see Chapter 7)	• Identify or rule out acute myocardial infarction as a cause of HF
Arterial blood gases	• Quantify the level of hypoxia and acid–base status
Thyroid function tests	• Hyper- and hypothyroidism increase the risk of incident HF (Kannan et al. 2018).
Transthoracic echocardiography (see Chapter 8)	• Assess cardiac structure and function (including measurement of LVEF – a surrogate measure of systolic function). • Assist in HF classification to guide management. *Echocardiography is the most useful investigation in patients with suspected or confirmed HF.* *EF does not always correlate with symptoms.*
Right heart catheterisation	• Determine CO, evaluate intracardiac shunts and valve dysfunction. • Gold standard method for diagnosing pulmonary hypertension (Callan & Clark 2016).
Tests to detect myocardial ischaemia: Stress echocardiography, SPECT, CTCA (see Chapter 8)	• Non-invasive tests for myocardial ischaemia

Basic investigations	Rationale
Coronary angiography (see Chapter 8) • with ventriculography	• Detect coronary artery disease to allow for revascularization in suitable patients of maximise pharmacotherapy in those with ischaemic cardiomyopathy • Determine LVEF • Detect wall motion abnormalities (aneurysm, pseudo-aneurysm, VSD, Takotsubo syndrome) • Detect apical filling defect (may indicate thrombus) • Assess regurgitant lesions
Cardiac magnetic resonance imaging (CMR) (see Chapter 8)	• High-resolution images without ionising radiation. • Provides useful functional, structural and valvular information • Identification of myocardial disease, whether infiltrative (sarcoidosis, haemochromatosis, amyloidosis), hypertrophic, fibrotic (acute and chronic infarction), ischaemic (myocardial viability, stress) • Helps to differentiate between acute myocarditis and Takotsubo syndrome. *Limitations to the use of MRI include access to machines, patient claustrophobia and presence of implanted metal devices.*

Tests for causes of dyspnoea other than HF:
- Lung function tests
- Ventilation/perfusion lung scan
- High-resolution CT chest
- D-Dimer

ECG = electrocardiogram; CXR = chest X-ray; HCM = hypertrophic cardiomyopathy; E = electrolytes, U = urea; Cr = creatinine; LFTs = liver function tests; CBE = complete blood examination; FBE = full blood examination; BNP=B-type natriuretic peptide; NTproBNP = N-terminal pro b-type natriuretic peptide; SPECT = single-photon emission computed tomography; CTCA = computed tomography coronary angiogram; VSD = ventricular septal defect

These include angiotensin-converting enzyme inhibitors (ACE-i), combined angiotensin receptor blocker/neprilysin inhibitor (ARN-i) or angiotensin receptor blockers (ARB), beta-blockers, diuretics, mineralocorticoid receptor antagonist, If channel blockers and vasodilators. These are discussed briefly below.

Angiotensin-Converting Enzyme Inhibitors (ACEi)

ACE-i inhibit the activity of angiotensin-converting enzyme (ACE), a component of the renin–angiotensin–aldosterone system (RAAS) resulting in venous and arterial vasodilatation with a subsequent reduction in preload and afterload, therefore reducing the workload of the heart.

Randomised controlled trials (RCTs) have shown that ACE inhibition leads to symptomatic improvement, reduced hospitalisation and enhanced survival in patients with HFrEF (McMurray 2011; Yancy et al. 2013; McMurray et al. 2014; McDonagh et al. 2021). All patients with HFrEF should be treated with an ACE-i to reduce the risk of HF hospitalisation and death (McDonagh et al. 2021). ACE-i are usually started at low doses and titrated by doubling the dose every 2 weeks until the target dose or maximum tolerated dose is reached. BP and biochemistry (renal function, potassium) should be monitored at commencement, with each dose escalation and 6 monthly long-term. If hypotension or decreased renal function occurs, volume status is reviewed and the need for concurrent medications not shown to improve outcomes in HF that lower BP or impact renal function assessed. The ACE-i may need to be reduced or ceased. Angioedema is a rare complication requiring cessation of the ACE-i. If a dry cough is attributed to the ACE-I, it may have to be replaced by an ARB (Atherton et al. 2018).

Angiotensin II Receptor Blockers (ARB)

If patients have a contraindication to, or cannot tolerate, an ACE-i an (ARB) should be considered as an alternative. This class of drugs work in a similar way to ACE inhibitors but block the terminal phase of the RAAS mechanism, inhibiting the effect of angiotensin II.

Angiotensin Receptor Blocker/ Neprilysin Inhibitor

The latest drug recommended to treat HF is the combination drug of *valsartan* (an ARB) and sacubitril (a neprilysin inhibitor). This drug combination has shown superior benefits in reduction in cardiovascular mortality, hospitalisation and all-cause mortality compared to enalapril (an ACE-i) (McMurray et al. 2014). Current guidelines recommend its use as a replacement for an ACE-inhibitor, in HF patients without a contraindication to the drug who remain symptomatic despite optimal therapy with NYHA Class II–IV HF and an EF of <40% (McDonagh et al. 2021).

Beta Blockers

A beta blocker, specifically bisoprolol, carvedilol, metoprolol (controlled release or extended release) or nebivolol, is recommended in all patients with HFrEF once they are stabilised with no or minimal clinical congestion on physical examination, unless contraindicated or not tolerated to decrease mortality and hospitalisations (Atherton et al. 2018).

Key Point

Beta blockers are only indicated in cases of compensated, stable HF. Beta blockers will likely worsen symptoms by decreasing contractility in patients with acute decompensated HF.

Beta blockers counteract the effects of prolonged sympathetic stimulation and lead to improvement in LV systolic and diastolic function, heart rate control, prevention of malignant arrhythmias, lowering of both cardiac afterload and preload and contribute to reversal of remodelling in patients with chronic HF (Prijic and Buchhorn 2014). As with ACE-I, beta blockers are started at a low dose and gradually titrated up to the target dose. If the patient has a symptomatic bradycardia, volume status is reviewed and the need for concurrent medications not shown to improve outcomes in HF that lower heart rate is assessed. The beta blocker may need to be reduced if no alternative management solution is identified. In a patient with increasing congestion, increasing the diuretic dose usually resolves the problem but if not, the beta blocker dose may need to be reduced or temporarily withdrawn, especially if recently commenced (Atherton et al. 2018).

Key Point

Clinicians should aim for the target drug doses of ACE-I and beta blockers used in the randomised controlled trial that showed the benefits of these drugs in HF patients (Atherton et al. 2018). In practice, this can require careful management to achieve patient concordance.

Diuretics

A diuretic should be considered in patients with HF and clinical symptoms, or signs of congestion, to improve symptoms and manage congestion (Atherton et al. 2018). Patients with HF are at risk of fluid retention, because of the neurohormonal compensatory mechanisms stimulated by reduced CO. Fluid retention leads to symptoms including dyspnoea and peripheral oedema. Patients with excess fluid are also at high risk of hospitalisation and death (Shoaib et al. 2014), treatments are therefore centred on the need to achieve normal fluid levels (*euvolaemia*). Reducing circulating volume must be undertaken carefully to avoid rebound electrolyte shifts and acute renal failure.

Loop diuretics such as furosemide (frusemide) or bumetanide cause a brisk and short-lived diuresis. Thiazide diuretics, such as bendroflumethiazide, are less potent diuretics when used as monotherapy, but when used in combination with a loop diuretic achieve profound diuresis.

> **Key Point**
>
> Caution should be taken when combining diuretics because it can produce rapid urinary output and profound electrolyte imbalance.

Diuretics were widely introduced into clinical practice from the 1960s and predate large clinical trials, so lack the robust evidence-base of more modern drugs. Use of diuretics in HF without combining them with disease-modifying drugs such as ACE-i can result in worse outcomes and should be avoided (Andries et al. 2019).

> **Key Point**
>
> Patients may also be educated to adjust the dose of diuretic (e.g. increase furosemide (frusemide) dose by 40 mg daily if weight increases over 2 kg).

Mineralocorticoid Antagonists (MRAs)

Aldosterone is a mineralocorticoid hormone secreted by the adrenal cortex that both exerts a direct vasoconstrictive effect on blood vessels and stimulates the renal tubules to increase the reabsorption of sodium (and consequently water), resulting in increased circulating volume. Mineralocorticoid antagonists (MRA) may be useful in HF as they block the effects of aldosterone and exert a diuretic effect, although this effect is not as rapid or powerful as loop diuretics. *Spironolactone* is the most widely used mineralocorticoid antagonist but *Eplerenone* may be used if the patient has recently had a MI or experiences the side effect of gynaecomastia. An MRA is recommended in all patients with HFrEF associated with a moderate or severe reduction in LVEF unless contraindicated or not tolerated, to decrease mortality and decrease hospitalisation for HF (Atherton et al. 2018).

> **Key Point**
>
> MRAs increase excretion of potassium and are usually used with a non-potassium sparing diuretic to reduce the risk of hyperkalaemia.

If Channel Blockers

Ivabradine blocks the channel responsible for the cardiac pacemaker current, I(f), which regulates heart rate. Ivabradine has been shown to decrease the combined end point of cardiovascular mortality and hospitalisation for patients with chronic HF, an LVEF of less than or equal to 35% and a sinus rate of 70 bpm or above on top of background HF therapy (Swedberg et al. 2010). Although both beta-blockers and *Ivabradine* reduce heart rate, the evidence for using a beta-blocker is stronger and the available evidence does not support use of *Ivabradine* as a preferential alternative for beta-blocker treatment of HF (Teerlink 2010; Ponikowski et al. 2016). Ivabradine is usually started at 2.5–5.0 mg twice daily and gradually uptitrated aiming for a target dose of 7.5 mg twice daily or the maximum tolerated dose, aiming for a sinus rate between 50 and 60 beats/min. Ivabradine should be ceased if the patient develops permanent AF and reconsidered if the patient reverts to sinus rhythm (Atherton et al. 2018).

Vasodilators

The combination of *hydralazine* and *isosorbide dinitrate* (ISDN) reduces cardiac preload by achieving arterial and venous dilatation. *Hydralazine* and *ISDN* provide an alternative in patients in whom ACE-I or ARB are contraindicated or not tolerated. If symptomatic hypotension develops, volume status should be assessed and the need for other drugs not shown to improve outcomes in HF that lower BP (e.g. calcium channel blockers, diuretics) reviewed (Atherton et al. 2018).

Digoxin

Digoxin has been shown to have no effect on mortality but decreased hospitalisation in patients with chronic HF associated with an LVEF of less than or equal to 45%, and sinus rhythm on top of background therapy. Digoxin should not be prescribed to the detriment of starting other drugs that have been shown to decrease mortality in patients with HFrEF (Atherton et al. 2018).

Sodium-Glucose Co-Transporter 2 Inhibitors

Recent clinical trials of sodium-glucose co-transporter 2 (SGLT2) inhibitors dapagliflozin (McMurray et al. 2019) and empagliflozin (Packer et al. 2020) added to therapy with ACE-I/ARNI/beta-blocker/MRA reduced the risk of CV death and worsening HF in patients with HFrEF (McDonagh et al. 2021). Unless contraindicated or not tolerated, dapagliflozin or empagliflozin are recommended for all patients with HFrEF already treated with an ACE-I/ARNI, a beta-blocker and an MRA. The diuretic/natriuretic properties of SGLT2 inhibitors may offer additional benefits in reducing congestion and may allow a reduction in loop diuretic requirement (McDonagh et al. 2021).

Key Point

Titration of drugs to the optimal dose is often an important role for HF nurse specialists and requires skill and careful monitoring

---

to implement without triggering adverse effects. Atherton et al. (2018) describe the role of nurses and nurse practitioners in nurse-led titration clinics. This information can be accessed via the publication by Atherton et al. (2018) in the reference list (p. 1163).

Adherence with Drug Regimens in HF

Medication adherence is an important component of self-care for HF patients; however, adherence to medications is a common problem among HF patients with the consequences of HF exacerbations, reduced physical function and higher risk for hospital admission and death (Ruppar et al. 2016). There are many published studies of interventions to improve medication adherence for HF patients leading to lower risk of hospital admission (Ruppar et al. 2016; Daliri et al. 2021).

Learning Activity 23.1

Poor adherence to medications is a common cause of worsened HF, particularly diuretics and beta blockers. Are there any strategies that are used in your place of practice to improve adherence to medication for patients with HF? Refer to the published systematic reviews and meta-analyses by Ruppar et al. (2016) and Daliri et al. (2021) in the reference list for this chapter for a summary of studies of interventions to improve medication adherence in patients with HF.

Key Points

Patients with HF are usually prescribed multiple medications and have complex dosing regimens. On average, HF patients take 6.8 prescription medications per day, resulting in 10.1 doses a day, and this estimate does not include over the counter or complementary medications (Page et al. 2016). Harm due to medications is common during the transition from hospital to home for patients with HF (Daliri et al. 2021).

Drugs that Cause Harm in Heart Failure

There is a long list of drugs that may cause or exacerbate HF by *causing* direct myocardial toxicity; impairing contractility, myocardial relaxation or decreasing heart rate; exacerbating hypertension; delivering a high-sodium load or by interactions with other drugs that limit the beneficial effects of HF medications (Page et al. 2016). Refer to the publication by Page et al. (2016) (found in the reference list for this chapter) for an extensive list of these.

Learning Activity 23.2

Review the medication charts of three patients with chronic HF in your care. Are their medications optimised as advised in the latest guidelines? If not, is there a clear reason why not? You should choose the guidelines that are followed in your country (listed below) but be aware that developing guidelines takes time and evidence changes rapidly, so some of the guideline's recommendations may be superseded prior to the development of new guidelines.

Cardiac Electronic Implantable Devices

Implantable Cardioverter Defibrillator

Patients with HFrEF have an increased risk of arrhythmia and around half of all HF patients will die of a sudden ventricular arrhythmia (Zhang et al. 2018). The transvenous implantable cardioverter defibrillator (ICD) was developed in the 1980s and in randomised clinical trials showed a significant survival benefit with an ICD implanted after cardiac arrest due to sustained ventricular arrhythmias (Mark et al. 2006). Subsequently, ICD use was expanded to include patients with no history of ventricular arrhythmia but who were identified to be at high risk for such events due to reduced LVEF.

A subcutaneous ICD is now available, but it does not have a pacing function and less functionality compared with the transvenous ICD and thus is only suitable for patients with an indication for an ICD but no indication for pacing.

Cardiac Resynchronisation Therapy

Around 20–30% of symptomatic HF patients exhibit an intraventricular conduction delay (Bristow et al. 2004; Eschalier et al. 2015). In other words, the normal electrical pacing impulse in the heart is delayed across the ventricles. This abnormality results in prolongation of LV activation time, ventricular dyssynchrony and impaired ventricular pumping function. Cardiac resynchronisation therapy (CRT), otherwise known as biventricular pacing, is recommended to eliminate ventricular conduction delays and reduce dyssynchrony and improve symptoms, QoL and mortality rate in HF patients (Ponikowski et al. 2016). (see Chapter 12).

Key Point

Not all HF patients will benefit from an ICD, CRT or CRT-D (a CRT device with a defibrillator function). Patients with the longest intraventricular conduction delays and those with a left bundle branch block pattern benefit most from cardiac devices (McDonagh et al. 2021).

Ventricular Assist Devices

Ventricular assist devices (VADs) may be considered for circulatory support in patients with advanced HF in the following circumstances:

- As a bridge to transplantation or a bridge to transplant candidacy who are ineligible at the time but expected to become suitable following a period of VAD support.
- As a bridge to recovery in patients with severe HF following cardiac surgery or reversible cause.
- As destination therapy to prolong life and reduce symptoms in patients who are not eligible for transplant (Atherton et al. 2018; McDonagh et al. 2021).

Surgical Interventions in Heart Failure

Ischaemic Heart Disease

Coronary artery bypass graft surgery (CABG) may be considered for selected patients with HF and CAD for relief of angina and HF symptoms, and decreased morbidity and long-term mortality (Atherton et al. 2018). The role of percutaneous coronary intervention (PCI) compared with either medical therapy alone or against CABG has not been well studied in patients with LV dysfunction to date (Velazquez 2020). PCI or surgical revascularisation may be considered for symptomatic relief of angina in HFpEF, but there is no clear evidence that these procedures improve outcomes for this group of patients (Ponikowski et al. 2016). Data on the benefit of myocardial revascularisation in patients with HF are limited (McDonagh et al. 2021).

Valvular Heart Disease

Valvular heart disease may cause or aggravate HF (Ponikowski et al. 2016). Surgical or percutaneous mitral valve (MV) repair or replacement may be considered in selected patients with severe mitral regurgitation (MR) to improve symptoms (Atherton et al. 2018). Surgical aortic valve replacement (SAVR) is recommended in patients with severe aortic stenosis (AS) or severe aortic regurgitation (AR) and HF in the absence of major comorbidities or frailty, to improve symptoms and decrease mortality (Atherton et al. 2018). Transcatheter aortic valve implantation (TAVI) may be considered for patients with severe AS and HF who are considered at high operative risk or inoperable for SAVR, and who are deemed suitable for TAVI following assessment by a heart team to improve symptoms and decrease mortality (Atherton et al. 2018, Ponikowski et al. 2016).

Cardiac Transplantation

Cardiac transplantation may be a surgical option for some patients with end-stage HF and severely impaired functional capacity despite receiving optimal HF treatment. Only a small minority of patients with end-stage HF will be suitable candidates for cardiac transplant and the small number of donor organs available means cardiac transplant remains a low-volume surgical procedure.

Comorbidities in Heart Failure

Most patients with HF who have comorbidities that may exacerbate both the disease process and the clinical severity of HF contribute to poorer outcomes and impact the ability to deliver optimal HF treatment. A more detailed management of these comorbidities can be found in HF guideline publications (Ponikowski et al. 2016; Atherton et al. 2018) included in the reference list for this chapter.

Anaemia

Anaemia and iron deficiency are common and often overlap in patients with HF. Iron deficiency is the most common cause of anaemia, but vitamin B12 and folate deficiency and chronic kidney disease (CKD) can contribute. Anaemia can be complicated by haemodilution, inflammation and the use of some medications. Reversible causes of anaemia should be treated to improve QoL for HF patients (Atherton et al. 2018).

Key Point

Iron deficiency is associated with a poor prognosis in HF (Ponikowski et al. 2016). Improvements in self-reported patient global assessment, QoL, exercise capacity, NYHA class and reduced hospitalisations have been demonstrated in two randomised controlled trials for HF patients with serum ferritin <100 ug/l, or ferritin between 100 and 299 ug/l with transferrin <20%, both with or without anaemia (Filippatos et al. 2013; Ponikowski et al. 2015).

Arrhythmias

People with HF have complex, interactive and dynamic changes in mechanical, structural, neurohumoral, metabolic and electrophysiological properties that together increase the risk of tachyarrhythmias (Masarone et al. 2017). For further information about arrhythmia identification and management, see Chapter 11.

Supraventricular Arrhythmias

Supraventricular arrhythmias can exacerbate the HF by decreasing CO and need to be controlled with pharmacological, electrical or catheter-based intervention (Masarone et al. 2017). Atrial fibrillation (AF) is a common precipitant of HF and conversely, HF is the strongest predictor for AF (Atherton et al. 2018). HF with AF increases the risk of stroke, hospitalisation and is associated with a higher mortality (Verma et al. 2017). In the setting of atrial flutter or AF, anticoagulation becomes paramount to prevent systemic or cerebral embolism (Maserone et al. 2017).

Ventricular Arrhythmias

Hypo- and hyperkalaemia are common in HF and often associated drugs used in HF treatment. Bothe hypo- and hyperkalaemia can potentiate ventricular arrhythmias (Ponikowski et al. 2016). Management of ventricular arrhythmias depends on the type of arrhythmia, underlying structural heart disease and severity of HF and includes correction of electrolyte abnormalities, withdrawal of agents that might provoke arrhythmias, optimisation of HF therapy and possibly catheter ablation or ICD insertion (Masarone et al. 2017). Amiodarone may be considered (often in combination with a beta-blocker) to suppress symptomatic ventricular arrhythmias where other treatment options have not been successful (Ponikowski et al. 2016).

Bradycardia

People with HF may develop bradycardia caused by sinus node dysfunction or atrio-ventricular block that may require the insertion of a permanent pacemaker (Masarone et al. 2017).

Cachexia

Cachexia refers to generalised wasting affecting skeletal muscle and fat and bone tissue that occurs most commonly in people with advanced HF. Cachexia is associated with more severe HF symptoms, impaired mobility, increased hospitalisations and decreased survival. Potential treatments may include appetite stimulants, nutritional supplements and exercise training (McDonagh et al. 2021).

Chronic Kidney Disease, Hyperkalaemia and Hypokalaemia

A systematic review and meta-analysis by Smith et al. (2006) suggest that CKD is present in over 60% of patients with HF, with moderate to severe CKD in around one-third. Acute kidney injury (AKI) is relatively rare in HF and is likely associated with the combination of diuretic therapy with other potentially nephrotoxic drugs or contrast media (Ponikowski et al. 2016).

Chronic Obstructive Pulmonary Disease and Asthma

Around 20% of patients with HF have coexisting chronic obstructive pulmonary disease (COPD). COPD is under-recognised in patients with HFre and negatively impacts prognosis (Atherton et al. 2018). Careful assessment is required to determine whether an acute presentation with breathlessness is due to an exacerbation of COPD or HF decompensation.

Cognitive Impairment

Evidence suggests that a substantial proportion of patients with HF have concomitant cognitive problems (Cameron et al. 2017; Cannon et al. 2017). Impaired cognition involving memory, attention, problem-solving and psychomotor speed may be associated with poor engagement in self-care (Cameron et al. 2017).

Coronary Artery Disease

CAD is the most common cause of HFrEF and is present in around half of all people with

HF. Angina is associated with greater functional limitation in HF patients. See section above on 'Surgical interventions in HF'.

Depression

Depression is common in HF and is both a risk factor for the development of HF and a marker of poor prognosis for patients with HF. Suicide risk has been found to be higher in patients with HF compared with those without HF and was associated with high levels of hopelessness, depression, low self-esteem (Korkmaz et al. 2019). Screening for depression should be undertaken using a validated questionnaire. Cognitive behavioural therapy, pharmacological treatment and exercise training may be considered in patients with HF associated with depression (Atherton et al. 2018).

Diabetes

Diabetes affects 30–40% of patients with HF and is associated with a poorer prognosis that is independent of associated comorbidities (Atherton et al. 2018).

Erectile Dysfunction

Some drugs used in the treatment of HF may contribute to erectile dysfunction in males. Treatment includes optimisation of therapies for underlying diseases and comorbidities including anxiety and depression. Phosphodiesterase type 5 inhibitors such as sildenafil (Viagra) may improve exercise capacity and QoL in patients with HFrEF but are contraindicated in patients taking nitrates (Ponikowski et al. 2016).

Gout and Arthritis

Hyperuricaemia and gout are common in HF and may be caused or aggravated by diuretic therapy. Gout attacks are better treated with colchicine rather than with NSAIDs if not contraindicated. Osteoarthritis and rheumatoid arthritis are common comorbidities in elderly patients with HF. Options for effective pharmacological pain relief are limited and associated pain and joint deformities contribute to physical inactivity which can worsen HF clinical status.

Hypertension

Hypertension (HT) is more commonly found in HFpEF than in HFrEF. Many prescribed HF medications have the effect of lowering BP. Optimally treated HFrEF is rarely associated with HT. BP targets in HF are those recommended in HT guidelines (see Chapter 5).

Hyponatraemia

Hyponatraemia (sodium <135 mmol/l) occurs in around 20% of HF patients and is predominantly dilutional secondary to water retention and fluid overload. Potential reversible causes should be addressed but hyponatraemia is often chronic and thus correction is rarely urgent (Atherton et al. 2018).

Sleep-Disordered Breathing

Sleep-disordered breathing (SDB) affects 50–75% of patients with HF and is an adverse prognostic marker (Atherton et al. 2018). SDB may take the form of obstructive sleep apnoea (OSA) or central sleep apnoea (CSA). OSA is characterised by periodic narrowing and obstruction of the pharyngeal airway during sleep that causes episodes of apnoea. Positive pressure ventilation (PPV) may improve QoL and decrease sleepiness in patients with predominant OSA, but it does not reduce mortality (Atherton et al. 2018). Lifestyle changes, such as losing weight and reducing alcohol intake, are the first line of treatment for OSA. OSA has significant implications for cardiovascular health, mental illness, QoL and driving safety (Slowik and Collen 2020). Central sleep apnoea (CSA) refers to pauses in breathing due to absent respiratory effort or drive to breathe that occurs in a cyclic or intermittent fashion during sleep. CSR with CSA occurs in patients with HF and is characterised by cyclical episodes of apnoea and hyperventilation (Rudrappa et al. 2020). The primary aim in CSA is to treat the HF (Atherton et al. 2018).

Systems of Care

Systems of care (SoC), known in the UK as *'care bundles'*, are groups of interventions that are implemented to improve service delivery. SoC for HF management usually include a multidisciplinary team with the primary aims of reducing hospitalisations, improving survival and containing the rising costs of HF and pressures on the health system. Hospital-initiated case management can be successful in reducing unplanned hospital readmissions for HF and length of hospital stay for people with HF (Huntley et al. 2016) and should include structured follow-up with patient education, optimisation of medical treatment, psychosocial support, and improved access to care (Ponikowski et al. 2016; Atherton et al. 2018). Specialist HF nurses have a major role in these teams and lead HF disease management programs and medication titration clinics.

Key Point

The term 'heart failure' may cause fear and a concern in those diagnosed with the condition that the heart may stop or that outlook is poor. Similarly, they need an explanation about the normal range of LVEF (Taylor et al. 2017). When people are diagnosed with HF, they need a careful explanation about their condition to allay fear and anxiety.

Remote Monitoring

A major focus of HF management has been to identify decompensation of HF before there is a need for emergency hospital admission. Remote monitoring strategies to improve communication and monitoring of the HF patient include a range of audio, video and other telecommunication technologies. Structured telephone support (typically provided by HF specialist nurses) is usually a component of a remote HF management programme. Technology for remote monitoring is continuously evolving and includes devices that can monitor a range of physiological variables such as BP, heart rate and rhythm, body weight, oxygen saturation, body temperature, fluid status, blood glucose concentration, body posture and electrocardiograph. Devices may be standalone for use at home, implantable for collection of data or therapeutic purposes but have a data collection function (pacemakers, ICDs), or wearable technologies such as watches or patches. Data is transmitted to an HF practitioner and the patient is contacted if clinical variables change beyond preset limits. The patient may be reviewed over the phone or advised to attend the clinic and necessary changes to care are implemented, or in concerning cases, the patient may be advised to attend the emergency department (Brahmbhatt and Cowie 2019).

Self-Care and Self-Management in Patients with Heart Failure

Self-care refers to the behaviours developed by people to maintain their health (self-care maintenance) and their response to worsening of symptoms should they occur (self-care management) (Riegel et al. 2009). In the context of HF, self-care maintenance involves daily monitoring body weight, signs or symptoms; adherence to pharmacological recommendations; consumption of a low-salt diet; cessation of tobacco use; limiting alcohol consumption; recognising and seeking appropriate care in the event of HF decompensation. Self-management interventions have a beneficial effect on all-cause death and HF-related hospitalisation; thus, educating HF patients and their carers about the self-management should commence soon after diagnosis and be 'patient-centred, appropriate to their level of health literacy, culturally appropriate, and revised continually throughout the person's life' (Atherton et al. 2018, p. 1165).

> **Key Point**
>
> Reliance on self-management interventions may increase the risk of all-cause mortality for patients with moderate/severe depression (Jonkman et al. 2016).

Non-pharmacological Management of Heart Failure

HF-specific cardiac rehabilitation and other disease management approaches including exercise, disease-specific education, dietary advice, social support and follow-up by a nurse may help to optimise functional status, enhance the patient's sense of control, reduce the risk of hospitalisation and improve health-related QoL (Davidson et al. 2010; Long et al. 2019). A recent updated Cochrane systematic review supports the benefits of exercise-based cardiac rehabilitation for patients with HF in terms of probable reductions in the risk of all-cause and HF-specific hospitalisation and improved health-related QoL in people with HF (Taylor et al. 2019b). The patient should be counselled about smoking cessation, alcohol moderation, weight reduction (for those who are overweight) and control of other cardiovascular risk factors. The benefits of salt and fluid restrictions are not well evidenced, especially in chronic HF populations (McDonagh et al. 2021). Fluid restriction should not be recommended to all patients with HF but may be used as a temporary measure in those with decompensated HF and/or those with hyponatraemia (Johansson et al. 2016).

End of Life

A diagnosis of HF does not necessarily mean the patient is imminently nearing the end of life, but HF is a common cause of death due to progressive pump failure or arrhythmia. Advance care planning is essential for patients with HF so that the patient and their family have an opportunity to express their concerns and preferences for end-of-life care. Patients with end-stage HF need the same expert care as anyone else nearing the end of life. Palliative care and community nursing services can provide support and avoid unwanted and futile hospital admissions. Recognising when patients with HF are approaching the end of their life can be difficult, as the progression of HF, unlike other palliative conditions, is unpredictable. Nonetheless, some important signs of deterioration can be used to guide care. These include declining renal function without a reversible cause, very high BNP levels, intractable symptoms and cognitive and psychological changes (Whellan et al. 2014). Without adequate treatment at home hospital admissions may also increase.

Traditionally the focus of end-of-life care shifts from active treatment to symptom palliation, but many HF drugs help to control symptoms and should be continued. Other treatments, such as statins, may become less significant. Many patients with HF will have had an ICD implanted in the earlier stages of HF. Repeated activation of the ICD in the final moments of life is inappropriate and distressing (Weterdahl et al. 2015); thus, it is sensible to wirelessly deactivate defibrillator functions on devices in the terminal phase of end of life. Where patients have a combined biventricular pacemaker and defibrillator (CRT-D), only the defibrillator function needs to be deactivated.

Acute Heart Failure

Acute HF (AHF) may occur as a first presentation of HF, but more often it is a result of decompensation in a patient with chronic HF. The causes of acute decompensated HF (ADHF) are multiple and varied, ranging from patient factors, disease state factors and comorbidities (Atherton et al. 2018). Factors known to be triggers for ADHF include acute coronary syndrome (ACS) and acute mechanical complications of ACS, tachy- and bradyar-rhythmias, severe hypertension, infection, toxic substances including medications (see Table 23.1), pulmonary disorders (exacerbation of chronic obstructive pulmonary disease, pulmonary embolism), surgery and perioperative complications, conditions associated with increased sympathetic drive, metabolic or hormonal derangements (see Table 23.1) or stroke (Atherton et al. 2018).

Key Point

Patients with AHF often constitute a medical emergency. Treating the precipitating factors for HF as well as the symptomatic acute decompensation has been shown to improve outcomes and response to therapy, but seeking a precipitating factor should not delay emergency management (Atherton et al. 2018).

The components of the history and physical examination may be used to classify a patient with AHF into one of four profiles reflecting congestion and systemic perfusion: dry and warm, wet and warm, cold and wet or cold and dry. Classification of patients into these profiles can be used to identify precipitants, tailor therapy and predict outcomes (Clerkin et al. 2019). See Figure 23.1.

Oxygen Therapy

Patients with AHF should have levels of peripheral arterial oxygen saturation monitored. Oxygen therapy is recommended in patients with oxygen saturation levels below 94% with oxygen delivery titrated to target levels of 94–98% unless the patient is at risk of hypercapnoea, in which case the target oxygen saturation should be 88–92%. Oxygen therapy should not be used in non-hypoxic patients as it causes vasoconstriction (including coronary

	No congestion (dry)	Congestion (wet)
Good perfusion (warm) **Compensated**	**Warm and dry** • PCWP normal • CI normal	**Warm and wet** • PCWP elevated • CI normal
Poor perfusion (cold)	**Cold and dry** • PCWP low-normal • CI decreased	**Cold and wet** • PCWP elevated • CI decreased

Markers of congestion
- Orthopnoea
- PND
- Elevated JVP
- Positive HJR
- S3 heart sound
- Ascites
- Hepatomegaly
- Peripheral oedema

Markers of low CO
- Cool extremities
- Narrow PPP
- Altered mental status
- Oliguria
- Hypotension*

PCWP = pulmonary capillary wedge pressure; CI = cardiac index; PND = paroxysmal nocturnal dyspnoea; JVP = jugular venous pressure; HJR = hepatojugular reflex; PPP = proportional pulse pressure

* Only 5–8% of all patients present with hypotensive AHF, which is associated with poor prognosis, particularly when hypoperfusion is also present (Ponikowski et al. 2016).

Figure 23.1 Profiles of acute heart failure.

vasoconstriction), a reduction in CO, and possible oxygen-free radical damage (Ponikowski et al. 2016; Atherton et al. 2018).

Ventilatory Support

In patients with pulmonary oedema or congestion with respiratory distress, ventilatory support with continuous positive airway pressure (CPAP) or bi-level positive pressure (BiPAP) ventilation may be required. Intubation may be required if the patient remains hypoxaemic (oxygen saturation < 94%) or hypercapnic ($PaCO_2 > 50$ mm Hg) and develops respiratory fatigue (Ponikowski et al. 2016; Atherton et al. 2018).

Circulation

In the 'wet and warm' patient, pharmacotherapy generally includes diuretics and vasodilators, whereas vasopressors may be considered for 'wet and cold' patients.

Key Point

Poor response to diuretic therapy (persistent signs and symptoms of congestion despite increasing doses of diuretic) is common in AHF (Trullàs et al. 2019). Causes of diuretic resistance include poor adherence to drug therapy or dietary sodium restriction, pharmacokinetic issues and compensatory

---

increases in sodium reabsorption in nephron sites that are not blocked by the diuretic (Hoorn and Ellison 2017). A combination of diuretics may be required to overcome diuretic resistance (Ponikowski et al. 2016).

Opiates

Opiates relieve dyspnoea and anxiety but routine use is not recommended in AHF. They may be considered with caution in patients who have severe dyspnoea, usually associated with pulmonary oedema. Opiates may cause bradycardia and hypotension as well as respiratory depression which may increase the risk of needing invasive ventilation. Opiates can cause nausea and vomiting which may increase the risk of aspiration for patients with non-invasive ventilation (McDonagh et al. 2021).

Conclusion

HF places a significant burden on health systems and individuals. In modern times diuretics, neurohormonal medication, cardiac devices and transplant offer patients a longer and better QoL after diagnosis. The management of failing hearts is likely to continue to progress and improve in the next few decades as new therapies emerge.

References

AlDabal, L. and BaHammam, A.S. (2010). Cheyne-stokes respiration in patients with heart failure. *Lung* **188** (1): 5–14.

Alpert, C.M., Smith, M.A., Hummel, S.L., and Hummel, E.K. (2017). Symptom burden in heart failure: assessment, impact on outcomes, and management. *Heart Failure Reviews* **22** (1): 25–39.

Andries, G., Yandrapalli, S., and Aronow, W.S. (2019). Benefit–risk review of different drug classes used in chronic heart failure. *Expert Opinion on Drug Safety* **18** (1): 37–49.

Atherton, J.J., Sindone, A., De Pasquale, C.G., Driscoll, A., MacDonald, P.S., Hopper, I., . . . & Thomas, L. (2018). National Heart Foundation of Australia and Cardiac Society of Australia and New Zealand: guidelines for the prevention, detection, and management of heart failure in Australia 2018. *Heart, Lung and Circulation*, **27** (10), 1123–1208. https://doi.org/10.1016/j.hlc.2018.06.1042.

Borlaug, B.A. & Colucci, S.W. (2019). Treatment and prognosis of heart failure with preserved ejection fraction. *UptoDate*. www.uptodate.com.

Bowman, B.N., Nawarskas, J.J., and Anderson, J.R. (2016). Treating diuretic resistance: an overview. *Cardiology in Review* **24** (5): 256–260.

Brahmbhatt, D.H., & Cowie, M.R. (2019). Remote management of heart failure: an overview of telemonitoring technologies. *Cardiac Failure Review*, **5** (2), 86. doi: https://doi.org/10.15420/cfr.2019.5.3.

Bristow, M.R., Saxon, L.A., Boehmer, J. et al. (2004). Cardiac-resynchronization therapy with or without an implantable defibrillator in advanced chronic heart failure. *New England Journal of Medicine* **350**: 2140–2150.

British Society for Heart Failure. (2017). National Heart Failure Audit 2015/16. www.ucl.ac.uk/nicor/audits/heartfailure/documents/annualreports/annual-report-2015-6-v8.pdf.

Butler, J., Anker, S.D., and Packer, M. (2019). Redefining heart failure with a reduced ejection fraction. *JAMA* **322** (18): 1761–1762.

Callan, P. and Clark, A.L. (2016). Right heart catheterisation: indications and interpretation. *Heart* **102** (2): 147–157.

Cameli, M., Pastore, M.C., De Carli, G. et al. (2019). ACUTE HF score, a multiparametric prognostic tool for acute heart failure: a real-life study. *International Journal of Cardiology* **296**: 103–108.

Cameron, J, Gallagher, R, & Pressler, S.J. (2017). Detecting and managing cognitive impairment to improve engagement in heart failure self-care. *Current Heart Failure Reports*, **14** (1), 13–22. https://doi.org/10.1007/s11897-017-0317-0.

Cannon, J.A., Moffitt, P., Perez-Moreno, A.C. et al. (2017). Cognitive impairment and heart failure: systematic review and meta-analysis. *Journal of Cardiac Failure* **23** (6): 464–475. https://doi.org/10.1016/j.cardfail.2017.04.007.

Clerkin, K.J., Mancini, D.M., and Lund, L.H. (2019). Chapter 6: Diagnosis of heart failure. In: *Heart Failure* (ed. D.S. Feldman and P. Mohacsi). Springer International Publishing Imprint: Springer. https://doi.org/10.1007/978-3-319-98184-0.

Colluci, W.S. (2020). Evaluation of the patient with suspected heart failure. *UpToDate*. www.uptodate.com.

Cook, C., Cole, G., Asaria, P. et al. (2014). The annual global economic burden of heart failure. *International Journal of Cardiology* **171** (3): 368–376.

Corotto, P., McCarey, M., Adams, S. et al. (2013). Heart failure patient adherence: epidemiology, cause and treatment. *Heart Failure Clinics* **9** (1): 49–58.

Dahlström, U. (2019). Chapter 1: Epidemiology of heart failure. In: *Heart Failure* (ed. D.S. Feldman and P. Mohacsi). Springer.

Daliri, S., Boujarfi, S., El Mokaddam, A. et al. (2021). Medication-related interventions delivered both in hospital and following discharge: a systematic review and meta-analysis. *BMJ Quality & Safety* **30** (2): 146–156.

Davidson, P.M., Cockburn, J., Newton, P.J. et al. (2010). Can a heart failure-specific cardiac rehabilitation program decrease hospitalizations and improve outcomes in high-risk patients? *European Journal of Cardiovascular Prevention and Rehabilitation* **17** (4): 393–402.

Eschalier, R., Ploux, S., Ritter, P. et al. (2015). Nonspecific intraventricular conduction delay: definitions, prognosis, and implications for cardiac resynchronization therapy. *Heart Rhythm* **12** (5): 1071–1079.

Filippatos, G., Farmakis, D., Colet, J.C. et al. (2013). Intravenous ferric carboxymaltose in iron-deficient chronic heart failure patients with and without anemia: a subanalysis of the FAIR-HF trial. *European Journal of Heart Failure* **15** (11): 1267–1276.

Hajouli, S. and Ludhwani, D. (2020). Heart Failure and Ejection Fraction. [Updated 2020 August 10]. In: StatPearls [Internet]. Treasure Island (FL): StatPearls Publishing; 2020 January-. https://www.ncbi.nlm.nih.gov/books/NBK553115/?report=reader#_NBK553115_pubdet.

Hoorn, E.J. and Ellison, D.H. (2017). Diuretic resistance. *American Journal of Kidney Diseases* **69** (1): 136–142.

Huntley, A.L., Johnson, R., King, A., Morris, R.W. & Purdy, S. (2016). Does case management for patients with heart failure based in the community reduce unplanned hospital admissions? A systematic review and meta-analysis. *BMJ Open*, **6** (5), [e010933]. https://doi.org/10.1136/bmjopen-2015-010933.

Johansson, P., van der Wal, M.H., Strömberg, A. et al. (2016). Fluid restriction in patients with heart failure: how should we think? *European Journal of Cardiovascular Nursing* **15** (5): 301–304.

Jonkman, N.H., Westland, H., Groenwold, R.H. et al. (2016). Do self-management interventions work in patients with heart failure? An individual patient data meta-analysis. *Circulation* **133** (12): 1189–1198.

Kannan, L., Shaw, P.A., Morley, M.P. et al. (2018). Thyroid dysfunction in heart failure and cardiovascular outcomes. *Circulation: Heart Failure* **11** (12): e005266.

Korkmaz, H., Korkmaz, S., and Çakar, M. (2019). Suicide risk in chronic heart failure patients and its association with depression, hopelessness and self esteem. *Journal of Clinical Neuroscience* **68**: 51–54.

Lavie, C., De Shutter, A., Alpert, M. et al. (2014). Obesity paradox, cachexia, frailty and heart failure. *Heart Failure Clinics* **10** (2): 319–326.

Levin, R., Dolgin, M., Fox, C., and Gorlin, R. (1994). The Criteria Committee of the New York Heart Association: nomenclature and criteria for diagnosis of diseases of the heart and great vessels. *LWW Handbooks* **9**: 344.

Long, L., Mordi, I.R., Bridges, C., Sagar, V.A., Davies, E.J., Coats, A.J., . . . & Taylor, R.S. (2019). Exercise-based cardiac rehabilitation for adults with heart failure. *Cochrane Database of Systematic Reviews*, (1): CD003331. doi: https://doi.org/10.1002/14651858.CD003331.pub5.

Mark, D.B., Nelson, C.L., and Anstrom, K.J. (2006). Cost-effectiveness of defibrillator therapy or amiodarone in chronic stable heart failure: results from the Sudden Cardiac Death in Heart Failure Trial (SCD-HeFT). *Circulation* **114** (2): 135–142.

Masarone, D., Limongelli, G., Rubino, M. et al. (2017). Management of arrhythmias in heart failure. *Journal of Cardiovascular Development and Disease* **4** (1): https://doi.org/10.3390/jcdd4010003.

McDonagh, T.A., Metra, M., Adamo, M., Gardner, R.S., Baumbach, A., Böhm, M., Burri, H., Butler, J., Čelutkienė, J., Chioncel, O., Cleland, J.G.F., Coats, A.J.S., Crespo-Leiro, M.G., Farmakis, D., Gilard, M., Heymans, S., Hoes, A.W., Jaarsma, T., Jankowska, E.A., & Lainscak, M. (2021). 2021 ESC Guidelines for the diagnosis and treatment of acute and chronic heart failure. *European Heart Journal*, **42** (36), 3599–3726. https://doi.org/10.1093/eurheartj/ehab368.

McMurray, J.J. (2011). CONSENSUS to EMPHASIS: the overwhelming evidence which makes blockade of the renin–angiotensin–aldosterone system the cornerstone of therapy for systolic heart failure. *European Journal of Heart Failure* **13** (9): 929–936.

McMurray, J.J.V., Packer, M., Desai, A.S. et al. (2014). Angiotensin – neprilysin inhibition versus enalapril in heart failure. *New England Journal of Medicine* **371** (11): 993–1004.

McMurray, J.J., Solomon, S.D., Inzucchi, S.E. et al. (2019). Dapagliflozin in patients with heart failure and reduced ejection fraction. *New England Journal of Medicine* **381** (21): 1995–2008.

Monza, K., Harris, D., and Shaw, C. (2015). The role of the nurse navigator in the management of the heart failure patient. *Critical Care Nursing Clinics* **27** (4): 537–549.

NICE (2018). Chronic Heart Failure in Adults: Diagnosis and management. www.nice.org.uk/guidance/ng106.

Packer, M., Anker, S.D., Butler, J. et al. (2020). Cardiovascular and renal outcomes with empagliflozin in heart failure. *New England Journal of Medicine* **383** (15): 1413–1424.

Page, R.L., O'Bryant, C.L., Cheng, D. et al. (2016). Drugs that may cause or exacerbate heart failure: a scientific statement from the American Heart Association. *Circulation* **134** (6): e32–e69.

Parenica, J., Spinar, J., Vitovec, J. et al. (2013). Long-term survival following acute heart failure: the Acute Heart Failure Database Main registry (AHEAD Main). *European Journal of Internal Medicine* **24** (2): 151–160.

Pfeffer, M.A., Shah, A.M., and Borlaug, B.A. (2019). Heart failure with preserved ejection fraction in perspective. *Circulation Research* **124** (11): 1598–1617.

Ponikowski, P., Van Veldhuisen, D.J., Comin-Colet, J. et al. (2015). Beneficial effects of long-term intravenous iron therapy with ferric carboxymaltose in patients with symptomatic heart failure and iron deficiency. *European Heart Journal* **36** (11): 657–668.

Ponikowski, P., Voors, A.A., Anker, S.D., Bueno, H., Cleland, J.G.F., Coats, A.J.S. . . . van der Meer, P. (2016). ESC Guidelines for the diagnosis and treatment of acute and chronic heart failure. *European Heart Journal*, http://eurheartj.oxfordjournals.org/content/ehj/early/2016/06/08/eurheartj.ehw128.full.pdf.

Prijic, S. and Buchhorn, R. (2014). Mechanisms of beta-blockers action in patients with heart failure. *Reviews on Recent Clinical Trials* **9** (2): 58–60.

Quach, S., Blais, C., and Quan, H. (2010). Administrative data have high variation in validity for recording heart failure. *The Canadian Journal of Cardiology* **26** (8): e306–e312.

Riegel, B., Lee, C.S., Dickson, V.V., and Carlson, B. (2009). An update on the self-care of heart failure index. *The Journal of Cardiovascular Nursing* **24** (6): 485.

Roberts, E., Ludman, A.J., Dworzynski, K. et al. (2015). NICE Guideline Development Group for Acute Heart Failure. The diagnostic accuracy of the natriuretic peptides in heart failure: systematic review and diagnostic meta-analysis in the acute care setting. *British Medical Journal* 350: h910.

Roger, V.L. (2013). Heart failure compendium: epidemiology of heart failure. *Circulation Research* 113 (6): 646–659.

Rudrappa, M., Modi, P., and Bollu, P.C. (2020). Cheyne Stokes Respirations. [Updated 2020 August 8]. In: StatPearls [Internet]. Treasure Island (FL): StatPearls Publishing; 2020 January-. https://www.ncbi.nlm.nih.gov/books/NBK448165.

Ruppar, T.M., Cooper, P.S., Mehr, D.R. et al. (2016). Medication adherence interventions improve heart failure mortality and readmission rates: systematic review and meta-analysis of controlled trials. *Journal of the American Heart Association* **5** (6): e002606. https://www.ahajournals.org/doi/pdf/10.1161/JAHA.115.002606.

Saenger, A., Rodriguez-Fraga, O., Ranka, L. et al. (2016). Specifity of B-type natriuretic peptide assays. *Clinical Chemistry* **63** (1): 351–358.

Sahle, B.W., Owen, A.J., Mutowo, M.P. et al. (2016). Prevalence of heart failure in Australia: a systematic review. *BMC Cardiovascular Disorders* **16** (1): 32.

Shoaib, A., Waleed, M., Khan, S. et al. (2014). Breathlessness at rest is not the dominant presentation of patients admitted with heart failure. *European Journal of Heart Failure* **16** (12): 1283–1291.

Sibetcheu, A.T., Agbor, V.N., Nyaga, U.F. et al. (2018). Epidemiology of heart failure in pediatric populations in low-and middle-income countries: a protocol for a systematic review. *Systematic Reviews* **7** (1): 52.

Slowik, J.M. and Collen, J.F. (2020). Obstructive Sleep Apnea. [Updated 2020 June 7]. In: StatPearls [Internet]. Treasure Island (FL): StatPearls Publishing; 2020 January-. https://www.ncbi.nlm.nih.gov/books/NBK459252.

Smith, G.L., Lichtman, J.H., Bracken, M.B. et al. (2006). Renal impairment and outcomes in heart failure: systematic review and meta-analysis. *Journal of the American College of Cardiology* **47** (10): 1987–1996.

Swedberg, K., Komajda, M., Borer, J.S. et al. (2010). Ivabradine and outcomes in chronic heart failure (SHIFT): a randomized placebo-controlled study. *The Lancet* **376** (9744): 875–885.

Taylor, C.J., Hobbs, F.D.R., Marshall, T. et al. (2017). From breathless to failure: symptom onset and diagnostic meaning in patients with heart failure – a qualitative study. *BMJ Open* 7: e013648.

Taylor, G.J., Ordonez-Mena, J.M., Roalfe, A.K., Lay-Flurrie, S., Jones, N.R., Marshall, T. & Hobbs, J.D.R. (2019a) Trends in survival after a diagnosis of heart failure in the United Kingdom 2000–2017: population based cohort study. *BMJ*, *364*, 1223. doi: https://doi.org/10.1136/bmj.l223.

Taylor, R.S., Long, L., Mordi, I.R. et al. (2019b). Exercise-based rehabilitation for heart failure: cochrane systematic review, meta-analysis, and trial sequential analysis. *JACC: Heart Failure* 7 (8): 691–705.

Teerlink, J.R. (2010). Ivabradine in heart failure – no paradigm SHIFT. . .yet. *The Lancet* **376**: 847.

Trullàs, J.C., Casado, J., Morales-Rull, J.L. et al. (2019). Prevalence and outcome of diuretic resistance in heart failure. *Internal and Emergency Medicine* 14 (4): 529–537.

Velazquez, E.J. (2020). Percutaneous coronary intervention or coronary artery bypass grafting to treat ischemic cardiomyopathy? *JAMA Cardiology* **5** (6): 641–642.

Verma, A., Kalman, J.M., & Callans, D.J. (2017). Treatment of patients with atrial fibrillation and heart failure with reduced ejection fraction. *Circulation*, **135** (16), 1547–1563. DOI: https://doi.org/10.1161/CIRCULATIONAHA.116.02605.

Viana, M., Laszczynska, O., Mendes, S. et al. (2014). Medication adherence to specific drug classes in chronic heart failure. *Journal of Managed Care and Speciality Pharmacy* **20** (10): 1018–1026.

Weterdahl, A., Sutton, R., and Frykman, V. (2015). Defibrillator patients should not be denied a peaceful death. *International Journal of Cardiology* **182**: 440–446.

Whellan, D.J., Goodlin, S.J., Dickinson, M.G. et al. (2014). End-of-life care in patients with heart failure. *Journal of Cardiac Failure* **20** (2): 121–134.

Yancy, C.W., Jessup, M., Bozkurt, B. et al. (2013). ACCF/AHA guideline for the management of heart failure: a report of the American College of Cardiology Foundation/American Heart Association Task Force on practice guidelines. *Journal of the American College of Cardiology* **62** (16): e147–e239.

Zhang, D., Tu, H., Wadman, M.C., and Li, Y.L. (2018). Substrates and potential therapeutics of ventricular arrhythmias in heart failure. *European Journal of Pharmacology* **15** (833): 349–356.

Ziaeian, B. and Fonarow, G.C. (2016). Epidemiology and etiology of heart failure. *Nature Reviews Cardiology* **13** (6): 368–378.

24

Congenital Heart Disease

Robyn Lotto, Christopher Nicholson, and Angela M. Kucia

Overview

This chapter will introduce the formation and management of congenital heart defects, valve abnormalities and genetic cardiomyopathies. Strictly speaking *congenital* refers to defects occurring at birth but is commonly used to describe defects that occur during foetal development, at birth or immediately after. Congenital heart disease is a complex sub-specialty of cardiac care. This chapter is presented as an introductory view to congenital heart disease, focusing on the continued needs of the congenital heart disease population into adulthood.

> **Learning Objectives**
>
> After reading this chapter, you should be able to:
>
> - Describe major congenital cardiac abnormalities.
> - Describe foetal blood flow and relationship to heart defect.
> - Discuss the anatomy and pattern of blood flood flow leading to cyanotic and acyanotic congenital heart disease.
> - Discuss specific health issues relating to adults with congenital heart disease.
> - Discuss the need for ongoing monitoring and follow-up for adults with congenital heart disease.

> **Key Concepts**
>
> Congenital heart disease; genetic heart disease; cyanotic and acyanotic heart disease; cardiac shunt; Eisenmenger syndrome

Background

Congenital heart defects are a heterogeneous group of abnormalities, ranging in severity and associated outcome. Critical cases of congenital heart disease (CHD) may be incompatible with survival without specific intervention in the newborn period/early infancy, whilst other forms may not require intervention until adulthood, and milder forms may not require any intervention at all (Patel et al. 2015). In some instances, an anomaly may be identified antenatally through screening, but others are not identified until after birth.

Epidemiology

CHD refers to a structural abnormality of the heart and great vessels present at birth that is, or could be, of functional significance. It is the most common birth defect and affects approximately 1% of all liveborn infants. In high-income countries, CHD has in part been attributed to maternal factors such as increased obesity and diabetes (Morris et al. 2018).

However, significant geographical variations exist, influenced by intrinsic maternal and environmental factors, as well as extrinsic factors such as access to antenatal screening, diagnostics and wider policies and laws (for example, options for termination) (Knowles et al. 2017).

Before the era of cardiac surgery, a serious congenital defect would usually result in death. Improved diagnostic techniques, as well as medical and surgical interventions, have resulted in 10-year survival rates exceeding 80% even in complex cases of CHD (Schwerzmann et al. 2017), but CHD remains the leading cause of mortality from birth defects in the developed world, and many patients with CHD have significant cardiac and extracardiac comorbidities that affect their quality of life, with neurodevelopmental disabilities having the largest impact (Zaidi and Brueckner 2017).

Antenatal detection of severe congenital heart defects is associated with a reduction in mortality and morbidity (Van Velzen et al. 2015; Thakur et al. 2016). In some instances, parents-to-be may make the decision to terminate the pregnancy (Smith et al. 2011), whilst for others, antenatal detection provides the opportunity to optimise follow-up and make plans for appropriate birthing procedures.

Key Point

Improved detection and management of CHD means that there are now more adults than children living with CHD (Zaidi and Brueckner 2017).

Risk Factors for the Development of Congenital Heart Disease

Various risk factors are associated with the development of a congenital heart defect. Many cases of CHD are multifactorial and result from a combination of genetic predisposition and environmental risk factors (Ossa Galvis et al. 2020). These include gene defects, chromosomal disorders, environmental factors or infections, teratogens or micronutrient deficiencies, but the anomaly cannot be attributed to a specific cause in around 80% of cases (Blue et al. 2012; Feldkamp et al. 2017). Several forms of CHD are associated with underlying syndromes including Down syndrome (also know as Trisomy 21), Turner syndrome, Klinefelter syndrome, Noonan syndrome, Williams syndrome, DiGeorge syndrome (velocardiofacial syndrome) and Holt-Oram syndrome (Stout et al. 2019). Down syndrome is the most common cause of chromosomal CHD.

Suggested Resource Website

If you would like to know more about genetic aspects of heart disease, read the following article:
Pierpont, M. E., Brueckner, M., Chung, W. K. et al. (2018). Genetic basis for congenital heart disease: revisited: a scientific statement from the American Heart Association. *Circulation* 138 (21): e653–e711. https://doi.org/10.1161/CIR.0000000000 000606

Maternal factors that have been associated with CHD include pregestational diabetes, phenylketonuria, obesity, exposure to smoking, alcohol and some drugs, infections such as rubella, whereas periconceptional folic acid supplementation or fortification has been found to have a protective effect (Roos-Hesselink and Johnson 2017; Dolk et al. 2020).

Key Point

The vast majority of foetal heart defects are seen in families <u>without</u> a known risk factor for CHD, which highlights the importance of having an effective screening program to detect foetal heart disease (Roos-Hesselink and Johnson 2017).

Embryology

The heart begins as a flat sheet of cells near the head of the embryo See Figure 24.1. By day 19 after conception, these cells form into two *endocardial tubes* with endothelial, myocardial and pericardial layers. Around day 22, these endocardial tubes merge into a single tube that forms the *primitive heart tube*. This tube has five regions from top to bottom: *truncus arteriosus, bulbus cordis, primitive ventricle, primitive atrium,* and *sinus venosus.* The heart develops by looping, ballooning and reforming these regions into atrial, ventricular and outflow tract areas, which then differentiate into the left and right heart structures seen in the mature heart (Moorman et al. 2003).

In the foetus, the heart is the first organ to begin functioning and beats by day 21 or 22 with the formation of the primitive heart. Cardiac cells (*myocytes*) spontaneously contract by electrical depolarisation. Specialised conducting tissue develops in the *primitive atrium* and *sinus venosus* into the *sinoatrial* and *atrioventricular* nodes, respectively. The foetal heart rate starts at a similar rate to the mother's

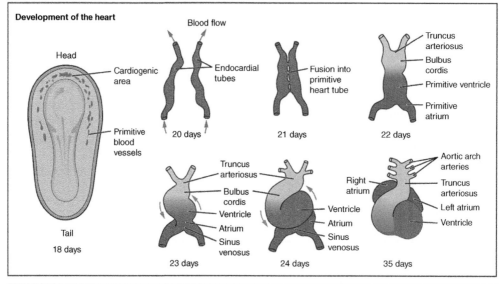

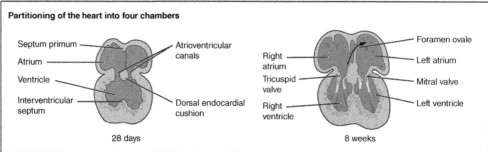

Figure 24.1 The developmental stages of a human heart beginning with the fusion of two endocardial tubes up to specific compartmentalisation. *Source:* Illustration of development of heart by OpenStax is licensed under a CC Attribution 4.0 International License. Accessed from https://openstax.org/books/anatomy-and-physiology/pages/19–5-development-of-the-heart#fig-ch20_05_01

but then increases in the second trimester before decelerating to the 120–160 bpm typically seen at birth (von Steinburg et al. 2013).

The walls of the heart form between day 27 and 37 as tissue grows and merges. In the atrioventricular area, the growth of the endocardial cushions forms the atrioventricular valves and the tracts for the aortic and pulmonary channels. In the atria, tissue growth leads to the closing of the original hole between the atria (ostium primum) and formation of a second hole (ostium secundum) with a slit (foramen ovale) through which blood can continue to flow from right to left during foetal circulation. Foetal gas exchange occurs in the placenta. Oxygenated blood travels through the umbilical vein into the inferior vena cava through the ductus venosus and bypasses the liver circulation. Oxygenated blood is shunted from the right atrium to the left atrium through the foramen ovale and then blood pumped to the left ventricle and into the aorta to reach systemic circulation. Only a small portion of blood is pumped from the right atrium to right ventricle and pulmonary artery (PA) where it is shunted to the aorta through the ductus arteriosus, thereby bypassing the lungs. Deoxygenated blood returns to the placenta via the umbilical arteries (Ossa Galvis et al. 2020). At birth, blood flow through the placenta stops and respiration begins, in normal circumstances, with a rise in right atrial pressure closing the foramen ovale and the ductus arteriosus beginning to close.

Patent Foramen Ovale (PFO)

In around 25% of the population, the foramen ovale fails to close (Homma et al. 2016). This anomaly is referred to as a patent foramen ovale. Of these, around 30% will be transient where the PFO is fused, opening only during high-pressure activities such as coughing. In these patients, no left-to-right shunt is visible on imaging. Patients with PFOs are usually asymptomatic, and therefore may not be diagnosed until later in life, when they present with neurological problems such as strokes, transient ischaemic attacks and migraines. Medical therapy subsequently may include antiplatelet or anticoagulant medication (Zhang et al. 2018). Where patients are symptomatic, PFOs can be closed using percutaneous devices or through open-heart surgery.

Suggested Resource Website

For a more comprehensive information about foetal development of the cardiovascular system, see the suggested resource below:
Development of the cardiovascular system- Teach Me Anatomy
https://teachmeanatomy.info/the-basics/embryology/cardiovascular-system

---

Congenital Heart Disease Classification

Classifying CHD is complex, with crossover between categories of classification, particularly in cases where patients present with different combinations of anomalies. At least 18 distinct types of CHDs have been recognised, with many additional anatomic variations (American Heart Association [AHA] 2020). CHD is traditionally classified according to presence of cyanosis, but patients with acyanotic defects may develop cyanosis. Acyanotic CHD includes congenital heart defects with dominant left-to-right shunt (see Box 24.1) and obstructive lesions. Cyanotic heart disease can be subdivided into conditions with decreased pulmonary blood flow and conditions with mixed blood flow.

Key Point

Cyanotic CHD is also known as critical congenital heart disease (CCHD). Approximately 25% of cases of CHD are considered to be CCHD (Ossa Galvis et al. 2020). Cyanosis occurs when deoxygenated blood bypasses the lungs and enters the systemic circulation resulting in low saturations and commonly a 'blue' colour.

Box 24.1 Cardiac shunts.

Foetal circulation

Shunts are crucial during foetal life as the placenta provides the exchange of gases and nutrients. Foetal circulation has four sites of shunting: the placenta, ductus venosus through which umbilical vein drains into inferior vena cava, foramen ovale within the interatrial septum, and the arterial duct through which blood in the PA flows into descending aorta. Shortly after birth, the placental circulation disappears, and pulmonary circulation is established. Interruption of the umbilical cord results in an increase in systemic vascular resistance and closure of the ductus venosus (Micheletti 2019).

Circulation following birth

Normal function of the heart involves the flow of blood from the atria to the respective ventricle and subsequently around the body or to the lungs. Pressures in the left side of a normal heart are persistently higher than those in the right. Patterns of blood flow that deviate from this normal circulation are called cardiac shunts. These may occur from left to right, right to left or bidirectional. The direction of the shunt is determined by pressure in the respective chamber, with blood shunted from areas of high pressure to low pressure. In a normal heart, the left heart pumps blood into circulation and therefore is a higher-pressure system. Conversely, the right heart has a smaller muscle mass and lacks the central constricting muscle fibres that are responsible for generating the force of contraction and is a lower-pressure system (Sheehan and Redington 2008). Therefore, shunt direction affects the status of pulmonary blood flow which can vary from normal, increased or decreased (Micheletti 2019).

The additional classification of blood flow patterns through the heart is also used and makes it easier to predict clinical manifestations. Congenital heart anomalies according to classification, blood flow patterns and clinical findings are shown in Table 24.1. Using this classification system, the clinical presentation and management of the most commonly encountered congenital heart defects are outlined in this chapter.

CHD with Shunt Between Systemic and Pulmonary Circulation

In conditions with left-to-right shunt, blood from the systemic arterial circulation mixes with systemic venous blood. The extent of flow through the shunt and its physiologic effects are impacted by multiple factors. An abnormal connection between the systemic and pulmonary circulations gives rise to potential excess volume of blood to flow from the systemic (left side) circulation to the pulmonary circulation (right side) resulting in the recirculation of already oxygenated pulmonary venous blood through the pulmonary vasculature. Left-to-right shunting can occur due to communications at the atrial, ventricular and arterial level, with blood preferentially shunting from a higher to lower resistance circulation (Kung and Triedman 2019). The clinical presentation of a patient with left-to-right shunt depends on the size of the shunt, the physiological effects of the shunt and presence of other cardiac anomalies. Any large left-to-right (L-R) shunt results in increased blood flow into the lungs associated with shortness of breath and prominent vascular markings on chest x-ray, volume overload of left ventricle (LV) associated with chamber dilatation and subsequently heart failure (Micheletti 2019). The most common CHD causes of left to right shunt include atrial septal defect (ASD), ventricular septal defect (VSD), patent ductus arteriosus (PDA) and atrioventricular septal defect (also known as atrioventricular canal defect). When pressure in the right side of the heart becomes higher than that in the left, Eisenmenger syndrome may develop (see Box 24.2).

Table 24.1 Classification of congenital heart disease by cyanosis/acyanosis, blood flow patterns and clinical findings.

	Acyanotic			Cyanotic
Blood flow pattern	Increased pulmonary blood flow (left to right shunt)	Obstruction to blood flow from ventricles	Decreased pulmonary blood flow	Mixed blood flow
Anomaly	• ASD • VSD • PDA • Complete AV canal defect	• Valvular AS • CoA • IAA • PVS	• TOF • Tricuspid atresia • Ebstein anomaly	• TGA • TAPVR • Truncus arteriosus • Hypoplastic left heart syndrome
Clinical findings	• ↑ PVR • ↑ right heart pressures • PH • HF • Reversal of shunt • ES (see Box 24.1)	• Left side: HF • Right side: cyanosis	• Cyanosis	• Variable based on the degree of mixing and amount of PBF. • Hypoxemia (with or without cyanosis) and HF usually occur together.

PVR = pulmonary vascular resistance; PH = pulmonary hypertension; HF = heart failure; ES = Eisenmenger syndrome; ASD = atrial septal defect; VSD = ventricular septal defect; PDA = patent ductus arteriosus; AV = atrioventricular; AS = aortic stenosis; CoA = coarctation of the aorta; IAA = interrupted aortic arch; PVS = pulmonic valve stenosis; TOF = Tetralogy of Fallot; TA = tricuspid atresia; TGA = transposition of the great arteries; TAPVR = total anomalous pulmonary venous return.

Box 24.2   Eisenmenger syndrome.

Eisenmenger syndrome (ES) is a rare progressive disorder. Whilst an increasing number of CHDs are diagnosed antenatally or soon after birth, complications can arise where an anomaly is not identified early. ES refers to any untreated congenital cardiac defect with intracardiac communication that over time leads to pulmonary hypertension (PH), reversal of flow and cyanosis. In the normal heart, the left side of the heart generates high pressure to supply the extensive high-resistance systemic circulation. The right side of the heart generates much lower pressures to allow blood to pass through the low-resistance and high-compliance pulmonary circulation. In the case of a defect that allows communication between the two sides of the heart, a shunt will develop causing blood to flow from the area of high pressure to lower pressure (left to right). The amount of blood shunted is proportional to the size of the defect. The abnormally high and pressure of blood directed through the shunt from the left side of the heart to the right side damages the pulmonary vasculature causing scar tissue and ultimately PH. The right side of the heart has to work harder to supply blood to the lungs, leading to hypertrophy of the right ventricle (RV) and increased right heart pressures. Once right heart pressures exceed those of the left side of the heart, the left-to-right shunt will reverse and deoxygenated blood returning to the right side of the heart will be shunted to the left, bypassing the lungs, and pumped to the systemic circulation leading to cyanosis and organ damage. The kidneys, sensing the decrease in oxygen saturation, try to compensate by increasing production of erythropoietin and red blood cells, leading to an increase in reticulocyte count and the risk of hyperviscosity syndrome. As reticulocytes are immature blood cells, they are not as efficient at carrying oxygen and changing shape compared with mature cells and are unable to transit easily through capillaries, leading to death of capillary beds. Patients with ES are at risk of both blood clots due to hyperviscosity and bleeding from their damaged lung capillaries. Clinically, ES manifests in cyanosis, desaturation, dyspnoea, syncope, and clubbing (Dakkak and Oliver 2020).

The natural history of ES is variable and depends upon the complexity of lesions, but it is typical for complications to start in the patient's third decade with high mortality in the third and fourth decades. Ventricular failure, haemoptysis, pregnancy complications, and strokes are common causes of death (Basit et al. 2020). Surgical repair is usually possible before PH becomes too high. Once severe PH is established, pulmonary vasodilators may help symptoms (D'Alto and Diller 2014). Surgical transplant of the lungs or heart–lungs is an option but usually only a viable treatment for a small number of people (Le Pavec et al. 2018).

Acyanotic CHD

Acyanotic CHD with Increased Blood Flow

Atrial Septal Defect (ASD)

An atrial septal defect (ASD) is the most common form of CHD found in adults. Most ASDs occur by chance, though familial transmission has also been reported. In the foetal circulation, there is normally an opening between the left and right atria to allow blood to bypass the lungs. This opening usually closes about the time the baby is born, but if the opening persists, it is called an ASD. Around 90% of ASDs occur in the central portion of the atrial septum and are referred to as secundum ASD (ASD II). An ASD may be managed conservatively or require closure using surgical or percutaneous device implantation.

ASD in Adults

Patients with an isolated ASDII often remain asymptomatic during childhood and adolescence, but supraventricular arrhythmias, right ventricular dysfunction, and PH increase with age, while exercise tolerance and life expectancy are reduced (Kuijpers et al. 2015). Conservative management includes reducing thromboembolic risks with anticoagulation or antiplatelet drugs. Risk of complications with ASD closure increases with age.

Key Point

Where the atrial shunt has reversed the sudden closure of the ASD can lead to the right ventricle having to overcome a high PA pressure, and this may result in HF.

Suggested Resource Reading

Oster, M., Bhatt, A. B., Zaragoza-Macias, E. et al. (2019). Interventional therapy versus medical therapy for secundum atrial septal defect: a systematic review (part 2) for the 2018 AHA/ACC guideline for the management of adults with congenital heart disease: a report of the American College of Cardiology/American Heart Association Task Force on Clinical Practice Guidelines. *Journal of the American College of Cardiology* 73 (12): 1579–1595. https://doi.org/10.1016/j.jacc.2018.08.1029

Ventricular Septal Defect (VSD)

Ventricular septal defect (VSD) refers to a hole in the septum dividing the right and left ventricle that occurs in the embryonic stage of heart development. It is the most common congenital cardiac anomaly in children, and the second most common congenital abnormality in adults (Dakkak and Oliver 2020; Mavroudis et al. 2020). Several genetic factors including Down syndrome have been identified to cause VSD, but non-inheritable factors have also been implicated. VSD may occur in isolation but can occur in association with other congenital heart defects and are a frequent component of complex CHD.

VSDs are classified according to location and size. Most VSDs are restrictive (<5 mm) and undergo spontaneous closure during the first year of life (Mavroudis et al. 2020). Small congenital VSDs may not need treatment but if a large VSD is not repaired children are likely to develop pulmonary vascular obstructive disease as early as 18 months to 2 years of age (Rao and Harris 2018). Management must be considered in the context of VSD size, location, coexisting congenital heart defects and clinical findings.

VSD in Adults

Adult patients with restrictive VSDs have about a 10% spontaneous closure rate during any decade of life, but there is a 25% chance of developing complications relating to the uncorrected VSD, including infective endocarditis, aortic regurgitation and symptomatic arrhythmias. Surgery is necessary if the VSD is large or associated with significant complications (Mavroudis et al. 2020). Percutaneous device VSD closure is reserved for those in whom surgery is very risky due to severe PAH, multiple comorbidities and those who had prior cardiothoracic surgery such as residual or recurrent VSD. Complications of VSD closure include residual or recurrent VSD, valvular incompetence such as tricuspid regurgitation and aortic insufficiency, arrhythmias (atrial fibrillation, complete heart block and uncommonly, ventricular tachycardia), LV dysfunction and progression of pulmonary hypertension (PH).

> **Key Point**
>
> Lifelong follow-up is recommended for patients with VSD whether they have had corrective surgery or not, as there is a measurable incidence of major complications during late follow-up of adult patients with restrictive VSDs regardless of operative status (Mavroudis et al. 2020).

Patent Ductus Arteriosus (PDA)

The *ductus arteriosus* is a foetal vessel that allows oxygenated blood from the placenta to bypass the lungs in utero (Gillam-Krakauer and Mahajan 2020). At birth, as lungs fill with air and normal circulation begins, the ductus arteriosus is redundant and functionally closes within 12–24 hours of birth, with permanent anatomic closure becoming complete within 2–3 weeks; 98% of infants will have a closed ductus by the time they are discharged from hospital. Preterm infants weighing less than 1000 g at birth are most at risk of PDA. Conservative management of a PDA with fluid restriction, supportive peak end-expiratory pressure to treat pulmonary oedema and indomethacin, ibuprofen or acetaminophen/paracetamol increasing peak expiratory may be sufficient to support the infant while awaiting spontaneous closure. In more severe cases, a PDA can result in blood flowing from the descending aorta across the PDA into the pulmonary circulation (left to right shunt) resulting in pulmonary oedema and pulmonary haemorrhage, intraventricular haemorrhage, congestive heart failure, bronchopulmonary dysplasia, with decreased blood flow to the lower body leading to renal failure and necrotising enterocolitis (Gillam-Krakauer and Mahajan 2020). PDAs are closed either using an open-heart surgery technique or, more commonly, percutaneously using a coil or plug (Baruteau et al. 2014). After closure of the PDA, most children have a normal life expectancy (Gillam-Krakauer and Mahajan 2020).

PDA in Adults

PDA is rare in adults as symptoms and signs usually occur in infancy and most cases are treated shortly after diagnosis. Untreated PDA can lead to PH, Eisenmenger syndrome, HF, and endarteritis. In adults, surgical closure of a PDA is always required as long as the patient has not developed fixed PH. Before the ductus is closed in an adult, the status of the pulmonary vasculature must be determined. Those with only mild PH have a normal life expectancy (Gillam-Krakauer and Mahajan 2020).

Atrioventricular Septal Defect (Atrioventricular Canal Defect; Endocardial Cushion Defect)

Atrioventricular septal defect (AVSD) accounts for around 5% of congenital heart anomalies. An AVSD may be complete, with a large non-restrictive inlet ventricular septal defect (VSD); transitional with a small- or moderate-sized restrictive VSD, or partial with no VSD. Patients with no VSD component or a small VSD and good AV valve function may be asymptomatic. In the case of a large VSD or significant AV valve regurgitation, patients often have signs of HF (Baffa 2018a). A complete AVSD (also called a complete common AV canal defect) may result in left-to-right shunt at the atrial and ventricular levels. AV valve regurgitation sometimes causes a direct left ventricle-to-right-atrial shunt. Over time, Eisenmenger syndrome may develop if not corrected (see Box 24.1). Complete AVSD heart failure is evident in an infant between 4 and 6 weeks old and requires surgical repair by age 2–4 months old. Symptoms in partial AVSD vary with the degree of mitral regurgitation: if mild or absent, symptoms may develop during adolescence or early adulthood (Baffa 2018a).

AVSD in Adults

Patients with milder disease may present in late childhood or early adulthood with congestive heart failure, PH with Eisenmenger syndrome, infective endocarditis, or arrhythmia. Surgical repair is indicated unless there is proven irreversible PH in which case medical management for PH with pulmonary vasodilators should be attempted (Kochav 2018).

Key Point

Most patients with the complete form of AVSD have Down Syndrome (Baffa 2018a).

Acyanotic CHD with Outflow Obstruction

This group of congenital heart defects all present with an obstruction to the outflow tract. A ventricular outflow tract is the section of left ventricle or right ventricle through which blood passes in order to reach the great arteries. Conditions associated with acyanotic obstructive CHD include aortic valve stenosis (AVS), coarctation of the aorta, interrupted aortic arch and pulmonic stenosis (PS).

Aortic Valve Stenosis

Aortic stenosis (AS) may be congenital or acquired. In pediatric patients, AS is almost always congenital. Congenital valvular AS (CVAS) accounts for approximately 3–6% of congenital heart defects and may be associated with other forms of CHD including patent ductus arteriosus, coarctation of the aorta and ventricular septal defects (Singh 2019). CVAS displays several morphologic types of abnormal valves: unicuspid, bicuspid, tricuspid and quadricuspid, and is a spectrum in which the degree of obstruction ranges from mild to severe. Clinical findings depend upon the age of the patient at the presentation, severity of the CVAS and the presence of associated cardiac lesions. The majority of infants with severe CVAS present with progressive congestive heart failure (HF) by 2 months of age.

Older children and adolescents are usually asymptomatic, but symptoms of dyspnoea, angina or syncope (particularly during exercise) should be investigated as there is a risk of sudden death in children aged 5–15 years with moderate-to-severe CVAS (Singh 2019). CVAS is a progressive disorder, and management is determined by the age of the patient at presentation, the severity of the obstruction and adequacy of left heart structures. Current therapeutic intervention options to relieve LVOT obstruction are percutaneous balloon aortic valvuloplasty, surgical aortic valvotomy and valve replacement (Singh 2019).

Congenital AVS in the Adult

Congenital aortic stenosis is a lifelong disease that often requires multiple interventions. Balloon aortic valvuloplasty is the intervention of choice in many centres, as it is seen to be a safer and a less invasive alternative to surgery, but surgical aortic valve repair may require less re-intervention (Donald et al. 2019). Patients may present with prior valve repair and symptoms resulting from patient-prosthesis mismatch due to the normally functioning valve prosthesis being too small in relation to the patient's body size, leading to high transvalvular pressure gradients (Dahou et al. 2016).

Key Point

The bicuspid aortic valve is the most common cause of aortic stenosis in patients less than the age of 70 years in developed countries (Pujari and Agasthi 2020). Aortic aneurysm formation and aortic dissection are the two major complications of bicuspid aortopathy, mostly encountered beyond paediatric age (Singh 2019).

Coarctation of the Aorta

Coarctation of the aorta (CoA) accounts for 6–8% of congenital heart anomalies.

No single cause has been identified, although evidence suggests a combination of genetic, environmental and haemodynamic factors. CoA involves a localised narrowing of the aortic lumen that results in upper-extremity hypertension (HT), left ventricular hypertrophy (LVH) and impaired perfusion of the abdominal organs and lower extremities (Baffa 2018b). It can occur in different sites in the aorta but usually occurs just beyond the branch of the left subclavian artery. The aorta can bulge either side of the narrowing and the subclavian artery can be dilated (Suradi and Hijazi 2015). CoA may occur alone or with various other congenital anomalies including bicuspid aortic valve, VSD, AS, patent ductus arteriosus and mitral valve disorders (Baffa 2018b). Neonates may present in shock and require prostaglandin E_1 to maintain ductal patency until the time of surgical repair. Older children usually present with upper extremity hypertension or murmur. Surgical repair in neonates and infants depends on the presence or absence of concomitant defects and the degree of associated arch hypoplasia (Nelson et al. 2019). Treatment is balloon angioplasty with stent placement, or surgical correction (Baffa 2018b).

Adults with CoA

CoA is commonly treated after birth or during childhood and is rarely seen in adults. Untreated CoA has a poor long-term prognosis, with a 75% mortality by the time the patient reaches their mid-forties (Suradi and Hijazi 2015). Adults may present with a history of a previous coarctation procedure, rupture of an old repair, heart failure, aortic aneurysm, aortic dissection, undersized grafts of previous repairs, intracranial haemorrhage, hypertension with exercise and infections (Shah and Shah 2018).

Key Point

CoA is more common in females than males (2 : 1 ratio) and occurs in 10–20% of patients with Turner syndrome (Baffa 2018b).

Interrupted Aortic Arch

Interrupted aortic arch (IAA) accounts for approximately 1.5% of all CHD. IAA differs from a coarctation because the aorta is not narrowed but discontinuous at a location between the ascending and descending aortic arch. IAA is associated with other cardiac anomalies, commonly VSD, PDA, and bicuspid aortic valve. In IAA, lower body perfusion is entirely PDA-dependent and in the absence of prenatal diagnosis, patients with IAA present in shock within the first few days to weeks of life when the PDA closes. PGE_1 infusion is usually given to keep the arterial duct open, and inotropic agents, diuretics and mechanical ventilation may be required to stabilise the patient in preparation for surgery. Mortality rate for patients with IAA is estimated to be 3.6% at 2 years and about 39% at 21 years (Micheletti 2019).

Adults with Interrupted Aortic Arch

IAA is associated with a significant burden in terms of the need for reintervention and deficits in exercise performance, health status and health-related quality of life (Micheletti 2019). Lifelong follow-up is needed for patients with repaired IAA, primarily to monitor for left ventricular outflow tract obstruction and recurrent aortic coarctation (Friedman 2018).

Pulmonary Valve Stenosis

Pulmonary valve stenosis (PVS) with normal cardiac connections accounts for 8–12% of all CHDs (McCarthy et al. 2019; Micheletti 2019) and is the most common cause of RV outflow tract obstruction (RVOTO). Concomitant presence of right ventricular hypertrophy (RVH) is dependent on the significance of the stenosis. PVS may occur as an isolated lesion but can coexist with other congenital heart lesions – notably it is one of the four cardinal features of tetralogy of Fallot (TOF). Isolated mild PVS is usually asymptomatic, and the probability of long-term survival is similar to the general population. Patients with severe PVS most often present during childhood with RV failure and cyanosis, most often in the presence of interatrial shunting (Fathallah and Krasuski 2017). Newborns with critical PVS need emergency treatment including PGE₁ infusion and cardiac catheterisation for percutaneous pulmonary when stabilised. If percutaneous balloon dilation is unsuccessful, surgical pulmonary valvotomy is urgently indicated in critically ill patients (Micheletti 2019). If PVS is successfully treated (balloon pulmonary valvuloplasty or pulmonic valve replacement), prognosis is generally excellent (Fathallah and Krasuski 2017). Treatment decisions are highly dependent on concomitant disease.

Adults with PVS

PVS is most often associated with the failure of the valvular leaflets to fuse and is clinically detected at different stages of life. The more severe the obstruction, the earlier the valvular abnormality is typically detected. Neonates with critical stenosis typically present with central cyanosis at birth. PVS may be recognised in infants and children by the presence of ejection murmurs auscultated in the pulmonic area. Symptoms of PVS progress with time. Adults present with symptoms of congestive HF and RVOT that is progressive in nature (Loewenthal 2016).

Key Point

Patients with Noonan's syndrome are often resistant to balloon dilatation due to the associated pulmonary trunk narrowing (Bellsham-Revell and Burch 2014). Surgery is usually the first-line treatment for this group.

Cyanotic CHD

Cyanotic CHD with Decreased Pulmonary Blood Flow

Tetralogy of Fallot

Tetralogy of Fallot (TOF) occurs in 10% of all CHD (Micheletti 2019) and is the most common cyanotic heart defect (McCarthy et al. 2019) occurring in 3–5 of every 10 000 live births (Diaz-Frias and Guillaume 2020). It is a complex condition defined by the presence of four conditions: (i) large malaligned VSD; (ii) pulmonary stenosis causing RVOT obstruction; (iii) RV hypertrophy resulting from RVOT obstruction; and (iv) an over-riding aorta above the VSD, which allows blood from both ventricles to enter the aorta (Micheletti 2019). The degree of patient cyanosis depends upon the degree of RVOT obstruction, which is variable. 'Pink TOF' is associated with mild pulmonary stenosis and has a similar presentation to that of VSD with high pulmonary blood flow, normal oxygen saturation and potential CHF symptoms early in life. All other forms of TOF may experience characteristic hypoxic or hypercyanotic spells that typically reach peak incidence in infants between 2 and 4 months of age. Immediate recognition and treatment is required to avoid severe complications including death.

TOF is typically treated by open heart surgery in the first year of life. The procedure involves reconstruction of the RVOT and repairing the VSD. Most patients undergoing surgery have a good long-term outcome, but residual post-surgical defects may affect life expectancy and increase the need for reoperation. Left untreated, TOF carries a 35% mortality rate in the first year of life, and a 50% mortality rate in the first 3 years of life (Diaz-Frias and Guillaume 2020).

Tricuspid Atresia

Failure of the tricuspid valve to grow during foetal development results in the right side of the heart developing without a connection between the atrium and ventricle. Whilst the left side of the heart functions normally, there is an underdeveloped right ventricle. Tricuspid atresia is a relatively rare anomaly, occurring in about two out of every 10 000 live births and accounting for around 1–2% of all cases of congenital heart disease (Murthy et al. 2019). Like many congenital cardiac conditions, tricuspid atresia is often associated with a series of additional defects in various combinations and with varying degrees of severity. ASD or VSD commonly occur alongside tricuspid atresia. This enables blood to shunt between the left and right side of the heart, allowing blood to mix, and therefore provide oxygen to the systemic circulation. Tricuspid atresia may also be classified as a univentricular (single ventricle) heart (discussed later in this chapter).

Ebstein Anomaly

Ebstein anomaly (EA) accounts for <1% of all CHD (Micheletti 2019) and is rare, with a prevalence of around 1 in 20 000 live births (Boyle et al. 2018). Patients with EA have an abnormal tricuspid valve (TV) with malformed leaflets leading to tricuspid regurgitation. The valve is also malpositioned, sitting lower in the RV than in normal anatomy. In addition, the right atrium (RA) is large and attached to a small RV. As with all CHD, this anomaly presents on a spectrum of severity depending on the precise anatomy (Geerdink et al. 2017). In some instances, the severity of the tricuspid regurgitation leads to raised pressures in the right atrium. This results in a right-to-left shunt across the PFO after birth, preventing the PFO closing, with deoxygenated blood then entering the systemic system. As a result, the baby may become cyanotic. Anomalies associated with EA include an ASD and less commonly a VSD or PDA. Complex forms of EA may be associated with pulmonary valve stenosis or atresia, tetralogy of Fallot, or left-sided abnormalities such as mitral valve stenosis or regurgitation (Micheletti 2019). It is common for these patients to have an accessory (extra) electrical conduction pathway in the heart, potentially leading to episodes of supraventricular tachycardia known as Wolff–Parkinson–White syndrome. As well as medical and surgical treatment, they may also require electrophysiology assessment.

EA in the Adult

Mortality and morbidity for children with EA have reduced with improved medical management and surgical techniques; most children live well into adulthood. Around 50% of patients will have required reoperation by 20 years after the initial procedure

Cyanotic CHD with Mixed Blood Flow

Transposition of the Great Vessels

Transposition of the great vessels (TGV) refers to a group of congenital heart in which there is abnormal arrangement of any of the great vessels (superior and/or inferior venae cavae, PA, pulmonary veins and aorta).

Transposition of the Great Vessels/ Transposition of the Great Arteries

Transposition of great arteries (TGA) accounts for 2–5% of all CHD with a prevalence of about 0.2–0.3 of 1000 births and is more common in males than in females (Micheletti 2019). There are two types of TGA. In dextro-transposition of the great arteries (d-TGA), the aorta arises from the RV, and the PA arises from the LV causing deoxygenated blood from the right heart to bypass the lungs and be pumped into the aorta and circulated throughout the body and the heart itself. The left heart continuously pumps oxygenated blood back into the lungs via the PA. This haemodynamic condition is incompatible with life unless a communication exists between the two circulations, which allows a mixing between oxygenated and deoxygenated blood (Micheletti 2019). VSD is present in 30–40% of d-TGA patients. Prostaglandin E_1 can be given to newborns to keep the ductus arteriosus open to allow mixing of the pulmonary and systemic circuits until surgery, though emergent balloon atrial septostomy may be required in some cases (Sarris et al. 2017). Prognosis for d-TGA is good following surgical intervention with survival rates greater than 90% (Szymanski et al. 2020).

Levo-transposition of the great arteries (also known as l-TGA) is a rare acyanotic form of TGA that is associated with transposed primary arteries, ventricles and atrioventricular valves. TGA can occur in isolation or as part of other complex CHD anomalies. Surgery is required to correct the defect for survival.

TGA in the Adult

In adolescents and adults, complications include coronary artery stenosis or occlusion that may lead to ventricular dysfunction, sinus node dysfunction, atrial arrhythmias and sudden death. Around 10% of patients will require reintervention or surgical revision (Micheletti 2019).

Total and Partial Anomalous Pulmonary Venous Connection (TAPVC/PAPVC)

The reported birth prevalence of TAPVC ranges from around 0.5% to 2.0% of live births (Tongsong et al. 2016) though some studies suggest that this may be an underestimate due to historical difficulties in antenatal detection (Tongsong et al. 2016).

The four pulmonary veins take oxygenated blood from the lungs back to the left atrium. In TAPVC, the veins are abnormally connected to the venous system – sometimes connected to the veins outside the heart and sometimes connecting with the right atrium. Oxygenated blood returns to the right atrium. The mixed blood moves across a PFO or ASD in order to reach the left atrium and then circulation. Surgery can reconnect the pulmonary veins to the left atrium and close shunts. In PAPVC, some but not all the pulmonary veins connect to the right atrium. In this case, the effects on the patient will depend upon the amount of blood flow through the abnormal circuit.

Total/Partial Anomalous Pulmonary Venous Connection (TAPVC/PAPVC)

The four pulmonary veins take oxygenated blood from the lungs back to the left atrium.

TAPVC

In TAPVC, the veins are abnormally connected – sometimes to the veins outside the heart and sometimes to the right atrium. Oxygenated blood from the lungs returns to the right atrium.

Communication between the left and right atrium is crucial for survival in TAPVC. Mixing of the oxygenated and deoxygenated blood occurs in the right atrium, which is then shunted right to the left at the level of atria. In most patients with TAPVC, an ASD is present, enabling the blood to shunt across until surgery is performed (Kim et al. 2014). The left atrium and aorta get mixed blood, which leads to cyanosis. In untreated patients, TAPVC is almost always fatal within the first few weeks of life. Surgery is offered soon after birth, in order to reconnect the pulmonary veins to the left atrium and close the shunts (Konduri and Aggarwal 2021).

PAPVC

In PAPVC, some but not all pulmonary veins connect into the right atrium (Sears et al. 2012).

The main physiologic effects of PAPVC are similar to those of ASD, which is left-to-right shunt at the atrial level leading to recirculation of oxygenated blood through the pulmonary vasculature. Untreated PAPVC in the long term can lead to PH and RV failure.

Patent Truncus Arteriosus

Truncus arteriosus (TA) occurs in 1–4% of all CHDs. During development, the TA should divide into a pulmonary trunk and an aorta. Rarely it does not, leaving a common arterial trunk and VSD and a mixture of oxygenated and deoxygenated blood entering the circulation. Clinical presentation depends on the amount of pulmonary blood flow.

TA in the Adult

Surgical repair is usually carried out within the first 6 months of life. Later presentation is often associated with PH and may lead to Eisenmenger syndrome (Micheletti 2019). Reoperation may be required later in life but has good survival rates.

Adults with Single Ventricle

Patients with single ventricle are at risk of multiple complications including cardiac, pulmonary, hepatic, gastrointestinal and neurological problems that may start from 5 to 10 years after the operative procedures. Heart transplantation may be the only effective option in some patients (Micheletti).

Whilst there have been significant developments in the treatment available to patients with CHD, not all lesions are correctable. Nonetheless, the offer of palliative procedures has seen a growing population of patients growing up with complex conditions. These lesions generally require multiple surgeries and patients will require lifelong follow-up.

Single Ventricle/Univentricular Hearts

Hearts with a functional single ventricle (functional univentricular heart) are rare, comprising 1–2% of all CHDs (Micheletti 2019) with a birth prevalence around 1 in 2000 births (Liu et al. 2019). The term 'single ventricle' is used to describe a heterogeneous group of anomalies with single atrioventricular connection (tricuspid atresia, mitral valve atresia, double-inlet LV) and/or severe hypoplasia of one ventricle and its own atrioventricular valve (hypoplastic left heart syndrome [HLHS], unbalanced complete AVSD). Although the anomalies may differ significantly from each other, they share the common feature that the patient develops with just one ventricle or one normal ventricle and a second undeveloped ventricle. The valves into the single functioning ventricle could be from both atria (*double inlet*), or from one atria, with the other valve being atresic, or have a single shared valve (*common inlet*). The developed ventricle chamber could be of either a right or a left ventricular type. Over the past four decades, the survival of these neonates has increased from 0 to nearly 90% (Ohye et al. 2016). Whilst predominantly a reflection of the development of surgical techniques, prenatal diagnosis is also associated with a higher survival in neonates with a single ventricle physiology (Weber et al. 2019). Mortality varies across the different anatomical presentations, with a lower mortality rate observed in patients with a dominant left ventricle and associated hyperplastic right ventricle (Beroukhim et al. 2015). Clinical findings will depend upon the amount of pulmonary blood flow and affected neonates may require PGE_1 infusion. Surgery is undertaken using a staged approach with several procedures, ultimately resulting in Fontan circulation.

Suggested Resource YouTube

Hypoplastic left heart syndrome (HLHS) Cincinnati Children's
https://youtu.be/3CP3xZVgpdg

Adults with Univentricular CHD

Most patients with single ventricle congenital heart disease are now expected to survive to adulthood. However, comorbidities are common (Collins et al. 2016).

Suggested Resource YouTube

The videos below from Cincinnati Children's outline the three operations undertaken for HLHS that result in Fontan circulation:

Norwood operation
https://youtu.be/u5VbSDp2qMU

Glenn repair
https://youtu.be/kBh8YDqcqxc

Fontan operation
https://youtu.be/hIpvCUwml3c

Dextrocardia

Dextrocardia refers to alignment towards the right rather than the left. In most cases, it is diagnosed incidentally, typically on routine radiological examination, which reveals an abnormal location of the heart (Nair and Muthukuru 2020). Dextrocardia is often associated with other development anomalies with several possible presentations. If the heart is on the right side of the chest but all other organs are in their normal position it is known as *situs solitus*; if the heart is in the opposite alignment facing the right with the abdominal organs also on the opposite side it is known as *situs inversus,* If the heart is turned to the right but the chamber positions are not changed and the abdominal organs stay in their usual position, it is known as *dextroversion*. If the heart stays in the left position but the heart chambers invert and the abdominal organs also switch position, it is known as *levoversion*. Both dextroversion and levoversion are almost always associated with additional heart defects such as transposition of the great vessels, pulmonary stenosis, VSDs and ASDs.

The Adult with Dextrocardia

Most patients with dextrocardia are asymptomatic and lead a normal life. The prognosis of patients with dextrocardia depends on the presence or absence of other accompanying congenital defects and the type of congenital anomalies (Nair and Muthukuru 2020).

Key Point

People with dextrocardia may have heterotaxy syndrome. Organs in the chest and abdomen normally have a particular location on the right or left side of the body, termed 'situs solitus'. Rarely, the orientation of the internal organs is reversed and is termed 'situs inversus'. Situs invertus does not normally cause problems unless it occurs as part of a syndrome affecting other parts of the body. 'Heterotaxy syndrome' refers to an arrangement of the organs somewhere between situs solitus and situs inversus, but unlike situs invertus, it is associated with serious health issues including alterations to the structure of the heart and other organs.

Adult Congenital Heart Disease

With the growing success of heart surgery in infancy, many children born with congenital heart defects now survive to adulthood. In addition, improvements in imaging techniques mean that less complex heart defects are being in adults. The ratio of adults to children living with CHD is now estimated to be 2 to 1 (DeMaso et al. 2017). Understanding the needs of this emergent population is therefore essential. Anatomy alone is not the best measure of severity of adult congenital heart disease (ACHD) severity as anatomy and physiology in ACHD are not always correlated. The severity of ADCH is determined by native anatomy, surgical repair and current physiology. The recently developed ACHD Anatomical and Physiological (AP) classification system captures CHD anatomic variables, as well as physiological variables, many of which have prognostic value in patients with ACHD. As with the New York Heart Association (NYHA) classification of functional status, patients may move from one ACHD AP classification to another over time (Stout et al. 2019). Physiological variables used in ACHD AP Classification include aortopathy (diameter of the aorta); presence and type of arrhythmia; severity of concomitant valvular heart disease; end-organ dysfunction (including renal, hepatic, pulmonary); exercise capacity, hypoxaemia/hypoxia/cyanosis; NYHA functional classification; presence of PH; shunt (haemodynamically significant); and venous and arterial stenosis.

Table 24.2 gives an overview of the range of various ACHD types and the variables that affect functional status (Stout et al. 2019).

Adult congenital heart disease (ACHD) patients require ongoing monitoring and sometimes further treatment. There is also a need for consideration of genetics and pregnancy issues for ACHD patients choosing to have children of their own. Other issues, such as the risk of infective endocarditis (IE), are particularly pertinent in some subgroups of

Table 24.2 ACHD AP classification (CHD anatomy + physiological stage = ACHD AP classification).

CHD anatomy[a]

I: Simple

Native disease
- Isolated small ASD
- Isolated small VSD
- Mild isolated pulmonic stenosis

Repaired conditions
- Previously ligated or occluded ductus arteriosus
- Repaired secundum ASD or sinus venosus defect without significant residual shunt or chamber enlargement
- Repaired VSD without significant residual shunt or chamber enlargement

II: Moderate complexity

Repaired or unrepaired conditions
- Aorto-left ventricular fistula
- Anomalous pulmonary venous connection, partial or total
- Anomalous coronary artery arising from the Pa
- Anomalous aortic origin of a coronary artery from the opposite sinus
- AVSD (partial or complete, including primum ASD)
- Congenital aortic valve disease
- Congenital mitral valve disease
- Coarctation of the aorta
- Ebstein anomaly (disease spectrum includes mild, moderate and severe variations)
- Infundibular right ventricular outflow obstruction
- Ostium primum ASD
- Moderate and large unrepaired secundum ASD
- Moderate and large persistently patent ductus arteriosus
- Pulmonary valve regurgitation (moderate or greater)
- Pulmonary valve stenosis (moderate or greater)
- Peripheral pulmonary stenosis
- Sinus of Valsalva fistula/aneurysm
- Sinus venosus defect
- Subvalvar aortic stenosis (excluding HCM; HCM not addressed in these guidelines)
- Supravalvar aortic stenosis
- Straddling atrioventricular valve

- Repaired tetralogy of Fallot
- VSD with associated abnormality and/or moderate or greater shunt

III: Great complexity (or complex)

- Cyanotic congenital heart defect (unrepaired or palliated, all forms)
- Double-outlet ventricle
- Fontan procedure
- Interrupted aortic arch
- Mitral atresia
- Single ventricle (including double inlet left ventricle, tricuspid atresia, hypoplastic left heart, any other anatomic abnormality with a functionally single ventricle)
- Pulmonary atresia (all forms)
- TGA (classic or d-TGA; CCTGA or l-TGA)
- Truncus arteriosus
- Other abnormalities of atrioventricular and ventriculoarterial connection (i.e. crisscross heart, isomerism, heterotaxy syndromes, ventricular inversion)

Physiological stage

A
- NYHA FC I symptoms
- No haemodynamic or anatomic sequelae
- No arrhythmias
- Normal exercise capacity
- Normal renal/hepatic/pulmonary function

B
- NYHA FC II symptoms
- Mild haemodynamic sequelae (mild aortic enlargement, mild ventricular enlargement, mild ventricular dysfunction)
- Mild valvular disease
- Trivial or small shunt (not haemodynamically significant)
- Arrhythmia not requiring treatment
- Abnormal objective cardiac limitation to exercise

C
- NYHA FC III symptoms
- Significant (moderate or greater) valvular disease; moderate or greater ventricular dysfunction (systemic, pulmonic or both)
- Moderate aortic enlargement
- Venous or arterial stenosis

Table 24.2 (Continued)

• Mild or moderate hypoxemia/cyanosis	• Arrhythmias refractory to treatment
• Haemodynamically significant shunt	• Severe hypoxemia (almost always associated with cyanosis)
• Arrhythmias controlled with treatment	
• PH (less than severe)	• Severe PH
• End-organ dysfunction responsive to therapy	• Eisenmenger syndrome
	• Refractory end-organ dysfunction
D	
• NYHA FC IV symptoms	
• Severe aortic enlargement	

ACHD indicates adult congenital heart disease; AP, anatomic and physiological; ASD, atrial septal defect; AVSD, atrioventricular septal defect; CCTGA, congenitally corrected transposition of the great arteries; CHD, congenital heart disease; d-TGA, dextro-transposition of the great arteries; FC, functional class; HCM, hypertrophic cardiomyopathy; l-TGA, levo-transposition of the great arteries; NYHA, New York Heart Association; TGA, transposition of the great arteries; and VSD, ventricular septal defect.

[a] This list is not meant to be comprehensive; other conditions may be important in individual patients.

Source: Reproduced with permission from Stout et al. (2019).

ACHD patients where risk of infection is significantly higher than the standard population. The lifelong nature of CHD means continuity of care is a priority. Specialist ACHD services are required for patients moving from the paediatric to adult phase of their lives (Hays 2015), with the term *transition* applied to this particular timeframe. This is the time at which young adults are likely to be leaving home and perhaps taking some risks in their lives, including with their health, and during this phase they are often lost to follow up.

Key Point
CHD is a lifelong condition, in some cases requiring multiple surgeries and lifelong monitoring.

Common issues associated with ACHD are briefly discussed below.

Pharmacotherapy

Patients with ACHD are commonly excluded from clinical trials, and there are few data to guide pharmacological therapies. Treatments used for HF patients may not have the same benefit in the heterogeneous population of patients with ACHD, and in some cases may cause harm. Pharmacological therapies in patients with ACHD are often directed to specific conditions, such as beta-blockers for arrhythmia treatment. Some pharmacological therapies affecting the pulmonary vasculature have a beneficial effect on long-term outcomes in patients with Eisenmenger syndrome. If new symptoms occur in a patient with ADHD, it is important to review the patient's symptoms in the context of their individual anatomy, prior surgical repair and physiology to assess whether there are any residual anatomical causes that may be amenable to intervention.

Infective Endocarditis

IE is an infection of the endocardium, or inner lining of the heart. It results from a complex interaction between a bloodstream pathogen (most commonly staphylococcus or streptococcus) and platelets at sites of endocardial cell damage. Turbulent blood flow that arises as a result of certain types of congenital or acquired heart disease, such as shunts or blood flow across a narrowed orifice (such as valvular disease), traumatise the endothelium that fosters deposition of platelets and fibrin on the surface of the endothelium (Wilson et al. 2007). Activities that risk introducing bacteria to the blood stream similarly increase the chance of developing IE. These include interventions such as haemodialysis, intravenous drug taking or administration, or dental procedures. Mucosal surfaces, such as those in the mouth, are populated by a dense endogenous microflora. Disturbance of this surface, particularly the gingival crevice around teeth, gastrointestinal tract, urethra, and vagina, transiently releases different microbial species into the bloodstream (Wilson et al. 2007). IE may present as an acute, subacute or chronic condition, and the clinical presentation is highly variable reflecting the variable causative microorganisms, underlying cardiac conditions and pre-existing comorbidities (Rajani and Klein 2020).

Infective Endocarditis in the ACHD Patient

IE is 15- to 30-fold higher in patients with CHD than in the general population (Ly et al. 2019).

Cardiac anatomy and previous interventions place some ACHD patients at higher risk of developing IE than others, and mortality is particularly high in patients with complex CHD (Ly et al. 2019). Whilst the difficulty in defining specific 'high risk' lesions are acknowledged, there is general agreement that the following conditions put CHD patients at 'high risk' for developing IE (Stout et al. 2019):

- previous IE;
- prosthetic valves (biological and mechanical, surgical and transcatheter);
- placement of prosthetic material within the previous 6 months;
- residual intracardiac shunts at the site of or adjacent to previous repair with prosthetic material or devices; or
- uncorrected cyanotic heart disease.

Recommendations for Treatment

Currently, here are no randomised controlled trials (RCTs) to support antibiotic prophylaxis to prevent IE following dental extraction (Cahill et al. 2017; Quan et al. 2020). Consequently, the National Institute for Health and Care Excellence (NICE) issued guidelines in 2008 recommending that antibiotic prophylaxis during invasive dental procedures should no longer be offered to people at risk of infective endocarditis in England. Subsequent epidemiological

studies undertaken have pointed to an increase in cases of IE in England (Dayer et al. 2015). The 2016 NICE guideline update reaffirms this position but inserts the word *routinely* to the recommendation that antibiotic prophylaxis should no longer be offered, stating that doctors and dentists should apply clinical judgement on a case-by-case basis (Chambers et al. 2016). In contrast, the American Heart Association and European Society of Cardiology guidelines continue to recommend antibiotic prophylaxis in certain high-risk cases such as those listed above (Quan et al. 2020).

Exercise and Sports

Historically, the focus has been on restriction of activity for adults with CHD due to fears of adverse events such as sudden cardiac death (SCD) or aortic dissection. More recently, it has been suggested that most patients with ACHD can safely engage in regular, moderate physical activity, but it is important to note that some conditions, such as systemic ventricular systolic dysfunction, systemic ventricular outflow tract obstruction, haemodynamically significant arrhythmias or aortic dilation, warrant more cautious recommendations (Stout et al. 2019). The level of sports participation recommended must be individualised to the particular patient and take into account the training and the competitive aspects of the activity, the patient's functional status and history of surgery. Non-invasive testing including exercise tolerance testing, Holter monitoring, echocardiography and cardiac magnetic resonance imaging may be useful in decision-making (Van Hare et al. 2015).

Suggested Resource Reading

The reading below provides recommendations for competitive athletes with particular types of heart disease including CHD: Pelliccia, A., Sharma, S., Gati, S. et al. (2020). ESC Guidelines on sports cardiology and exercise in patients with cardiovascular disease: the task force on sports cardiology and exercise in patients with cardiovascular disease of the European Society of Cardiology (ESC). *European Heart Journal* ehaa605. https://doi.org/10.1093/eurheartj/ehaa605.

> **Key Point**
>
> Physical activity is widely recognised as being beneficial for physical and mental health. Activity recommendations for people with ACHD should be individualised according to clinical status and the patient's interests (Stout et al. 2019).

Sexual Health

Guidance on sexual functioning and reproductive health issues has largely been neglected for patients with ACHD. Sexuality is an important element of quality of life (QoL) and though sexual function is an issue that affects QoL for both women and men with ACHD, there appears to be minimal evidence to guide interventions (Stout et al. 2019) or advice on the safety of sexual activity. Most patients with ACHD have a reduced exercise capacity. It is uncertain to what extent this is caused by the heart defect per se or a sedentary life style because of restrictions and/or overprotection (Sandberg et al. 2016). There is evidence to suggest that adults with CHD have fears regarding the safety of performing sexual activities triggered by anecdotal reports of sudden deaths occurred during sexual arousal and 15% of men (and 9% of women reported cardiac symptoms (dyspnoea, perceived arrhythmia, increased fatigue, syncope, chest pain) during sexual activity, with symptoms being more common in those with more severe disease (Vigl et al. 2009, 2010). Concerns with sexual health are present in 20–40% of men with CHD and erectile dysfunction is reported by up to 42% of men with CHD (Stout et al. 2019). The prevalence of sexual dysfunction in ACHD patients is high and the aetiology appears to be multifactorial. Psychological

health, cardiac medications, clinical symptoms, and delay in psychosexual development may all play a part in sexual dysfunction for people with ACHD (Huang and Cook 2018).

> **Key Point**
>
> Patients often feel do not feel confident in voicing concerns about sexual health. Nurses should create an environment in which the patient with ACHD feels comfortable addressing concerns about their sexuality.

Early discussion and counselling about reproductive risk is essential. This includes information on the individual risk of inherited cardiac disease, and for women, the risks associated with pregnancy itself. These risks vary significantly depending on the defect and whether there has been surgical repair. Ideally, discussions should take place before the woman becomes pregnant.

Pregnancy

Pregnancy is frequently more complicated in women with CHD and requires specialty management (Stout et al. 2019). Women with CHD have greater rates of comorbidities that may complicate delivery, including cardiomyopathy, valvular heart disease, PH, systemic HT, cardiac conduction disorder, anaemia, and non-gestational diabetes (Schlichting et al. 2019). The risk of adverse pregnancy outcomes is much higher in women with CHDs due to the strain pregnancy places on the cardiovascular system, including increased blood volume, heart rate, and cardiac output, which may lead to HF, stroke, arrhythmias and myocardial infarction. Women with CHD are also have a higher frequency of adverse obstetric events including pre-term labour, maternal death, operative vaginal delivery, and caesarean delivery. Babies born to women with CHDs are also at higher risk of including premature birth, being small for gestational age and CHD or other congenital anomalies (Schlichting et al. 2019).

Suggested Resource Reading

Canobbio, M.M., Warnes, C.A., Aboulhosn, J. et al. (2017). Management of pregnancy in patients with complex congenital heart disease: a scientific statement for health-care professionals from the American Heart Association. *Circulation* 135 (8): e50–e87. https://www.ahajournals.org/doi/pdf/10.1161/cir.0000000000000458

Pre-Pregnancy Counselling

Women with ACHD who are considering pregnancy should have an individualised risk assessment individual patient's anatomy and physiology, followed by discussion about maternal risks during pregnancy, delivery and the postpartum period, as well as foetal risk in regard to CHD transmission and overall risk to the health of the foetus. Ideally, this should be undertaken with a cardiologist who specialises in ACHD. Women at extremely high risk of maternal mortality or severe morbidity include (but are not limited to) those with PH, LV EF <30% and/or NYHA III–IV symptoms, severe left heart obstruction or severe native coarctation. In pregnant women with these conditions, the option of pregnancy termination should be discussed (Stout et al. 2019).

Key Point

If the patient with CHD or their partner is pregnant, there is an increased risk of CHD in the offspring. Foetal echocardiography can be useful in determining whether CHD is present, and if so, helps to inform the course of action at the time of delivery (Stout et al. 2019).

Birthing in high-risk women should take place in a specialist centre with multidisciplinary input and close monitoring (Brennan and Hatch 2018).

CHD in Older Adults

Many people with CHD are now living to middle-age and some into the geriatric age range leading to increased use of the medical system for both routine and episodic care. CHD and the sequelae of previous interventions must be treated in the setting of late complications, acquired cardiac disease and the general effects of aging on other body systems.

Suggested Resource Reading

Bhatt, A.B., Foster, E., Kuehl, K. et al. (2015). Congenital heart disease in the older adult: a scientific statement from the American Heart Association. *Circulation* 131 (21): 1884–1931. https://doi.org/10.1161/CIR.0000000000000204

Genetic Heart Disease

Advances in family screening and human gene profiling have led to increased recognition of genetic abnormalities that can lead to congenital heart defects. Certain established patterns of gene disorders, often called by eponymous syndromes, are closely associated with heart defects. Where there are congenital birth defects, a family history should look to identify possible genetic causes. Family screening should be considered and where particular genes are identified as disordered family members can have genotype screening. Certain physical characteristics and developmental delays or learning disabilities can suggest certain syndromes.

Psychosocial Considerations

Whilst there have been marked improvements in understanding and subsequent support and care provision, patients with CHD remain at higher risk of psychological problems compared with a healthy population (Kronwitter et al. 2019). The risk and severity of psychological impairment, encompassing cognitive deficits, mood and anxiety disorders and post-traumatic stress disorder increase with greater complexity of the cardiac lesion (Wilson et al. 2015; Kovacs 2019). In particular, depression in adults with CHD is highly prevalent and is strongly associated with poor prognosis (Huntley et al. 2019; Ladak et al. 2019). Similar patterns are observed within the paediatric and adolescent CHD population, in particular in those with single ventricle anatomy (DeMaso et al. 2017).

Learning Activity 24.1

When patients (or their children) are diagnosed with CHD, most will seek information online about the condition. Identify some reliable resources to which you could direct patients. Consider also organisations that may relate to CHD-related complications. Some examples are provided below but there are many more.

Suggested Resource YouTube

Adult Congenital Heart Disease Association
http://www.achaheart.org
Arrhythmia Alliance
www.heartrhythmcharity.org.uk
British Heart Foundation
www.bhf.org.uk
Canadian Congenital Heart Alliance
http://www.cchaforlife.org
Cardiomyopathy Association
http://www.cardiomyopathy.org
Heart Kids Australia
www.heartkids.org.au
Heart Kids New Zealand
http://heartnz.org.nz
The Somerville Foundation
www.thesf.org.uk

Conclusion

Congenital heart defects are the most common form of congenital anomaly. They are a heterogeneous group of defects affecting the structure of the heart or great vessels. Due to developments in technology and surgery, the majority of patients now survive into adulthood. The needs of this group of patients differ to those with acquired heart disease, and therefore, understanding the underlying pathophysiology of this group of conditions is essential in order to optimise care.

Learning Activity 24.2

There are several video resources available on YouTube on the topic of CHD. As you read about the various types of CHD in this chapter, locate a video on YouTube that relates to the anomaly and describes surgical or percutaneous repair procedures.

Suggested Resource

The Cincinnati Children's Heart Encyclopedia provides detailed information on the congenital heart defects described in this chapter, including signs and symptoms, diagnoses and treatment options. A list can be found at:
Cincinnati Children's Heart Encyclopedia
https://www.cincinnatichildrens.org/patients/child/encyclopedia

---

Suggested Resource YouTube

Congenital heart disease
Joseph Alpert – Lecturio Medical (2018)
https://youtu.be/pNn7pICPAvU

Suggested Resource YouTube

An approach to congenital heart disease
R. Kannan Mutharasan (2018)
https://youtu.be/t0rJOIb10PQ

Suggested Resource website

American Heart Association
Congenital heart defects (2020)
https://www.heart.org/en/health-topics/congenital-heart-defects

References

American Heart Association (AHA) (2020). Common Types of Heart Defects. https://www.heart.org/en/health-topics/congenital-heart-defects/about-congenital-heart-defects/common-types-of-heart-defects.

Baffa, J.M. (2018a). Atrioventricular septal defect. MSD Manual. https://www.msdmanuals.com/professional/pediatrics/congenital-cardiovascular-anomalies/atrioventricular-septal-defect.

Baffa, J.M. (2018b). Coarctation of the aorta. MSD Manual. https://www.msdmanuals.com/professional/pediatrics/congenital-cardiovascular-anomalies/coarctation-of-the-aorta.

Baruteau, A.E., Hascoët, S., Baruteau, J. et al. (2014). Transcatheter closure of patent ductus arteriosus: past, present and future. *Archives of Cardiovascular Diseases* **107** (2): 122–132.

Basit, H., Wallen, T.J., and Sergent, B.N. (2020). Eisenmenger Syndrome. [Updated 2020 June 30]. In: StatPearls [Internet]. Treasure Island (FL): StatPearls Publishing; 2020 January-. https://www.ncbi.nlm.nih.gov/books/NBK507800.

Bellsham-Revell, H. and Burch, M. (2014). Congenital heart disease in infancy and childhood. *Medicine* **42** (11): 650–655.

Beroukhim, R.S., Gauvreau, K., Benavidez, O.J. et al. (2015). Perinatal outcome after prenatal diagnosis of single-ventricle cardiac defects. *Ultrasound in Obstetrics and Gynecology* **45** (6): 657–663.

Blue, G.M., Kirk, E.P., Sholler, G.F. et al. (2012). Congenital heart disease: current knowledge about causes and inheritance. *The Medical Journal of Australia* **197** (3): 155–159.

Boyle, B., Addor, M.C., Arriola, L. et al. (2018). Estimating Global Burden of Disease due to congenital anomaly: an analysis of European data. *Archives of Disease in Childhood-Fetal and Neonatal Edition* **103** (1): F22–F28.

Brennan, K. and Hatch, D.M. (2018). Eisenmenger's syndrome. In: *Consults in Obstetric Anesthesiology* (ed. S.K.W. Mankowitz), 185–187. Cham: Springer.

Cahill, T.J., Baddour, L.M., Habib, G. et al. (2017). Challenges in infective endocarditis. *Journal of the American College of Cardiology* **69** (3): 325–344.

Chambers, J., Thornhill, M., Dayer, M., and Shanson, D. (2016). Antibiotic prophylaxis for dental procedures. *British Journal of General Practice* https://bjgp.org/content/antibiotic-prophylaxis-dental-procedures.

Collins, R.T. II, Doshi, P., Onukwube, J. et al. (2016). Risk factors for increased hospital resource utilization and in-hospital mortality in adults with single ventricle congenital heart disease. *The American Journal of Cardiology* **118** (3): 453–462.

Dahou, A., Mahjoub, H., and Pibarot, P. (2016). Prosthesis-patient mismatch after aortic valve replacement. *Current Treatment Options in Cardiovascular Medicine* **18** (11): 67.

D'Alto, M. and Diller, G.P. (2014). Pulmonary hypertension in adults with congenital heart disease and Eisenmenger syndrome: current advanced management strategies. *Heart* **100** (17): 1322–1328.

Dakkak, W. and Oliver, T.I. (2020). Ventricular Septal Defect. [Updated 2020 June 7]. In: StatPearls [Internet]. Treasure Island (FL): StatPearls Publishing; 2020 January-. https://www.ncbi.nlm.nih.gov/books/NBK470330.

Dayer, M.J., Jones, S., Prendergast, B. et al. (2015). Incidence of infective endocarditis in England, 2000–2013: a secular trend, interrupted time-series analysis. *The Lancet* **385** (9974): 1219–1228.

DeMaso, D.R., Calderon, J., Taylor, G.A. et al. (2017). Psychiatric disorders in adolescents with single ventricle congenital heart disease. *Pediatrics* **139** (3): e20162241.

Diaz-Frias, J. and Guillaume, M. (2020). Tetralogy of Fallot. [Updated 2020 June 7]. In: StatPearls [Internet]. Treasure Island (FL): StatPearls Publishing; 2020 January-. https://www.ncbi.nlm.nih.gov/books/NBK513288.

Dolk, H., McCullough, N., Callaghan, S. et al. (2020). Risk factors for congenital heart disease: the baby hearts study, a population-based case-control study. *PLoS One* **15** (2): e0227908.

Donald, J.S., Wallace, F.R., d'Udekem, Y., and Konstantinov, I.E. (2019). Congenital aortic valve stenosis: to dilate or operate? *Heart, Lung and Circulation* **28** (4): 519–520.

Fathallah, M. and Krasuski, R.A. (2017). Pulmonic valve disease: review of pathology and current treatment options. *Current Cardiology Reports* **19** (11): 108.

Feldkamp, M.L., Carey, J.C., Byrne, J.L. et al. (2017). Etiology and clinical presentation of birth defects: population based study. *BMJ* **357**: j2249.

Friedman, K. (2018). Preoperative physiology, imaging, and management of interrupted aortic arch. In: *Seminars in Cardiothoracic and Vascular Anesthesia*, vol. **22**, No. 3, 265–269. Sage CA: Los Angeles, CA: SAGE Publications https://journals.sagepub.com/doi/abs/10.1177/1089253218770198.

Geerdink, L.M., du Marchie Sarvaas, G.J., Kuipers, I.M. et al. (2017). Surgical outcome in pediatric patients with Ebstein's anomaly: a multicenter, long-term study. *Congenital Heart Disease* **12** (1): 32–39.

Gillam-Krakauer, M. and Mahajan, K. (2020). Patent Ductus Arteriosus. [Updated 2020 June 24]. In: StatPearls [Internet]. Treasure Island (FL): StatPearls Publishing; 2020 January-. https://www.ncbi.nlm.nih.gov/books/NBK430758.

Hays, L. (2015). Transition to adult congenital heart disease care: a review. *Journal of Pediatric Nursing* **30** (5): e63–e69.

Homma, S., Messe, S.R., Rundek, T. et al. (2016). Patent foramen ovale. *Nature Reviews Disease Primers* **2** (1): 1–16.

Huang, S. and Cook, S.C. (2018). It is not taboo: addressing sexual function in adults with congenital heart disease. *Current Cardiology Reports* **20** (10): 93.

Huntley, G.D., Tecson, K.M., Sodhi, S. et al. (2019). Cardiac denial and expectations associated with depression in adults with congenital heart disease. *The American Journal of Cardiology* **123** (12): 2002–2005.

Kim, C., Cho, Y.H., Lee, M. et al. (2014). Surgery for partial anomalous pulmonary venous connections: modification of the warden procedure with a right atrial appendage flap. *The Korean Journal of Thoracic and Cardiovascular Surgery* **47** (2): 94.

Knowles, R.L., Ridout, D., Crowe, S. et al. (2017). Ethnic and socioeconomic variation in incidence of congenital heart defects. *Archives of Disease in Childhood* **102** (6): 496–502.

Kochav, J. (2018). Patent ductus arteriosus. In: *Adult Congenital Heart Disease in Clinical Practice* (ed. D.D. Yeh and A. Bhatt), 91–105. Cham: Springer.

Konduri, A. and Aggarwal, S. (2021). Partial and Total Anomalous Pulmonary Venous Connection. In: *StatPearls*. Treasure Island (FL): StatPearls Publishing. https://www.ncbi.nlm.nih.gov/books/NBK560707/ (accessed January 2022).

Kovacs, A.H. (2019). Neuropsychological outcomes and posttraumatic stress disorder in adults with congenital heart disease. In: da Cruz, E., Macrae, D., & Webb, G. *Intensive Care of the Adult with Congenital Heart Disease* (pp. 507–519). Springer, Cham.

Kronwitter, A., Mebus, S., Neidenbach, R. et al. (2019). Psychosocial situation in adults with congenital heart defects today and 20 years ago: any changes? *International Journal of Cardiology* **275**: 70–76.

Kuijpers, J.M., Mulder, B.J., and Bouma, B.J. (2015). Secundum atrial septal defect in adults: a practical review and recent developments. *Netherlands Heart Journal* **23** (4): 205–211.

Kung, G.C. and Triedman, J.K. (2019). Pathophysiology of left to right shunts. www.uptodate.com.

Ladak, L.A., Hasan, B.S., Gullick, J., and Gallagher, R. (2019). Health-related quality of life in congenital heart disease surgery in children and young adults: a systematic review and meta-analysis. *Archives of Disease in Childhood* **104** (4): 340–347.

Le Pavec, J., Hascoët, S., and Fadel, E. (2018). Heart-lung transplantation: current indications, prognosis and specific considerations. *Journal of Thoracic Disease* **10** (10): 5946.

Liu, Y., Chen, S., Zühlke, L. et al. (2019). Global birth prevalence of congenital heart defects 1970–2017: updated systematic review and meta-analysis of 260 studies. *International Journal of Epidemiology* **48** (2): 455–463.

Loewenthal, M.A. (2016). Pulmonic valvular stenosis. *Medscape*. https://emedicine.medscape.com/article/759890-overview#a4.

Ly, R., Pontnau, F., Lebeaux, D. et al. (2019). Management and outcome of Infective endocarditis in adults with congenital heart disease. *Archives of Cardiovascular Diseases Supplements* **11** (1): 126–127.

Mavroudis, C., Dearani, J.A., and Anderson, R.H. (2020). Ventricular septal defect. In: *Atlas of Adult Congenital Heart Surgery* (ed. C. Mavroudis and J.A. Dearani), 91–115. Cham: Springer.

McCarthy, K., Franklin, R., Slavik, Z., and Ho, S.Y. (2019). Simplified guide to understanding the anatomy of congenital heart disease. In: *Critical Heart Disease in Infants and Children*, 3ee (ed. R.M. Ungerleider, J.N. Meliones, K.N. McMillan, et al.), 100–110. Elsevier.

Micheletti A. (2019) Congenital heart disease classification, epidemiology, diagnosis, treatment, and outcome. In: Flocco S., Lillo A., Dellafiore F., Goossens E. (eds) Congenital Heart Disease. Springer, Cham. https://link.springer.com/chapter/10.1007/978-3-319-78423-6_1.

Moorman, A., Webb, S., Brown, N.A. et al. (2003). Development of the heart: (1) Formation of the cardiac chambers and arterial trunks. *Heart* 89 (7): 806–814.

Morris, J.K., Springett, A.L., Greenlees, R. et al. (2018). Trends in congenital anomalies in Europe from 1980 to 2012. *PLoS One* **13** (4): e0194986.

Murthy, R., Nigro, J., and Karamlou, T. (2019). Tricuspid atresia. In: *Critical Heart Disease in Infants and Children*, 3ee (ed. R.M. Ungerleider, J.N. Meliones, K.N. McMillan, et al.), 765–777. Elsevier.

Nair, R. and Muthukuru, S.R. (2020). Dextrocardia. [Updated 2020 August 10]. In: StatPearls [Internet]. Treasure Island (FL): StatPearls Publishing; 2020 January-. https://www.ncbi.nlm.nih.gov/books/NBK55607.

National Institute of Clinical Excellence (2008). Prophylaxis against infective endocarditis: antimicrobial prophylaxis against infective endocarditis in adults and children undergoing interventional procedures. In: Department of Health U, editor.: National Institute of Clinical Excellence.

Nelson, J.S., Stone, M.L., and Gangemi, J.J. (2019). Coarctation of the aorta. In: *Critical Heart Disease in Infants and Children*, 3ee (ed. R.M. Ungerleider, J.N. Meliones, K.N. McMillan, et al.), 551–564. Elsevier.

Ohye, R.G., Schranz, D., and D'Udekem, Y. (2016). Current therapy for hypoplastic left heart syndrome and related single ventricle lesions. *Circulation* **134** (17): 1265–1279.

Ossa Galvis, M.M., Bhakta, R.T., Tarmahomed, A. et al. (2020). Cyanotic Heart Disease. [Updated 2020 July 2]. In: StatPearls [Internet]. Treasure Island (FL): StatPearls Publishing; 2020 January-. https://www.ncbi.nlm.nih.gov/books/NBK500001.

Patel, V., D. Chisholm., T. Dua, R. Laxminarayan, and M.E. Medina-Mora, Eds. 2015. *Mental, Neurological, and Substance Use Disorders. Disease Control Priorities*, 3, Vol **4**. Washington, DC: World Bank. doi:https://doi.org/10.1596/978-1-4648-0426-7.

Pujari, S.H. and Agasthi, P. (2020). Aortic Stenosis. [Updated 2020 May 30]. In: StatPearls [Internet]. Treasure Island (FL): StatPearls Publishing; 2020 January-. https://www.ncbi.nlm.nih.gov/books/NBK557628.

Quan, T.P., Muller-Pebody, B., Fawcett, N. et al. (2020). Investigation of the impact of the NICE guidelines regarding antibiotic prophylaxis during invasive dental procedures on the incidence of infective endocarditis in England: an electronic health records study. *BMC Medicine* **18** (1): 1–17.

Rajani, R. and Klein, J.L. (2020). Infective endocarditis: a contemporary update. *Clinical Medicine* **20** (1): 31.

Rao, P.S. and Harris, A.D. (2018). Recent advances in managing septal defects: ventricular septal defects and atrioventricular septal defects. *F1000Research* 7: F1000 Faculty Rev-498. doi: https://doi.org/10.12688/f1000research.14102.1.

Roos-Hesselink, J.W. and Johnson, M.R. (ed.) (2017). *Pregnancy and Congenital Heart Disease*. Switzerland: Springer International Publishing.

Sandberg, C., Pomeroy, J., Thilén, U. et al. (2016). Habitual physical activity in adults with congenital heart disease compared with age-and sex-matched controls. *Canadian Journal of Cardiology* **32** (4): 547–553.

Sarris, G.E., Balmer, C., Bonou, P. et al. (2017). Clinical guidelines for the management of patients with transposition of the great arteries with intact ventricular septum. *European Journal of Cardio-Thoracic Surgery* **51** (1): e1–e32.

Schlichting, L.E., Insaf, T.Z., Zaidi, A.N. et al. (2019). Maternal comorbidities and complications of delivery in pregnant women with congenital heart disease. *Journal of the American College of Cardiology* **73** (17): 2181–2191.

Schwerzmann, M., Schwitz, F., Thomet, C. et al. (2017). Challenges of congenital heart disease in grown-up patients. *Swiss Medical Weekly* **147** (w14495): w14495.

Sears, E.H., Aliotta, J.M., and Klinger, J.R. (2012). Partial anomalous pulmonary venous return presenting with adult-onset pulmonary hypertension. *Pulmonary Circulation* **2** (2): 250–255.

Shah, S.N. and Shah, A.N. (2018). Aortic coarctation. *Medscape*. https://emedicine.medscape.com/article/150369-overview.

Sheehan, F. and Redington, A. (2008). The right ventricle: anatomy, physiology and clinical imaging. *Heart* **94** (11): 1510–1515.

Singh, G.K. (2019). Congenital aortic valve stenosis. *Children* **6** (5): 69.

Smith, L.K., Budd, J.L., Field, D.J., & Draper, E.S. (2011). Socioeconomic inequalities in outcome of pregnancy and neonatal mortality associated with congenital anomalies: population based study. *BMJ*, **343**: d4306. doi: https://doi.org/10.1136/bmj.d4306.

Stout, K.K., Daniels, C.J., Aboulhosn, J.A. et al. (2019). 2018 AHA/ACC guideline for the management of adults with congenital heart disease: a report of the American College of Cardiology/American Heart Association Task Force on Clinical Practice Guidelines. *Journal of the American College of Cardiology* **73** (12): e81–e192.

Suradi, H. and Hijazi, Z.M. (2015). Current management of coarctation of the aorta. *Global Cardiology Science and Practice* **44**: 1–11.

Szymanski, M.W., Moore, S.M., and Kritzmire, S.M. et al. (2020) Transposition of The Great Arteries. [Updated 2020 April 28]. In: StatPearls [Internet]. Treasure Island (FL): StatPearls Publishing; 2020 January-. https://www.ncbi.nlm.nih.gov/books/NBK538434.

Thakur, V., Munk, N., Mertens, L., and Nield, L.E. (2016). Does prenatal diagnosis of hypoplastic left heart syndrome make a difference? – a systematic review. *Prenatal Diagnosis* **36** (9): 854–863.

Tongsong, T., Luewan, S., Jatavan, P. et al. (2016). A simple rule for prenatal diagnosis of total anomalous pulmonary venous return. *Journal of Ultrasound in Medicine* **35** (7): 1601–1607.

Van Hare, G.F., Ackerman, M.J., Evangelista, J.A.K. et al. (2015). Eligibility and disqualification recommendations for competitive athletes with cardiovascular abnormalities: task force 4: congenital heart disease: a scientific statement from the American Heart Association and American College of Cardiology. *Circulation* **132** (22): e281–e291.

Van Velzen, C.L., Haak, M.C., Reijnders, G. et al. (2015). Prenatal detection of transposition of the great arteries reduces mortality and morbidity. *Ultrasound in Obstetrics and Gynecology* **45** (3): 320–325.

Vigl, M., Hager, A., Bauer, U. et al. (2009). Sexuality and subjective wellbeing in male patients with congenital heart disease. *Heart* **95** (14): 1179–1183.

Vigl, M., Kaemmerer, M., Niggemeyer, E. et al. (2010). Sexuality and reproductive health in women with congenital heart disease. *The American Journal of Cardiology* **105** (4): 538–541.

Von Steinburg, S.P., Boulesteix, A.L., Lederer, C. et al. (2013). What is the 'normal' fetal heart rate? *PeerJ* **1**: e82.

Weber, R.W., Stiasny, B., Ruecker, B. et al. (2019). Prenatal diagnosis of single ventricle physiology impacts on cardiac morbidity and mortality. *Pediatric Cardiology* **40** (1): 61–70.

Wilson, W., Taubert, K.A., Gewitz, M. et al. (2007). Prevention of infective endocarditis: guidelines from the American heart association: a guideline from the American heart association rheumatic fever, endocarditis, and Kawasaki disease committee, council on cardiovascular disease in the young, and the council on clinical cardiology, council on cardiovascular surgery and anesthesia, and the quality of care and outcomes research interdisciplinary working group. *Circulation* **116** (15): 1736–1754.

Wilson, W.M., Smith-Parrish, M., Marino, B.S., and Kovacs, A.H. (2015). Neurodevelopmental and psychosocial outcomes across the congenital heart disease lifespan. *Progress in Pediatric Cardiology* **39** (2): 113–118.

Zaidi, S. and Brueckner, M. (2017). Genetics and genomics of congenital heart disease. *Circulation Research* **120** (6): 923–940.

Zhang, X.L., Kang, L.N., Wang, L., and Xu, B. (2018). Percutaneous closure versus medical therapy for stroke with patent foramen Ovale: a systematic review and meta-analysis. *BMC Cardiovascular Disorders* **18** (1): 45.

25

Structural Heart Disease

Christopher Nicholson, Salimah Hassan, Robyn Lotto, and Angela M. Kucia

Overview

Structural heart disease is the term used to describe conditions that affect the valves, muscles or walls of the heart. Structural heart disease may be present from birth (congenital), but they often can develop with ageing or result from other diseases (acquired). This chapter provides an overview of common structural heart diseases. Congenital heart disease is discussed in detail in Chapter 24.

Learning Objectives

After reading this chapter and completing the learning activities, the reader will be able to:

- Describe cardiac conditions classed as acquired and hereditary structural heart disease.
- Discuss the relationship between rheumatic heart disease and valvular disease.
- Identify the most common forms of cardiomyopathy and their causes.
- Discuss the role of the nurse in a multidisciplinary team caring for patients with structural heart disease.
- Identify sources of information for patients with structural heart disease and their families.

Key Concepts

Valvular disease; valve stenosis; valve regurgitation; cardiomyopathy; rheumatic heart disease

Valvular Heart Disease

The most common form of structural heart disease is valvular disease. The prevalence of VHD is estimated to be around 2.5% in developed countries (Lung and Vahanian 2014). With the decline of rheumatic heart disease (RHD) (see Box 25.1), degenerative aetiologies have become the predominant cause of VHD in developed countries resulting in a marked increase in diagnosis in patients over the age of 65 (Lung and Vahanian 2014).

Valvular heart disease (VHD) is caused by either damage or defect in one of the four heart valves: aortic; mitral; tricuspid or pulmonary. VHD may present as valvular stenosis, regurgitation or a combination of both. A stenotic valve is one where the valve acts as an obstruction to blood leaving the heart chamber, whilst regurgitation, or valve insufficiency, refers to leakage of blood through the valve as it closes. Aortic stenosis and mitral regurgitation are the most common diagnoses, continuing to account for about three in four cases of VHD

Cardiac Care: A Practical Guide for Nurses, Second Edition. Edited by Angela M. Kucia and Ian D. Jones.

Box 25.1   Rheumatic heart disease.

Acute rheumatic fever (ARF) and its sequel rheumatic heart disease (RHD) are under-recognised conditions that are associated with significant morbidity and mortality in developing countries and in some sub-populations in developed countries (Watkins et al. 2017). Infections such as strep throat, scarlet fever, or skin sores, pyoderma, impetigo that are associated with Group A β-haemolytic streptococcus (GAS) can lead to ARF. In a susceptible host, GAS may trigger an autoimmune response that results in a generalised inflammatory illness (ARF). Generalised inflammatory symptoms that involve the skin and joints may resolve, but if the heart has been affected (acute carditis), damage to the heart valves may remain once the acute carditis has resolved, leading to chronic RHD. Recurrent GAS infections and episodes of ARF can further damage the heart valves, making RHD progressively worse over time (He et al. 2016). Prevention of RHD at the time of a first attack of acute rheumatic fever is the best strategy. In the case of infection, antibiotic treatment of group A streptococcus sore throat is key in primary prevention. The management of GAS infection is a simple shot of Benzathine Penicillin G (BPG), which can prevent the development of RHD at a rate of 80%, but many countries have been affected by a worldwide shortage of penicillin (Yellapu et al. 2019). Even in developed countries, some subsections of the population bear a higher burden of RHD. Rates of RHD among Indigenous (Aboriginal and Torres Strait Islander) Australians, many of whom live in poverty in overcrowded conditions, are among the highest rates reported worldwide (He et al. 2016).

---

valvular disease, it is recommended that you consult the appropriate national/international guidelines used in your country.

Suggested Resources

- Writing Committee Members, Otto, C.M., Nishimura, R.A., Bonow, R.O., Carabello, B.A., Erwin III, J.P., Gentile, F., Jneid, H., Krieger, E.V., Mack, M.n and McLeod, C. (2021). 2020 ACC/AHA guideline for the Management of Patients with Valvular Heart Disease: a report of the American College of Cardiology/American Heart Association Joint Committee on Clinical Practice Guidelines. *Journal of the American College of Cardiology*, 77(4), e25–e197. https://doi.org/10.1016/j.jacc.2020.11.018
- Vahanian, A., Beyersdorf, F., Praz, F., Milojevic, M., Baldus, S., Bauersachs, J., ... & Wojakowski, W. (2022). 2021 ESC/EACTS Guidelines for the management of valvular heart disease: developed by the Task Force for the management of valvular heart disease of the European Society of Cardiology (ESC) and the European Association for Cardio-Thoracic Surgery (EACTS). *European Heart Journal*, 43(7), 561–632. https://doi.org/10.1093/eurheartj/ehab395

Key Point

Secondary national or international guidelines for management of RHD (see suggested resource guidelines for management of valvular disease above) provide advice on secondary prophylaxis regimes, antibiotic choice, dose, frequency, and duration of secondary prophylaxis.

(Lung and Vahanian 2011; Bravo-Jaimes et al. 2018). Valvular abnormalities may be congenital or acquired. This section focusses on acquired valve disease. For in-depth information on current management strategies for

Aortic Valve Disease

The aortic valve lies between the left ventricle and the aorta. During the cardiac cycle, the left ventricle contracts and the blood is expelled through the aortic valve into the aorta and around the systemic circulation.

Aortic Valve Stenosis

Aortic valve stenosis (AVS) is the most common primary valve disease that leads to surgery or catheter intervention in Europe and North America (Vahanian et al. 2021). In patients with aortic stenosis, the afterload (the amount of resistance the heart must overcome to open the aortic valve and push the blood volume out into the systemic circulation) steadily increases as the aortic valve narrows. As a result, the left ventricle is required to generate an increasingly high systolic pressure to pump the blood through the valve. To compensate for this, the left ventricular (LV) muscle wall thickens. This is known as concentric hypertrophy (Carabello and Paulus, 2009). The thickened myocardium enables the LV systolic contraction to strengthen, thus initially maintaining an adequate stroke volume (SV) and cardiac output (CO). However, over time, compensatory mechanisms start to fail, heart failure (HF) develops (see Chapter 22 for the pathophysiology of HF). The hypertrophic myocardium may also compress the coronary arteries, thereby reducing coronary blood flow and potentially causing ischaemia.

Aortic valve replacement (AVR) is the only 'curative' intervention for AVS, but the decision to offer intervention must be carefully considered: to intervene too early may unnecessarily expose patients to the risks of valve replacement; to intervene too late may cause irreversible cardiac damage that is associated with an increased risk of HF and death (Bing and Dweck 2020). AVR may be performed using transcatheter aortic valve implantation (TAVI) or surgical AVR according to the patient risk profile and availability of the intervention. A recent meta-analysis of trials comparing surgical AVR with TAVI suggests that in patients with symptomatic, severe AS, TAVI was associated with a reduction in all-cause mortality and stroke up to 2 years compared with surgical AVR (Siontis et al. 2019). However, long-term durability data for TAVI beyond 5 years are still limited (Okutucu et al. 2020).

Durability and structural valve deterioration are the main limitations for bioprosthetic heart valves, whereas an increased risk of bleeding due to the requirement for oral anticoagulation is a limitation of mechanical valves (Head et al. 2017).

Aortic Regurgitation

Aortic regurgitation (AR) can be caused by primary disease of the aortic valve cusps and/or abnormalities of the aortic root and ascending aortic geometry. In developed countries, AR is more commonly due to degenerative causes. Acute AR may occur secondary to infective and rheumatic endocarditis, and less commonly, aortic dissection, blunt chest trauma or iatrogenic causes following transcatheter procedure (Otto et al. 2020). Asymptomatic patients with severe aortic regurgitation require careful follow-up of symptomatic status and LV size and function (Vahanian et al. 2021). Valve surgery is indicated for symptomatic patients (spontaneous or on exercise testing) and/or LVEF <50% and/or end-systolic diameter > 50 mm. Medical therapy can provide some symptomatic improvement in individuals with chronic severe AR in whom surgery is not feasible (Otto et al. 2020). In patients with acute severe aortic regurgitation from aortic dissection or infective endocarditis, medical therapy to reduce LV afterload may be required, especially if hypotension, pulmonary oedema, or evidence of low flow is present (Otto et al. 2020).

Key Point

Intra-aortic balloon counterpulsation (IABP) is contraindicated in patients with acute severe AR (Otto et al. 2020). IABP will increase diastolic pressure in the aorta and will augment forward flow to the body and organs, but it will also increase back flow. If the aortic valve does not close properly, IABP will increase the amount of blood flowing back into the LV through the incompetent aortic valve, thereby increasing the workload of the LV.

Mitral Valve Disease

The mitral valve sits between the left atrium and left ventricle. In a normal cardiac cycle, the mitral valve is open as the atrium contracts and blood flows through into the ventricle. The valve then closes during systole as the left ventricle contracts. The mitral valve is functionally and anatomically complex and consists of several components: the annulus, the leaflets and the sub-valvular apparatus including the chordae tendineae, the papillary muscles and the ventricular wall (Del Forno et al. 2020).

Mitral Regurgitation

Mitral regurgitation (MR) is the second-most frequent indication for valve surgery in Europe (Vahanian et al. 2021). It is essential to distinguish primary from secondary MR as the two diseases have different aetiologies, pathophysiology, natural history, and thus different indications and responses to medical, transcatheter, and surgical therapies. Primary MR is caused by inherent lesions that impair the function of the mitral apparatus, including the leaflets, chordae tendineae, papillary muscles or annulus, and is the most common cause of primary MR is mitral valve prolapse. Up to 70% of patients with primary MR have a Class 1 indication for surgery (Monteagudo Ruiz et al. 2018). As primary MR is due to disease of the valve itself, treating the valve can be curative (Izquierdo-Gómez et al. 2018).

In secondary MR, the mitral valve is morphologically normal, but disease of the left ventricle has led to abnormal anatomy and function that causes displacement of one or both papillary muscles, leaflet tethering, inadequate closure of the valve and often annular dilatation. Secondary MR may result from ischaemic or non-ischaemic ventricular disease including ischaemic cardiomyopathy, idiopathic dilated cardiomyopathy, atrial functional MR or hypertrophic cardiomyopathy. Atrial fibrillation with left atrial enlargement may be the underlying mechanism of secondary MR when LV structure and function are normal (Del Forno et al. 2020). In secondary MR, the mitral valve itself is not the origin of the disease; therefore, therapy directed only at MR may reduce regurgitation but cannot cure the basic underlying pathology (Izquierdo-Gómez et al. 2018). The therapeutic approach for secondary MR remains uncertain (Monteagudo Ruiz et al. 2018).

Key Point

Acute MR classically occurs with a spontaneous chordae tendineae or papillary muscle rupture secondary to myocardial infarction. Other causes include rupture of these structures due to mitral valve prolapse, endocarditis, and trauma. Acute pulmonary edema and cardiogenic shock often complicate the course of acute MR. The operative mortality in these cases approaches 80% (Chin 2020). In chronic MR, the left ventricle adapts for some time, and symptoms may be delayed for years (Lung 2003). However, in acute MR, the left ventricle is unable to adequately compensate, and the patient is likely to present with severe symptoms. This is reflected in increased mortality and morbidity rates (Nishino et al. 2016.)

Mitral Stenosis

Mitral stenosis (MS) is characterised by obstruction of blood flow across the mitral valve from the left atrium to the left ventricle. Mitral stenosis has a variable presentation. RHD has been a frequent cause of mitral stenosis (MS) worldwide, though the incidence is low in high-income countries, and slowly declining elsewhere. In regions with a high prevalence of RHD, patients usually present at a younger age (10–30 years) (Otto et al. 2020). Another infrequent form of MS may result from congenital heart disease. Non-rheumatic degenerative calcific mitral valve disease is encountered mainly in elderly patients (Vahanian et al. 2021). Calcific MS results from calcification of the mitral valve annulus that extends to the base of the leaflets resulting in narrowing of the annulus and rigidity of the leaflets (Gaasch 2020).

One of the most common complications of MS is atrial fibrillation (AF) (Lung et al. 2018). AF is associated with an increased risk of morbidity, in particular stroke (see Chapter 11).

Key Point

Medical management of atrial fibrillation (AF) in patients with MS does not differ significantly from routine AF guidelines, but as AF often has exaggerated haemodynamic effects in MS, prompt therapy is often necessary (Gaasch 2020).

Periodic monitoring is recommended in asymptomatic patients with MS to assess for disease progression and development of indications for intervention (Gaasch 2020). Diuretics, beta-blockers, digoxin or heart-rate-regulating calcium-channel blockers can transiently improve symptoms. The timing and type of intervention is decided based on clinical characteristics, valve anatomy and local expertise. Percutaneous mitral commissurotomy should be considered as an initial treatment for selected patients with mild to moderate disease who have otherwise favourable clinical characteristics and surgery, usually for valve replacement, is indicated in the other patients (Percutaneous mitral commissurotomy).

Tricuspid Valve Disease

The tricuspid valve sits between the right atrium and right ventricle. It opens at the end of systole, then closes as the ventricles contract, to ensure that blood flows in a forward direction. This enables blood to be pumped from the right side of the heart to the lungs for oxygenation.

Tricuspid Regurgitation

The more common form of tricuspid disease is tricuspid regurgitation (TR). This occurs when the valve cannot close adequately, resulting in the backward leakage of blood into the right atrium with each heart contraction. Causes of tricuspid regurgitation include HF (which can be a cause or a consequence of TR), cardiomyopathies, ventricular dilation secondary to high blood pressure in the pulmonary circulation (pulmonary hypertension), and less commonly, trauma, infective endocarditis, RHD, carcinoid syndrome and congenital heart defects (Harris et al. 2017). For further information on congenital heart defects, refer to Chapter 24.

Tricuspid Stenosis

In tricuspid stenosis (TS), the valve becomes stiff and narrowed, preventing the forward flow of blood from the atrium to the ventricle (Harris et al. 2017). TS most commonly results from RHD, which causes the leaflets of the valve to become thick, hardened and less able to open widely, thus restricting forward blood flow. Infective endocarditis on the right side of the heart is relatively rare (Shrestha et al. 2015). But around 90–95% of cases involve the tricuspid valve (Murdoch et al. 2009). Many of these infections result from IV drug use, accounting for approximately 30–40% of tricuspid valve endocarditis (Edmond et al. 2001; Hussain et al. 2017).

Key Point

Patients with TS tend to present only when the valve disease is severe.

Symptoms reflect those of right-sided HF and include fatigue, shortness of breath, raised central venous pressure and potentially an enlarged pulsating liver. Management of tricuspid valve disease will depend on the severity of the disease and symptoms, as well as the underlying cause. Treatment of the underlying HF with medication can relieve symptoms. Valve repair or replacement may be an option depending on co-morbidities (Harris et al. 2017).

Pulmonary Valve Disease

The pulmonary valve sits between the right ventricle and the pulmonary artery. Abnormalities of the pulmonary valve may lead to an obstruction to the right ventricle outflow tract.

Pulmonary Valve Stenosis

Pulmonary valve stenosis (PVS) is predominantly associated with congenital cardiac disease, but in rare instances, acquired disorders such as carcinoid or rheumatic fever affect the pulmonary valve (Fathallah and Krasuski 2017). PVS results in overload of the right ventricle, which in turn leads to compensatory right ventricular hypertrophy. Increased muscle mass is a compensatory mechanism to assist the right ventricle to maintain a normal CO. Over time, progressive right ventricular hypertrophy can give rise to right ventricular dysfunction. Treatment options for PVS include surgical valvotomy, balloon pulmonary valvuloplasty (BPV) and pulmonary valve replacement. Balloon pulmonary valvuloplasty (BPV) is the procedure of choice for PVS as it is less invasive and has a very high success. Long-term complications following BPV are progressive PR and restenosis (Fathalla and Krasuski 2017).

Pulmonary Valve Regurgitation

Pulmonary regurgitation (PR) is rarely seen as a primary pathology. Primary causes of PR have some overlap with causes of PS, but PR is most often the result of prior intervention on the pulmonary valve (Ruckdeschel and Kim 2019). Iatrogenic PR may occur after surgical valvotomy, percutaneous valvuloplasty or Tetralogy of Fallot-related surgery (Fathalla and Krasuski 2017).

Key Point

Pulmonary valvular issues resulting in stenosis and/or regurgitation established long-term consequences of mediastinal radiation (Ky et al. 2020).

Key Point

Endocarditis prophylaxis with antibiotics should be considered for high-risk procedures in patients with prosthetic valves, including transcatheter valves, or with repairs using prosthetic material, and for those with previous episodes of infective endocarditis (IE) (Vahanian et al. 2021). For more information on endocarditis prophylaxis, see Chapter 24.

Cardiomyopathy

Cardiomyopathies are disorders of the cardiac muscle that are characterised by mechanical and/or electrical dysfunction that result in dilated, hypertrophic or restrictive pathophysiology (Schultheiss et al. 2019). Cardiomyopathy can be classed as being primary or secondary. Primary cardiomyopathy does not result from another disease or condition that leads to a weakened heart muscle. In some cases, the cardiomyopathy is inherited and may be passed down to other family members. Secondary cardiomyopathy may result from a medical condition such as hypertension, valve disease, congenital heart disease, coronary artery disease, illicit drug use, excessive alcohol use, chemotherapy and other medications. The goal of therapy for patients with secondary cardiomyopathy is to identify and correct the medical condition(s) that are responsible for the condition.

Initially, patients with a cardiomyopathy may experience few or no symptoms. However, longer-term patients are likely to experience symptoms associated with HF. Many develop arrhythmias and are subsequently at higher risk of sudden cardiac death (Bagnall et al. 2016).

Primary cardiomyopathies are classified into several general categories depending upon their respective disorders of structure and function. The most common of which are dilated cardiomyopathy (DCM), hypertrophic cardiomyopathy (HCM) and arrhythmogenic right ventricular dysplasia cardiomyopathy (ARVD/C).

Dilated Cardiomyopathy

Dilated cardiomyopathy (DCM) is one of the most common causes of HF and the most common indication for heart transplantation worldwide (Weintraub et al. 2017). DCM is characterised by LV or biventricular dilation and impaired contraction that is not explained by abnormal loading conditions (such as hypertension and valvular heart disease) or coronary artery disease. There are several causes of DCM. Around 50% of cases are idiopathic and around half of these patients will have familial disease. DCM can be a component of an inherited disorder, such as neuromuscular diseases (muscular dystrophies and myotonic dystrophy), hereditary haemochromatosis, and hereditary sideroblastic anaemias and thalassaemias. There are currently no clinical or histologic criteria, other than family history that distinguish familial from non-familial disease (Weigner and Morgan 2020). Secondary causes include myocarditis, ischaemic heart disease, infiltrative disease (amyloidosis, sarcoidosis and haemochromatosis), peripartum cardiomyopathy, autoimmune conditions, endocrine disorders (thyroid dysfunction, pheochromocytoma), hypertension, HIV infection, connective tissue disease, chemotherapy agents, and illicit drug and heavy alcohol use (Japp et al. 2016; Schultheiss et al. 2019; Weigner and Morgan 2020). Standard approaches to prevent or treat HF are the first-line treatment for patients with DCM (see Chapter 23), including cardiac resynchronisation therapy and implantable cardioverter–defibrillators (see

Chapter 12) to prevent life-threatening arrhythmias if required (Schultheiss et al. 2019). Identification of the probable cause of DCM helps tailor-specific therapies to improve prognosis (Schultheiss et al. 2019).

Genetic Testing

Genetic testing in patients with DCM facilitates screening, and all first-degree relatives of patients with familial DCM should undergo clinical screening. Pre-test counselling needs to be provided to all patients with DCM, ideally by a person with knowledge of DCM genetics, such as a genetic counsellor. Pre-test counselling helps to facilitate patient understanding of the rationale for testing, increase empowerment and improve communication and dynamics within families. Patients must also understand issues relating to the privacy of their genetic testing results and how it may impact on aspects of their lives in areas such as employment and insurability for themselves and their family members (Rosenbaum et al. 2020).

Hypertrophic Cardiomyopathy

Hypertrophic cardiomyopathy (HCM) is the most common heritable cardiomyopathy though the underlying genetic cause of disease is only found in 34% of patients (Bos et al. 2014). The LV becomes hypertrophic (thickened), non-dilated in HCM and left ventricular (LV) function is preserved (Marian and Braunwald 2017). Patient may be asymptomatic or present with HF or sudden cardiac death (SCD). HCM can be classified as obstructive or non-obstructive depending on whether the heart anatomy causes left ventricular outflow obstruction (LVOT) (Geske et al. 2018). Symptoms relate to the type of structural or functional abnormalities and include fatigue, dyspnoea, chest pain, palpitations and presyncope or syncope (Maron 2020). Therapy is aimed at reduction of LVOT and includes lifestyle modifications, pharmacotherapies and septal reduction therapies. Most patients experience little or no disability, and life expectancy is normal. However, a small subset of patients with HCM will experience SCD (around 1% annually), with risk stratification a significant clinical challenge (Geske et al. 2018) and concordance in international guidelines is lacking. High-risk patients may be treated effectively with the implantable cardioverter–defibrillator. Genetic testing in HCM largely centres on family screening; if a causative genetic mutation is identified, testing for this mutation is the preferred method of family screening (Geske et al. 2018).

Restrictive Cardiomyopathy

Restrictive cardiomyopathy is rare condition. Restrictive cardiomyopathy may occur secondary to causes such as amyloidosis, haemochromatosis and sarcoidosis, but the cause is often idiopathic. Characteristics of restrictive cardiomyopathy that distinguish it from other forms of cardiomyopathy include a non-dilated ventricle with typically normal wall thicknesses, rigid ventricular walls that result in severe diastolic dysfunction and dilated atria, and generally normal LV systolic function (Ammash and Tajik 2020). Some people with this condition have no symptoms or minor symptoms, but others may develop symptoms of HF and arrhythmia. There is no specific therapy for idiopathic restrictive cardiomyopathy. Management includes lifestyle modifications and standard approaches to HF management. Treatment of the disease may be beneficial in patients with secondary restrictive cardiomyopathy (Ammash and Tajik 2020).

Key Point

Incidental radiation therapy to myocardial tissues during treatment for diseases such as breast or lung cancer can result in a restrictive cardiomyopathy (Ky et al. 2020).

Arrhythmogenic Right Ventricular Dysplasia Cardiomyopathy

ARVD/C is a rare inherited form of cardiomyopathy in which the right ventricular heart muscle is gradually replaced by fat or fibrous tissue. As a result, the right ventricle becomes dilated, with reduced contractility. ARVD is characterised by ventricular tachyarrhythmia, predominant right ventricular dysfunction and sudden cardiac death (Wang et al. 2019). The estimated prevalence of ARVD ranges from 1 in 5000 to 1 in 2000 in some European countries (Coelho et al. 2019). Patients typically present in the second to fourth decade of life (Wang et al. 2019), usually with palpitations (30–60%), light-headedness (20%) and syncope (10–30%) linked to the presence of non-sustained or sustained ventricular arrhythmias. Up to 19% of ARVD/C patients present with cardiac arrest. Atrial arrhythmias and atrial fibrillation have also been associated with ARVD/C (Wang et al. 2019). ARVD is one of the leading causes of arrhythmic cardiac arrest in young people and in particular, athletes (Basso et al. 2009). Whilst over 50% of diagnoses have a genetic origin, ARVD may also occur due to non-genetic causes such as myocarditis, or congenital abnormalities affecting the right ventricle.

The clinical approach to managing patients with ARVD/C patients consists of establishing an accurate diagnosis; risk stratification for sudden death; prevention of sustained ventricular arrhythmia; preventing the development of HF; cardiac transplant; and screening and follow-up of family members. ICD implantation with anti-tachycardia pacing (ATP) may be recommended following a discussion about the risk-benefits of having/not having and ICD. The use of anti-arrhythmic drugs rarely eliminates the risk of sudden death and is mainly to reduce the arrhythmia burden (Wang et al. 2019). See Chapter 12 for further information on AVRD.

Learning Activity 25.1

When patients receive a serious diagnosis such as arrhythmogenic right ventricular dysplasia cardiomyopathy, they generally go to the internet for information. Identify at least three reliable and evidence-based sources of information that are suitable for patients with conditions discussed in this chapter.

Other Forms of Cardiomyopathy

Some types of cardiomyopathy do not fit well into the general classifications. These are discussed briefly below.

Takotsubo Syndrome

Takotsubo syndrome (TTS), previously known as 'takotsubo cardiomyopathy', 'stress cardiomyopathy' or apical ballooning syndrome' is a condition that is usually associated with an emotional or physical stressor that leads to transient LV wall motion abnormalities and reduced EF that may lead to HF (see Chapter 26).

Peripartum Cardiomyopathy

Peripartum cardiomyopathy is a relatively rare form of cardiomyopathy with systolic dysfunction that typically presents in late pregnancy and up to 6 months postpartum. The cause of PPCM is unknown and the diagnosis of PPCM is one of exclusion of other causes of HF. PPCM incidence is highest in women of African

descent, and other associated factors include age > 25 years, pregnancy-associated hypertensive disorders and anaemia (Rodriguez Ziccardi and Siddique 2020). The LV ejection fraction (EF) is almost always below 45% and the left ventricle may or may not be dilated. PPCM is associated with HF, an increased risk of atrial and ventricular arrhythmias, thromboembolism and sudden cardiac death. The initial medical management of PPCM is like that for other causes of HF, with the special consideration of how the pregnancy will be affected.

Therapeutic considerations may include arrhythmia management, anticoagulation therapy, inotropes (with close monitoring and weaning off as soon as practical), mechanical support and possible transplant (Rodriguez Ziccardi and Siddique 2020). More than half of affected women recover systolic function, although some are left with a chronic cardiomyopathy, and a minority require mechanical support or cardiac transplantation (Honigberg and Givertz 2019). Women with a minimal decrease in EF tend to have a good prognosis, whereas those with a poor EF and those requiring mechanical support have a higher risk of death (Rodriguez Ziccardi and Siddique 2020). Information, education and support are critical for patients with PPCM. As management of PPCM involves input from various specialties (obstetrics, midwifery, cardiology, heart failure teams; social work, community health and possibly mental health), coordinated multidisciplinary support is essential for these patients. Many will face significant physical and psychological challenges in caring for a newborn whilst they are ill.

Key Point

A recent study has suggested that around one third of pregnancy-associated cardiomyopathy patients had TTS. Peripartum takosubo syndrome should be considered as a differential diagnosis of HF during peripartum (Kim et al. 2020).

Chemotherapy/Radiotherapy-Induced Cardiomyopathy

Cancer therapy may result in damage to multiple cardiac structures as a late complication that may not be manifested for years after treatment has completed. The outcomes of cancer survivors who develop cardiomyopathy (whether due to chemotherapy or radiation therapy) are generally poor. Anthracycline analogues, particularly doxorubicin (Adriamycin), are the chemotherapeutic agents most associated with cardiotoxicity, but there are several others (Ky et al. 2020). Historically, it has been thought that cardiotoxicity related to anthracyclines is irreversible, but more recent evidence demonstrates that early identification of cardiotoxicity and prompt therapy for HF can lead to substantial improvement in LVEF. Early detection of cardiac dysfunction and provision of cardiac-specific therapy is imperative to prevent progression of cardiac dysfunction (Ky et al. 2020).

Key Point

It has been suggested that chemotherapy accounts for 1–2% of TTS triggers (Storey and Sharkey 2019). Fluorouracil (5FU) is the most reported, though there are many others (Coen et al. 2017). The onset of TTS relative to chemotherapy initiation is quite variable and may occur at any time from the initial administration to several weeks beyond initiation. TTS in the setting of treatment for malignancy is associated with substantial mortality (Storey and Sharkey 2019).

The Multidisciplinary Team Caring for Patients with Acquired Structural Heart Disease

A multidisciplinary team approach inclusive of cardiologists, surgeons, specialist nurses, physiologists or clinical scientists is recommended for all types of valve disease and infective endocarditis (Chambers et al. 2017). Roles of the nurse may include providing information and education for the patient about their condition, monitoring of the patient for symptoms, physical examination, review of medication, lifestyle advice about smoking cessation, weight control and dental surveillance and communicate the results of follow-up with the general practitioner and referring physician. Nurses often coordinate outpatient clinics, manage appointments, maintain audit databases, follow-up laboratory results, and run the telephone and email helplines. Multidisciplinary valve clinics have been found to be patient-focused and cost-effective (Chambers et al. 2020).

Patients with cardiomyopathy complicated by HF are also best managed by a multidisciplinary team with health care professionals that specialise is various aspects of care, including primary physicians (general practitioners), HF nurse specialist, cardiologist, dietician, pharmacist, psychologist, physical and occupational therapists, exercise physiologist and social worker. Additionally, patients with familial DCM and their families may needed additional support from geneticists and councillors.

Conclusion

Structural heart disease encompasses a broad range of congenital, hereditary, and acquired conditions with a wide variation in morbidity and mortality. Structural heart disease can present across the lifespan and occur as a primary condition or secondary to other disease processes, environmental and lifestyle factors. Heart failure is a common feature of many structural heart diseases and early identification and intervention are needed to halt the progression of disease and maximise cardiac function to improve survival and quality of life.

References

Ammash, N.M. and Tajik, A.J. (2020). Idiopathic restrictive cardiomyopathy. In: (ed. W.J. McKenna), *UpToDate*. https://www.uptodate.com/contents/idiopathic-restrictive-cardiomyopathy (accessed 14 January 2021).

Bagnall, R.D., Weintraub, R.G., Ingles, J. et al. (2016). A prospective study of sudden cardiac death among children and young adults. *New England Journal of Medicine* **374** (25): 2441–2452.

Basso, C., Corrado, D., Marcus, F.I. et al. (2009). Arrhythmogenic right ventricular cardiomyopathy. *The Lancet* **373** (9671): 1289–1300.

Bing, R. and Dweck, M.R. (2020). Management of asymptomatic severe aortic stenosis: check or all in? *Heart* http://dx.doi.org/10.1136/heartjnl-2020-317160.

Bos, J.M., Will, M.L., Gersh, B.J. et al. (2014). Characterization of a phenotype-based genetic test prediction score for unrelated patients with hypertrophic cardiomyopathy. *Mayo Clinic Proceedings* **89** (6): 727–737. Elsevier.

Bravo-Jaimes, K., Tankut S. & Mieszczanska, H.Z. (2018). Diagnosis and management of valvular heart disease in Mieszczanska H.Z. & Budzikowski, A.S. (Eds.), *Cardiology Consult Manual* (pp. 159–189). Springer International Publishing.

Carabello, B.A. and Paulus, W.J. (2009). Aortic stenosis. *The Lancet* **373** (9667): 956–966.

Chambers, J.B., Prendergast, B., Iung, B. et al. (2017). Standards defining a "Heart Valve Centre": ESC Working Group on valvular heart disease and European Association for cardiothoracic surgery viewpoint. *European Heart Journal* **38** (28): 2177–2183.

Chambers, J.B., Parkin, D., Rimington, H., Subbiah, S., Campbell, B., Demetrescu, C., . . . & Rajani, R. (2020). Specialist valve clinic in a cardiac centre: 10-year experience. *Open Heart*, **7** (1): e001262. https://doi.org/10.1136/openhrt-2020-001262.

Chin, M.M. (2020) Acute mitral regurgitation. Medscape. https://emedicine.medscape.com/article/758816-overview (accessed 18 April 2022).

Coelho, S.A., Silva, F., Silva, J., and António, N. (2019). Athletic training and arrhythmogenic right ventricular cardiomyopathy. *International Journal of Sports Medicine* **40** (5): 295–304.

Coen, M., Rigamonti, F., Roth, A., and Koessler, T. (2017). Chemotherapy-induced Takotsubo cardiomyopathy, a case report and review of the literature. *BMC Cancer* **17** (1): 1–5.

Del Forno, B., De Bonis, M., Agricola, E. et al. (2020). Mitral valve regurgitation: a disease with a wide spectrum of therapeutic options. *Nature Reviews Cardiology* **17** (12): 807–827.

Edmond, J.J., Eykyn, S.J., and Smith, L.D. (2001). Community acquired staphylococcal pulmonary valve endocarditis in non-drug users: case report and review of the literature. *Heart* **86** (6): E17.

Fathallah, M. and Krasuski, R.A. (2017). Pulmonic valve disease: review of pathology and current treatment options. *Current Cardiology Reports* **19** (11): 108.

Gaasch, W.H. (2020). Overview of the management of mitral stenosis. In: (ed. S.B. Yeon), *UpToDate*. https://www.uptodate.com/contents/overview-of-the-management-of-mitral-stenosis (accessed 3 January 2021).

Geske, J.B., Ommen, S.R., and Gersh, B.J. (2018). Hypertrophic cardiomyopathy: clinical update. *JACC: HF* **6** (5): 364–375.

Harris, C., Croce, B., and Munkholm-Larsen, S. (2017). Tricuspid valve disease. *Annals of Cardiothoracic Surgery* **6** (3): 294–294.

He, V.Y., Condon, J.R., Ralph, A.P. et al. (2016). Long-term outcomes from acute rheumatic fever and rheumatic heart disease: a data-linkage and survival analysis approach. *Circulation* **134** (3): 222–232.

Head, S.J., Çelik, M., and Kappetein, A.P. (2017). Mechanical versus bioprosthetic aortic valve replacement. *European Heart Journal* **38** (28): 2183–2191.

Honigberg, M.C., & Givertz, M.M. (2019). Peripartum cardiomyopathy. *BMJ*;364:k5287. https://doi.org/10.1136/bmj.k5287.

Hussain, S.T., Witten, J., Shrestha, N.K. et al. (2017). Tricuspid valve endocarditis. *Annals of Cardiothoracic Surgery* **6** (3): 255.

Izquierdo-Gómez, M.M., Marí-López, B., and Lacalzada-Almeida, J. (2018). Ischaemic mitral valve regurgitation. *E-Journal of Cardiology Practice* 16: 12.

James, C.A., Bhonsale, A., Tichnell, C. et al. (2013). Exercise increases age-related penetrance and arrhythmic risk in arrhythmogenic right ventricular dysplasia/ cardiomyopathy – associated desmosomal mutation carriers. *Journal of the American College of Cardiology* **62** (14): 1290–1297.

Japp, A.G., Gulati, A., Cook, S.A. et al. (2016). The diagnosis and evaluation of dilated cardiomyopathy. *Journal of the American College of Cardiology* **67** (25): 2996–3010.

Kim, D.Y., Kim, S.R., Park, S.J. et al. (2020). Clinical characteristics and long-term outcomes of peripartum takotsubo cardiomyopathy and peripartum cardiomyopathy. *ESC Heart Failure* **7** (6): 3644–3652.

Ky, B., Kondapalli, L. & Lenihan, D.J. (2020). Cancer survivorship: Cardiovascular and respiratory issues. In: (ed. P.A. Ganz), *UpToDate*. https://www.uptodate.com/ contents/cancer-survivorship-cardiovascular- and-respiratory-issues (accessed 14 January 2021).

Lung, B. (2003). Management of ischaemic mitral regurgitation. *Heart* **89** (4): 459–464.

Lung, B. and Vahanian, A. (2011). Epidemiology of valvular heart disease in the adult. *Nature Reviews Cardiology* **8** (3): 162–172.

Lung, B. and Vahanian, A. (2014). Epidemiology of acquired valvular heart disease. *Canadian Journal of Cardiology* **30** (9): 962–970.

Lung, B., Leenhardt, A., and Extramiana, F. (2018). Management of atrial fibrillation in patients with rheumatic mitral stenosis. *Heart* **104** (13): 1062–1068.

Marian, A.J. and Braunwald, E. (2017). Hypertrophic cardiomyopathy: genetics, pathogenesis, clinical manifestations, diagnosis, and therapy. *Circulation Research* **121** (7): 749–770.

Maron, M. (2020). Hypertrophic cardiomyopathy: Clinical manifestations, diagnosis, and evaluation. In: (ed. W.J. McKenna), *UpToDate*. https://www.uptodate.com/contents/ hypertrophic-cardiomyopathy-clinical- manifestations-diagnosis-and-evaluation (accessed 14 January 2021).

Monteagudo Ruiz, J.M., Galderisi, M., Buonauro, A. et al. (2018). Overview of mitral regurgitation in Europe: results from the European Registry of mitral regurgitation (EuMiClip). *European Heart Journal-Cardiovascular Imaging* **19** (5): 503–507.

Murdoch, D.R., Corey, G.R., Hoen, B. et al. (2009). Clinical presentation, etiology, and outcome of infective endocarditis in the twenty-first century: the International Collaboration on Endocarditis-Prospective Cohort Study. *Archives of Internal Medicine* **169** (5): 463–473.

Nishino, S., Watanabe, N., Kimura, T. et al. (2016). The course of ischemic mitral regurgitation in acute myocardial infarction after primary percutaneous coronary intervention: from emergency room to long-term follow-up. *Circulation: Cardiovascular Imaging* **9** (8): e004841.

Okutucu, S., Niazi, A.K., Oliveira, D. et al. (2020). A systematic review on durability and structural valve deterioration in TAVR and surgical AVR. *Acta Cardiologica* **76** (9): 921–932.

Otto, C.M., Gaasch, W.H., & Yeon, S.B. (2020). Acute aortic regurgitation in adults. *UpToDate*. www.uptodate.com (accessed February)

Rodriguez Ziccardi, M. and Siddique, M.S. (2020). Peripartum Cardiomyopathy.

[Updated 2020 July 24]. In: StatPearls [Internet]. Treasure Island (FL): StatPearls Publishing; 2020 January-. https://www.ncbi.nlm.nih.gov/books/NBK482185.

Rosenbaum, A.N., Agre, K.E., and Pereira, N.L. (2020). Genetics of dilated cardiomyopathy: practical implications for heart failure management. *Nature Reviews Cardiology* **17** (5): 286–297.

Ruckdeschel, E. and Kim, Y.Y. (2019). Pulmonary valve stenosis in the adult patient: pathophysiology, diagnosis and management. *Heart* **105** (5): 414–422.

Schultheiss, H.P., Fairweather, D., Caforio, A.L. et al. (2019). Dilated cardiomyopathy. *Nature Reviews Disease Primers* **5** (1): 1–19.

Shrestha, N.K., Jue, J., Hussain, S.T. et al. (2015). Injection drug use and outcomes after surgical intervention for infective endocarditis. *Annals of Thoracic Surgery* **100** (3): 875–882.

Siontis, G.C.M., Overtchouk, P., Cahill, T.J. et al. (2019). Transcatheter aortic valve implantation vs surgical aortic valve replacement for treatment of symptomatic severe aortic stenosis: an updated meta-analysis. *European Heart Journal* **40** (38): 3143–3153.

Storey, K. and Sharkey, S.W. (2019). Clinical features and outcomes of patients with chemotherapy-induced takotsubo syndrome. *US Cardiology Review* **13** (2): 74–82. https://doi.org/10.15420/usc.2019.10.1.

Vahanian, A., Beyersdorf, F., Praz, F., Milojevic, M., Baldus, S., Bauersachs, J., ... & Wojakowski, W. (2022). 2021 ESC/EACTS Guidelines for the management of valvular heart disease: developed by the Task Force for the management of valvular heart disease of the European Society of Cardiology (ESC) and the European Association for Cardio-Thoracic Surgery (EACTS). *European heart journal*, **43** (7), 561–632.

Wang, W., James, C.A., and Calkins, H. (2019). Diagnostic and therapeutic strategies for arrhythmogenic right ventricular dysplasia/cardiomyopathy patient. *Ep Europace* **21** (1): 9–21.

Watkins, D.A., Johnson, C.O., Colquhoun, S.M. et al. (2017). Global, regional, and national burden of rheumatic heart disease, 1990–2015. *New England Journal of Medicine* **377** (8): 713–722.

Weigner, M. and Morgan, J.P. (2020). Causes of dilated cardiomyopathy. In: (ed. W.J. McKenna), *UpToDate*. https://www.uptodate.com/contents/causes-of-dilated-cardiomyopathy (accessed 14 January 2021).

Weintraub, R.G., Semsarian, C., and Macdonald, P. (2017). Dilated cardiomyopathy. *The Lancet* **390** (10092): 400–414.

Yellapu, V., Malik, Q.Z., Perez Figueroa, I. et al. (2019). Global burden of rheumatic heart disease and the shortage of penicillin. *Circulation* **140** (Suppl_1): A15479–A15479.

26

Takotsubo Syndrome

Angela M. Kucia

Overview

Takotsubo syndrome (TTS) is a condition that has gained increasing interest in the past two decades. TTS was first identified in by Sato et al. in 1990, which is an acute form of heart failure with reversible left ventricular (LV) systolic function that predominantly affects postmenopausal women but can be found in males and females throughout the lifespan. The onset of TTS in most cases is preceded by an acute stressor that may be emotional or physical in nature, but in around one third of cases, no acute stressor is identified. The pathophysiological mechanisms of TTS are incompletely understood, but increased levels of catecholamines have a central role in its development. Unlike other forms of cardiomyopathy, the RWMA and EF in TTS appear to return to normal in 2–4 weeks post onset, but more advanced imaging techniques have demonstrated that in some women, LV contractile function was abnormal for up to 4 months after the acute event. TTS was initially believed to be a benign condition due to the transient nature of associated LV dysfunction, but accumulating evidence shows that TTS is anything but benign. A recent review suggests that life-threatening acute complications have been described in around half of all patients with TTS and n-hospital death rate ranges from 2.4 to 4.1% (Santoro et al. 2021).

Learning Objectives

After reading this chapter and completing the learning activities, the reader will be able to:

- Describe the clinical presentation of takotsubo syndrome.
- Discuss the populations affected by takotsubo syndrome.
- Identify risks associated with takotsubo syndrome in the acute phase.
- Discuss the current management of takotsubo syndrome and the rationale for various treatments.
- Describe information support needs for people with takotsubo syndrome during hospitalisation and after hospital discharge.

Key Words

Takotsubo syndrome; stress cardiomyopathy; apical ballooning; regional wall motion abnormalities; brain–heart axis

Background

The condition now referred to as 'takotsubo syndrome' (TTS) was first reported by a Japanese cardiologist (Sato et al. 1990) who described a female with a clinical presentation consistent with acute coronary syndrome (ACS) but subsequently found to have normal coronary arteries and LV dysfunction associated with an unusual regional wall motion abnormality (RWMA). The LV appeared to have a narrowed neck at the base and apical ballooning during systole and resembled a Japanese pot used to catch octopus (takotsubo in Japanese) – hence the initial nomenclature of 'takotsubo cardiomyopathy' that reflected the shape of the LV and the associated LV dysfunction and decreased ejection fraction (EF). The apical wall motion abnormality was for some time the only recognised form of RWMA, and so TTS was sometimes referred to as 'apical ballooning syndrome'. TTS was initially recognised following a stressful event and, hence, has also been called 'stress cardiomyopathy', and as in many cases the stressor was loss or grief, and thus it has often been called 'broken heart syndrome'. It is now known that TTS can also be triggered by physical stress, and in some cases, no trigger is identified. Approximately one third of people have no identifiable trigger at the time of presentation. It may be that in some people without a clear trigger, illness may be present, but the person is unaware of it at the time of TTS onset. As understanding of the condition evolved, so did the nomenclature (see Table 26.1).

Epidemiology

TTS may occur in males and females of all age groups, including children and neonates. Women with a mean age of 67–70 years account for most published cases of TTS (Lyon et al. 2016), and most of these women are above 50 years of age (Ghadri et al. 2018a). It is estimated that between 1 and 3% of all patients presenting with presumed ST-segment elevation myocardial infarction (STEMI) will be identified as having TTS (Bybee et al. 2004; Prasad et al. 2014). If women only are considered, TTS will account for approximately 5–10% of cases (Ghadri et al. 2018a; Lyon et al. 2019).

The reason for the large sex disparity in the incidence of TTS is not well understood. Currently, there is little data regarding the potential impact of race and/or ethnicity in TTS presentation and outcomes (Dias et al. 2019a).

Key Point

It is likely that subclinical TTS cases remain undetected, particularly in centres without percutaneous coronary intervention capability (Ghadri et al. 2018a). The overall incidence of TTS is almost certainly higher than is currently reported (Lyon et al. 2019).

Prognosis

TTS was initially thought to be a benign condition from which most people recovered within a few weeks. With increasing clinical recognition of TTS, it has been found that TTS is in fact a serious condition with an in-hospital mortality of 4–5%, which is similar to that of ST-elevation myocardial infarction (STEMI) (Ghadri et al. 2018b). Furthermore, all-cause mortality at 5 years is higher for TTS than for STEMI. Men have a less favourable prognosis compared with women. As men with TTS are more likely to have acute illness as the trigger for TTS, it is unclear whether the poorer prognosis is due to the severity of the underlying illness or the TTS presentation (Lyon et al. 2019).

On long-term follow-up in the International Takotsubo Registry (InterTAK), the rate of major adverse cardiac and cerebrovascular events was 9.9% per patient-year and death (all cause) was 5.6% per patient-year (Templin et al. 2015). Excess mortality on long-term follow-up appears to occur predominantly in the first 4 years after TTS diagnosis and is partially related to concomitant non-cardiac illnesses including malignancy (Nguyen et al. 2019).

Recovery of the LVEF on echocardiography has led to an erroneous belief by many medical community that TTS is transient and

Table 26.1 Names used for takotsubo syndrome (TTS).

Pre-1990	Neurogenic stunned myocardium	Acute heart failure in neurologic events has been recognised for more than a century (Shanahan 1908). Neurogenic stunned myocardium and TTS share the same features and clinical course and are likely the same entity (Guglin and Novotorova 2011; Win et al. 2011; Tavazzi et al. 2017).
	Reversible LV dysfunction	Case reports and series have been published prior to 1990 describing acute reversible left ventricular dysfunction that was not attributed to existing cardiac disease (Cebelin and Hirsch 1980; Y-Hassan and Yamasaki 2013).
1990	Takotsubo cardiomyopathy	Sato et al. (1990) described five cases of 'takotsubo-type cardiomyopathy'.
	Broken heart syndrome	Early cases of TTS tended to be noted in older women who had experienced an emotionally stressful event, such as bereavement: hence, TTS was sometimes called 'broken heart syndrome'.
	Stress cardiomyopathy	Emotional stress was thought to be the primary trigger for TTS, and so many cases escaped diagnosis in the early years. It was subsequently recognised that physical stressors commonly cause TTS, and in some cases, no trigger can be identified. Anxiety or depressive disorders or chronic stress may be present.
	Apical ballooning syndrome	Apical ballooning (affecting the LV apex) is the most common form of TTS and for some time, the only recognised form.
	Global TTS	Global hypokinesis presenting with classic findings and clinical course for TTS been described (Win et al. 2011).
	Reverse and midventricular takotsubo cardiomyopathy	With time it was recognised that TTS could also affect the base of the LV (called 'reverse TTS' or 'basal TTS') (or the mid LV mid-ventricle (called 'midventricular TTS'). Midventricular TTS can occur alone or with apical or basal TTS.
	Focal TTS	New research suggests that TTS can affect a smaller area of the left ventricle, known as 'localised' or 'focal' TTS' (Kato et al. 2015).
	Happy heart syndrome	Excitement, or a happy event such as a lottery win, can cause TTS (Ghadri et al. 2016).
	Takotsubo Syndrome (TTS)	Most cardiomyopathies are long-term conditions. Unlike a classic cardiomyopathy, a heart affected by TTS appears to return to normal shape and function within a few weeks though some people have ongoing symptoms even after the shape and function of the heart appear to have returned to normal. It is thought that this may be due to persistent inflammation. The name "takotsubo syndrome" better reflects the range of symptoms and varying degrees of recovery from the condition.
2020		

Source: Adapted with permission. Kucia (2019).

self-limiting (Dawson 2018). Data now exists to show that in the longer term, patients with TTS have symptoms and objective findings compatible with a heart failure syndrome that has a significant impact on quality of life (Scally et al. 2018).

> **Key Point**
>
> The acute and longer-term phases of TTS may be associated with various complications and conditions that carry a significant mortality risk.

Pathophysiology

Several pathophysiological mechanisms for the myocardial stunning that typifies TTS have been proposed. Among these were plaque rupture with rapid lysis, multivessel coronary artery spasm and genetic predisposition, but these have not been consistently evident in patients with TTS.

Microvascular Dysfunction

Macrovascular and microvascular dysfunction (MVD) with abnormal vasomotor reactivity are common findings in patients with TTS, but it is uncertain whether they are a cause or a result of the acute TTS episode. It has been suggested that myocardial oedema and inflammation that are hallmark findings in TTS could also involve the coronary microvasculature and may also lead to acquired MVD. MVD tends to be transient, and recovery of MVD correlates with improved myocardial function (Lyon et al. 2021).

Catecholamines

There is general acceptance that sympathetic hyperactivity via activation of the hypothalamic–pituitary–adrenal (HPA) axis resulting in the release of supraphysiological levels of circulating catecholamines play a major role in the development of TTS (Rawish et al. 2021). In support of this theory, (i) there are many published reports of TTS following exogenous administration of adrenalin (epinephrine), noradrenalin (norepinephrine), isoprenaline (isoproteranol), and dobutamine (Kido and Guglin 2017); (ii) clinical conditions associated with acute severe sympathetic neural activation or adrenal catecholamine release such as acute subarachnoid haemorrhage, phaeochromocytoma and acute thyrotoxicosis have been associated with TTS (Y-Hassan and Tornvall 2018); and (iii) morphological changes seen in the myocardium in TTS match those seen after catecholamine-induced cardiotoxicity (Kido and Guglin 2017; Y-Hassan and Tornvall 2018).

The exact mechanism by which a catecholamine surge causes myocardial stunning in the diverse patterns of the RWMAs seen is not entirely clear, but findings from preclinical studies suggest that adrenergic receptor pathway activation in response to high catecholamine levels are important in the pathophysiology of TTS (Lyon et al. 2021). Transient LV dysfunction known as neurogenic or catecholaminergic stunning has been demonstrated due to the direct effects of catecholamines on the ventricular myocardium and is associated with cardiomyocyte dysfunction, arrhythmias and irreversible cellular injury due to calcium overload, reactive oxidative species production and mitochondrial dysfunction following intense activation of β-adrenergic receptors (βARs) that activate a pathway to switch from a positive inotropic effect to a negative inotropic effect. Epinephrine (one of the major catecholamines released in response to stress) improves contractility at lower levels; at high levels it paradoxically exerts a negative inotropic effect through a process known as 'stimulus trafficking' that involves β-adrenergic receptors (βARs) that control neuronal and cardiovascular responses to catecholamines during stress. It has been suggested that the transient wall motion abnormalities may be a protective mechanism to preserve myocardial integrity (Lyon et al. 2021).

The Brain–Heart Axis

> **Key Point**
>
> There is increasing interest in the brain–heart axis in people with TTS following a finding that functional connectivity in the limbic system of the brain, which controls emotion and the autonomic system, is reduced in patients with TTS compared with healthy individuals.

Recent studies have found evidence of abnormalities in functional structure and activity in areas of the brain related to both emotions and the sympathetic nervous system in TTS survivors (Templin et al. 2019). It is uncertain whether these changes were pre-existing and predisposed the person to TTS, or alternately were the consequences of a major catecholamine storm and TTS episode (Lyon et al. 2021).

Inflammation

Inflammation is a fundamental part of the pathophysiology of TTS (Rawish et al. 2021), with evidence of persistent inflammation found more than 12 months after the initial event in some patients (Lyon et al. 2021). Endomyocardial biopsy shows mononuclear infiltrates and contraction band necrosis, a unique form of myocyte injury that has been described in clinical states of endogenous and exogenous catecholamine excess (Wittstein et al. 2005). Slowly resolving global myocardial oedema is present on magnetic resonance imaging (Neil et al. 2012) and as this subsides, a process of global microscopic fibrosis develops in its place (Schwarz et al. 2017).

> **Key Point**
>
> The pathophysiological mechanism of TTS appears to be complex and multifactorial. To date, there is no single unifying explanation, but it is possible that TTS may result from more than one pathophysiological pathway (Akashi et al. 2015).

Triggers for TTS

Typically, there is a history of an acute physical or emotional stressor within the preceding hours/few days that triggers TTS. Emotional triggers usually involve grief, panic, fear, anxiety, anger or frustration. Triggers vary in nature, ranging from what may be perceived by others to be a trivial event (loss of a personal item) to a life-changing event (death of a loved one). TTS can also be triggered by positive emotional events such as winning a prize, or

happiness at a celebration of a birthday, wedding or family reunion. The magnitude of the event does not appear to be the determinant of TTS occurrence. Any event that causes acute emotional stress or excitement in a susceptible individual can trigger TTS.

Physical stressors, including acute illness, trigger around 40% of TTS cases. Physical triggers are more common in males and younger women (Nyman et al. 2019). As with emotional stressors, there is a wide range of physical stressors that have been associated with TTS, and commonly this is an underlying illness. When TTS occurs secondary to physical illness, it is known as *secondary TTS*.

> **Key Point**
>
> Women are more likely to have an emotional trigger for TTS, whereas TTS in men tends to be triggered by physical stress as severe critical medical illnesses (Y-Hassan and Tornvall 2018).

> **Suggested Resource**
>
> For examples of events that have triggered TTS in people who have self-reported their TTS, go to the webpage below:
> Takotsubo Wall
> Takotsubo Network 2019
> https://takotsubo.net/takotsubo-wall-results

Several drugs have been associated with the development of TTS.

Catecholamines

Exogenous catecholamines including adrenaline (epinephrine), noradrenaline, (norepinephrine), isoprenaline (isoproterenol), dopamine and dobutamine and can cause TTS. Adrenaline and noradrenaline are the drugs most associated with causing TTS (Kido and Guglin 2017). Dobutamine-induced TTS is increasingly reported during pharmacological stress testing (Hajsadeghi et al. 2018).

Serotonin Norepinephrine Reuptake Inhibitors (SNRIs)

Serotonin norepinephrine re-uptake inhibitors (SNRIs) (desvenlafaxine, venlafaxine, duloxetine and milnacipran) used to treat depression, anxiety and chronic pain disorders have been associated with the development of TTS.

Drugs Used to Treat Cancer

In addition to the significant emotional stress associated with a cancer diagnosis, several chemotherapeutic agents, monoclonal antibodies and tyrosine kinase inhibitors have been identified as possible culprits for TTS. The most common chemotherapy drugs associated with TTS are 5-fluorouracil (5-FU) and its oral pro-drug capecitabine, but many other chemotherapy drugs have been associated with the development of TTS (Coen et al. 2017). The significant emotional stress associated with a cancer diagnosis cannot be discounted as also being a trigger or contributor to the development of TTS. There is a significantly higher mortality for cancer patients with TTS compared with those without TTS (Joy et al. 2018; Desai et al. 2019).

Drugs Used in Obstetrics

TTS can occur throughout pregnancy or later in the peripartum period, but the risk is greatest during or soon after birthing. The development of TTS within 24 hours of delivery may be multifactorial. Peripartum TTS is more common following caesarean section (Kucia et al. 2015; Citro et al. 2018). In cases where hypotension is induced by spinal anaesthesia, the drugs given to counteract hypotension are the likely trigger for TTS. These include adrenaline, noradrenaline, dopamine, dobutamine, phenylephrine and ephedrine. Uterotonics that have been linked with the development of TTS include oxytocin, ergot alkaloids and prostaglandins (PGE_2 or $PGF2\alpha$). Ritodrine, used as a tocolytic, has also been reported as a possible trigger in TTS cases (Kucia et al. 2015).

Key Point

TTS should be considered as a possible diagnosis if symptoms of chest pain, shortness of breath and signs of haemodynamic compromise occur in pregnancy, particularly during or soon after birthing.

Asthma Medications

Medications used in the treatment of respiratory diseases including β_2 adrenergic receptor agonists albuterol (salbutamol),[167–173] terbutaline[174] and salmeterol[175] likely have a role in the development of TTS, but in some cases TTS onset appears to be associated with higher than recommended doses of these drugs.

Other Drugs/Medications

Cocaine, methamphetamines and cannabis have been associated with TTS. TTS may be triggered by withdrawal from alcohol, methadone, opioids, baclofen, buprenorphine and sudden cessation of beta-blockers. See the website below for other drugs that have been associated with TTS.

Suggested Resource

Drugs that may cause Takotsubo Takotsubo Network 2019 https://takotsubo.net/drugs-that-may-cause-takotsubo

---

Clinical Presentation

The clinical presentation for TTS is much the same as that for acute coronary syndrome (ACS). Chest pain and dyspnoea are the most common symptoms. Less commonly, a patient may present with syncope. Sudden death due to cardiac arrest is an underestimated threat in TTS. A recent study by Gili et al. (2019) found that cardiac arrest occurred in 5.9% of patients with TTS, typically at presentation, and was associated with worse outcomes.

ECG in TTS

The 12-lead ECG is not helpful in distinguishing between TTS and ACS in the first 24–48 hours of onset. Various ECG criteria have been proposed to differentiate between TTS and ACS but thus far have not found to be reliable in the clinical setting (Guerra et al. 2017). The ECG in early TTS may show various abnormalities, and in some cases, no abnormalities at all. ECG features of TTS tend to be dynamic and characterised by different evolutionary patterns over time, some of which can extend a few months after the acute event (Guerra et al. 2017).

ST-Segment Abnormalities

ST-segment elevation may be present in the initial stages of TTS. It is uncertain as to what percentage of patients with TTS present with ST-segment elevation. Initially, it was hypothesised that it occurred in all patients initially but may have resolved by presentation. It has become increasingly clear that this is not the case and is probably present in less than half of TTS cases. TTS is more frequently recognised early in the presence of ST-segment elevation as these patients will have early coronary angiography. ST-segment depression is less frequently observed in TTS.

T-Wave Inversion

T-wave inversion is the most common finding on the ECG in TTS. T-wave inversion in TTS often differs from that found in STEMI in that it tends to be deep and widespread and is usually not limited to the territory of a single coronary artery (see Figure 26.1). T-wave inversion usually manifests around 24–48 hours following symptom onset. If a patient presents with TTS T-wave inversion, it is likely a late presentation. T-wave inversion persists for some weeks after LVEF appears to have recovered to within normal range and is thought to be associated with myocardial oedema (Park 2020).

QT Interval Prolongation

QT interval prolongation is common in TC and can persist up to 6 months after complete recovery of both systolic dysfunction and cardiac biomarkers.

QRS Abnormalities

Low QRS voltage in the admission ECG and attenuation of the amplitude of the QRS complexes in serial ECGs have been shown to be prevalent ECG signs of TTS and are probably due to myocardial oedema (Madias 2014). QRS amplitude decreases during the acute phase of TTS and its recovery appears to relate to the normalisation of cardiac biomarkers levels and left ventricular ejection fraction, suggesting recovery of cardiac function (Guerra et al. 2017).

Q-Waves

Q-waves in ACS are generally persistent and an ECG marker of myocardial necrosis. Q-waves are a rare finding in TTS and interestingly are usually transient. Q-waves in TTS usually disappear in the subacute phase of TTS following R-wave reappearance and normalisation of QRS voltage. This seems to be associated with resolution of myocardial oedema seen on cardiac magnetic resonance imaging (Guerra et al. 2017).

Key Point

Serial ECGs should be performed at least daily on patients with suspected or known TTS. The evolution of T-wave inversion and QTc prolongation may be helpful in diagnosis is a patient with suspected TTS.

Bundle Branch Block/Axis Deviation

The initial presenting ECG in TTS may show bundle branch block or axis deviation. These are often transient.

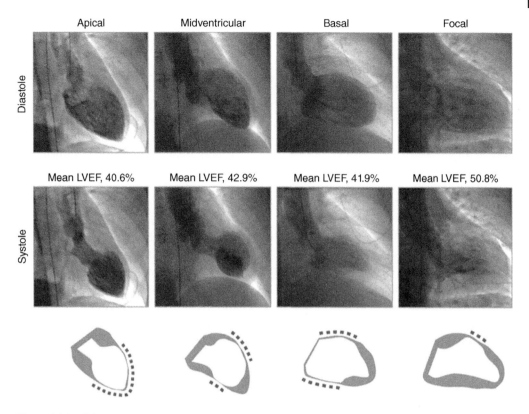

Figure 26.1 Takotsubo phenotypes. *Source:* Ghadri (2014).

Arrhythmia

The prevalence of adverse rhythm disorders (defined as ventricular tachycardia, ventricular fibrillation, torsade de pointes asystole, or complete atrioventricular block) in TTS is between 7 and 10% (El-Battrawy et al. 2020). Adverse rhythm disorder in TTS is short- and long-term mortality rate of TTS patients presenting with an adverse rhythm disorder was significantly higher than in TTS patients presenting without it (El-Battrawy et al. 2020). New onset atrial tachyarrhythmias (atrial fibrillation and atrial flutter) occur in around 25% of patients with TTS and are associated with a poorer short- and long-term prognosis (Stiermaier et al. 2017; Jesel et al. 2019).

Key Point

Cardiac arrest in TTS is usually due to ventricular fibrillation and tends to occur at or

---

soon after presentation. This leads to the question of whether VF was a cause or consequence of TTS (Ong et al. 2020). Moreover, it raises the possibility that TTS may be the cause of sudden death in some patients where no cause was found at autopsy.

Wall Motion Abnormalities in TTS

Apical ballooning is still considered to be the typical phenotype of TTS and is found in around 80% of patients. With an expanded understanding of TTS, it is evident that TTS can affect regions of the left ventricle other than the apex, including the base, the midventricle, focal areas, or there may be global involvement. Moreover, right ventricular (RV) involvement is present in approximately 33% of TTS patients and is a predictor for poorer prognosis (Rawish et al. 2021).

Key Point

The basal phenotype of TTS occurs more frequently in younger patients and has been related to adrenaline-induced TTS, the presence of pheochromocytoma and subarachnoid haemorrhage (Rawish et al. 2021).

Cardiac Biomarkers

Troponin

Cardiac troponin is almost always elevated in TTS. However, it tends to be lower than in acute myocardial infarction and is disproportionately low considering the area of myocardial ballooning, suggesting largely preserved myocardial viability (Dawson 2018).

Brain Natriuretic Peptides

In contrast to mildly elevated troponin levels, brain natriuretic peptide (BNP) and N-type pro-brain natriuretic peptide (NTproBNP) tend to be very high (Nguyen et al. 2011). It is likely that the disproportionate rise in BNP/NT-proBNP reflects inflammation rather than heart failure (Visvanathan et al. 2021).

Diagnostic Criteria

Various sets of diagnostic criteria for TTS have been proposed over the years, but as more becomes known about the condition some of the criteria have become outdated. The most current of these are the InterTak diagnostic criteria (see Box 26.1) (Ghadri et al. 2018).

Diagnostic Imaging

Coronary Angiography

Coronary angiography (CA) with left ventriculography is considered to be the gold standard diagnostic tool for diagnosis of TTS, but TTS is

---

Box 26.1   International Takotsubo Diagnostic Criteria (InterTAK Diagnostic Criteria).

1) Patients show transient[a] left ventricular dysfunction (hypokinesia, akinesia or dyskinesia) presenting as apical ballooning or midventricular, basal or focal wall motion abnormalities. Right ventricular involvement can be present. Besides these regional wall motion patterns, transitions between all types can exist. The regional wall motion abnormality usually extends beyond a single epicardial vascular distribution; however, rare cases can exist where the regional wall motion abnormality is present in the subtended myocardial territory of a single coronary artery (focal TTS).[b]

2) An emotional, physical or combined trigger can precede the takotsubo syndrome event, but this is not obligatory.

3) Neurologic disorders (e.g. subarachnoid haemorrhage, stroke/transient ischaemic attack or seizures) as well as pheochromocytoma may serve as triggers for takotsubo syndrome.

4) New ECG abnormalities are present (ST-segment elevation, ST-segment depression, T-wave inversion, and QTc prolongation); however, rare cases exist without any ECG changes.

5) Levels of cardiac biomarkers (troponin and creatine kinase) are moderately elevated in most cases; significant elevation of brain natriuretic peptide is common.

6) Significant coronary artery disease is not a contradiction in takotsubo syndrome.

7) Patients have no evidence of infectious myocarditis.[b]

8) Postmenopausal women are predominantly affected.

[a]Wall motion abnormalities may remain for a prolonged period of time or documentation of recovery may not be possible. For example, death before evidence of recovery is captured.
[b]Cardiac magnetic resonance imaging is recommended to exclude infectious myocarditis and diagnosis confirmation of takotsubo syndrome.

Source: Ghadri et al. (2018b).

usually diagnosed by way of CA that is performed for suspected ACS. Typically, the angiogram will show non-critical coronary artery disease (CAD), but a recent study has shown co-existing obstructive CAD in 23% of patients and non-obstructive CAD in 41% of patients with TTS (Napp et al. 2020). The ventriculogram will show typical RWMAs associated with TTS. In most cases, apical and mid-ventricular regional wall motion abnormalities (termed apical ballooning) are seen, often with hyperkinetic basal segments. In fewer cases, basal (inverted TTS), localised or even global wall motion abnormalities are seen. Approximately one third of patients will have concomitant wall motion abnormalities of the right ventricle (Rawish et al. 2021). Multimodality imaging is helpful for establishing the diagnosis, guiding therapy, and stratifying prognosis of TTS patients in both the acute and post-acute phase (Citro et al. 2020).

Key Point

Co-existence of coronary artery disease does not rule out co-existence of takotsubo syndrome.

Echocardiography

Transthoracic echocardiography (TTE) is useful in identifying wall motion abnormalities that typify TTS and monitoring functional recovery. The key echocardiographic feature in distinguishing TTS from ACS is the large area of myocardial systolic dysfunction that extends beyond the territory of a single coronary artery and symmetrical regional abnormalities in TTS (Izumo and Akashi 2018). TTE is also used to detect potential TTS complications including left ventricular outflow obstruction (LVOTO), mitral regurgitation, right ventricular involvement, apical thrombus formation, pericardial effusion and ventricular rupture (Izumo and Akashi 2018),

as well as monitoring the recovery of LV function.

Key Point

Return to normal LVEF does not necessarily reflect full recovery. Despite apparent normalisation of LVEF and of most other echocardiographic indexes, subtle but clinically relevant impairment of LV systolic function, as measured by global longitudinal strain, persists for months after an acute episode of TTS (Neil et al. 2015).

Cardiac Magnetic Resonance Imaging

Cardiac magnetic resonance (CMR) imaging constitutes the gold standard for the qualitative and quantitative assessment of structural and functional abnormalities in patients with TTS. CMR can identify the presence of reversible and irreversible myocardial damage (myocardial oedema or scarring). Thus, CMR is useful in distinguishing TTS from acute myocardial infarction or myocarditis. CMR can also identify potential complications of TTS, including left ventricular outflow tract obstruction (LVOTO), valve disease, pericardial effusion and LV thrombus (Bratis 2017).

Key Point

There are some groups of patients, including critically ill ICU patients, for whom emergency CA or CMRI is not a practicable option. For these patients, TTE can provide a presumptive diagnosis of TTS (Visvanathan et al. 2021).

Clinical Course

In-hospital mortality for TTS is estimated to be between 3 and 5%, with the mode of death attributed to ventricular arrhythmias, intractable pump failure, cardiac rupture or thromboembolic stroke (Dawson 2018). A syndrome resembling cardiogenic shock occurs in up to 10% of TTS patients and is associated with a significant increase in 28-day mortality compared with patients without CS (Stiermaier et al. 2017). In the setting of poor LV function, LVOTO, transient MR and RV may contribute to shock. Intraventricular thrombosis is reported to occur in around 3% of patients in the acute phase of TTS (Ding et al. 2018) with the attendant risk of embolic complications, including stroke. Ventricular tachyarrhythmias (monomorphic and polymorphic ventricular tachycardia and ventricular fibrillation) occur in an estimated 10% of patients with TTS and are linked to worsened survival in both acute and convalescent phases of TTS (Möller et al. 2018). New onset of atrial arrhythmia (atrial fibrillation and atrial flutter) occurs in up to 25% of patients with TTS and is associated with a worsened short (El-Battrawy et al. 2020; Berthon and Jesel 2018) and long-term prognosis (El-Battrawy et al. 2020; Stiermaier et al. 2017; Berthon and Jesel 2018). Atrio-ventricular block has less frequently been described in the setting of TTS but leads to torsade de pointes in some cases (Oshima et al. 2015). Cardiac arrest at the time of TTS presentation or during the acute phase of the syndrome is associated with increased in-hospital and long-term mortality compared with TTS patients without cardiac arrest (Gili et al. 2019)ˊ A physical trigger for TTS (such as acute illness or medical procedures) has been found to be an independent predictor for in-hospital complications, with TTS secondary to neurologic disease having the worst short- and long-term prognosis (Ghadri et al. 2018b, part II).

In the longer term, many with TTS continue to experience pain, shortness of breath and fatigue for months after the acute phase (Dawson 2018; Scally et al. 2019), and an estimated 10–15% of patients go on to have single or multiple occurrences of TTS. The interval of time to a recurrence is unpredictable.

Management

Medical Management

There are no randomised clinical trials to guide the management of TTS to date: thus, treatment recommendations are based on expert opinion. Consequently, as Lyon et al. (2021, p. 918) state '. . .the most important doctrine that should guide decision-making is the fundamental ethical principle in medicine: primum non nocere (first, do no harm)'. Acute management is based on supportive care and prevention of complications. The clinical course of TTS may be mild with swift recovery in which case no treatment or a short course of medical therapy will suffice. At the other end of the spectrum, TTS may be complicated by severe circulatory failure in which case mechanical support may be required as a bridge to recovery. For patients with an LVEF less than 40%, the patient should be treated with an angiotensin converting enzyme inhibitor (ACEi) and beta-blocker (preferably carvedilol, unless significant left ventricular outflow tract obstruction is present in which case a beta-1 selective beta-blocker such as bisoprolol is preferred). The ACEi and beta-blocker can be weaned off when the LVEF recovers unless there are other indications for treatment with these agents (Lyon et al. 2021).

Key Point

The treatment plan post TTS is often poorly understood by General Practitioners, which means that people are left on ACEi and beta-blockers far longer than necessary. This often contributes to fatigue and lethargy for people with TTS.

Cardiac Rehabilitation

Currently, there is no consistent approach to cardiac rehabilitation (CR) for people with TTS and no evidence that supports or negates referral to CR in TTS. CR begins in hospital with education, followed by exercise-based outpatient CR and secondary prevention that focuses on cardiac risk factor reduction for patients with ACS. While there are well-established guidelines for management and secondary prevention of acute coronary syndrome (ACS) following hospital discharge, this is not the case for people with TTS. TTS is not associated with a suite of modifiable risk factors to prevent recurrence other than (potentially) stress management. To date there is no evidence of benefit for exercise programs following TTS, and it is not clear at what timepoint following the initial event that exercise should be undertaken. Symptoms of fatigue, chest pain and breathlessness may persist for some months after the acute TTS episode are often exacerbated by physical activity. Physical activity may have a benefit given its effects on general health and stress reduction. Recent evidence suggests that women with TS do need for support and education similar to that offered in CR programs, but it appears that this is not routinely available to them (Dahlviken et al. 2015; Schubert et al. 2018). A recent study by Gobeil et al. (2021) suggests that CR is inconsistently utilised for TTS patients, and that enrolment and adherence to cardiac rehabilitation is low. However, there appeared to be gains in exercise capacity for TTS patients that did attend CR. CR programs should have a tailored approach for people recovering from TTS that focuses on the particular needs of this group.

Key Point

As the recognition of TTS is relatively new and much is still not known, people with TTS, particularly women, often report difficulty in finding information and support. The cardiac nurse should have a good understanding of TTS to support patients with this condition.

Learning Activity 26.1

Visit the Takotsubo Network website www.takotsubo.net and locate the resources for health professionals and people with TTS. Read the 'Voices of Takotsubo' page and read about the experiences that people with TTS have had. Identify ways in which the people in these stories could have been better supported following the event.

Learning Activity 26.2

Read the following article that is written from the perspective of women affected by TTS. What do you think the salient messages are in this article? As health professionals, how can we endeavour to overcome some of these concerns?
Curragh, C., Rein, M., and Green, G. (2020). Takotsubo syndrome: voices to be heard. *European Journal of Cardiovascular Nursing* 19 (1): 4–7. https://journals.sagepub.com/doi/full/10.1177/1474515119886078

Conclusion

TTS is a serious condition that predominantly affects older women and is in most cases associated with an acute emotional or physical stressor. Currently, in the absence of evidence from randomised trials, the management of this condition is based upon expert opinion. In contrast to earlier beliefs that TTS was a quickly resolving condition, many people with TTS, particularly women, experience ongoing symptoms and fatigue due to persistent myocardial inflammation. The support needs of people with TTS are often poorly understood. Nurses are well placed to provide information for patients with TTS providing they keep up to date with evolving evidence.

References

Akashi, Y.J., Nef, H.M., & Lyon, A.R. (2015). Epidemiology and pathophysiology of Takotsubo syndrome. *Nature Reviews Cardiology*, **12** (7), 387. https://doi.org/10.1038/nrcardio.2015.39.

Berthon, C. and Jesel, L. (2018). Atrial arrhythmias in Takotsubo cardiomyopathy: Incidence, predictive factors and prognosis. *Archives of Cardiovascular Diseases Supplements* **10** (1): 100.

Bratis, K. (2017). Cardiac magnetic resonance in Takotsubo syndrome. *European Cardiology Review* **12** (1): 58.

Bybee, K.A., Kara, T., Prasad, A. et al. (2004). Systematic review: transient left ventricular apical ballooning: a syndrome that mimics ST-segment elevation myocardial infarction. *Annals of Internal Medicine* **141** (11): 858–865.

Cebelin, M.S. and Hirsch, C.S. (1980). Human stress cardiomyopathy: myocardial lesions in victims of homicidal assaults without internal injuries. *Human Pathology* **11** (2): 123–132.

Citro, R., Lyon, A., Arbustini, E. et al. (2018). Takotsubo syndrome after cesarean section: rare but possible. *Journal of the American College of Cardiology* **71** (16): 1838–1839.

Citro, R., Okura, H., Ghadri, J.R. et al. (2020). Multimodality imaging in takotsubo syndrome: a joint consensus document of the European Association of Cardiovascular Imaging (EACVI) and the Japanese Society of Echocardiography (JSE). *European Heart Journal-Cardiovascular Imaging* **21** (11): 1184–1207.

Coen, M., Rigamonti, F., Roth, A., and Koessler, T. (2017). Chemotherapy-induced Takotsubo cardiomyopathy, a case report and review of the literature. *BMC Cancer* **17** (1): 1–5.

Dahlviken, R.M., Fridlund, B., and Mathisen, L. (2015). Women's experiences of T akotsubo cardiomyopathy in a short-term perspective – a qualitative content analysis. *Scandinavian Journal of Caring Sciences* **29** (2): 258–267.

Dawson, D.K. (2018). Acute stress-induced (takotsubo) cardiomyopathy. *Heart* **104** (2): 96–102.

Desai, R., Abbas, S.A., Goyal, H. et al. (2019). Frequency of Takotsubo cardiomyopathy in adult patients receiving chemotherapy (from a 5-year nationwide inpatient study). *The American Journal of Cardiology* **123** (4): 667–673.

Dias, A., Gil, I.J.N., Santoro, F. et al. (2019a). Takotsubo syndrome: state-of-the-art review by an expert panel–part 1. *Cardiovascular Revascularization Medicine* **20** (1): 70–79.

Ding, K.J., Cammann, V.L., Gili, S. et al. (2018). P4742 Clinical correlates and outcome of thromboembolism in takotsubo syndrome. *European Heart Journal* **39** (suppl_1): ehy563-P4742.

El-Battrawy, I., Santoro, F., Stiermaier, T. et al. (2020). Prevalence, management, and outcome of adverse rhythm disorders in takotsubo syndrome: insights from the international multicenter GEIST registry. *Heart Failure Reviews* **25** (3): 505–511.

Ghadri, J.R., Ruschitzka, F., Lüscher, T.F., and Templin, C. (2014). Takotsubo cardiomyopathy: still much more to learn. *Heart* **100** (22): 1804–1812. https://doi.org/10.1136/heartjnl-2013-304 691. Epub 2014 Apr 7. PMID: 24711482.

Ghadri, J.R., Wittstein, I.S., Prasad, A. et al. (2018). International expert consensus document on Takotsubo syndrome (part I): clinical characteristics, diagnostic criteria, and pathophysiology. *European Heart Journal* **39** (22): 2032–2046.

Ghadri, J.R., Sarcon, A., Diekmann, J. et al. (2016). Happy heart syndrome: role of positive emotional stress in takotsubo syndrome. *European Heart Journal* **37** (37): 2823–2829.

Ghadri, J.R., Wittstein, I.S., Prasad, A. et al. (2018a). International expert consensus document on Takotsubo syndrome (part I): clinical characteristics, diagnostic criteria, and pathophysiology. *European Heart Journal* **39** (22): 2032–2046.

Ghadri, J.R., Wittstein, I.S., Prasad, A. et al. (2018b). International expert consensus document on Takotsubo syndrome (part II): diagnostic workup, outcome, and management. *European Heart Journal* **39** (22): 2047–2062.

Gili, S., Cammann, V.L., Schlossbauer, S.A. et al. (2019). Cardiac arrest in takotsubo syndrome: results from the InterTAK Registry. *European Heart Journal* **40** (26): 2142–2151.

Gobeil, K., White, K., Bhat, A. et al. (2021). Cardiac rehabilitation in Takotsubo cardiomyopathy: predictors of utilization and effects of exercise training. *Heart and Lung* **50** (2): 230–234.

Guerra, F., Giannini, I., and Capucci, A. (2017). The ECG in the differential diagnosis between takotsubo cardiomyopathy and acute coronary syndrome. *Expert Review of Cardiovascular Therapy* **15** (2): 137–144.

Guglin, M. and Novotorova, I. (2011). Neurogenic stunned myocardium and takotsubo cardiomyopathy are the same syndrome: a pooled analysis. *Congestive Heart Failure* **17** (3): 127–132.

Hajsadeghi, S., Rahbar, M.H., Iranpour, A. et al. (2018). Dobutamine-induced takotsubo cardiomyopathy: a systematic review of the literature and case report. *Anatolian Journal of Cardiology* **19** (6): 412.

Izumo, M. and Akashi, Y.J. (2018). Role of echocardiography for takotsubo cardiomyopathy: clinical and prognostic implications. *Cardiovascular Diagnosis and Therapy* **8** (1): 90.

Jesel, L., Berthon, C., Messas, N. et al. (2019). Atrial arrhythmias in Takotsubo cardiomyopathy: incidence, predictive factors, and prognosis. *Ep Europace* **21** (2): 298–305.

Joy, Parijat Saurav, Guddati, Achuta Kumar, & Shapira, Iuliana. (2018). Outcomes of Takotsubo cardiomyopathy in hospitalized cancer patients. *Journal of Cancer Research and Clinical Oncology.*, **144** (8), 1539–1545. https://doi.org/10.1007/s00432-018-2661-1.

Kato, K., Sakai, Y., Ishibashi, I., and Kobayashi, Y. (2015). Transient focal left ventricular ballooning: a new variant of Takotsubo cardiomyopathy. *European Heart Journal-Cardiovascular Imaging* **16** (12): 1406–1406.

Kido, K. and Guglin, M. (2017). Drug-induced takotsubo cardiomyopathy. *Journal of Cardiovascular Pharmacology and Therapeutics* **22** (6): 552–563.

Kucia, A.M. (2019). Takotsubo syndrome overview. *Takotsubo Network*. https://takotsubo.net/information/about-takotsubo-syndrome.

Kucia, A.M., Dekker, G., and Arstall, M. (2015). Peripartum takotsubo cardiomyopathy. *Journal of the American College of Cardiology* **65** (10S): A926–A926.

Lyon, A.R., Bossone, E., Schneider, B. et al. (2016). Current state of knowledge on Takotsubo syndrome: a Position Statement from the Taskforce on Takotsubo Syndrome of the Heart Failure Association of the European Society of Cardiology. *European Journal of Heart Failure* **18** (1): 8–27.

Lyon, A., Sweeney, M., and Omerovic, E. (2019). Takotsubo syndrome. In: *The ESC Handbook on Cardiovascular Pharmacotherapy* (ed. J.C. Kaski and K.P. Kjeldsen), 123. Google Books.

Lyon, A.R., Citro, R., Schneider, B. et al. (2021). Pathophysiology of Takotsubo syndrome: JACC State-of-the-Art review. *Journal of the American College of Cardiology* **77** (7): 902–921.

Madias, J.E. (2014). Transient attenuation of the amplitude of the QRS complexes in the diagnosis of Takotsubo syndrome. *European Heart Journal: Acute Cardiovascular Care* **3** (1): 28–36.

Möller, C., Eitel, C., Thiele, H. et al. (2018). Ventricular arrhythmias in patients with Takotsubo syndrome. *Journal of arrhythmia* **34** (4): 369–375.

Napp, L.C., Cammann, V.L., Jaguszewski, M. et al. (2020). Coexistence and outcome of coronary artery disease in Takotsubo syndrome. *European Heart Journal* **41** (34): 3255–3268.

Neil, C., Nguyen, T.H., Kucia, A. et al. (2012). Slowly resolving global myocardial inflammation/oedema in Tako-Tsubo cardiomyopathy: evidence from T2-weighted cardiac MRI. *Heart* **98** (17): 1278–1284.

Neil, C.J., Nguyen, T.H., Singh, K. et al. (2015). Relation of delayed recovery of myocardial function after takotsubo cardiomyopathy to subsequent quality of life. *The American Journal of Cardiology* 115 (8): 1085–1089.

Nguyen, T.H., Neil, C.J., Sverdlov, A.L. et al. (2011). N-terminal pro-brain natriuretic protein levels in takotsubo cardiomyopathy. *The American Journal of Cardiology* 108 (9): 1316–1321.

Nguyen, T.H., Stansborough, J., Ong, G.J. et al. (2019). Antecedent cancer in Takotsubo syndrome predicts both cardiovascular and long-term mortality. *Cardio-Oncology* 5 (1): 1–9.

Nyman, E., Mattsson, E., and Tornvall, P. (2019). Trigger factors in takotsubo syndrome–a systematic review of case reports. *European Journal of Internal Medicine* 63: 62–68.

Ong, G.J., Nguyen, T.H., Kucia, A. et al. (2020). Takotsubo syndrome: finally emerging from the shadows? *Heart, Lung and Circulation* 30 (1): 36–44.

Oshima, T., Ikutomi, M., Ishiwata, J. et al. (2015). Takotsubo cardiomyopathy associated with complete atrioventricular block and torsades de pointes. *International Journal of Cardiology* 181: 357–359.

Park, Y.H. (2020). Time course of functional recovery and ECG change in Takotsubo cardiomyopathy. *Journal of Cardiovascular Imaging* 28 (1): 61.

Prasad, A., Dangas, G., Srinivasan, M. et al. (2014). Incidence and angiographic characteristics of patients with apical ballooning syndrome (takotsubo/stress cardiomyopathy) in the HORIZONS-AMI trial: An analysis from a multicenter, international study of ST-elevation myocardial infarction. *Catheterization and Cardiovascular Interventions* 83 (3): 343–348.

Rawish, E., Stiermaier, T., Santoro, F. et al. (2021). Current knowledge and future challenges in Takotsubo syndrome: part 1 – pathophysiology and diagnosis. *Journal of Clinical Medicine* 10 (3): 479.

Santoro, F., Mallardi, A., Leopizzi, A. et al. (2021). Current knowledge and future challenges in Takotsubo syndrome: part 2 – treatment and prognosis. *Journal of Clinical Medicine* 10 (3): 468. doi: https://doi.org/10.3390/jcm10030468.

Sato, H., Tateishi, H., Uchida, T. et al. (1990). Takotsubo-type cardiomyopathy due to multivessel spasm. In: *Clinical Aspect of Myocardial Injury: From Ischemia to Heart Failure* (ed. K. Kodama, K. Haze and M. Hori), 56–64. Tokyo: Kagakuhyouronsha Publishing Co.

Scally, C., Rudd, A., Mezincescu, A. et al. (2018). Persistent long-term structural, functional, and metabolic changes after stress-induced (Takotsubo) cardiomyopathy. *Circulation* 137 (10): 1039–1048.

Scally, C., Abbas, H., Ahearn, T. et al. (2019). Myocardial and systemic inflammation in acute stress-induced (Takotsubo) cardiomyopathy. *Circulation* 139 (13): 1581–1592.

Schubert, S.C., Kucia, A., and Hofmeyer, A. (2018). The gap in meeting the educational and support needs of women with Takotsubo syndrome compared to women with an acute coronary syndrome. *Contemporary Issues in Education Research* 11 (4): 133–144.

Schwarz, K., Ahearn, T., Srinivasan, J. et al. (2017). Alterations in cardiac deformation, timing of contraction and relaxation, and early myocardial fibrosis accompany the apparent recovery of acute stress-induced (takotsubo) cardiomyopathy: an end to the concept of transience. *Journal of the American Society of Echocardiography* 30 (8): 745–755.

Shanahan, W.T. (1908). Acute pulmonary oedema as a complication of epileptic seizures. *NY Medical Journal* 37: 54–56.

Stiermaier, T., Santoro, F., Eitel, C. et al. (2017). Prevalence and prognostic relevance of atrial fibrillation in patients with Takotsubo syndrome. *International Journal of Cardiology* 245: 156–161.

Tavazzi, G., Zanierato, M., Via, G. et al. (2017). Are neurogenic stress cardiomyopathy and Takotsubo different syndromes with common pathways?: etiopathological insights on dysfunctional hearts. *JACC. Heart Failure* 5 (12): 940–942.

Templin, C., Ghadri, J.R., Diekmann, J. et al. (2015). Clinical features and outcomes of Takotsubo (stress) cardiomyopathy. *New England Journal of Medicine* **373** (10): 929–938.

Templin, C., Hänggi, J., Klein, C. et al. (2019). Altered limbic and autonomic processing supports brain-heart axis in Takotsubo syndrome. *European Heart Journal* **40** (15): 1183–1187.

Visvanathan, V., Kucia, A., Reddi, B., and Horowitz, J. (2021). Late development of Takotsubo syndrome following intensive care unit discharge. *Netherlands Journal of Critical Care* **29** (1): 14–21.

Win, C.M., Pathak, A., and Guglin, M. (2011). Not Takotsubo: a different form of stress-induced cardiomyopathy – a case series. *Congestive Heart Failure* **17** (1): 38–41.

Wittstein, I.S., Thiemann, D.R., Lima, J.A. et al. (2005). Neurohumoral features of myocardial stunning due to sudden emotional stress. *New England Journal of Medicine* **352** (6): 539–548.

Y-Hassan, S. and Tornvall, P. (2018). Epidemiology, pathogenesis, and management of takotsubo syndrome. *Clinical Autonomic Research* **28** (1): 53–65.

Y-Hassan, S. and Yamasaki, K. (2013). History of takotsubo syndrome: is the syndrome really described as a disease entity first in 1990? Some inaccuracies. *International Journal of Cardiology* **166** (3): 736–737.

27

Non-Obstructive Coronary Artery Disease (*MINOCA/INOCA*)

Angela M. Kucia and John F. Beltrame

Overview

Over the past few decades, there has increasing recognition of myocardial infarction/myocardial ischaemia with no obstructive coronary artery disease (MINOCA/INOCA). MINOCA carries a risk of adverse outcomes including stroke, heart failure and death. MINOCA can be a debilitating condition in the long term due to persistent angina resulting in socioeconomic, personal and societal burden. Conditions that can cause MINOCA are diverse and have varying pathophysiological causes. Diagnosis and treatment of these conditions is critical to reduce morbidity and mortality associated with MINOCA.

Learning Objectives

After reading this chapter and completing the learning activities, the reader will be able to:

- Identify populations most at risk of developing MINOCA.
- Describe the diagnostic criteria for conditions that are associated with MINOCA.
- Discuss management options for MINOCA.
- Discuss the potential impact on quality-of-life for those who experience MINOCA.

Key Concepts

MINOCA; INOCA; coronary microvascular disease; coronary artery spasm; vasospastic angina

Myocardial Infarction with Non-Obstructive Coronary Arteries (MINOCA)

Background

Myocardial infarction with non-obstructive coronary arteries (MINOCA) encompasses a heterogeneous group of conditions resulting in myocardial damage that is not due to obstructive coronary artery disease (CAD) (Beltrame 2013; Singh et al. 2021). The prognosis of patients presenting with MINOCA depends on the underlying cause (Tamis-Holland et al. 2019).

Epidemiology

The prevalence of MINOCA ranges between 1 and 14% in several large trials with an overall estimated prevalence around 6% (Pasupathy et al. 2015a). Compared with patients who have MI due to obstructive CAD, MINOCA is diagnosed more frequently in younger patients (mean age 55 years) and more often in women (Pasupathy et al. 2015a, b; Pacheco Claudio et al. 2018). The cardiovascular risk profile for

Cardiac Care: A Practical Guide for Nurses, Second Edition. Edited by Angela M. Kucia and Ian D. Jones.
© 2022 John Wiley & Sons Ltd. Published 2022 by John Wiley & Sons Ltd.

MINOCA differs from that for obstructive CAD in that patients are less likely to have hyperlipidaemia and diabetes but have a higher reported prevalence of hypertension (Pacheco Claudio et al. 2018).

Key Point

Compared with men, women with symptoms and signs of myocardial ischaemia are more likely to have no obstructive CAD on coronary angiography in the setting of both chronic and acute coronary syndromes (ACS) (Bairey Merz et al. 2017).

Prognosis

A recent study suggests that in-hospital outcomes for people diagnosed with MINOCA are better than for those diagnosed with myocardial infarction (MI) due to obstructive CAD (Jung et al. 2020). However, compared with the general population, people with MINOCA have an elevated risk for a cardiovascular event including death, acute coronary syndrome (ACS), MI, stroke and heart failure (HF). Furthermore, they have recurrent hospitalisations repeated cardiac investigations (including angiography) (Pacheco Claudio et al. 2018), and an impaired angina-related quality of life, with more dissatisfaction in their medical management compared to patients with obstructive CAD (Grodzinsky et al. 2015). Hence, it is important to identify the underlying cause for the clinical presentation in these patients and initiate appropriate therapy (Pasupathy et al. 2016).

Pathophysiology

Conditions that can cause MINOCA are diverse and have varying pathophysiological causes. MINOCA may result from conditions that affect the coronary arteries such as coronary artery spasm, coronary microvascular disease (CMD), plaque disruption, spontaneous coronary thrombosis/emboli and spontaneous coronary artery dissection (SCAD); conditions that affect the myocardium including myocarditis, takotsubo

syndrome (TTS) (see Chapter 26) and some cardiomyopathies; and non-cardiac causes such as kidney disease and pulmonary embolism (Pasupathy et al. 2017).

Presentation

Patients with MINOCA are less likely to experience angina prior to MI (Pacheco Claudio et al. 2018). Distinguishing a patient with MINOCA from those with obstructive CAD based on the clinical presentation and characteristics alone is not possible.

Diagnosis

Initial diagnosis is usually made following invasive coronary angiography to evaluate an apparent AMI. MINOCA is clinically defined by the presence of MI as specified by the Fourth Universal Definition of Acute MI (Thygesen et al. 2018) (see Chapter 13), absence of obstructive coronary artery disease (no epicardial stenoses ≥50%) and no overt cause for the clinical presentation at the time of angiography (Agewall et al. 2017). Although the diagnostic criteria for MINOCA are specific, it should not be considered a final diagnosis, but rather a 'working diagnosis' whose underlying aetiology requires further evaluation (Pasupathy et al. 2015b).

An important step in the assessment of patients with MINOCA is to exclude non-coronary causes of elevated troponin such as kidney disease or pulmonary embolus (PE), both of which are associated with an elevation of cardiac enzymes. Investigations for PE may include plasma D-dimer levels, a thoracic CT scan or ventilation/perfusion scintigraphy is critical in guiding treatment and improving patient outcome (Poku and Noble 2017).

Key Point

D-dimers are one of the fragments produced when plasmin cleaves fibrin to break down clots. Any process that increases fibrin production or breakdown, such as deep vein thrombosis or pulmonary embolism, also increases serum plasma D-dimer levels. D-dimer levels are routinely measured in clinical diagnosis algorithms for venous thromboembolism (VTE) using D-dimer cut-off values in a test that is sensitive, but non-specific for VTE (Yao et al. 2020).

Management

Patients without obstructive CAD are not candidates for coronary revascularisation and are less aggressively managed with secondary prevention and less likely to be referred to cardiac rehabilitation compared with patients with obstructive CAD. Non-interventional strategies are needed to improve outcomes and reduce hospital readmissions for people with MINOCA/INOCA. Potential targets for improvement of angina burden may include addressing psychosocial issues and examining strategies for improving medication adherence (Grodzinsky et al. 2015).

Epicardial Vascular Causes of MINOCA

Coronary Artery Spasm/Vasospastic Angina

Coronary artery spasm (CAS) refers to the sudden, intense vasoconstriction of an epicardial coronary artery that causes vessel occlusion or near occlusion. Vasospastic angina (VSA) is a form of myocardial ischaemia due to spasm in one or more epicardial coronary arteries that may be multifocal, multivessel or diffuse involving one or more coronary branches (Poku and Noble 2017). Prevalence varies widely across ethnic populations, with higher prevalence in Asian populations. VSA is caused by hyper-reactivity of large coronary arteries in response to vasoconstrictor stimuli including inflammation, endothelial dysfunction, oxidative stress, autonomic nervous system deregulation, respiratory alkalosis, magnesium deficiency, physical or mental stress, exposure to cold temperatures and smoking (Kaski et al. 1986; Poku and Noble 2017). VSA usually occurs at rest and can be precipitated by hyperventilation but not usually exertion. VSA symptoms may exhibit a circadian pattern, typically worse in the mornings.

Although VSA (previously called Prinzmetal or variant angina) has been a recognised clinical entity for more than 55 years, it has received limited attention because the diagnosis is easily overlooked (Beltrame et al. 2015). There are several reasons why it is important to consider a diagnosis of VSA, with the most important being the prevention of cardiac events including MI and sudden cardiac death (SCD) (Beltrame et al. 2017). Patients with VSA often have a negative or equivocal exercise stress test and coronary angiography reveals no significant CAD (Poku and Noble 2017). Unfortunately, ECG abnormalities during spontaneous episodes of rest angina are rarely documented and provocative testing may be required. International diagnostic criteria have been established for vasospastic angina (Beltrame et al. 2017), which should facilitate its diagnosis in the future. Table 27.1 outlines diagnostic criteria for VAS.

The gold standard method for provocative spasm testing involves the administration of a provocative stimulus (typically intracoronary acetylcholine or alternatively intracoronary or intravenous ergonovine) during invasive coronary angiography while monitoring for patient symptoms, ECG abnormalities and angiographic evidence of coronary artery spasm. A positive provocative test for coronary artery spasm must induce all the following in response to the provocative stimulus: (i) reproduction of the usual chest pain, (ii) ischaemic ECG changes and (iii) >90% vasoconstriction on angiography (Beltrame et al. 2017).

The conventional management of VSA involves lifestyle changes including smoking cessation and aerobic exercise training. VSA normally responds promptly to short-acting nitrates and typically suppressed by calcium-channel blockers (Beltrame et al. 2017).

Table 27.1 Coronary artery vasospastic disorders Summit diagnostic criteria for vasospastic angina[a].

Vasospastic angina diagnostic criteria elements

1) *Nitrate-responsive angina* – during spontaneous episode, with at least one of the following:
   a) Rest angina – especially between night and early morning
   b) Marked diurnal variation in exercise tolerance – reduced in morning
   c) Hyperventilation can precipitate an episode
   d) Calcium-channel blockers (but not β-blockers) suppress episodes
2) *Transient ischaemic ECG changes* – during spontaneous episode, including any of the following in at least two contiguous leads:
   a) ST-segment elevation ≥0.1 mV
   b) ST-segment depression ≥0.1 mV
   c) New negative U waves
3) *Coronary artery spasm* – defined as transient total or subtotal coronary artery occlusion (>90% constriction) with angina and ischaemic ECG changes either spontaneously or in response to a provocative stimulus (typically acetylcholine, ergot or hyperventilation)

[a] 'Definitive vasospastic angina' is diagnosed if nitrate-responsive angina is evident during spontaneous episodes and either the transient ischaemic ECG changes during the spontaneous episodes or coronary artery spasm criteria are fulfilled. 'Suspected vasospastic angina' is diagnosed if nitrate-responsive angina is evident during spontaneous episodes but transient ischaemic ECG changes are equivocal or unavailable and coronary artery spasm criteria are equivocal.
Source: Reprinted with permission. Beltrame et al. (2017).

Calcium-channel blockers are the first-line therapy for VSA and have been shown to reduce episodes of symptomatic angina, suppress inducible CAS and reducing major adverse cardiovascular events. Nitrates and nicorandil are effective in reducing episodes of angina and ameliorating symptoms. However, less than 40% achieve complete resolution of symptoms despite pharmacotherapy, leaving many with refractory VSA that impacts on quality of life. PCI is not usually indicated in VSA unless it is associated with a concomitant atherosclerotic lesion (Beltrame et al. 2017).

Key Point

Drugs that may predispose to vasospasm, including β-blockers, ergots, and sympathomimetics, must be avoided in patients with VSA (Beltrame et al. 2017).

Spontaneous Coronary Artery Dissection (SCAD)

Spontaneous coronary artery dissection (SCAD) is a sudden tear in wall of one or more coronary arteries, creating a false lumen within the coronary artery wall that may lead to flow limitation by compressing the true coronary lumen leading to limited blood flow. The left anterior descending artery is the most commonly affected vessel (Adlam et al. 2018; Hayes et al. 2018). Coronary dissections that are secondary to atherosclerotic disease, extension of an aortic dissection, iatrogenic (such as during percutaneous catheter interventions) or related to a trauma are not classed as SCAD (Garcia-Guimarães et al. 2020). SCAD is a relatively infrequent cause of acute coronary syndrome that predominantly affects young to middle-aged women, but the true prevalence is not known due to under-diagnosis (Hayes et al., 2018). SCAD has been associated with several disorders including fibromuscular dysplasia, collagen vascular disorders, chronic inflammatory systemic diseases, pregnancy.

Key Point

SCAD is the most common cause of pregnancy-associated MI (Hayes et al. 2018).

Precipitating factors include emotional or physical stressors. Invasive coronary angiography is still the main technique used in the diagnosis of SCAD (Garcia-Guimarães et al. 2020), but to date, observational studies have shown that percutaneous coronary intervention (PCI) with balloon or stent has a high complication rate. Management of SCAD may be conservative in stable patients who are not at high risk. High-risk patients such as those with dissection of the left main coronary artery, ongoing ischaemia or haemodynamic instability may require PCI or coronary artery bypass surgery (CABG).

Suggested Resource

Patient resource:
Spontaneous coronary artery dissection (SCAD)
British Heart Foundation
www.bhf.org.uk/informationsupport/conditions/spontaneous-coronary-artery-dissection

---

Plaque Disruption

A proposed cause of MINOCA is plaque disruption (erosion, ulceration, rupture or intraplaque haemorrhage) in non-obstructive coronary lesions or in coronary arteries that appear angiographically normal. It is thought that the cause may be transient thrombus formation on a disrupted plaque, which totally or partially occludes the coronary artery for a sufficient to cause myocardial injury before spontaneous thrombolysis. Evaluation for plaque disruption may include intravascular ultrasound and optical coherence tomography in selected patients. Once plaque disruption is confirmed, it is recommended that statin therapy be considered and dual antiplatelet therapy be prescribed for 1 year, followed by lifelong mono-antiplatelet therapy (Poku and Noble 2017).

Microvascular Causes of MINOCA

Coronary Microvascular Dysfunction

Coronary microvascular dysfunction (CMD) refers to disorders affecting the structure and function of the coronary microcirculation. CMD is associated with an increased risk of adverse events (Taqueti and Di Carli 2018).

Key Point

CMD may be a cause of ischaemia but may also be caused by myocardial injury.

The coronary arterial system is comprised of a continuous network of functionally distinct vessel segments of decreasing size. The primary function of the large epicardial arteries is to conduct blood to the myocardium and under normal conditions (in the absence of obstructive coronary disease), there is minimal resistance to coronary flow. In contrast, the pre-arterioles and arterioles function as a resistance circuit and regulate and distribute blood flow to match the dynamic needs of local tissue metabolism via the coronary capillaries (Taqueti and Di Carli 2018). Structural and/or functional abnormalities of the coronary microvessels may impair their ability to modulate blood flow in response to the functional needs of myocardial cell in response to changing demands, such as during exercise. Endothelial dysfunction may result in an impaired vasodilatory response leading to inadequate blood flow and reduced myocardial perfusion. Functional abnormalities of smooth muscle cells regulating arteriolar tone are also present in many patients with CMD (Taqueti and Di Carli 2018).

Key Point

CMD is commonly associated with conditions that cause MINOCA (Tamis-Holland et al. 2019).

CMD is more prevalent in women, particularly those who are postmenopausal. Cardiovascular risk factors in patients with MVA are like those in CAD (Ong et al. 2018).

The clinical presentation for CMD, microvascular angina (MVA), is like that of obstructive cardiac disease in that patients may present with typical angina pectoris, atypical symptoms or angina-equivalent symptoms during exertion or at rest. Symptoms may also occur soon after the exercise has ceased. Patients with MVA do not appear to respond as well to sublingual or oral nitrates as those with obstructive CAD (Ong et al. 2018).

Clinical criteria for suspecting MVA are shown in Table 27.2.

Table 27.2 Clinical criteria for suspecting microvascular angina (MVA)[a].

---

1) Symptoms of myocardial ischaemia
   a) Effort and/or rest angina
   b) Angina equivalents (i.e. shortness of breath)
3) Absence of obstructive CAD (<50% diameter reduction or FFR > 0.80) by
   a) Coronary CTA
   b) Invasive coronary angiography
3) Objective evidence of myocardial ischaemia
   a) Ischaemic ECG changes during an episode of chest pain
   b) Stress-induced chest pain and/or ischaemic ECG changes in the presence or absence of transient/reversible abnormal myocardial perfusion and/or wall motion abnormality
4) Evidence of impaired coronary microvascular function
   a) Impaired coronary flow reserve (cut-off values depending on methodology use between ≤2.0 and ≤2.5)
   b) Coronary microvascular spasm, defined as reproduction of symptoms, ischaemic ECG shifts but no epicardial spasm during acetylcholine testing.
   c) Abnormal coronary microvascular resistance indices (e.g. IMR > 25).
   d) Coronary slow flow phenomenon, defined as TIMI frame count >25.

ECG = electrocardiogram, CAD = coronary artery disease, CTA = computed tomographic angiography, FFR = fractional flow reserve, IMR = index of microcirculatory resistance, TIMI = thrombolysis in myocardial infarction.
[a] Definitive MVA is only diagnosed if all four criteria are present for a diagnosis of microvascular angina. Suspected MVA is diagnosed if symptoms of ischaemia are present (criteria-1) with no obstructive coronary artery disease (criteria-2) but only (a) objective evidence of myocardial ischaemia (criteria-3), or (b) evidence of impaired coronary microvascular function (criteria-4) alone.
Source: Reprinted with permission. Ong et al. (2018).

> **Key Point**
>
> A diagnosis of MVA must be made using standardised diagnostic criteria and cannot be made based on symptoms alone (Ong et al. 2018).

Treatment of MVA includes management of cardiovascular risk factors and conditions such as inflammatory disease, oestrogen deficiency or high adrenergic activity that might impair clinical outcomes. A primary goal of treatment is to reduce angina symptoms and improve quality of life (Lanza et al. 2018).

A suggested therapeutic approach to MVA is shown in Figure 27.1.

> **Key Point**
>
> Quality of life can be severely affected by MVA. Frequent and unpredictable episodes of pain necessitate significant change to lifestyle, work and family commitments and social activities for many patients.

Non-ischaemic Causes of MINOCA

Myocarditis

Myocarditis is inflammation of the myocardium that is usually caused by a viral infection, though it may be caused by some drugs and cancer treatments. Clinical manifestations of myocarditis include chest pain, elevation of myocardial necrosis biomarkers and ST-segment changes on ECG in the absence of significant vascular stenosis. However, endothelial cell injury and microvascular dysfunction may result from myocarditis (Abdu et al. 2020).

> **Suggested resource**
>
> What you should know: MyocarditisWebMD (2020)
> URL: https://www.webmd.com/heart-disease/myocarditis

Takotsubo Syndrome

The clinical presentation of takotsubo syndrome is the same as that for an acute coronary syndrome. Takotsubo syndrome is discussed in Chapter 26.

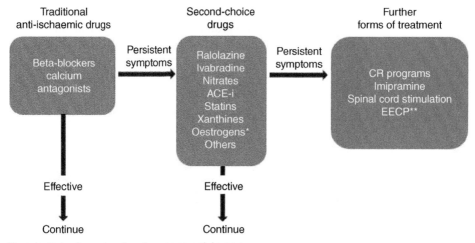

*In selected subgroups of post-menopausal women.

**EECP = Enhanced External Counter Pulsation (EECP)

Figure 27.1 Therapeutic approach in patients with primary stable microvascular angina. Adapted with permission. Lanza et al. (2018). Awaiting permission.

Ischaemia and no obstructive coronary artery disease (INOCA).

Whereas MINOCA represents an acute coronary syndrome with non-obstructive coronary arteries, INOCA includes chronic coronary syndromes in the absence of obstructive CAD. Cases of ischaemia and no obstructive coronary artery disease (INOCA) are increasing, but it is likely that many cases remain undiagnosed (Beltrame et al. 2021). It is not a benign condition and is associated with elevated rates of readmission and repeat cardiac investigations, including angiography, due to recurring symptoms (Bairey Merz et al. 2017). As for MINOCA, CAS or CMD may be underlying pathologies in INOCA. Other conditions mimicking INOCA include hypertensive heart disease, severe aortic stenosis, severe anaemia, heart failure or cardiogenic shock, myocarditis, congenital heart disease, shunts, coronary anomalies, myocardial bridging, and some drugs. Most patients with INOCA and chronic angina have some degree of coronary atherosclerosis suggesting that it is a key mediator of the syndrome (Bairey Merz et al. 2017). INOCA is often associated with chronic stable angina

symptoms that produces functional limitations (eg, reduce exercise capacity), and impacts upon quality of life (Beltrame et al. 2021). Currently there are no evidence-based guidelines to direct a management strategy for INOCA other than treating underlying conditions. Further research is required to address knowledge gaps and to formulate evidence-based approaches to the definition, diagnostic evaluation, risk stratification, and management of patients with INOCA (Bairey Merz et al. 2017).

Conclusion

MINOCA and INOCA are conditions associated with myocardial ischaemia or infarction that are not as well understood or managed as conditions related to obstructive cardiac disease. MINOCA and INOCA are not benign conditions and impact on quality of life for those who are affected. While progress has been made in developing diagnostic criteria for MINOCA, there is a need for further progress in addressing knowledge gaps in INOCA.

References

Abdu, F.A., Mohammed, A.Q., Liu, L., Xu, Y., & Che, W. (2020). Myocardial Infarction with Nonobstructive Coronary Arteries (MINOCA): A Review of the Current Position. *Cardiology*, **145** (9), 543–552. https://doi.org/10.1159/000509100.

Adlam, D., Alfonso, F., Maas, A., Vrints, C., & Writing Committee. (2018). European Society of Cardiology, acute cardiovascular care association, SCAD study group: a position paper on spontaneous coronary artery dissection. *European Heart Journal*, **39** (36), 3353. https://doi.org/10.1093/eurheartj/ehy080.

Agewall, S., Beltrame, J.F., Reynolds, H.R. et al. (2017). ESC working group position paper on myocardial infarction with non-obstructive coronary arteries. *European Heart Journal* **38** (3): 143–153.

Bairey Merz, C.N., Pepine, C.J., Walsh, M.N. et al. (2017). Ischemia and no obstructive coronary artery disease (INOCA) developing evidence-based therapies and research agenda for the next decade. *Circulation* **135** (11): 1075–1092.

Beltrame, J.F. (2013). Assessing patients with myocardial infarction and nonobstructed coronary arteries (MINOCA). *Journal of Internal Medicine*, **273** (2), 182–185. https://doi.org/10.1111/j.1365-2796.2012.02591.x.

Beltrame, J.F., Crea, F., Kaski, J.C., Ogawa, H., Ong, P., Sechtem, U., . . . & Coronary Vasomotion Disorders International Study Group. (2015). The who, what, why, when, how and where of vasospastic angina. *Circulation Journal* **80** (2): 289–298. https://doi.org/10.1253/circj.CJ-15-1202.

Beltrame, J.F., Crea, F., Kaski, J.C. et al. (2017). Coronary Vasomotion Disorders International Study Group (COVADIS). International standardization of diagnostic criteria for vasospastic angina. *European Heart Journal* **38** (33): 2565–2568.

Beltrame, J.F., Tavella, R., Jones, D., and Zeitz, C. (2021). Management of ischaemia with non-obstructive coronary arteries (INOCA). *BMJ 375*: e060602. doi: https://doi.org/10.1136/bmj-2021-060602.

Garcia-Guimarães, M., Bastante, T., Antuña, P. et al. (2020). Spontaneous coronary artery dissection: mechanisms, diagnosis and management. *European Cardiology Review* **15**: 1.

Grodzinsky, A., Arnold, S.V., Gosch, K. et al. (2015). Angina frequency after acute myocardial infarction in patients without obstructive coronary artery disease. *European Heart Journal–Quality of Care and Clinical Outcomes* **1** (2): 92–99.

Hayes, S.N. et al. (2018). Spontaneous coronary artery dissection: current state of the science: a scientific statement from the American Heart Association. *Circulation*, **137** (19), e523–e557. https://doi.org/10.1161/CIR.0000000000000564.

Jung, R.G., Parlow, S., Simard, T., Chen, C., Ghataura, H., Kishore, A., . . . & Singh, K. (2020). Clinical features, sex differences and outcomes of myocardial infarction with nonobstructive coronary arteries: a registry analysis. *Coronary Artery Disease*, **32** (1), 10–16. https://doi.org/10.1097/MCA.0000000000000903.

Kaski, J.C., Crea, F., Meran, D. et al. (1986). Local coronary supersensitivity to diverse vasoconstrictive stimuli in patients with variant angina. *Circulation* **74** (6): 1255–1265.

Lanza, G.A., De Vita, A., and Kaski, J.C. (2018). 'Primary' microvascular angina: clinical characteristics, pathogenesis and management. *Interventional Cardiology Review* **13** (3): 108.

Ong, P., Camici, P.G., Beltrame, J.F. et al. (2018). International standardization of diagnostic criteria for microvascular angina. *International Journal of Cardiology* **250**: 16–20.

Pacheco Claudio, C., Quesada, O., Pepine, C.J., and Noel Bairey Merz, C. (2018). Why names matter for women: MINOCA/INOCA (myocardial infarction/ischemia and no obstructive coronary artery disease). *Clinical Cardiology* **41** (2): 185–193.

Pasupathy, S. and Beltrame, J.F. (2018). Refining the diagnosis of myocardial infarction with nonobstructive coronary arteries. *Coronary Artery Disease* **29** (6): 528–529.

Pasupathy, S., Air, T., Dreyer, R.P. et al. (2015a). Systematic review of patients presenting with suspected myocardial infarction and nonobstructive coronary arteries. *Circulation* **131** (10): 861–870.

Pasupathy, S., Tavella, R., McRae, S., and Beltrame, J.F. (2015b). Myocardial infarction with non-obstructive coronary arteries– diagnosis and management. *European Cardiology Review* **10** (2): 79.

Pasupathy, S., Rodgers, S., Tavella, R. et al. (2016). Risk of Thrombosis in Myocardial Infarction with Non Obstructive Coronary Arteries (MINOCA). *Heart, Lung and Circulation* **25**: S64.

Pasupathy, S., Tavella, R., and Beltrame, J.F. (2017). Myocardial Infarction With Nonobstructive Coronary Arteries (MINOCA) The Past, Present, and Future Management. *Circulation* **135** (16): 1490–1493.

Poku, N. and Noble, S. (2017). Myocardial infarction with non obstructive coronary arteries (MINOCA): a whole new ball game.

Expert Review of Cardiovascular Therapy **15** (1): 7–14.

Safdar, B., Spatz, E.S., Dreyer, R.P. et al. (2018). Presentation, clinical profile, and prognosis of young patients with myocardial infarction with nonobstructive coronary arteries (MINOCA): results from the VIRGO study. *Journal of the American Heart Association* **7** (13): e009174.

Singh, T., Chapman, A.R., Dweck, M.R. et al. (2021). MINOCA: a heterogenous group of conditions associated with myocardial damage. *Heart* **107** (18): 1458–1464.

Tamis-Holland, J.E., Jneid, H., Reynolds, H.R. et al. (2019). Contemporary diagnosis and management of patients with myocardial infarction in the absence of obstructive coronary artery disease: a scientific statement from the American Heart Association. *Circulation* **139** (18): e891–e908.

Taqueti, V.R. and Di Carli, M.F. (2018). Coronary microvascular disease pathogenic mechanisms and therapeutic options: JACC state-of-the-art review. *Journal of the American College of Cardiology* **72** (21): 2625–2641.

Thygesen, K., Alpert, J.S., Jaffe, A.S. et al. (2018). Fourth universal definition of myocardial infarction (2018). *Journal of the American College of Cardiology* **72** (18): 2231–2264.

Yao, Y., Cao, J., Wang, Q. et al. (2020). D-dimer as a biomarker for disease severity and mortality in COVID-19 patients: a case control study. *Journal of Intensive Care* **8** (1): 1–11.

Index

Cardiac Care: A Practical Guide for Nurses, Second Edition. Edited by Angela M. Kucia and Ian D. Jones.
© 2022 John Wiley & Sons Ltd. Published 2022 by John Wiley & Sons Ltd.